LABORATORY TESTS

LABORATORY TESTS

Implications for Nursing Care

SECOND EDITION

C. Judith Byrne, BS, MT (ASCP)
Dolores F. Saxton, RN, EdD
Phyllis K. Pelikan, RN, MA
Patricia M. Nugent, RN, MS

 Addison-Wesley Publishing Company

Health Sciences Division, Menlo Park, California
Reading, Massachusetts • Don Mills, Ontario • Wokingham, UK
Amsterdam • Sydney • Singapore • Tokyo • Mexico City
Bogotá • Santiago • San Juan

Sponsoring Editor: Katherine Pitcoff
Production Supervisor: Glenda Epting
Copy Editor: Dori Bingham
Cover Designer: Richard Kharibian
Interior Designer: Richard Kharibian
Cover Photo: An inside view of the Cetus Pro/Pette® automated liquid handling system. Pro/Pette®
is a registered trademark of the Cetus Corporation, Emeryville, California.

Library of Congress Cataloging in Publication Data
Main entry under title:

Laboratory tests.
    Includes bibliographies and index.
    1. Diagnosis, Laboratory.   2. Nursing.
I. Byrne, C. Judith (Claire Judith), 1944– .
[DNLM: 1. Diagnosis, Laboratory—nurses' instruction.
QY 4 L1235]
RB37.L276   1986   616.07′5   85-13555
ISBN 0-201-12670-2

DEFGHIJKL-MA-898

The authors and publishers have exerted every effort to ensure that drug selection and dosage set
forth in this text are in accord with current recommendations and practice at the time of publication. However, in view of ongoing research, changes in government regulations and the constant
flow of information relating to drug therapy and drug reactions, the reader is urged to check the
package insert for each drug for any change in indications of dosage and for added warnings and
precautions. This is particularly important where the recommended agent is a new and/or infrequently employed drug.

Addison-Wesley Publishing Company
Health Sciences Division
2725 Sand Hill Road
Menlo Park, California 94025

This book is dedicated to Claire and Frank Byrne, whose faith, love, and support sustained me through this edition as in life itself.

"If the Lord does not build a house, then in vain do the builders labor."   Psalm 127

Contents

Preface   vii

1 Urinalysis   1

FORMATION OF URINE   2

COLLECTION AND HANDLING OF URINE   4

Procedures for Collecting Specimens   4

Times for Collecting Specimens   5

Preservation of Urine   6

PHYSICAL EXAMINATION OF URINE   7

Volume   7

Odor   9

Color   9

Turbidity   12

ROUTINE URINALYSIS   13

Specific Gravity   14

pH Reaction   16

Glucose and Nonglucose Sugars   18

Protein   21

Ketones   24

Occult Blood   26

Bilirubin   29

Urobilinogen   31

Nitrite   33

MICROSCOPIC EXAMINATION   37

Red Blood Cells   38

White Blood Cells   39

Epithelial Cells   40

Casts   40

Crystals   42

Bacteria   43

Miscellaneous Constituents   43

SPECIAL URINE TESTS   44
Porphobilinogen and Porphyrins   44
Calcium   47
KIDNEY FUNCTION STUDIES   49
Creatinine Clearance Test   50
Concentration Test   51
Phenolsulfonphthalein Test   53
RENAL CALCULI   55
AMINOACIDURIA   57
Homogentisic Acid   58
Phenylpyruvic Acid   59
OTHER URINE STUDIES   60

2 Hematology   62
SPECIMEN COLLECTION AND HANDLING   63
Capillary Blood   63
Venipuncture   64
COMPLETE BLOOD COUNT   65
Hemoglobin   66
Hematocrit   68
Erythrocyte Count   70
Leukocyte Count   73
Differential White Blood Cell Count   75
Stained Red Blood Cell Examination   85
ERYTHROCYTE INDICES   89
ERYTHROCYTE SEDIMENTATION RATE   93
RETICULOCYTE COUNT   96
ERYTHROCYTE OSMOTIC FRAGILITY TEST   98
PLATELET COUNT   100
EOSINOPHIL COUNT AND THORN TEST   102
LUPUS ERYTHEMATOSUS CELL TEST   104
LEUKOCYTE ALKALINE PHOSPHATASE STAIN   106
**GLUCOSE-6-PHOSPHATE DEHYDROGENASE
    DEFICIENCY TEST   188**
HEMOGLOBIN ELECTROPHORESIS   109
SICKLE CELL TEST   113
**ALKALI DENATURATION TEST FOR
    FETAL HEMOGLOBIN   114**
BONE MARROW EXAMINATION   116
OTHER TESTS OF HEMOGLOBIN METABOLISM   120

3 Chemistry: Tests of Hemoglobin
Metabolism   122

HEMOGLOBIN SYNTHESIS AND BREAKDOWN   123
Hemoglobin Synthesis   123
Hemoglobin Breakdown   123
TESTS OF HEMOGLOBIN SYNTHESIS   125
Vitamin B_{12} 125
Folic Acid   127
Porphyrins and Their Precursors   128
Serum Iron   132
Transferrin, Total Iron-Binding Capacity, and Percent Saturation   134
Serum Ferritin   137
TESTS OF HEMOGLOBIN BREAKDOWN   139
Plasma Hemoglobin   139
Haptoglobin   141
Bilirubin   143
Urobilinogen   148
OTHER HEMOGLOBIN TESTS   149

4 Chemistry: Routine Studies   151

SPECIMEN COLLECTION AND HANDLING   152
Specimen Types   152
Anticoagulants Used to Prevent Clotting   152
Collection Times   153
Collection Tubes   153
Order of Specimen Draw   154
Performing a Venipuncture   154
Preserving and Processing Blood Specimens   156
**AUTOMATION IN THE CHEMISTRY
LABORATORY   157**
CARBOHYDRATES   157
Fasting Blood Glucose   159
Two-Hour Postprandial Glucose   161
Glucose Tolerance Test   163
Glycohemoglobin Test   168
D-Xylose Absorption Test   170
Lactose Tolerance Test   171
ENZYMES   172
Amylase   173
Lipase   176
Acid Phosphatase   178

Alkaline Phosphatase   180
Cholinesterase and Pseudocholinesterase   182
Aldolase   183
Creatine Phosphokinase (Creatine Kinase)   185
Lactic Dehydrogenase   189
Hydroxybutyric Dehydrogenase   192
Aspartate Aminotransferase   194
Alanine Aminotransferase   196
Gamma-Glutamyl Transferase   198
5'-Nucleotidase   200

LIPIDS   201
Cholesterol   202
Triglycerides   205
Lipoproteins   207
Free Fatty Acids, Phospholipids, and Total Lipids   211

LIVER FUNCTION TESTS   213
MISCELLANEOUS TESTS   214
Ascorbic Acid   214
Carotene and Vitamin A   215
Copper   217
Zinc   218

NONPROTEIN NITROGEN COMPOUNDS   219
Blood Ammonia   220
Blood Urea Nitrogen   222
Creatinine   224
Blood Urea Nitrogen/Creatinine Ratio   227
Uric Acid   228

SERUM PROTEINS   230
Total Protein, Albumin, and Globulins   231
Immunoglobulins   235
Serum Protein Electrophoresis and Immunoelectrophoresis   237

TUMOR MARKERS   241
α-Fetoprotein   242
Carcinoembryonic Antigen   243

5 Chemistry: Serum Electrolytes and Blood Gas Studies   247

FLUID AND ELECTROLYTE BALANCE   248
Total Body Fluid   248
Electrolyte Studies   248
Sodium   250
Potassium   257

Carbon Dioxide   260
Chloride   263
Calcium   265
Phosphorus   268
Magnesium   270
Anion Gap   272
Osmolality   275

ACID-BASE BALANCE AND BLOOD GASES   278

Bicarbonate-Carbonic Acid Buffers   278
Blood Gas Studies   279
Blood Gas Specimen Collection and Handling   279
pH   283
Partial Pressure of Carbon Dioxide   285
Base Excess   286
Partial Pressure of Oxygen   287
Oxygen Saturation   288
Acid-Base Imbalance   289

6   Chemistry: Tests of Endocrine Function   294

ADRENAL HORMONE STUDIES   295

Aldosterone   297
Catecholamines   298
Cortisol   301
17-Hydroxycorticosteroids   303
17-Ketogenic Steroids   305
17-Ketosteroids   307
Vanillylmandelic Acid   310

MISCELLANEOUS HORMONE STUDIES   312

Calcitonin   312
5-Hydroxyindoleacetic Acid   313
Parathyroid Hormone   314
Renin   316
Vitamin D   317

PITUITARY HORMONE STUDIES   319

Adrenocorticotropic Hormone   320
Follicle-Stimulating Hormone   321
Growth Hormone   323
Luteinizing Hormone   324
Prolactin   326
Thyroid-Stimulating Hormone   329

REPRODUCTIVE HORMONE STUDIES   330

Estrogens   331
Human Chorionic Gonadotropin   335

Human Placental Lactogen   338
Pregnanediol   339
Progesterone   341
Testosterone   342

THYROID HORMONE STUDIES   344

Triiodothyronine   346
Thyroxine   347
T₃ Uptake and T₃ Uptake Ratio   350
Free Thyroxine Index   352

7   Chemistry: Clinical Toxicology and Therapeutic Drug Monitoring   355

CLINICAL TOXICOLOGY   356

Specimen Collection and Handling   356
Medicolegal Specimen Collection and Handling   357

THERAPEUTIC DRUG MONITORING   358

Factors Affecting Drug Response   358
Test Interpretation   359
Specimen Collection and Handling   360

ALCOHOL   360

Ethanol   360
Isopropanol   363
Methanol   364

AMINOGLYCOSIDES   366

AMPHETAMINES   367

ANALGESICS   369

Acetaminophen   369
Acetylsalicylic Acid   370

ANTICONVULSANTS   372

Carbamazepine   372
Ethosuximide   374
Phenobarbital   374
Phenytoin   376
Primidone   377
Valproic Acid   378

BARBITURATES   379

CARDIAC DRUGS   382

Digitoxin and Digoxin   382
Lidocaine   385
Disopyramide   386
Procainamide   387

Propranolol   389
Quinidine   390

HEMOGLOBIN DERIVATIVES   391

Carbon Monoxide   391
Methemoglobin   394
Sulfhemoglobin   396

HEAVY METALS   397

Arsenic   397
Iron   398
Lead   400
Mercury   402

MISCELLANEOUS SUBSTANCES   404

Bromide   404
Methotrexate   405
Theophylline   407

PSYCHOTHERAPEUTIC DRUGS   409

Lithium   409
Phenothiazines   411
Tricyclic Antidepressants   412

MINOR TRANQUILIZING AGENTS   414

Benzodiazepines   414
Other Sedative/Tranquilizing Agents   416

DRUG ABUSE   418

DRUG SCREENING   420

8 Chemistry: Body Fluid Analysis   423

AMNIOTIC FLUID ANALYSIS   424

Specimen Collection and Handling   424
Physical Examination   426
α-Fetoprotein   427
Bilirubin   429
Creatinine   431
Lecithin/Sphingomyelin Ratio   432

CEREBROSPINAL FLUID ANALYSIS   434

Specimen Collection and Handling   434
Physical Examination   437
Cell Counts   439
Glucose   442
Lactic Acid   443
Protein   444
Microbiologic Examination   448
Tests for Syphilis   448

FECAL ANALYSIS 449
Specimen Collection and Handling 449
Physical Examination 450
Fecal Fat 452
Occult Blood 454
Trypsin 456
Urobilinogen 456
Microbiologic Examination 458

GASTRIC ANALYSIS 458
Specimen Collection and Handling 458
Physical Examination 460
Gastric Acidity 462

PLEURAL FLUID ANALYSIS 464
Specimen Collection and Handling 465
Physical Examination 465
Cell Counts 466
Glucose 467
pH 467
Specific Gravity and Total Protein 468
Microbiologic Examination 469

SYNOVIAL FLUID ANALYSIS 469
Specimen Collection and Handling 470
Physical Examination 470
Cell Counts 475
Crystals 476
Glucose 477
Microbiologic Examination 478

9 Microbiology   480

SPECIMEN COLLECTION AND HANDLING 482
Specimens for General Examination 482
Specimens for the Examination of Stained Smears 484
Specimens for Anaerobic Examination 485
Specimens for Fungus Examination 485
Specimens for Virus Examination 486

MICROSCOPIC EXAMINATION OF STAINED SMEARS 486
Gram's Stain 487
Acid-Fast Stain 487

CULTURES 488
Anaerobic Cultures 488
Fungus Cultures 489

**SPECIMENS FOR MICROBIOLOGIC
EXAMINATION 489**
Blood 489
Cerebrospinal Fluid 491
Ear 496
Eye 497
Genitourinary Tract Secretions and Discharges 500
Hair, Skin, and Nails 501
Nasopharynx and Throat Secretions and Discharges 506
Sputum 512
Stool 514
Synovial Fluid 520
Urine 521
Wound Exudates and Drainage 524
ANTIBIOTIC SUSCEPTIBILITY TESTING 528
Antibiotic Activity 529
Disk Diffusion Tests 529
Quantitative Dilution Tests 530

10 Hemostasis and Coagulation   532
HEMOSTASIS 533
COAGULATION 534
Stage I 534
Stage II 536
Stage III 536
Stage IV 536
COAGULATION FACTORS 537
Factor I (Fibrinogen) 537
Factor II (Prothrombin) 538
Factor III (Thromboplastin) 538
Factor IV (Calcium) 538
Factor V (Proaccelerin) 539
Factor VII (Proconvertin) 539
Factor VIII (Antihemophilic Factor) 539
Factor IX (Plasma Thromboplastin Component) 540
Factor X (Stuart-Prower Factor) 541
Factor XI (Plasma Thromboplastin Antecedent) 541
Factor XII (Hageman Factor) 542
Factor XIII (Fibrin Stabilizing Factor) 542
Fletcher Factor (Prekallikrein) 542
COAGULATION PROFILE 543
SPECIMEN COLLECTION AND HANDLING 543

TESTS OF VASCULAR AND PLATELET FUNCTION   544
Bleeding Time   544
Tourniquet Test   546
Clot Retraction   547
Platelet Count   548
Platelet Adhesion and Aggregation   550

TESTS OF OVERALL COAGULATION   553
Whole Blood Clotting Time   553
Circulating Anticoagulants   555
Partial Thromboplastin Time   556
Plasma Recalcification Time   557

TESTS TO EVALUATE STAGE I COAGULATION   558
Prothrombin Consumption Time   558
Thromboplastin Generation Time   560

**TESTS TO EVALUATE STAGE II AND III
COAGULATION   561**
Prothrombin Time   561
Stypven Time   563
Thrombin Time   564
Antithrombin III   565
Fibrinogen Assay   567

TESTS TO EVALUATE STAGE IV COAGULATION   568
Fibrin-Fibrinogen Degradation Products   568
Euglobulin Lysis Time   570
Paracoagulation Tests   571
Plasminogen   572

**ANTICOAGULANT THERAPY AND
ASSOCIATED TESTS   573**
Heparin   573
Coumarin Derivatives   575

11 Serology/Immunology   578

ANTIGEN-ANTIBODY REACTIONS   579
T- and B-Lymphocytes   579
Immunoglobulins   580
Complement   581

**SPECIMEN COLLECTION FOR SEROLOGIC
STUDIES   585**

SEROLOGIC TESTS FOR AUTOIMMUNITY   586
Test for Antinuclear Antibodies   586
Tests for Deoxyribonucleic Acid Antibodies   588

Tests for Antimitochondrial and Anti-Smooth Muscle Antibodies   589
Test for the Rheumatoid Factor   591
Tests for Thyroid Antibodies   592

SEROLOGIC TESTS FOR FEBRILE AGGLUTININS   593
Widal's Test for Typhoid and Paratyphoid Fevers   594
Weil-Felix Test for Rickettsial Diseases   596
Agglutination Test for Brucellosis   597
Agglutination Test for Tularemia   598

SEROLOGIC TESTS FOR FUNGAL INFECTIONS   599
SEROLOGIC TESTS FOR MYCOPLASMAL INFECTIONS   602
Test for Cold Agglutinins   602
Test for Mycoplasmal Antibodies   603
Test for *Streptococcus* MG Agglutinins   604

SEROLOGIC TESTS FOR PARASITIC INFECTIONS   605
Test for Toxoplasmosis   605
Tests for Other Parasitic Infections   607

SEROLOGIC TESTS FOR STREPTOCOCCAL INFECTIONS   609
Test for Antistreptolysin O Titer   609
Tests for Antideoxyribonuclease B and Antihyaluronidase   611
Test for C-Reactive Protein   612

SEROLOGIC TESTS FOR SYPHILIS   614
Tests for Nontreponemal Antibodies   615
Tests for Treponemal Antibodies   618

SEROLOGIC TESTS FOR TORCH DISEASES   619
SEROLOGIC TESTS FOR VIRAL INFECTIONS   620
Tests for Cytomegalovirus   620
Tests for Viral Hepatitis   621
Test for Herpes Simplex Virus   625
Tests for Infectious Mononucleosis   627
Test for Rubella   629

12 Immunohematology and Transfusion Therapy   633
BLOOD TYPES   634
ABO System   634
Rh System   637
Other Blood Group Systems   640
ANTIBODY DETECTION   642
Direct Antiglobulin Test (Direct Coombs' Test)   643

Antibody Screen (Indirect Coombs' Test)   644
Antibody Identification   645

COMPATIBILITY TESTING   646

Specimen Collection and Handling   647
Routine Crossmatch   647
Emergency Crossmatch   648
Crossmatching Blood for Newborns and Infants   648

TRANSFUSION THERAPY   649

Selection of Blood and Alternate Donor Groups   649
Administration of Blood   650
Massive Transfusions   651

COMPONENT THERAPY   652

Whole Blood   652
Red Blood Cells   652
Granulocytes   656
Platelets   657
Cryoprecipitated Antihemophilic Factor   659
Plasma   660

TRANSFUSION REACTIONS   661

Investigation of Transfusion Reactions   662
Acute Hemolytic Transfusion Reactions   663
Bacterial Reactions   664
Circulatory Overload   665
Febrile Reactions   665
Hypersensitivity Reactions   666
Transmission of Disease Via Transfusion   667

**SELECTION AND SCREENING OF
BLOOD DONORS   669**

Criteria for Selecting Blood Donors   669
Criteria for Excluding Blood Donors   670

Appendix A—Organ Panels and
Disease Profiles   673

Appendix B—Blood Specimen Tube
Requirements   679

Appendix C—Normal Values   683

Glossary   713

Index   731

Preface

RATIONALE AND PHILOSOPHY

LABORATORY TESTS: IMPLICATIONS FOR NURSING CARE is an interdisciplinary text designed to assist health team members in their understanding of the purpose, clinical significance, necessary preparations, procedure, precautions, findings, and subsequent nursing interventions for current laboratory tests.

Because it is prepared by a medical technologist and nursing educators, this text provides firsthand discussions of the common problems associated with performing laboratory tests and applying their results. While the nurse's role before, during, and after testing is emphasized wherever appropriate, the basic physiologic information and understandable explanations provided in this text will enable all health professionals to expand their knowledge of laboratory medicine.

When using this book it is important to remember that ranges of normal values vary depending on the laboratory, and that those ranges provided in this book are useful guidelines. However, it is always important to check normal ranges from the lab where the values are obtained.

AUDIENCE

The detailed material presented in this text is designed to provide nursing and allied health students, instructors, and practitioners as well as other health care professionals with applicable, practical information at all stages of their careers.

Students.
This text is a valuable complement to the program of learning in nursing and allied health curricula. Basic terminology, thorough background discussion of each test, clear descriptions, concise conclusions, and step-by-step instructions for many procedures make this book an indispensable companion in the classroom and during the clinical experience. To increase the usefulness of this text for students, we have included a glossary of common terms in laboratory medicine, as well as numerous figures and tables summarizing test significance and implications.

Instructors.
Use of this text during presentation of curriculum content provides the basis for discussion of the physiology and pathophysiology underlying changes in test results. Investigation of why laboratory tests result in the appearance of recognizable patterns for certain disorders

enhances the student's understanding of disease process. Titles of specialty texts in each field are included in the extensive bibliography for each chapter and can be used as a resource by student and instructor.

Practitioners.

This text promotes the rapid and efficient identification of information to provide more complete fulfillment of the patient's needs. Application of test implications and critical reference values can alert the practitioner to potentially serious changes in the patient's test results. As a special feature to practitioners, the appendix includes material on laboratory test panels, disease profiles, required specimen collection tubes for specific tests, and an extensive table of normal values to facilitate sufficient extraction of data.

ORGANIZATION

Since laboratory tests are generally performed to help formulate a diagnosis or to monitor the effects of specific therapy, we have tried to reflect these aspects in the organization of the text.

All test discussions are presented, whenever possible, according to the clinical laboratory department that usually performs the test and the laboratory request form on which each study is normally listed. For example, basic chemistry procedures such as glucose tolerance, BUN, protein, lipids, and liver function studies, which are generally listed on a routine chemistry laboratory slip, are included in Chapter 4 (Routine Chemistry). In addition, this convenient format groups certain tests that are commonly performed as part of a unit or single request. Thus, all the observations and determinations included in a urinalysis are arranged consecutively in Chapter 1 (Urinalysis) in the order they routinely appear on the test request slip. Similarly, all procedures that compose a CBC are discussed and interpreted in Chapter 2 (Hematology). Presentation of tests in this manner, rather than by disease or body system, is designed to facilitate practical use of the book and accelerate on-the-job application of specific test results.

The format of Chapter 12 (Immunohematology and Transfusion Therapy) differs somewhat from the other chapters. In addition to significant laboratory information, this chapter discusses the use of blood and its component parts, monitoring of the recipient, identification of transfusion reactions, and the appropriate intervention in the hospital and in the laboratory.

FORMAT

Our approach to the study of laboratory tests is unlike most other textbooks of this type. *A comprehensive, uniform format for presentation of similar material throughout promotes quick and easy location of desired information.* Each chapter or major unit begins with a clear, thorough introduction to the body component or physiologic process being measured. Topics such as the role of enzymes and hormones, urine formation, fluid and acid-base balance, coagulation mechanism, and hemoglobin metabolism are presented in sufficient detail to provide an understanding of the test.

To facilitate learning, individual test discussions are set up in a consistent format and include the following information:

- Definition of that procedure
- Why or when the test is ordered
- Clinical significance of the findings
- Application of the findings to patient care
- Normal values
- Interpretation of test values and various test interrelationships (when indicated)
- Extensive list of pathologic and physiologic causes for variations from normal
- Specific test precautions

This format provides information for determining if abnormal test values result from an existing condition, reflect altering factors such as certain medications and previous diagnostic studies, or signal the presence of an unsuspected disorder. Detailed procedures are consistently included for the collection, handling, and preservation of blood, urine, stool, spinal fluid, and specimens for gastric and microbiologic analysis, along with the necessary directions to prepare the individual for testing.

NEW MATERIAL

The second edition of LABORATORY TESTS is totally revised, expanded, and updated to reflect recent advances in laboratory technology and current emphasis on such topics as clinical immunology, hormonal studies, and drug monitoring. Four new chapters: Chapter 3 (Tests of Hemoglobin Metabolism), Chapter 5 (Serum Electrolytes and Blood Gas Studies), Chapter 6 (Tests of Endocrine Function), and Chapter 7 (Clinical Toxicology and Therapeutic Drug Monitoring) have been added to aid understanding and interpretation of test results. All other chapters, particularly Chapter 8 (Body Fluid Analysis) and Chapter 11 (Immunology/Serology), have been completely reorganized and rewritten to include new tests and to emphasize their clinical significance.

Some tests that were previously popular but have been replaced by newer procedures and those tests that were too experimental for widespread use at the time of writing are not included. For completeness, however, we have retained as many once commonly performed procedures as possible. We have not included discussions of other diagnostic tests (such as EEG, ECG, fiberoptics, nuclear medicine, and radiologic studies) in favor of concentrating on the primary topics and presenting a more in-depth discussion of commonly performed laboratory tests.

Acknowledgments

A special word of thanks is due to Claire and Francis Byrne for their help, encouragement, and support, not only with this task, but with all things, and to Neil, Kelly, and Heather Nugent and the rest of our families for their support and love.

C. J. B.
D. F. S.
P. K. P.
P. M. N.

1

Urinalysis

FORMATION OF URINE 2

COLLECTION AND HANDLING OF URINE 4
Procedures for Collecting Specimens · Times for Collecting Specimens
· Preservation of Urine

PHYSICAL EXAMINATION OF URINE 7
Volume · Odor · Color · Turbidity

ROUTINE URINALYSIS 13
Specific Gravity · pH Reaction · Glucose and Nonglucose Sugars
· Protein · Ketones · Occult Blood · Bilirubin · Urobilinogen
· Nitrite

MICROSCOPIC EXAMINATION 37
Red Blood Cells · White Blood Cells · Epithelial Cells · Casts
· Crystals · Bacteria · Miscellaneous Constituents

SPECIAL URINE TESTS 44
Porphobilinogen and Porphyrins · Calcium

KIDNEY FUNCTION STUDIES 49
Creatinine Clearance Test · Concentration Test
· Phenolsulfonphthalein Test

RENAL CALCULI 55

AMINOACIDURIA 57
Homogentisic Acid · Phenylpyruvic Acid

OTHER URINE STUDIES 60

Urine is a complex aqueous solution of various organic and inorganic substances that are the waste products of metabolism or products derived directly from ingested foods and fluids. The most important organic constituents are urea, uric acid, and creatinine; the chief inorganic constituents are the chlorides, phosphates, sulfates, and ammonia.

Urine is a valuable index to many normal and pathologic processes because most intrinsic kidney diseases, as well as many extrarenal conditions, can alter its composition. Certain substances appear in the urine only when pathologic conditions are present. The most important of these are sugars, proteins, ketone bodies, hemoglobin, bilirubin, urobilinogen, porphyrins, and porphobilinogen. Various additional microscopic structures such as cells, casts, crystals, and bacteria also may be present during many disorders.

FORMATION OF URINE

Formation of urine in the kidney is a complex, vital process necessary to rid the body of its metabolic waste products. Adequate renal performance depends on the functional units of the kidney known as **nephrons**. These microscopic structures vary the volume, concentration, and constituents of urine on a minute-to-minute basis according to the needs of the body. Each nephron consists of a glomerular capillary bed, the proximal convoluted tubule, the loop of Henle, the distal convoluted tubule, and the collecting duct, which leads to the renal pelvis (Figure 1-1). Each kidney contains approximately 1 million nephrons.

Urine formation involves three distinct processes: glomerular filtration, tubular reabsorption, and tubular secretion.

Glomerular Filtration
In the normal adult, approximately 1200 mL of blood pass through the kidneys each minute, exposing the blood to the semipermeable membranes of the functioning glomeruli. The principal activity of the glomerular capillary loop is filtration, which causes approximately 120 mL of plasma and its solutes to filter from the blood per minute for further processing, leaving behind most of the plasma proteins. The ultrafiltrate received in the capsule surrounding the glomerulus (**Bowman's capsule**) contains similar concentrations of most of the organic and inorganic chemicals found in the blood (glucose, amino acids, urea, uric acid, sodium, potassium, and others). The specific gravity of this almost protein-free glomerular filtrate is 1.010.

Tubular Reabsorption
As the glomerular filtrate passes through the proximal tubule, 80%−85% of its water and electrolytes and virtually all its glucose, amino acids, and other substances useful to the body are reabsorbed into the blood through the tubule cells. By varying the amounts of electrolytes reabsorbed, the kidney regulates their concentrations in the body fluids. The most important of these reclaimed electrolytes are sodium, potassium, calcium, chloride, magnesium, sulfate, and phosphate.

This selective reabsorptive process leaves metabolic waste products such as urea, uric acid, and creatinine to be excreted ultimately with the urine. Thus, the body actively reabsorbs from the glomerular filtrate those substances it needs and refuses to reabsorb those that would be harmful.

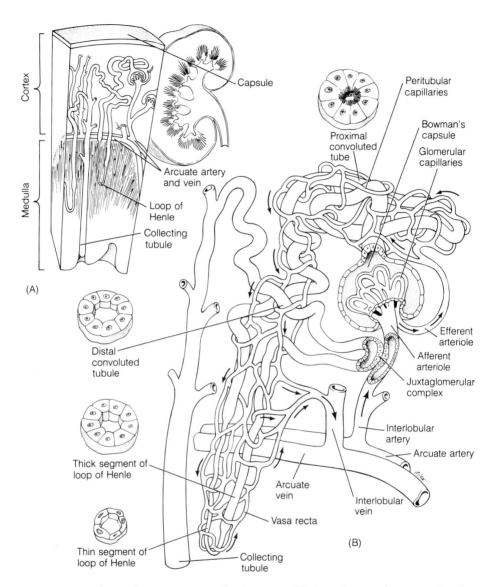

Figure 1-1   The nephron. **A**, Longitudinal section of kidney showing location of nephrons. **B**, Enlargement of nephron and its blood supply. Cross sections illustrate types of cells that are characteristic of each region of the nephron. Arrows indicate general direction of blood flow. (From Spence, A. P., and Mason, E. B. 1979. HUMAN ANATOMY AND PHYSIOLOGY. Menlo Park, Calif.: Benjamin/Cummings Publishing Co., Inc., p. 710.)

Tubular Secretion

The renal tubular cells also permit substances from the blood to enter the filtrate flowing within the tubule. Molecules of creatinine and synthetic substances such as penicillin move from the blood into the filtrate in the proximal tubule, whereas molecules of water, ammonia, and potassium move from the blood into the filtrate within the distal tubule.

By the time the filtrate reaches the loop of Henle, the original rate of flow of 120 mL/min has been reduced to about 20 mL/min because of the absorption of most of the electrolytes. The filtrate is further reduced to a flow rate of about 1 mL/min as it reaches the end of the distal tubule. This final tubule fluid, which now may be called **urine**, drips through the collecting ducts into the renal pelvis.

This continuous adjustment of urine volume and electrolyte content within the tubules is controlled by antidiuretic hormone (ADH) from the neurohypophysis and the sodium-retaining hormone aldosterone. Many additional factors such as renal blood flow, type and amount of solute load, and acid-base status influence these adjustments.

COLLECTION AND HANDLING OF URINE

Procedures for Collecting Specimens

Urine collection and handling techniques are critical to the interpretation of laboratory test results. All specimens should be collected in chemically clean, preferably sterile, containers with tight-fitting lids. A clean-voided specimen is adequate for routine examination, and a clean-catch (midstream) specimen is usually adequate for a bacteriologic culture unless otherwise ordered. Catheterizations for collecting specimens present an unnecessary risk of genitourinary tract infections and pyelonephritis.

▶▶ *Nursing Responsibilities and Implications—Voided Specimens*
To obtain a voided specimen, the following procedure should be used and/or taught to the patient:

1. Void into a clean, dry container; a clean, dry bedpan may be used and the specimen transferred into an appropriate container; a disposable specimen collection bag can be applied to the genitals of infants and young children and the specimen transferred.

2. Obtain another specimen if the original specimen is contaminated by feces; voided specimens should not be used from a woman with a vaginal discharge or one who is menstruating (obtain a clean-catch specimen).

3. Label the container with the patient's name, identification number, and room number and the date and time.

▶▶ *Nursing Responsibilities and Implications—*
Clean-Catch Specimens
To obtain a clean-catch (midstream) specimen, the following procedure should be used and/or taught to the patient:

1. Saturate three or four sterile cotton balls with an antiseptic solution such as povidone-iodine complex (Betadine).

2. With one hand, spread the female labia or retract the male foreskin, if present.

3. With the meatus exposed, use saturated sterile cotton balls to cleanse the area.

4. Start at the meatus and make only one downward stroke with each cotton ball. Repeat three times.

5. Still exposing the meatus, start urinating.

6. After a few seconds, place a sterile container under the stream to collect urine, touching only the outside of the container.

7. Cover tightly and rinse the outside of the container.

8. Affix a label with the patient's name, identification number, and room number and the date and time.

▶▶ *Nursing Responsibilities and Implications—Specimen From a Closed Urinary Drainage System*

Urine from an indwelling catheter must be collected carefully to ensure proper test interpretation. The catheter and drainage system need not be disconnected. The nurse should proceed as follows:

1. Cleanse the special collection portal on the drainage tubing with an iodine-type antiseptic solution.

2. Insert a 1-inch, 25-gauge needle of a large sterile syringe into the collection portal.

3. Gently withdraw a minimum of 10–20 mL of urine. Exerting strong suction when withdrawing the urine specimen can cause discomfort and bladder spasms.

4. Cleanse the tubing with an antiseptic solution after the needle is withdrawn.

5. Put the specimen in a sterile container.

6. Affix a label with the patient's name, identification number, and room number and the date and time.

Times for Collecting Specimens

First-Morning Specimen.   A specimen obtained during the first urination of the day is recommended for routine urine examination because it has a higher, more uniform concentration and a more acid pH than specimens obtained later in the day. Therefore, this specimen is more likely to reveal abnormalities. Because chemical tests measure the concentration of substances, significant abnormalities may be missed in dilute urine. An acid pH is also necessary to ensure better preservation of casts and other formed elements.

Random Specimen.   Random urine samples are suitable only for qualitative examinations because the concentration of any solute in urine varies widely depending on the volume of water being excreted at the time. It is misleading to compare the concentrations of substances in separate random tests.

Postprandial Specimen.   The postprandial urine specimen is obtained 2 hours after a meal and therefore is more likely to contain protein and glucose.

Afternoon Specimen.   Specimens obtained between 2 and 4 PM are best for evaluating urobilinogen.

Twenty-Four-Hour Specimen.   Quantitative estimations of urinary solutes such as total urine protein, creatinine, and electrolytes require 24-hour specimens. The 24-hour time period provides comparable urine samples for measurement when a series of tests is needed to assess the progress of disease or the efficacy of treatment.

▶▶ *Nursing Responsibilities and Implications*
Because the composition of urine changes on standing, urine should be collected when the laboratory is open or it should be refrigerated until that time. The nurse should tell the patient and other staff at what time the specimen is required and how it is to be collected. The patient who can assume responsibility should be taught how to collect the specimen.

When collecting a timed specimen, uniform collection procedures must be followed. The following procedure should be used and/or taught to the patient:

1. Ask the patient to empty the bladder at the beginning of the time period (e.g., 8 AM) and discard this urine.

2. Post a notice of the timed collection on the chart at the nursing station, in the patient's bathroom, and on the bedpan hopper.

3. Save all urine voided during the allotted time (e.g., 24 hours), including the urine voided at the end of the time period.

4. Collect the total specimen in a clean, wide-mouthed, covered container and keep on ice or refrigerated the entire time, unless otherwise specified.

5. Add special preservatives to the container as required at the beginning of the collection period.

6. Label the container, indicating the test, date, time the collection is started and when it should end, and the patient's name, identification number, and room number.

7. If any part of the specimen is accidently discarded, the laboratory should be notified of the amount because the test may need to be restarted.

Preservation of Urine

Urine should be examined within 30 minutes after it is passed because some urinary components are unstable. Allowing urine to stand at room temperature can cause the precipitation of phosphates in an alkaline urine and the growth of bacteria with a resulting change to an alkaline pH.

If a urine specimen cannot be examined immediately, it must be refrigerated. Bacteriologic culture also should be done within 30 minutes, but the specimen may be refrigerated for up to 2 hours if necessary.

Preservation of urine prevents bacterial proteins from interfering with tests for proteins, instability of urinary solutes, degeneration of organized sediments (pus, blood, and casts), bacterial growth, and degradation of glucose by bacteria or yeasts. In addition, preservation of urine helps maintain an acid pH by preventing alkaline fermentation (conversion of urea to ammonium carbonate) caused by urea-splitting organisms.

Refrigeration.   Refrigeration is the most satisfactory method of preservation and is necessary regardless of whether chemical preservatives are added.

Toluene.   When enough toluene is added to form a thin layer over the surface, it preserves acetone, diacetic acid, reducing substances, and protein. It does not interfere with other tests nor effectively stop the growth of microorganisms.

Thymol.   A small crystal (5 mm diameter of thymol) per 100 mL of urine is a good preservative for most chemical tests. However, excess amounts give a false-positive protein (albumin) reading and interfere with bile tests.

Formalin 40%.   One drop of 40% formalin per 30 mL of urine or 10 mL per 24-hour volume preserves formed elements of urinary sediment. Excess amounts precipitate urea, which interferes with microscopic examinations. Formalin causes positive Clinitest and Fehling results and interferes with tests for indican.

Formaldehyde Tablets.   One tablet of formaldehyde per 60 mL of urine is an excellent preservative for routine chemical tests and for formed elements. However, it interferes with sodium, potassium, and hormone studies and slightly increases the specific gravity of urine.

Special Preservatives.   Certain tests require special preservatives, which are added to the container before urine collection, including the following:

Epinephrine (Adrenalin), nor-adrenaline, catecholamines, vanillyl-mandelic acid: 10 mL of concentrated pH 2.0 hydrochloric acid in a brown bottle (to protect from light)

Aldosterone: 10 mL of pH 4.5 glacial acetic acid

Porphyrins: 10 g of sodium carbonate

Serotonin: 10−15 g boric acid

Steroids: 10 mL of concentrated hydro-chloric acid

PHYSICAL EXAMINATION OF URINE

Volume

Urine volume depends on the amount of solutes to be excreted, loss of fluid in perspiration and exhaled air, cardiac and renal status of the patient, and hormonal influences, as well as the amount of fluid ingested. Young children usually excrete three to four times more urine per kilogram of body weight than adults.

Normal Values

The normal values for urine volume are:

Children	300−1500 mL/24 hours
Adults	800−2000 mL/24 hours
Overnight	<400 mL
Day-to-night ratio	2:1−3:1

Variations

Polyuria.   Urine excretion of more than 2000 mL/day or 55 mL/hr when fluid intake is restricted (no fluid for 14 hours) constitutes **polyuria**. Polyuria must be distinguished from the small, frequent voidings associated with cystitis and pyelonephritis.

Increased urine volume may be associated with:

Increased amount of circulating blood

  Administration of large amounts of intravenous fluids

  Burns (48–72 hours after injury)

  Chilling of the skin

  Correction of cardiac decompensation

  Excessive fluid intake (**polydipsia**), as in some pathologic or psycho-neurotic states

Increased solutes in the filtrate

  Diabetes mellitus

  Excess calcium intake

  Excess salt intake

  High-protein diet

  Hyperparathyroidism

  Infections

Pathologic states

  Hormone dysfunction

    Addison's disease (decreased adrenal corticoids)

    Adrenalectomy

    Diabetes insipidus (decreased ADH)

    Primary aldosteronism (increased aldosterone)

    Secondary adrenal insufficiency

  Renal disorders (chronic, progressive)

    Potassium depletion (prolonged and severe)

    Renal insufficiency (early)

    Salt-depleting nephritis

    Tubular damage

Pharmacologic preparations

  Administration of potassium chloride, sodium sulfate, and urea

  Alcohol

  Caffeine

  Diuretics (mercurial and thiazide)

  Intravenous glucose or saline solutions

Oliguria or Anuria. Even under conditions of severe water restriction, an individual usually excretes at least 30 mL of urine per hour. Therefore, an excretion of less than 30 mL of urine per hour or 500 mL/24 hours indicates definite **oliguria**. **Anuria** is the excretion of less than 10 mL of urine per hour or 125 mL/24 hours caused by the suppression of urine formation or obstruction of the urinary tract.

Decreased urine volume may be associated with:

Decreased amount of circulating blood

  Congestive heart failure

  Dehydration (prolonged vomiting, diarrhea, diaphoresis, or fever without adequate fluid replacement)

  Edema

  Shock

  Water deprivation, diminished fluid intake

Decreased sodium in the filtrate

Renal pathology

  Acute glomerulonephritis

  Acute pyelonephritis

  Crush syndrome (symptoms of renal failure following the crushing of a part)

  Obstruction—bilateral hydronephrosis

  Terminal chronic nephritis

  Transfusion reaction

  Toxic agents (carbon tetrachloride, diethylene glycol, mercury bichloride, and sulfonamides)

Odor

Fresh urine from most healthy patients has an aromatic odor. This odor may be modified after standing for any length of time by bacterial decomposition, which produces the characteristic pungency of ammonia.

Variations
Additional odors may be due to a variety of causes:

Certain ingested foods (garlic and asparagus) and medications (menthol, antibiotics, paraldehyde, and vitamins) give characteristic odors

Acetone and acetoacetic acid formed in starvation, diabetes mellitus, or dehydration are easily recognized by their sweet or fruity smell

Maple syrup urine disease, an inherited metabolic disorder in infants, gains its name from the passage of urine with that odor

Phenylketonuria produces urine described as smelling "mousey"

The bacterial action on pus in heavily infected urine results in a particularly offensive odor

Color

Freshly voided urine ranges in color from light straw to dark amber because of a mixture of pigments referred to as urochromes (uroerythrin, urochrome, and urobilin). The color varies with specific gravity: dilute urine is pale yellow; concentrated urine appears almost deep orange.

Variations
Numerous metabolic products, pigments, drugs, and foods influence urine color, but these seldom have real diagnostic importance. In other circumstances urine color may have great diagnostic significance (Table 1-1).

The most common abnormal urine color is **red or red-brown**. Although the color may result from many causes, when it is seen in females, the possibility of menstrual contamination should immediately be considered.

Yellow-brown or green-brown urine most often is associated with bile pigments, chiefly bilirubin. Bilirubin oxidizes on standing to green biliverdin, so with severe obstructive jaundice, the urine may be dark green. Urine with bilirubin may be distinguished from normal dark, concentrated urine by the appearance of yellow foam when a sample is shaken. Normal urine has a white foam.

Urine that contains large amounts of urobilin resembles dark concentrated normal urine and is **orange-red or orange-brown**. When excreted, urobilinogen is colorless, but in the presence of light and acid it is converted to urobilin, which is light yellow or orange. Unlike bilirubin, urobilin does not color foam on shaking.

Acid urine that contains hemoglobin becomes **dark brown or black** on standing because of the formation of methemoglobin. The black color also may be caused by melanin, which is seen in association with extensive melanotic sarcoma or ochronosis.

TABLE 1-1   Color and Appearance of Urine

Appearance	Cause
Almost colorless (very pale greenish yellow)	Alcohol ingestion
	Chronic kidney disease
	Diabetes insipidus
	Diabetes mellitus
	Diuretic therapy
	Large fluid intake
	Nervousness
	Severe iron deficiency
Yellow	Acriflavine
	Anisindione (Miradon [in alkaline urine])
	Cascara
	Fluorescein sodium (given IV)
	Food color
	Mepacrine
	Nitrofurantoin (Furadantin)
	Phenacetin
	Phenindione (Hedulin [in alkaline urine])
	Quinacrine hydrochloride (Atabrine)
	Riboflavin
	Salicylazosulfapyridine (Azulfidine [in alkaline urine])
Orange	Azo Gantrisin
	Bilirubin
	Carotene
	Concentrated urine
	Ethoxazene
	Excess sweating
	Fever
	Food color
	Furazolidone (Furoxone)
	Multivitamins
	Nitrofurantoin
	Phenazopyridine hydrochloride (Pyridium)
	Restricted fluid intake
	Rhubarb, senna, santonin, cascara (in acid urine)
	Sulfasalazine
	Sulfonamides
	Thiamine hydrochloride
	Urobilin in excess
Pink, red, or reddish orange	Amidopyrine
	Azo Gantrisin
	Beets
	Cascara (in alkaline urine)
	Chlorzoxazone

TABLE 1-1 Color and Appearance of Urine (*continued*)

Appearance	Cause
Pink, red, or reddish orange (*continued*)	Chlorpromazine hydrochloride (Thorazine)
	Chromogenic bacteria (*Serratia marcescens*)
	Deferoxamine (Desferal)
	Dorbantyl
	Doxidan
	Emodin (in alkaline urine)
	Ex-Lax
	Food color
	Fuscin
	Hemoglobin
	Methemoglobin
	Modane
	Myoglobin
	Neotropin
	Phenindione
	Phenolphthalein (in alkaline urine)
	Phenolsulfonphthalein (in alkaline urine)
	Phenothiazine
	Phenytoin (Dilantin)
	Porphyrin
	Pyrvinium pamoate (Povan)
	Rhubarb, santonin, senna (in alkaline urine)
	Rifampin
	Selenium
	Sulfobromophthalein sodium (Bromsulphalein [in alkaline urine])
Green or blue-green (often blue mixed with yellow urine)	Amitriptyline (Elavil hydrochloride)
	Azuresin (Diagnex Blue)
	Bilirubin-biliverdin
	Blutene
	Evans blue
	Guiacol
	Indican
	Indigo-carmine
	Methocarbamol (Robaxin)
	Methylene blue
	Phenylsalicylate
	Pseudomonas toxemia
	Vitamin B complex
	Yeast concentrate
Pale blue	Pyrenium
Brown or black	Alkapton bodies (homogentisic acid)
	Bilirubin-biliverdin
	Cascara

TABLE 1-1 Color and Appearance of Urine (*continued*)

Appearance	Cause
Brown or black (*continued*)	Chloroquine phosphate (Aralen)
	Furazolidone (Furoxone)
	Hematin
	Iron compounds (injectable)
	Levodopa (L-dopa)
	Lysol poisoning
	Melanin
	Metronidazole
	Methemoglobin
	Nitrofurantoin
	Phenol
	Phenylhydrazine
	Porphyrin
	Rhubarb, senna, santonin, cascara (in acid urine)
	Sinemet
Cloudy	Bacteria
	Calculi "gravel"
	Clumps, pus, tissue
	Fecal contamination
	Leukocytes
	Mucin, mucous threads
	Phosphates, carbonates
	Prostatic fluid
	Red blood cells (smoky)
	Spermatozoa
	Urates, uric acid
	X-ray contrast media
Milky	Fat (lipuria, opalescent; chyluria, milky)
	Pyuria

Turbidity

Freshly voided urine is usually clear but may appear cloudy, a feature that generally has no pathologic significance. When clear urine stands at room temperature for several days, a hazy sediment of mucous threads, phosphates, and bacteria may appear in the bottom of the container. The mucous threads originate from the bladder, prostate, and kidney and have little clinical significance. A sediment of urates or phosphates may appear in a postprandial specimen. This turbidity usually disappears from specimens collected 2–3 hours after a meal. Cellular contamination in female patients is a common cause of turbidity. However, pathologic urine specimens are often turbid, so a careful microscopic examination of urine sediment must be performed to detect the cause.

Variations

Cloudy urine may be ascribed to the following:

Amorphous phosphates form a white sediment in neutral or alkaline urine that disappears when acid is added. The amount of phosphates increases when urine stands because it becomes more alkaline due to the formation of ammonia. Phosphates are very common and have little clinical significance.

Amorphous urates are less common and form a pink sediment that disappears with heating.

Pus (**pyuria**) is grossly indistinguishable from amorphous phosphates, but it does not disappear when acid is added. Pus appears mucoid in alkaline urine, but it is crumbly in acid urine.

Blood, which produces a reddish brown or smoky color, must be confirmed by microscopic or chemical tests. About 200 white blood cells per cubic millimeter or 500 red blood cells per cubic millimeter are sufficient to produce turbidity.

Bacteria that produce a uniform cloud or opalescence usually multiply in the urine after voiding and have no clinical significance.

Fat (**lipuria**) gives a milky appearance or a "greasy" cloudiness.

Chyle (**chyluria**), which gives urine a cream color, may be caused by filarial parasites, thoracic duct obstruction, trauma, or tumor.

ROUTINE URINALYSIS

Urinalysis is important from two general standpoints: diagnosis and management of renal or urinary tract disease and detection of metabolic or systemic diseases not directly related to the kidneys. Urinalysis is a valuable screening aid for detecting diabetes mellitus; acid-base, fluid, or electrolyte imbalance; and genitourinary tract inflammation. A few simple tests such as those for sugar, protein, ketones, and others, along with examination of urinary sediment, provide much helpful information. When combined with a specific gravity reading and microscopic examination of the urinary sediment (routine urinalysis), much important information can be obtained.

▶▶ Nursing Responsibilities and Implications

Basic chemical screening can be done quickly and routinely using reagent strips and tablets to replace the classic individual wet or bench methods. Most reagent strips contain six to eight separate test areas for the estimation of pH and the detection of protein, glucose, ketones, bilirubin, urobilinogen, nitrite, and blood. Regardless of the reagent strip being used (see Table 1-2), the nurse should proceed as follows:

1. Obtain a freshly voided specimen.

2. Use the clean-catch method if the patient is menstruating or has a vaginal or urethral discharge.

3. Record the product being used; use the same product that has been used previously or note the change.

4. Dip the reagent stick or tape into the urine to completely cover the testing area.

5. Hold the stick or tape horizontally and tap the side of the container to remove excess urine and prevent the chemicals from mixing.

6. Read the results sequentially in good light at the time specified by the manufacturer.

7. Use only the color chart supplied with the product.

8. Record the results on the patient's chart.

9. Notify the physician of any unexpected or significant deviations.

10. Do not use strips or tapes that are discolored because they produce inaccurate results.

Specific Gravity

Although the renal glomeruli filter approximately 170 L of fluid daily, an average of only 1.5 L is voided as urine. This volume reduction is due to reabsorption of water and solutes in the renal tubules, which is regulated by the antidiuretic hormone (ADH). A healthy kidney varies the volume of excreted urine and solute concentration to maintain homeostasis of body fluids and electrolytes. The kidney does this by selectively reabsorbing or excreting electrolytes, salts, and water. The specific gravity of the urine indicates the amount of dissolved solids in the fluid. The most important urine solutes are urea, sodium, and chloride, but uric acid, creatinine, sulfates, and phosphates also are excreted in the urine.

In the healthy person, the ingestion of large quantities of water produces a large volume of dilute, low-solute-content urine. On the other hand, water deprivation produces a reduced volume of concentrated, high-solute-content urine as water is conserved by the kidneys. The most convenient way of measuring the concentrating and diluting functions of the kidney is to measure the specific gravity, which is an indicator of the concentration of dissolved solids in the urine.

Clinical Significance

The consistent inability of the kidneys to concentrate or dilute urine indicates severe involvement of the renal tubules or ADH deficiency. Accurate measurement of specific gravity is valuable in differentiating prerenal causes of oliguria, such as dehydration, from renal causes, such as acute renal necrosis, because concentrated urine yielding a high specific gravity is found in dehydration. Differentiation is important because of the need to restrict fluids in patients with acute tubular necrosis and to give fluids and electrolytes to patients who are dehydrated.

Normal Values
The normal values for urine specific gravity are:

Normal diet and fluid intake	1.016–1.022
First-morning specimen	1.007–1.030
Under stress conditions	1.001–1.040

Variations

Increased urine specific gravity (values over 1.020 [hyperosthenuria]) may result from:

Congestive heart failure

Decreased fluid intake

Dehydration (caused by fever, vomiting, diarrhea, or excessive sweating)

Diabetes mellitus

Intravenous albumin

Liver disorders

Nephrosis

Urine preservatives

X-ray contrast media

Decreased urine specific gravity (values less than 1.009 [hyposthenuria]) may result from:

Acute renal failure

Alkalosis

Diabetes insipidus

Hypercalcemia (resulting from sarcoidosis, bone disease, hyperparathyroidism, vitamin D intoxication)

Hypothermia

Increased fluid intake

Renal parenchymal disease (pyelonephritis, polycystic disease, hydronephrosis)

Severe potassium deficiency

Methodology

Specific gravity most commonly is measured by the urinometer method, which indicates the buoyancy of a special hydrometer plummet calibrated for urine. Urinometers are calibrated to read 1.000 in water at 20 C. However, room temperature and therefore urine temperature are usually much higher than this, so exact specific gravity readings should be temperature corrected by subtracting 0.001 from the specific gravity reading for each 2 degrees above 20 C.

Specific gravity also may be measured with a refractometer calibrated in specific gravity units. This method is rapid and requires only one large drop of urine as compared with the 15 mL needed for the urinometer.

A specific gravity reading higher than 1.040 suggests the presence of abnormal substances such as glucose, proteins, or x-ray contrast media. For the specific gravity measurement to better reflect the concentrating ability of the kidneys, the readings should be corrected by subtracting 0.001 from the specific gravity reading for every 0.4 g of protein per deciliter of urine and 0.004 from the specific gravity reading for every 1.0 g of glucose per deciliter of urine.

▶▶ ## Nursing Responsibilities and Implications

The nurse usually is asked to measure the specific gravity of urine with the urinometer, using a glass cylinder to hold the urine. The nurse should proceed as follows:

1. Use a fresh specimen of urine that has been well mixed.

2. Fill the cylinder with enough urine to freely float the urinometer.

3. Gently spin the urinometer so it does not adhere to the sides of the cylinder.

4. Read the scale at eye level at the lowest point of the meniscus.

5. Remember that the scale is calibrated in units of 0.0001 ranging from 1.001 to 1.060 and is read from top to bottom.

6. Monitor intake and output if values are increased or decreased.

7.   Encourage fluid intake, if permitted, when the specific gravity is increased.

8.   Observe the patient for signs of circulatory overload caused by excessive intravenous fluid intake, impending renal failure, and diabetes insipidus when the specific gravity is decreased.

pH Reaction

Urinary pH is a measure of the amount of free hydrogen ions excreted by the body. It is controlled by the renal tubules, excretion of metabolic acids by the glomerulus, ammonia formation, bicarbonate reabsorption, changes in the glomerular filtration rate, and renal blood flow. The renal tubules, together with the lungs, play a central role in maintaining a normal hydrogen ion concentration in plasma and extracellular fluid. Changes in urinary pH depend largely on the acid-base composition of the blood.

Clinical Significance
The metabolic activity of the body (mainly protein and fat metabolism) produces excess nonvolatile acids, which are principally sulfuric, phosphoric, and hydrochloric acids, with small amounts of pyruvic, lactic, and citric acids. Small amounts of ketone bodies also are formed. The glomerulus normally excretes these nonvolatile metabolic acids because the lungs are unable to expel them from the body.

   During sleep, decreased pulmonary ventilation causes mild respiratory acidosis, and the urine becomes highly acid. Immediately following a meal the urine becomes less acid (the "alkaline tide"), only to become more acid again a few hours later. Because of these physiologic changes, the urinary pH varies widely in healthy individuals. The kidneys' ability to vary urine pH is one of the first physiologic mechanisms lost in patients with pyelonephritis or necrosis of the distal tubular epithelium.

Normal Values
The normal values for urine pH are:

Random specimen	4.6–8.0
Average	6.0
During sleep	<6.0
After eating	>6.0

Variations
Persistently low urine pH (below 6) may be associated with:

Administration of ammonium chloride, ascorbic acid, diazoxide, hippuric acid, methenamine mandelate, metolazone

High-protein diet

Ingestion of certain fruits (cranberries)

Metabolic acidosis (diabetes mellitus, diarrhea, starvation)

Metabolic diseases (alkaptonuria, phenylketonuria)

Pyrexia

Respiratory acidosis (anesthesia, emphysema, methyl alcohol poisoning)

Tuberculosis, renal

Urine pH should be kept low (acid) in patients during treatment for:

Urinary calculi that develop in alkaline urine (calcium phosphate, calcium carbonate, and magnesium ammonium phosphate stones)

Urinary tract infections and persistent bacteriuria, particularly those involving urea-splitting organisms

Persistently high urine pH (above 6) may be associated with:

Administration of acetazolamide, aldosterone, amphotericin B, mafenide, parathyroid extract, potassium citrate, prolactin, sodium bicarbonate

Excessive ingestion of vegetables and citrus fruits

Metabolic alkalosis (prolonged gastric suction, intractable vomiting, overdose of alkali, constant diuretic therapy, hyperaldosteronism, Cushing's disease)

Potassium depletion (renal insufficiency, prolonged therapy with cortisone or carbonic anhydrase inhibitors)

Respiratory alkalosis (hyperventilation and some cases of cardiac failure)

Urinary tract infections (caused by urea-splitting organisms)

Urine pH should be kept high (alkaline) in patients during:

Blood transfusion therapy (because blood pigments are more soluble in an alkaline media, the alkaline urine is thought to offer some protection to the kidneys should hemolytic transfusion reactions occur)

Mecamylamine therapy for hypertension

Streptomycin, neomycin, kanamycin

therapy (effective in genitourinary tract infections only if the urine is alkaline)

Sulfonamide therapy (alkaline urine helps to prevent sulfonamide crystallization in the urinary tract)

Treatment of salicylate intoxication

Treatment for urinary calculi that can develop in acid urine (uric acid, calcium oxalate, or cystine stones)

Methodology
Precise pH measurements require freshly voided specimens because pH tends to rise on standing due to loss of carbon dioxide and ammonia production from bacterial growth (see Table 1-2).

▶▶ Nursing Responsibilities and Implications
Before sending a urine specimen to the laboratory for pH measurement, the nurse should fill the container to minimize the amount of dead air space and cover the container tightly.

The nurse may be required to measure urinary pH on the unit instead of sending the specimen to the laboratory. Several commercial stick or paper products are available for this purpose that vary little in methodology. In addition to following the manufacturer's specific directions for using the product, the nurse should proceed as follows:

1. Use a freshly voided specimen.

2. Test the specimen; see the guidelines for reagent strip use under Routine Urinalysis—Nursing Responsibilities and Implications.

3. Read the results immediately in good light using only the color chart supplied with the product.

4. Record the results.

5. If the urinary pH is acid, monitor the patient for metabolic or respiratory acidosis.

6. If the urinary pH is alkaline, monitor the patient for the presence of a urinary tract infection; encourage fluid intake.

Glucose and Nonglucose Sugars

Routine screening of urine samples for the presence of glucose (**glycosuria**) is included in the basic examination for any patient. The primary goal of tests for glucose is the detection of diabetes mellitus. However, because glycosuria may have other causes, such as recent ingestion of large amounts of carbohydrate or impaired renal tubular activity, further studies are required to confirm the diagnosis of diabetes mellitus. Screening tests for glycosuria are best done on postprandial specimens.

Clinical Significance
In the healthy kidney, the glucose filtered through the glomerulus from the blood is reabsorbed in the proximal tubule. The renal tubules have a maximum reabsorptive capacity (renal threshold) of about 160–180 mg/dL of blood. At blood concentrations above this value, glucose appears in the urine in concentrations high enough to be detected by the usual screening methods. Glucose also may appear in the urine at normal blood levels if the ability of the renal tubules to reabsorb it is decreased.

Glucose usually appears in the urine when blood levels are only moderately elevated. However, many diabetics, especially those with long-standing diabetes or atherosclerosis, have an increased renal threshold for glucose that prevents its appearance in the urine until the blood glucose level is quite elevated. Therefore, establishing the blood glucose level at which glycosuria occurs is an important guide for individualized diabetic management. (Blood glucose levels are discussed in Chapter 4.)

Normal Values

Normal urine glucose values are:

Reagent strip screening test	Negative
Quantitative measurement	Approximately 15 mg/dL*

*May be influenced by many drugs and nonglucose sugars, which can cause false-positive results on screening tests (see Methodology).

Variations
Glycosuria may be associated with:

Administration of aminosalicylic acid (aspirin), ammonium chloride, asparaginase, carbamazepine, corticosteroids, dextrothyroxine, ephedrine, furosemide, lithium carbonate, nicotinic acid, phenothiazines, phenytoin, thiazide diuretics

Alimentary glycosuria (occurs after the ingestion of large amounts of sugar, especially following gastrectomy)

Anesthesia (also following morphine or strychnine administration and asphyxia)

Diabetes mellitus (accompanied by hyperglycemia)

Disease or damage of the central nervous system (meningitis, cerebrovascular accidents)

Endocrine disturbance (hyperthyroidism, acromegaly, Cushing's disease)

Epinephrine (whether injected or released from the adrenal glands)

Excitement and stress

Fanconi's syndrome (lowered renal tubular reabsorptive capacity for glucose)

Glucose infusions

Infections

Intracranial injury (especially subarachnoid hemorrhage)

Liver damage (due to the liver's inability to convert glucose to glycogen)

Pancreatitis (due to disturbed carbohydrate utilization)

Pregnancy

Renal tubular damage (resulting from mercury, uranium, or Lysol disinfectant poisoning, myelomatosis, or acute glomerulonephritis)

Occasionally, the demonstration of sugars other than glucose is highly significant. The presence of these additional sugars may signify dietary peculiarities or congenital metabolic abnormalities.

Galactosuria may occur in patients with advanced liver disease. In infants galactosuria is a more significant finding than glycosuria. It may signal the presence of galactosemia, a potentially life-threatening hereditary disease. Unless detected early and treated by the elimination of lactose and galactose from the diet, it may lead within several months to the development of cataracts, mental retardation, and cirrhosis and may progress to an early death. Galactose excretion occurs only if the child is ingesting moderate amounts of milk, so tests performed during the immediate newborn period before milk is included in the diet cannot detect galactosuria.

Fructosuria may result from severe liver disease, or it may occur with a very rare inherited metabolic defect. Early detection is important because complete fructose elimination from the diet results in total recovery. Fructosuria also may appear in patients with diabetes mellitus.

Pentosuria appears in a rare inherited disease that affects metabolism. It also may occur following the ingestion of certain fruits such as plums or cherries. Pentosuria has been reported in morphine addicts.

Lactosuria normally occurs in women during pregnancy and lactation. Lactose intolerance associated with lactosuria is a rare metabolic disorder.

Methodology

Reagent strip screening tests for urine sugar (N-Multistix and Chemstrip) are specific for glucose and indicate the degree of glycosuria (see Table 1-2). However, these methods will not reveal the presence of nonglucose sugars and can be a liability when used as a general screening test for urinary sugars. They are therefore not appropriate for pediatric screening, certain diabetics with marked glycosuria, or patients receiving parenteral nutrition with fructose. In these situations Clinitest tablets should be used to detect and measure glycosuria. Clinitest tablets also should be used when the reagent strip test for glucose is positive in the presence of a moderate amount of ketone.

Clinitest tablets detect glucose as well as a variety of additional nonglucose reducing substances that may be found in the urine. Specific identification of these nonglucose sugars requires thin-layer or paper chromatographic techniques. The nonglucose substances that may cause a false-positive result when Clinitest tablets are used include:

Amidopyrine	Galactose	Para-aminobenzoic acid
Ampicillin	Glucosamine	Para-aminosalicylic acid
Ascorbic acid	Glucuronic acid	Paraldehyde
Camphor	Homogentisic acid	Penicillin
Cephalosporins	Isoniazid	Pentose
Cephalothin	Lactose	Phenol
Chloral hydrate	L-Dopa	Probenecid
Chloramphenicol	Menthol	Salicylates
Chloroform	Metaxalone	Streptomycin
Creatinine	Nalidixic acid	Tetracyclines
Formaldehyde	Nitrofurantoin	Turpentine
Fructose	Oxytetracycline	Uric acid

▶▶ *Nursing Responsibilities and Implications*

The nurse often is asked to test urine for glucose. In addition to following the manufacturer's specific directions for the product being used, the nurse should proceed as follows:

1. Use a freshly voided specimen.

2. Use the same method that has been used previously or chart any change in the method being used.

3. Make certain all equipment such as the collection container, graduate, and test tubes are clean.

4. If the nurse is testing the urine to provide coverage with regular insulin 30 minutes before meals and at bedtime, the patient should be taught to empty the bladder 30 minutes before the specimen is due, encouraged to drink fluids, and to void again at the specified time (double-voided specimen).

5. If a reagent strip method is used, see the guidelines for reagent strip use under Routine Urinalysis—Nursing Responsibilities and Implications.

6. If the Clinitest method is used, the nurse should:
   a. Place the proper number of drops of urine into a test tube (two-drop method or five-drop method).
   b. Rinse the dropper and place ten drops of water into the test tube.
   c. Drop one Clinitest tablet into the test tube; avoid touching the tablet to prevent contamination; a burn may be sustained if the hands are wet.
   d. Do not touch the test tube during the reaction to prevent burns.

7. Read the results in good light at the specific time directed by the manufacturer, using only the color chart supplied with the product.

8. Remember that the same glucose content in the urine may be indicated by different colors or number of plus signs in different products.

Protein

The presence of protein in the urine (**proteinuria**), in sufficient quantities to be detected by most screening tests, is a very sensitive indicator of renal disorders. Because the degree of proteinuria varies depending on the type and severity of the disease, measuring the amount of protein excreted aids in diagnosis and directs therapy.

A benign transitory proteinuria that is unrelated to organic disease can occur following nonpathologic activities such as strenuous exercise, severe emotional stress, or prolonged exposure to cold. However, continued proteinuria in an apparently healthy person usually is a sign of at least minimal kidney damage.

In pathologic states the degree of proteinuria, although continuous, is rarely constant. Because protein concentration depends on many factors, including urine concentration, every random urine sample may not contain abnormal amounts of protein. Therefore, a 24-hour protein determination is the most accurate indicator of the severity of the condition. Although normal glomeruli prevent most albumin and the larger plasma globulins from entering the glomerular filtrate, it usually contains 10−25 mg of protein per deciliter or about 18−45 g/24 hours. Tubular epithelial cells reabsorb most of this protein, making the normal amount of protein too small to be detected in random samples.

Clinical Significance

Theoretically, proteinuria may be associated with:

Passage of excess proteins across a glomerular filter injured by disease

Disturbance of normal renal tubular protein reabsorption

Abnormal secretion of protein from the plasma by renal tubular cells

The most common pathologic cause of proteinuria involves increased passage through a damaged glomerular capillary filter rather than decreased reabsorption by the renal tubules. In most kidney diseases involving proteinuria, albumin is the most predominant fraction because its relatively small molecular weight allows it to be filtered most easily. As kidney damage increases, proteins of increasingly higher molecular weight escape into the urine; therefore, not only albumin but also many of the larger globulins may be present. Even in diseases in which albumin is the predominant fraction, the term proteinuria is preferred to the older albuminuria because these other proteins also may be present.

Normal Values

The normal values for urine protein are:

Reagent strip screening test	Negative
Quantitative measurement	2−8 mg/dL
	40−80 mg/24 hours
Upper limits of normal	20 mg/dL
	150 mg/24 hours
Following strenuous exercise	50 mg/dL

Variations

Proteinuria may occur in varying degrees and result from many causes.

    Heavy proteinuria (more than 4 g/24 hours) may be associated with:

Acute and chronic glomerulonephritis

Amyloid disease

Lupus erythematosus

Nephrotic syndrome

Severe venous congestion of the kidney

    Moderate proteinuria (0.5 – 4.0 g/24 hours) may be associated with all of the conditions listed under heavy proteinuria, as well as:

Abdominal tumors and intestinal obstruction

Acute infectious diseases due to the irritant effect of bacterial toxins (diphtheria, scarlet fever, pneumonia, typhoid fever, acute streptococcal infections)

Cardiac disease

Central nervous system lesions

Convulsions

Drugs such as amphotericin B, ampicillin, aspirin, bacitracin, barbiturates, cephaloridine, corticosteroids, gentamicin, gold, kanamycin, mercurial diuretics, neomycin, phenylbutazone, polymyxin B, streptomycin, sulfonamides

Hematologic disorders (severe anemia, leukemia, purpura)

Hepatic disease with jaundice and ascites

Hyperthyroidism

Irritation of the kidneys from radiation

Multiple myeloma

Nephrogenic diabetes insipidus

Nephrosclerosis

Pyelonephritis with hypertension

Septicemia

Subacute bacterial endocarditis

Toxemia of pregnancy (due to preeclampsia or primary hypertensive disease or preexisting renal disease)

Toxic irritation of the kidney from the ingestion of substances such as arsenic, carbon tetrachloride, ether, lead, mercury, mustard, opiates, phenol, phosphorus, propylene glycol, sulfosalicylic acid, turpentine

    Minimal proteinuria (less than 0.5 g/24 hours) may be associated with:

Chronic pyelonephritis (however, in the presence of progressive renal involvement, proteinuria and pyuria may be absent; therefore, a negative screening test for proteinuria does not completely rule out pyelonephritis)

Polycystic kidney disease

Renal tubular disease (acute tubular necrosis, Butler-Albright syndrome, Bright's disease, Fanconi's syndrome, Bartter's syndrome)

    Transient proteinuria (usually benign but may indicate incipient renal damage) may be associated with:

Dehydration

Emotional stress

Exposure to cold

Fever

Hemorrhage (post)

High-protein diet

Injections of epinephrine or norepinephrine

Orthostatic proteinuria (proteinuria found during the day while the patient is upright but not at night while reclining because it is apparently related to an exaggerated lordotic position that results in changes in renal circulation)

Salt depletion

Strenuous and unaccustomed exercise (may persist for as long as 3 days)

False proteinuria results from the accidental mixture of urine with such protein-containing substances as pus, blood, or vaginal discharge. About 80–100 red blood cells per cubic millimeter will give 0.1% albumin. This contamination occurs most frequently in pyelitis, cystitis, chronic vaginitis, and prostatitis and during menstruation.

Abnormal proteins in the urine are rare but may appear under certain conditions. The most prominent of these is the Bence-Jones protein, which is highly suggestive but not absolutely diagnostic of multiple myeloma; it occurs in 50%–80% of patients with this disease. The Bence-Jones protein originates from plasma cells in the bone marrow and is filtered by the glomerular capillary membrane. Large amounts of the Bence-Jones protein are excreted by patients with bone tumors and certain other conditions, causing degeneration of renal tubular cells and an overall decrease of renal function. The classic urine heat and acid test uses characteristic physical properties to screen for the Bence-Jones protein. This protein forms a heavy precipitate at temperatures between 45 and 60 C that disappears at higher or lower temperatures.

The presence of the **Bence-Jones protein** in the urine is associated with:

Amyloidosis	Malignant lymphoma
Chronic lymphocytic leukemia	Metastatic bone tumor
Hyperparathyroidism	Multiple myeloma
Macroglobulinemia	Osteomalacia

Other abnormal proteins or direct protein components such as globulin fragments, myoglobin, and mucoprotein also may be present in urine, indicating heavy chain disease, macroglobulinemia, or various tubular defects. However, routine reagent strip or heat screening tests may miss as many as one-third of these dysproteinurias. A special electrophoretic technique is needed to detect and identify abnormal urine proteins as well as to differentiate the individual proteins and protein components. (Urine and serum protein electrophoresis are discussed in Chapter 4.)

Methodology

Reagent strip screening tests for urine protein (N-Multistix, Chemstrip) are most sensitive to albumin, but they are inadequate for detecting the presence of globulins, mucoproteins, or the Bence-Jones protein (see Table 1-2). The color chart accompanying these test strips lists a grading of the nuances of test colors with approximate protein levels ranging from negative to 4+ concentrations. These grades are as follows:

Negative = Under 10 mg/dL
Trace   = 15–25 mg/dL
1+   = 30 mg/dL
2+   = 100 mg/dL
3+   = 300 mg/dL
4+   = 1000 mg/dL (or more)

The classic tests for proteinuria involve precipitating all proteins with an acid, which allows the amount present in the specimen to be estimated. However, x-ray contrast media and drugs such as cephaloridine, chlorpromazine, promazine, thymol, tolbutamide, sulfisoxazole, massive doses of penicillin, and para-aminosalicylic acid (PAS) may cause false-positive results. On the other hand, false-negative results occur in highly buffered alkaline urine specimens and with severe urinary tract infections caused by urea-splitting organisms.

▶▶ *Nursing Responsibilities and Implications*
The nurse often is asked to test urine for albumin (protein). In addition to following the manufacturer's specific directions for the product being used, the nurse should proceed as follows:

1. Teach the patient the procedure for obtaining a clean-catch specimen (see Collection and Handling of Urine—Nursing Responsibilities and Implications) to avoid contamination by the protein in blood, feces, and vaginal or urethral discharge.

2. Instruct the patient to collect the specimen the first thing in the morning after standing upright if this activity is permitted. The test often is repeated later in the morning after the patient has been upright for some time.

3. Test the specimen; see the guidelines for reagent strip use under Routine Urinalysis—Nursing Responsibilities and Implications.

4. If the test result is a trace or higher, it should be recorded and the physician notified so that a 24-hour urine collection can be initiated; any protein in the urine is abnormal.

Ketones

Ketonuria is the presence in the urine of ketone bodies, which are substances originating in the liver as a result of incomplete fat metabolism. If these substances are present, they usually consist of acetoacetic acid or diacetic acid (20%), acetone (2%), and β-hydroxybutyric acid (78%). The presence of acetone, which comprises the smallest number of ketone bodies, is used as an indicator of ketonuria.

Ketonuria commonly occurs in uncontrolled diabetes mellitus when ketone bodies accumulate in the blood and are excreted in the urine. The accumulation of these ketone bodies in diabetics often results in acidosis, which can progress to diabetic coma. Tests for ketonuria are valuable in differentiating between coma caused by ketosis and coma caused by uremia, hypoglycemia, cerebral vascular disease, or other disorders. Routine screening for ketonuria should be performed for any patient showing increased excretion of glucose or other reducing substances. These screening tests also aid in assessing the severity of acidosis and in evaluating the effects of its treatment.

Clinical Significance
When the needs of the body surpass the available glucose supply, as in conditions of abnormal carbohydrate metabolism, fat combustion is used as an alternate energy source. However, fat metabolism is less efficient and results in the accumulation of ketone bodies, the end products of fatty acid oxidation. The formation of these ketones correlates with the amount of available glycogen in the liver. When glycogen is depleted, fatty acid oxidation accelerates, increasing the level of ketones in the blood and resulting in ketonuria.

Usually, only negligible amounts of ketones appear in the urine because they are almost totally metabolized. Any condition increasing metabolic demand that is accompanied by reduced carbohydrate intake can produce ketonuria. In general the degree of ketonuria roughly reflects the severity of the metabolic stress. Symptomatic ketosis occurs at levels of 50 mg/dL or above, although levels of 20−30 mg/dL are high enough to signify a moderately severe metabolic imbalance. Current medical management suggests that all patients with diabetes be regularly tested for ketonuria as well as glycosuria, especially in the presence of infection.

Normal Values

The normal values for total ketone bodies are:

Reagent strip screening test	Negative
Quantitative measurement	0.3−2.0 mg/dL

Variations

Ketonuria, in varying degrees of severity, may result from:

Administration of anesthesia

Cachexia

Cyclic vomiting in children

Dietary imbalance or digestive disturbances

Eclampsia

Excessive exogenous insulin

Exposure to cold

Febrile diseases

Isoniazid intoxication

Isopropyl alcohol intoxication

Pernicious vomiting of pregnancy

Pyloric stenosis

Severe diarrhea

Starvation

Strenuous exercise

Treatment with ketogenic diet (high-fat, low-carbohydrate diet, which is used in the treatment of epilepsy)

Uncontrolled diabetes mellitus

Von Gierke's disease (a glycogen storage disease caused by an inborn error of carbohydrate metabolism)

Methodology

Screening tests generally used for ketonuria are most sensitive to the presence of acetoacetic acid, less sensitive to acetone, and do not detect the presence of hydroxybutyric acid at all. Fortunately, all three ketone bodies have equal significance, so individual determinations are unnecessary. A positive test reaction indicates the presence of all three ketone bodies.

Reagent strip tests (N-Multistix, Chemstrip) may yield false-positive reactions in some patients taking L-dopa when large amounts of phenylpyruvic acid are present (congenital phenylketonuria) and following BSP (bromsulphthalein) or PSP (phenolsulfonphthalein) tests. Drugs that can cause false-positive ketone test results include ether, insulin, isopropyl alcohol, L-dopa, metformin, paraldehyde, phenformin, and pyridium. (See Table 1-2.)

▶▶ *Nursing Responsibilities and Implications*
The nurse often is asked to test urine for ketones (acetone), usually along with the test for glucose. In addition to following the manufacturer's specific directions for the product being used, the nurse should proceed as follows:

1. Use a freshly voided specimen.

2. Use a second voided specimen when testing in the morning.

3. Test within 1 hour of voiding or refrigerate the specimen to prevent the release of acetone and a false-negative result.

4. Permit a refrigerated specimen to return to room temperature before testing.

5. Test the specimen using a reagent strip; see the guidelines for reagent strip use under Routine Urinalysis—Nursing Responsibilities and Implications.

6. Test the specimen using an Acetest tablet by:
   a. Putting a tablet on a clean paper towel.
   b. Placing one drop of urine on the tablet.
   c. Waiting a timed 30 seconds.
   d. Not using tablets that are darkened because this produces inaccurate results.

7. Compare the results using only the color chart supplied with the product.

8. A positive result may indicate ketoacidosis, starvation, or weight loss.

Occult Blood

The occult blood test chemically screens urine for the presence of free hemoglobin (**he-moglobinuria**) or red blood cells in amounts too small for visual detection. This test is a complementary procedure to the microscopic examination of urine sediment for red blood cells (**hematuria**). Although hematuria occurs more often than hemoglobinuria, both tests should be performed in a routine urinalysis.

In strongly alkaline or very hypotonic (dilute) urine specimens, all the red blood cells present lyse, resulting in a negative microscopic examination for red blood cells and a positive test for free hemoglobin. Hemoglobinuria caused by the lysis of red blood cells is accompanied by red blood cell envelopes or "ghosts" in the urine sediment. Reagent strip screening tests are most sensitive to free hemoglobin but also give a positive result when **myoglobin** (a muscle pigment) is present. Myoglobin does not originate in the kidney but appears in the urine (**myoglobinuria**) after it is filtered from the blood following muscle injury.

Clinical Significance
Red blood cells can enter the urine from trauma, hemorrhage, infarction, or infection at any level in the urinary system.

Hemoglobin in the urine usually results from renal clearance of excess free hemo-globin from the plasma. When extensive or rapid destruction of red blood cells takes place in the bloodstream, the body cannot metabolize or store the excessive amounts of hemo-globin released. Acute hemolysis results in free hemoglobin appearing in the plasma (**hemoglobinemia**) and ultimately in the urine when concentrations exceed the renal threshold. Hemoglobinuria begins 1–2 hours after an acute hemolytic event and usually does not persist beyond 24 hours.

Myoglobin is released during acute skeletal muscle destruction, rapidly cleared from the blood, and excreted in the urine. Only the breakdown of skeletal muscle fibers releases sufficient myoglobin to produce myoglobinuria. When large amounts of myoglobin are filtered by the kidneys, anuria may be caused by the resulting renal damage.

Normal Values
Normal urine values for occult blood are:

Reagent strip screening test   Negative*

*Urine should not contain red blood cells, hemoglobin, or myoglobin.

Variations
A variety of factors can cause positive reagent strip test results for occult blood in the urine. **Hematuria** is discussed under Microscopic Examination—Red Blood Cells. **Hemoglobinuria** may be caused by lysis of the red blood cells present in voided urine. Hemoglobinuria also may result from:

Autoimmune hemolytic anemia (associated with lupus erythematosus, lymphomas, viral pneumonia)

Blackwater fever

Clostridium perfringens infections

Drug ingestion (arsenic, bacitracin, coumarin, indomethacin, nitrofurantoin, phenacetin, phenothiazines, phenylbutazone, quinine)

Hemolytic anemia (hereditary spherocytosis, sickle cell anemia, thalassemia)

Irrigation of surgical prostatic bed with water (continuous bladder irrigation)

Malaria (Plasmodium falciparum infections)

Paroxysmal nocturnal hemoglobinuria (Donath-Landsteiner antibodies)

Toxin (poisonous mushrooms)

Transfusion reaction (severe intravascular hemolysis)

Various venoms

Myoglobinuria may occur with:

Alcoholic polymyopathy

Convulsions

Electrical shock

Extensive burns

Familial myoglobinuria

Hyperthermia (malignant hyperthermia with anesthesia)

Infarction of muscle

Infection (acute polymyositis)

"March" myoglobinuria (prolonged strenuous or unaccustomed exercise)

Progressive muscle diseases

Toxin (fish poisoning)

Trauma (crush injury, beating, bullet wound)

Various venoms

Methodology
Hemoglobinuria and hematuria cannot be detected visually if the blood is diluted more than 1 part in 1000 parts of urine. Chemical tests for occult blood are considerably more sensitive. Test reagents react more readily in urine containing free hemoglobin than in urine containing intact red blood cells. Red blood cells must have hemolyzed to be de-

tected; therefore, the microscopic examination of urine for red blood cells is the best method for indicating their presence in small numbers. Reagent strip tests detect the presence of red blood cells and myoglobin as well as hemoglobin. These methods (N-Multistix, Chemstrip) react to blood diluted 1 part in 8000 parts of urine, which corresponds to 0.02 mg of hemoglobin per deciliter or 0.3 mg of myoglobin per deciliter (see Table 1-2). Occultest tablets are specific for hemoglobin and are the most sensitive test, detecting as little as 1 part of blood in 32,000 parts of urine, which corresponds to 0.05−0.1 mg of hemoglobin per deciliter.

Precautions

To ensure accurate results when testing for hematuria, myoglobinuria, or hemoglobinuria, the following precautions should be observed:

1. Refrigerate the specimen if the test cannot be performed immediately or send the specimen to the laboratory as soon as it is collected because red blood cells are destroyed when the specimen is permitted to stand at room temperature.

2. Do not use the reagent strip method when the patient is receiving ascorbic acid because it may retard or inhibit the test strip reaction; certain antibiotics that use ascorbic acid as a preservative (Terramycin, Achromycin, Panmycin, Tetracyn, tetracycline) may contain sufficient amounts to inhibit the test results.

3. Do not use the reagent strip method when the patient is receiving bromides, copper, iodides, and oxidizing agents because they may produce false-positive results.

▶▶ Nursing Responsibilities and Implications

If the urine is to be tested for occult blood in the laboratory, the nurse should send the specimen to the laboratory as soon as the patient voids. Care should be taken not to shake or agitate the specimen. When testing urine for hemoglobinuria, hematuria, or myoglobinuria, the nurse should proceed as follows:

1. Obtain a freshly voided specimen; a clean-catch specimen may be adequate during menstruation to limit contamination with exogenous blood, although a catheterized specimen may be necessary; indicate on the laboratory slip that the patient is menstruating.

2. Test the specimen using a dipstick; see the guidelines for reagent strip use under Routine Urinalysis—Nursing Responsibilities and Implications.

3. Test the specimen using occult tablets by:
   a. Placing one drop of urine on the filter paper supplied by the manufacturer.
   b. Putting a tablet on the urine.
   c. Placing two drops of water on the tablet.
   d. Inspecting the color of the filter paper after 2 timed minutes; a positive reaction is indicated by a blue color; *or*

4. Test the specimen using an occult blood test solution by:
   a. Placing one drop of urine on the filter paper in the package supplied by the manufacturer.
   b. Closing the package and opening the side opposite to that containing urine.
   c. Putting two drops of occult blood test solution in this side.
   d. Inspecting the filter paper after 30 seconds; a positive reaction is indicated by a blue color.

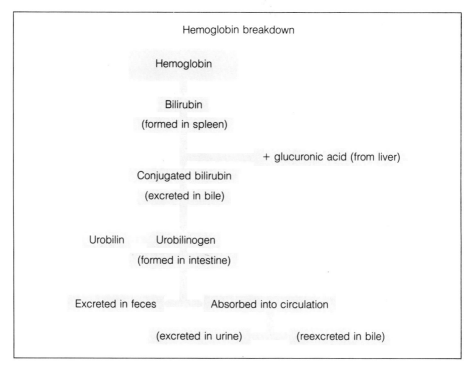

Figure 1-2 Progression of hemoglobin breakdown to urine urobilinogen and bile.

Bilirubin

Bilirubin, the chief bile pigment, is derived from the breakdown of red blood cells by the reticuloendothelial cells of the liver and spleen. This free bilirubin travels to the liver, where it is linked (conjugated) with glucuronic acid and excreted with bile into the gastrointestinal tract (Figure 1-2). Normally, only very small amounts of conjugated bilirubin are found in the blood, although any obstruction to the flow of bile causes this concentration to increase. (Serum bilirubin levels are discussed in Chapter 3.)

Conjugated bilirubin is water-soluble and easily passes the glomerular barrier of the kidney and appears in the urine (**bilirubinuria**). The presence of bilirubin in the urine may occur before jaundice becomes visible and has the same significance as jaundice in the detection of liver disease. Laboratory screening tests for urine bilirubin frequently are included in routine urinalysis to detect latent or unsuspected liver disease, especially disorders that do not produce recognizable jaundice. Tests for the presence and degree of bilirubinuria also help to guide clinical management of liver or biliary tract disorders such as obstruction, periportal fibrosis or inflammation, and hepatocellular damage.

Clinical Significance

Tests to detect urine bilirubin aid in the differential diagnosis of jaundice because bilirubinuria does not occur with hemolytic jaundice but usually accompanies obstructive and hepatic jaundice. Hemolytic disorders cannot cause bilirubinuria because the increased amounts of plasma bilirubin are in the water-insoluble free form that is not filtered by the kidney. Bilirubinuria is indicated by a urine color that ranges from yellow-orange to brown or by a yellow foam that results when the urine specimen is shaken.

Normal Values

Normal values for urine bilirubin are:

Reagent strip screening test   Negative

Quantitative measurement   0.02 mg/dL

Variations
Bilirubinuria may result from:

Alcoholic hepatitis

Chronic and acute hepatitis (persistent bilirubinuria following hepatitis signals serious liver dysfunction)

Cirrhosis

Drug-induced hepatitis (many drugs, such as chlordiazepoxide, erythromycin, ethacrynic acid, ethionamide, imipramine, methotrexate, nitrofurantoin, oxyphenisatin, phenothiazine, and phenylbutazone, are hepatotoxins capable of causing liver damage)

Hyperthyroidism

Infectious mononucleosis

Liver or biliary tract tumors

Septicemia

Methodology
There are several common screening methods for bilirubinuria, including Ictotest tablets and reagent strips such as N-Multistix and Chemstrip (see Table 1-2). Ictotest tablets detect bilirubin levels as low as 0.05−0.1 mg/dL, which is just above the upper limit of normal. False-positive reactions may occur in the presence of salicylates, whereas large amounts of ascorbic acid can interfere with the color reaction and produce a false-negative result.

Reagent strip screening tests (N-Multistix, Chemstrip) yield false-positive reactions in urine containing phenazopyridine or phenothiazines and false-negative reactions if bacterial overgrowth destroys the conjugated bilirubin.

Precautions
To ensure accurate results when testing for bilirubinuria, the following precautions should be observed:

1. Protect the test reagent tablets from exposure to strong light, moisture, high humidity, and prolonged temperatures above 37.7 C because these conditions cause the tablets to decompose.

2. Test the urine for bilirubin within 1 hour after specimen collection because bilirubin is unstable in urine, especially when the specimen is exposed to light.

3. Note on the laboratory slip if the patient is taking salicylates, ascorbic acid, phe-

nazopyridine, or phenothiazines because these agents can interfere with the test results.

▶▶ *Nursing Responsibilities and Implications*

If testing for bilirubinuria is to be done in the laboratory, the urine specimen should be sent immediately, marked for special handling by laboratory personnel. If the testing is to be done by the nurse, the following steps should be taken:

1. Obtain a freshly voided urine specimen.

2. Test the specimen using a reagent strip; see the guidelines for reagent strip use under Routine Urinalysis—Nursing Responsibilities and Implications.

3. Test the specimen using tablets and a cellulose test mat by:
    a. Placing five drops of urine on the test mat.
    b. Putting one tablet on the moistened area of the mat.
    c. Placing two drops of water on the tablet.
    d. Inspecting the mat for a change in color within 30 timed seconds using the manufacturer's color chart; a positive reaction is indicated by a blue to purple hue; a negative reaction is indicated by a pink to red color.

4. If bilirubinuria is present, observe the patient for jaundice in the sclera and mucous membranes; assess the stool color for a loss of bile pigment (pale to clay color).

Urobilinogen

Urobilinogen is a substance produced by the degradation of bilirubin. Its formation in the intestines results from bacterial activity on the conjugated bilirubin excreted in the bile (Figure 1-2). Intestinal bacteria reduce the bilirubin to a series of colorless compounds known collectively as urobilinogen, which are further oxidized to orange-brown urobilin.

About half of the urobilinogen formed in the intestine is excreted with the feces. The remainder passes into the bloodstream via the portal system. Most of this reabsorbed urobilinogen returns to the liver for reexcretion with the bile, but a minute amount enters the urine as the blood passes through the kidneys. (Urine urobilinogen also is discussed in Chapter 3; fecal urobilinogen is discussed in Chapter 3 and Chapter 8.)

If obstruction or severe liver disease prevents or interrupts the flow of bile, bilirubin cannot reach the intestine, preventing the formation of urobilinogen and causing urobilinogen levels to decrease. Conversely, urine urobilinogen levels increase when abnormally large amounts accumulate in the intestine or when the liver cannot adequately dispose of the reabsorbed urobilinogen. Laboratory tests for urine urobilinogen help to differentiate obstructive jaundice from the jaundice associated with hemolytic anemia.

Clinical Significance

Urobilinogen appears in the urine in increased amounts in individuals with hemolytic diseases or hepatic problems. Urobilinogen levels in the urine are a sensitive gauge of hepatic damage and are helpful in the differential diagnosis of the cause of jaundice. Elevated urobilinogen levels are often the first indication of incipient liver disease, rising before the serum or urine bilirubin level. Maximum urobilinogen excretion occurs between noon and early evening.

Normal Values

The normal values for urine urobilinogen are:

Reagent strip screening test	Negative
Quantitative measurement	0.3−1.0 Ehrlich units/2 hours
	0.5−4.0 Ehrlich units/24 hours
	0.05−2.5 mg/24 hours

Variations

Increased urine urobilinogen may be associated with:

Alkaline urine	Hepatitis—infectious and toxic
Bacterial colonization of the small intestine	Infectious mononucleosis
	Malaria
Cirrhosis	Portal-systemic venous shunt
Erythropoietic porphyria	Prolonged intestinal transit time
Hemolytic anemia	

Decreased urine urobilinogen may be associated with:

Absence of intestinal bacteria	Probenecid
Acid urine	Rapid intestinal transit time
Antibiotic administration	Reduced renal function
Biliary obstruction	Starvation
Hepatitis with cholestasis	

Methodology

A fresh random urine specimen is required for reagent strip screening tests for urine urobilinogen (N-Multistix, Chemstrip; see Table 1-2). False-positive test results are obtained when urine specimens contain porphobilinogen and frequently occur in patients receiving such drugs as para-aminosalicylic acid, sulfisoxazole, or phenazopyridine. However, such interfering substances react immediately with the test reagent, whereas the red-orange color develops gradually during the 60-second reaction time in the presence of elevated amounts of urobilinogen. Urine specimens that test negative by qualitative dipstick methods also should be checked for the presence of urobilin, which has the same diagnostic significance.

Many quantitative methods used to measure urine urobilinogen are nonspecific because the Ehrlich reagent reacts with all chromogens in the urine, including porphobilinogen, indole, and bilirubin. Therefore, an additional extraction procedure may be used to separate urobilinogen from these other compounds. When this extraction is performed, results are reported as milligrams of urobilinogen; when this extraction process is not carried out, results are reported in Ehrlich units.

Precautions

To ensure accurate results when testing for urobilinogen, the specimen should be collected in a brown bottle containing 5 g of anhydrous sodium carbonate, refrigerated, and examined as soon as possible because urobilinogen is oxidized to urobilin when exposed to room temperature, light, and air.

Nursing Responsibilities and Implications

Urobilinogen may be detected by testing a random or 24-hour urine specimen. If any urine is inadvertently discarded during the 2- or 24-hour collection period, the nurse should discard the previously collected urine and begin the test anew. If the testing for urobilinogen is to be done by the nurse, the following steps should be taken:

1. Obtain a freshly voided specimen, preferably in the afternoon because this is the time of maximum excretion.

2. Test the urine immediately using a reagent strip; see the guidelines for reagent strip use under Routine Urinalysis—Nursing Responsibilities and Implications.

3. Match the color of the strip to the manufacturer's chart exactly 60 seconds after the stick is removed from the specimen; the color varies from yellow (normal) to yellow-orange to brown-orange depending on the amount of urobilinogen present.

Nitrite

Nitrite determinations are performed to detect the presence of asymptomatic bacteriuria. Because the only way nitrite can appear in the urine is through the bacterial metabolism of nitrates, positive test results always indicate significant bacterial infection. Laboratory tests for urinary nitrite are used to determine if urine culture and identification of organisms are needed.

Clinical Significance

Positive nitrite results, indicated by any uniform color development on the reagent test strip, suggest bacterial infection of 100,000 organisms or more per milliliter. However, the degree of color development is not proportional to the number of bacteria present. Negative test results do not always prove that significant bacteriuria is absent.

Nitrite determinations are significant only when performed on urine that was retained in the bladder long enough for nitrate to be reduced to nitrite. Thus, nitrite tests are most accurate when performed on a first-morning specimen or on urine that has incubated in the bladder for 4 hours or more. Bacterial infection is less likely to be detected when urine output is high. Urine specimens that remain at room temperature for several hours before testing produce inaccurate test results because contaminating organisms may generate nitrite even in the absence of clinical bacteriuria.

Normal Values

Normal values for urine nitrite are:

Reagent strip screening test	Negative
Quantitative measurement	<100,000 organisms/mL

Variations

Positive urine nitrite may be associated with bacterial infection (>100,000 organisms/mL) or a contaminated specimen.

Negative urine nitrite may be associated with the absence of urinary nitrates, diuresis, or infection with non-nitrite–forming bacteria (*Enterococcus*).

TABLE 1-2   Summary of Methods for Urine Screening

Test	Method	Specificity	Sensitivity	Comments
pH	N-Multistix*	Measures pH of 5–8.5	Series of distinct colors through yellow and green to blue	Bacterial growth leads to alkaline urine
Sugar	N-Multistix* Diastix*	Specific for glucose	Identifies 0.1–2 g/dL with colors from blue to brown	Report as positive or negative at 10 seconds; quantitate at 30 seconds. Large amounts of ketones and ascorbic acid decrease color development
	Chemstrip[†]	Specific for glucose	Detects levels as low as 40 mg/dL with a color change from yellow to green	Report as positive or negative at 30–60 seconds. Large amounts of ascorbic acid decrease sensitivity
	Clinitest*	Measures all reducing sugars	Five-drop test: identifies 0.25–2 g/dL with colors from dark green to orange Two-drop test: identifies 0.25–5 g/dL with colors from green to orange-brown	Used for pediatric patients and when large amounts of ascorbic acid are present. False-positive results are caused by many substances. Heat and humidity destroy the reagent; keep in an airtight, dark bottle
Protein	N-Multistix* Chemstrip[†]	Specific for albumin	Detects levels as low as 5–20 mg/dL with shades of yellow to green	Read at 30–60 seconds. Highly buffered or alkaline urine caused by factors such as bacterial contamination, pyuria, or quaternary ammonium compounds produces false-positive results
	Heat and acid	Measures all proteins	Detects levels as low as 5–10 mg/dL by varying degrees of turbidity	False-positive results are produced by x-ray contrast media, tolbutamide, penicillin, sulfisoxazole, paraaminosalicylic acid, cephaloridine and cephalothin, nafcillin, tolmetin, sodium bicarbonate, and high uric acid levels. Highly buffered alkaline urine produces false-negative results

Ketones	N-Multistix* Chemstrip† Ketostix*	Specific for diacetic acid	Detects levels as low as 5–10 mg/dL by shades of buff-pink to maroon	Read at 15* or 60+ seconds. False-positive results are produced by bromsulphthalein (BSP), phenolsulfonphthalein (PSP), L-dopa, phenazopyridine, and phenylpyruvic acid. Bacterial growth may produce a false-negative result. Moisture destroys the sensitivity of strips. Keep in an airtight container
	Acetest*	Measures both diacetic acid and acetone	Detects levels as low as 5–10 mg/dL by shades of lavender to deep purple	Melanogens, cystine, and creatinine may produce false-positive results. Excess light and moisture destroy the reagent; keep in an airtight, dark container
Blood	N-Multistix*	Measures red blood cells, myoglobin, and hemoglobin	Detects levels as low as 0.015–0.045 mg/dL of free hemoglobin (5–15 RBCs/μL) with colors from orange to dark blue	Read at 30 seconds. False-positive results may be caused by hypochlorite solutions. False-negative results may occur with high ascorbic acid or nitrite concentrations. Heat and moisture destroy the reagent; keep in an airtight container
	Chemstrip†	Measures red blood cells, myoglobin, and hemoglobin	Detects levels as low as 0.05–0.3 mg/dL of free hemoglobin with colors from yellow to green	Read at 60 seconds; 0.3 mg/dL of hemoglobin equals 10 lysed RBCs/μL. Heat and moisture destroy the reagent; keep in an airtight container
	Occultest*	Specific for hemoglobin	Detects levels as low as 1 part of blood per 32,000 parts of urine (20 red blood cells per high-power field) by the appearance of a blue color	May decompose, lose effervescence, and become less sensitive

TABLE 1-2 Summary of Methods for Urine Screening (*continued*)

Test	Method	Specificity	Sensitivity	Comments
Bilirubin	N-Multistix* Chemstrip[†]	Specific for bilirubin	Detects levels as low as 0.2–0.5 mg/dL with various shades of tan	Read at 20* or 30–60[+] seconds. False-positive results occur with large doses of chlorpromazine, phenazopyridine, phenothiazines, and ethoxazene. Bacterial growth and ascorbic acid may produce false-negative results
	Ictotest*	Specific for bilirubin	Detects levels as low as 0.05–0.1 mg/dL by the appearance of a blue to purple color	Light and moisture decompose the reagent; keep in an airtight, dark container
Urobi-linogen	N-Multistix*	Measures uro-bilinogen and porpho-bilinogen	Detects levels as low as 0.1 mg/dL with shades of light yellow to brown-orange	False-positive results occur with sulfisoxazole, para-aminosalicylic acid, and indole
	Chemstrip[†]	Specific for urobilinogen	Detects levels as low as 0.4 mg/dL with a color change to red	Read at 10–30 seconds. False-positive results occur with phenazopyridine
Nitrite	N-Multistix* Chemstrip[†]	Specific for nitrite	Detects levels as low as 0.05–0.075 mg/dL (<100,000 organisms/mL) by a color change to pink-violet	Read at 30 seconds. False-positive results occur with phenazopyridine. False-negative results occur with high specific gravity and ascorbic acid levels. A negative result does not exclude significant bacteriuria

* Ames Company, Elkhart, Ind.

[†] Lilly Company, Indianapolis, Ind.

Methodology

Urinary nitrite determinations require a first-morning urine specimen or urine collected at least 4 hours after the patient last voided. Urine specimens with a high specific gravity reduce the sensitivity of reagent strip nitrite tests (N-Multistix; see Table 1-2). False-negative test results occur with ascorbic acid concentrations of 25 mg/dL or more in specimens containing less than 0.03 mg/dL of nitrite ions.

▶▶ Nursing Responsibilities and Implications

Urine specimens should be delivered to the laboratory immediately for prompt testing to prevent the growth of contaminating organisms and false-positive test results. If immediate testing is not possible, the specimen must be refrigerated. If the testing for nitrite is to be done by the nurse, the following steps should be taken:

1. Obtain a freshly voided specimen.

2. Test the specimen immediately using a reagent strip (Microstix-nitrite); see the guidelines for reagent strip use under Routine Urinalysis—Nursing Responsibilities and Implications.

3. If the test is positive for nitrites, obtain a clean-catch or sterile urine specimen for culture and sensitivity tests.

MICROSCOPIC EXAMINATION

Microscopic examination of the urine sediment allows some of the constituents of the urinary tract to be sampled directly and indicates the status of the urinary tract. A microscopic examination identifies such constituents as red and white blood cells, epithelial cells, casts, crystals, bacteria, and miscellaneous elements such as parasites and yeasts. A microscopic examination reveals problems that otherwise would be difficult to identify. Close attention to the urine sediment yields a great deal of information important to the diagnosis and prognosis of renal parenchymal disease. Larger numbers of red and white blood cells may appear in healthy individuals after strenuous exercise or exposure to severe cold; otherwise, the presence of abnormal constituents always signals renal disease.

Normal Values

Microscopic examination of normal urine sediment reveals:

Red blood cells	0−2 RBCs/hpf*
White blood cells	0−4 WBCs/hpf
Epithelial cells	0−10 cells/hpf
Casts	Occasional hyaline
Crystals	Variety†
Bacteria	<1000 organisms/mL

*hpf = high-power field.

†Depends on urine pH (see Normal Values under Crystals).

Methodology

Microscopic examination should be performed on a fresh, concentrated, first-morning, clean-catch specimen within 1 or 2 hours of collection because concentrated urine contains more formed elements than a dilute specimen. Refrigerating acid urine preserves almost all formed constituents fairly well for a few hours.

Red Blood Cells

Clinical Significance

Hematuria varies from gross amounts with obvious "smoky" or bloody urine to minute amounts detectable only by microscopic examination or chemical tests for occult blood. Blood cells may be imperceptible microscopically if the urine specimen is hypotonic (dilute) or alkaline because red blood cell lysis occurs under these conditions. Therefore, when hemoglobin is found during urine screening and no red blood cells can be seen microscopically, specific gravity and pH should be measured to rule out hemoglobinuria.

Occasional red blood cells (two to three per high-power field) may have no pathologic significance. However, persistent findings of even small numbers of erythrocytes warrant further investigation. Almost any disease of the kidneys or urinary tract causes hematuria. When red blood cells are accompanied by red blood cell casts, the pathologic process probably originates in the kidneys. A lower urinary tract origin is indicated when red blood cell casts are not found with the red blood cells and there is little proteinuria.

Normal Values
(See Normal Values under Microscopic Examination.)

Variations

Hematuria may be associated with:

Anticoagulants (urine should be examined daily for the presence of red blood cells)

Calculi

Cystitis

Glomerulonephritis (blood leakage caused by glomerular capillary damage)

Hydronephrosis

Hypertension or arteriosclerosis with renal involvement

Invading tumors from the colon, rectum, or pelvis

Lupus nephritis

Malaria and acute febrile infections

Parasites of the urinary bladder

Polyarteritis nodosa

Pyelonephritis

Renal tuberculosis

Renal vein thrombosis

Scurvy

Subacute bacterial endocarditis (hematuria may occur intermittently)

Thrombocytopenia and other hemorrhagic disorders

Toxic reaction to drugs such as salicy-lates, methenamine, mandelic acid, sulfonamides, coumarin, amphotericin B, methicillin, bacitracin, acetanilid, phenacetin, and barbiturates

Trauma (including renal biopsy and catheterization)

Tumors of the kidney or bladder

Vaginal contamination during menstruation

White Blood Cells

Clinical Significance
Increased numbers of white blood cells (pus cells) in the urine (**pyuria**) indicate acute infection at some point in the urinary tract. Leukocytes associated with white blood cell casts, granular casts, bacteria, and renal epithelial cells originate in the kidney and strongly suggest the kidney as the site of infection. The degree of pyuria does not necessarily reflect the severity of inflammation but only how closely the infection impinges on functioning nephrons, collecting ducts, and the renal pelvis. Occasionally, a microscopic report includes "glitter cells," which are altered neutrophils that exhibit brownian movement. These cells, if large, are thought to originate in the renal tubules and may be associated with pyelonephritis.

Infections originating in the bladder do not produce casts because the inflammation occurs below the renal tubules where casts are formed. Pyuria caused by cystitis usually is accompanied by red blood cells, bladder epithelial cells, and bacteria.

When pus is visible to the naked eye or the number of white blood cells exceeds 50 per high-power field, a urinary tract infection is certainly present. However, leukocytes may not be present in urine even when significant infection is demonstrated by persistent bacteriuria. A large number of leukocytes in the urine can contribute significantly to the protein content of the urine.

Pyuria and clumps of leukocytes in urine sediment usually indicate acute or chronic renal and urinary tract infections and warrant urine culture. Acute pyelonephritis usually is characterized by pyuria, but chronic pyelonephritis is not.

Normal Values
(See Normal Values under Microscopic Examination.)

Variations
Pyuria may result from:

Acute Bright's disease

Acute glomerulonephritis

Bladder tumor

Drug therapy (allopurinol, ampicillin, kanamycin, methicillin)

Fever

Pathogenic bacteria

Salicylate toxicity

Strenuous exercise

Systemic lupus erythematosus (lupus nephritis)

Tuberculosis infection

Epithelial Cells

Clinical Significance

The few epithelial cells routinely found in normal urine represent the sloughing off of aging tissue. Most frequently, these are squamous cells originating from the superficial layers of the urethra or vagina and have no pathologic significance.

The presence of renal cells or transitional cells from the lining of the renal pelvis, ureters, or bladder indicates pathologic or inflammatory conditions in the upper urinary tract. Large numbers of renal epithelial cells or casts containing renal cells strongly suggest active degeneration of the renal tubules. When the cells are too numerous to count individually, they are reported from 1+ to 4+.

Normal Values

(See Normal Values under Microscopic Examination.)

Variations

Large numbers of epithelial cells may result from:

Active pyelonephritis	Acute renal transplant rejection
Active tubular necrosis	Glomerulonephritis

Casts

Clinical Significance

Casts are cylinderlike structures with parallel sides that are formed from gelled protein that has precipitated and molded to the lumen of the renal tubules. They usually are formed in the narrow distal portion of the tubule, vary in diameter according to the portion of the tubule in which they originate, break away, and are flushed out with the flow of urine.

Casts are composed of a homogeneous mucoprotein material in which structures such as red blood cells, pus cells, or epithelial cells may be incorporated. Casts are named for the predominant cellular element contained within them. As the cellular elements degenerate, casts appear coarsely granular, finely granular, or waxy, which usually indicates renal parenchymal damage.

Casts are a valuable aid in the differential diagnosis of renal and lower urinary tract disease. Increased numbers of any type of casts in the urine (**cylindruria**) usually accompany proteinuria and indicate renal disease. However, casts also may accompany the administration of amphotericin B, bacitracin, ethacrynic acid, furosemide, gentamicin, griseofulvin, isoniazid, kanamycin, neomycin, penicillin, radiographic agents (x-ray contrast media), streptomycin, and sulfonamides.

Normal Values

(See Normal Values under Microscopic Examination.)

Variations

Several types of casts may be identified, each having a unique significance.

Hyaline casts are the most common casts found in the urine, occurring when urine flow in the renal tubules is diminished. They usually indicate the mildest tubular damage and may be found in small numbers in normal persons following strenuous exercise, fever, or postural proteinuria. Hyaline casts also may be associated with:

Acute glomerulonephritis	Congestive heart failure	Malignant hypertension
Acute pyelonephritis	Diabetic nephropathy	Shock
Chronic renal disease	Inflammation	

Red blood cell casts suggest damage to glomerular capillaries or ruptured tubular walls. They may be associated with:

Acute glomerulonephritis	Polyarteritis nodosa
Acute inflammation	Glomerular infarction (subacute bacterial endocarditis, sickle cell disease, scurvy, vascular disorders, thrombocytopenic purpura)
Collagen diseases	
Lupus erythematosus	
Renal thromboembolism	

White blood cell casts generally indicate a kidney infection. They are commonly associated with:

Glomerulonephritis	Pyogenic infection
Pyelonephritis, acute and chronic	Nephrotic syndrome

Renal epithelial casts characteristically occur during or following:

Acute renal transplant rejection	Eclampsia
Acute tubular necrosis (heavy metal poisoning)	Malignant nephrosclerosis
	Advanced glomerulonephritis
Amyloidosis	Pyelonephritis

Granular or waxy casts are believed to be any type of cellular casts that have degenerated and thus have basically the same significance. They are rarely found in normal urine and may occur with:

Acute renal transplant rejection	Orthostatic proteinuria
Acute or chronic renal disease	Pyelonephritis
Chronic lead intoxication	Viral diseases
Congestive heart failure	

Broad casts are also known as renal-failure casts because they originate in dilated collecting tubules during advanced renal insufficiency. Normally, urine flows so rapidly in these ducts that cast formation is prevented. The development of these casts therefore indicates a severe slowing of the urinary stream and pronounced renal malfunction. Broad casts indicate a grave prognosis.

Fatty casts contain lipid droplets and characteristically occur with diabetes mellitus, chronic renal disease, and the nephrotic syndrome.

Cylindroids resemble casts and indicate mild kidney irritation. They are believed to be early or abortive casts because they frequently appear before actual casts are identified and may remain after the casts have disappeared.

Crystals

Clinical Significance

Crystals in the urine (**crystalluria**) are not present at the time of voiding but form as the specimen stands and cools. Most crystals have little clinical significance. Crystalluria becomes important in patients with some amino acid metabolic disorders, patients with renal lithiasis, and patients taking sulfa drugs or other medications that are not very soluble. The type of crystals seen on microscopic examination of urine depends on the pH of the freshly voided specimen. The presence of albumin in the specimen often interferes with the crystallization process.

Normal Values
Crystals normally found in urine include:

Acid urine	Amorphous urates
	Calcium oxalates
	Sodium urates
	Uric acid
Alkaline urine	Amorphous phosphates
	Ammonium magnesium phosphate (triple phosphate)
	Ammonium urates
	Calcium carbonate
	Calcium phosphate

Variations
An **increased number of normal crystals** may be associated with:

Calcium oxalate	Immobilization (bone fractures, central nervous system injuries)	Leukemia
Acetazolamide therapy		Liver disease
		Lymphoma
Excessive milk intake	Oxaluria	Polycythemia
Glycogen metabolism (diabetes mellitus)	Uric acid	Theophylline therapy
	Gout	Thiazide therapy

Abnormal crystals may appear in patients with:

Sulfonamide intoxication (sulfonamides and other sulfa-based drugs, such as tolbutamide, chlorothiazide, and other thiazide diuretics, may precipitate in acid urine and block the renal tubules)

Cystinuria (cystine crystals appear in the urine of patients with cystinosis, transient acute phase of chronic pyelonephritis, and aciduria such as occurs in Wilson's disease)

Leucinuria and tyrosinuria (leucine and tyrosine crystals are seen in the urine of patients with hepatic necrosis during advanced liver failure)

Xanthinuria (xanthine crystals appear in the urine of patients with large amounts of purine or who have received allopurinol)

Bacteria

Clinical Significance

Bacteria in a urine specimen may or may not be significant, depending on how the urine was collected and how soon after collection it was examined. The presence of large numbers of bacteria in fresh urine is definitely abnormal. Significant numbers of bacteria reported in a microscopic examination suggest infection.

Normal Values
(See Normal Values under Microscopic Examination.)

Variations

Pyuria frequently accompanies bacterial infection caused by most organisms. This does not always apply with *Escherichia coli* infections, in which the inflammatory response may be minimal. Therefore, urine cultures are indicated for all specimens containing significant bacteria, regardless of whether pyuria is present.

Miscellaneous Constituents

Urine specimens also may contain miscellaneous constituents such as:

Mucous strands or fibers are usually present in small numbers. Increased numbers indicate chronic inflammation of the urethra and bladder.

Spermatozoa in the urine of males are not significant but should be reported to account for the presence of protein.

Yeast can occur as a common contaminant from skin and air. *Candida albicans* is a common urinary finding in patients with diabetes mellitus.

Parasites such as *Trichomonas vaginalis*, resulting from vaginal contamination, and *Schistosoma haematobium* or *Schistosoma mansoni* ova are occasionally seen in urinary sediment.

Contaminants and artifacts such as partially digested muscle fibers or vegetable cells, cotton, hair, fibers, starch, or powder granules result from improper cleansing techniques and fecal contamination.

SPECIAL URINE TESTS

Porphobilinogen and Porphyrins

Porphobilinogen, the first structure formed in the synthesis of heme pigment, is produced in the liver and normally appears in the urine in very small amounts. It is one of the precursors of the **porphyrins**, a group of several compounds also involved in the formation of hemoglobin. Porphyrins occur in the urine of healthy individuals mainly in the form of coproporphyrin, although small amounts of uroporphyrin also are present.

The porphyrins are synthesized in living cells from porphobilinogen. When several molecules of porphobilinogen and its precursors combine, they produce uroporphyrin, which becomes transformed into coproporphyrin. Both of these forms have a red fluorescent appearance in urine when viewed under ultraviolet light. Coproporphyrin in turn is further modified to form protoporphyrin, which becomes the heme portion of hemoglobin when it combines with iron. (Porphobilinogen and porphyrins also are discussed in Chapter 3.)

Clinical Significance
Increased amounts of the porphyrins in the urine (**porphyrinuria**) may be secondary to a number of unrelated conditions or associated with a group of metabolic disorders known as the **porphyrias**. Secondary porphyrinuria can result from cirrhosis, hepatitis, biliary obstruction, infectious mononucleosis, rheumatic fever, anemias, and chemical poisoning. The porphyrias, on the other hand, are congenital conditions in which porphyrin production and excretion are abnormally increased. These relatively rare diseases produce a rather complex pattern of symptoms that often mimics more common diseases, and unnecessary surgical procedures often are performed unless the correct diagnosis is established in time.

Normal Values
The normal values for the urine porphyrins are:

Coproporphyrin	50–160 µg/24 hours
Porphobilinogen	0–2.0 mg/24 hours
Uroporphyrin	10–30 µg/24 hours

Variations
Increased porphobilinogen excretion may result from acute intermittent porphyria, carcinomatosis, and hepatitis.

Increased uroporphyrin excretion may result from:

Acute porphyrias	Hemochromatosis
Cirrhosis	Lead poisoning

Increased coproporphyrin excretion may result from:

Acute poliomyelitis	Acute rheumatic fever
Acute porphyrias	Alcoholic cirrhosis

Chemical toxicity following arsenic, mercury, sedative, sulfonamide, ethyl alcohol, carbon tetrachloride, chloroform, and hypervitaminosis ingestion or inhalation

Hepatitis, infectious

Hodgkin's disease

Increased erythropoietic activity accompanying anemia

Infections

Lead poisoning (coproporphyrin levels are used to monitor the course of the disease)

Malignancy

Myocardial infarction

Obstructive jaundice

Thyrotoxicosis

The porphyrias are divided into two different groups according to the main organs involved: erythropoietic and hepatic (Table 1-3).

The rare disease **porphyria erythropoietica**, usually found in infancy or early childhood, produces extreme sensitivity to ultraviolet light (photosensitivity) that results in blistering and scarring of the skin. Patients with this disease develop hemolytic anemia and porphyrin deposits in their bones and teeth that cause them to become deep brown. Their urine characteristically appears pink to dark burgundy and contains large amounts (up to 50 mg/24 hours) of uroporphyrin and smaller amounts of coproporphyrin.

Five types of hepatic porphyria generally are recognized: acute intermittent porphyria, porphyria cutanea tarda, acquired porphyria hepatica, variegate porphyria, and hereditary coproporphyria. Urine specimens frequently exhibit a red-orange fluorescence when exposed to ultraviolet light.

Acute intermittent porphyria, the most common type, usually occurs in women and is caused by an inherited defect of porphyrin metabolism in the liver. Patients experience intermittent attacks of abdominal pain, constipation, and vomiting along with neurologic and psychiatric manifestations that mimic acute abdominal emergencies and mental disorders. These attacks may be induced by drugs and chemicals such as alcohol, arsenic, barbiturates, chlordiazepoxide, chloroquine, glutethimide, griseofulvin, meprobamate, methyldopa, methyprylon, phenytoin, and sulfa drugs. Acute attacks also may be triggered by menstruation or pregnancy and are accompanied by the excretion of normal-appearing urine that turns red on standing. Urine specimens contain markedly increased amounts of porphobilinogen and its precursors (diagnostic of the condition), moderately increased amounts of uroporphyrin, and mildly elevated amounts of coproporphyrin.

Porphyria cutanea tarda attacks later in life and is thought to be caused by a metabolic liver defect or a complication of alcoholic cirrhosis. Patients experience symptoms similar to those associated with acute intermittent porphyria, as well as skin photosensitivity, with blisters and scarring occurring after exposure to sunlight. The urine of individuals with this condition is red and contains markedly elevated amounts of uroporphyrin and coproporphyrin but normal amounts of porphobilinogen and its precursors.

Variegate porphyria, caused by enzyme defects that block normal heme synthesis, produces a mild to moderate photosensitivity as well as abdominal and neurologic symptoms. Variegate porphyria is indicated by a markedly increased excretion of all porphyrins and their precursors.

Hereditary coproporphyria is usually a mild disorder, but anticoagulants, barbiturates, and tranquilizers may induce acute attacks of mental disturbances and photosensitivity. Urine specimens contain increased amounts of all porphyrin precursors.

TABLE 1-3 Summary of Clinical and Laboratory Findings in Porphyria

Name	Porphyria Erythropoietica	Acute Intermittent Porphyria	Variegate Porphyria	Porphyria Cutanea Tarda	Hereditary Coproporphyria	Acquired Porphyria Hepatica
Age at clinical onset	Birth to 5 years	After puberty	After puberty; peaks at 30–40 years	40–60 years	Adult	Adult
Symptoms	Extreme photosensitivity; cutaneous scarring; ulceration; hyperpigmentation	Acute abdominal pain; hypertension; tachycardia; psychologic disturbances; barbiturate sensitivity	Photosensitivity; hyperpigmentation; occasional acute abdominal pain; barbiturate sensitivity	Mild to severe photosensitivity; mild to severe attacks of abdominal pain	Occasional acute abdominal pain; mild to severe photosensitivity	Mild photosensitivity
Laboratory findings	CP ↑ PBG N UP ↑↑	Acute phase: CP ↑ PBG ↑↑ UP ↑–↑↑ Remission: CP ↑–↑↑ PBG N–↑ UP N–↑	Acute phase: CP ↑–↑↑ PBG ↑↑ UP ↑↑ Remission: CP N–↑↑ PBG N UP N–↑	CP ↑↑ PBG N UP ↑↑	Acute phase: CP ↑↑ PBG ↑↑ UP ↑↑	CP ↑–↑↑ PBG N UP ↑↑

Legend:
CP = Coproporphyrin
PBG = Porphobilinogen
UP = Uroporphyria

N = Normal
↑ = Increased
↑↑ = Large increase

Acquired porphyria hepatica is a frequent complication of alcoholic cirrhosis, syphilis, diabetes, or heavy metal intoxication (such as from exposure to gold, lead, or arsenic). A variety of drugs also produce this porphyrialike clinical picture in the presence of a previously damaged liver parenchyma, including alcohol, barbiturates, penicillin G, procaine, sedatives, hypnotics, sulfonamides, and diethylstilbestrol. Urine specimens contain increased amounts of uroporphyrin and coproporphyrin.

Methodology

Urine screening methods for porphobilinogen and the porphyrins are nonspecific because the reagents used also react with any urobilinogen present. When any of these screening tests are positive, appropriate quantitative determinations should be performed.

Porphobilinogen converts slowly to porphobilin and uroporphyrin in the presence of light and air, and any coproporphyrin present decreases in amount. Substances such as para-aminosalicylic acid, chlorpromazine hydrochloride, and phenazopyridine produce strong colors that interfere with the interpretation of test results.

▶▶ Nursing Responsibilities and Implications

1. Protect the urine specimens from exposure to light and have them examined as soon as possible after collection.

2. Collect 24-hour specimens in a container to which 5 g of sodium bicarbonate has been added.

3. Indicate on the laboratory slip if the patient is pregnant or menstruating because porphyrins may normally be increased in these conditions.

Calcium

The presence of calcium in the urine (**calciuria**) directly reflects dietary calcium intake, skeletal weight, equilibrium between circulating calcium and phosphate levels, or one of several hormonal factors. Dietary intake is an important factor in evaluating calcium excretion during a 24-hour period, but serum calcium levels are far more important in evaluating the significance of the findings. (Serum calcium levels are discussed in Chapter 5.)

Clinical Significance

Patients with normal kidneys reabsorb as much as 99% of the 9 g of calcium filtered through their tubules daily. Thus, patients with normal serum calcium levels (9–11 mg/dL) excrete only small amounts of calcium in the urine. Serum calcium levels below 7.5 mg/dL cause the kidneys to reabsorb most of the filtered calcium and return it to the bloodstream, leaving practically none in the urine. Serum calcium levels exceeding 11.5 mg/dL cause increased amounts of calcium to be excreted in the urine.

Calcium excretion also varies according to the intake of other dietary ions as the body attempts to maintain electrolyte equilibrium. Increased calcium excretion accompanies high sodium and magnesium intake, whereas decreased excretion follows high phosphate intake.

Normal Values
The normal values for urine calcium are:

Average diet (200–500 mg of
calcium daily)

Sulkowitch test	1+ to 2+ turbidity
Random	10 mg/dL
24-hour	50–250 mg/24 hours

Low-calcium diet (<200 mg of
calcium daily)

Sulkowitch test	Negative
Random	1–3.5 mg/dL
24-hour	<150 mg/24 hours

High-calcium diet (0.5–1.0 g of
calcium daily)

Sulkowitch test	3+ to 4+ turbidity
Random	30–40 mg/dL
24-hour	250–300 mg/24 hours

Variations
Increased urine calcium levels (**hypercalciuria** [urinary excretion greater than 400 mg/24 hours with a normal diet]) may result from:

Cushing's disease

Elevated serum calcium

Hyperparathyroidism

Hyperthyroidism

Metastatic malignancies, primarily of bone, breast, or lung

Multiple myeloma

Osteolytic bone disease (Paget's disease)

Osteoporosis

Prolonged immobilization

Renal tubular acidosis with excessive loss of base

Sarcoidosis

Vitamin D intoxication caused by increased intestinal absorption

Wilson's disease

Decreased urine calcium levels (**hypocalciuria** [urinary excretion of less than 50 mg/24 hours with a normal diet]) may result from:

Hypoparathyroidism

Low serum calcium

Malabsorption syndromes such as sprue or celiac disease

Nephrosis

Vitamin D deficiency

False-positive urine calcium levels occur with androgens and anabolic steroids, cholestyramine, and parathyroid injections.

False-negative urine calcium levels may be caused by sodium phytate, thiazide diuretics, and viomycin.

Methodology

The Sulkowitch test is a simple semiquantitative screening of random urine specimens that measures calcium excretion by varying the degrees of turbidity reported from 0 (no precipitate) to 4+ (heavy, flocculent precipitate). This test is a reliable urine calcium screening tool for laboratory use and home control of parathyroid disorders. Specific quantitative determinations of calciuria also may be performed by atomic absorption, flame photometry, and titration techniques.

▶▶ ### Nursing Responsibilities and Implications

1. Indicate on the laboratory request slip if calcium intake has been normal or restricted for 3 days prior to testing; list any drugs the patient is taking that might interfere with the test results.

2. Obtain a 24-hour specimen for quantitative evaluation of total calcium excretion.

3. Collect the 24-hour specimen in a container to which 10 mL of concentrated hydrochloric acid has been added; this prevents the precipitation of calcium salts, which would give falsely decreased results.

4. Obtain an early morning urine specimen when testing for hypercalciuria because calcium excretion reaches its lowest point at this time; obtain a postprandial specimen when testing for hypocalciuria because calcium excretion reaches its maximal level after a meal.

KIDNEY FUNCTION STUDIES

Kidney function tests are an important method of evaluating damage or destruction of renal tissue that results in renal dysfunction. This renal pathology frequently causes materials that are normally excreted to accumulate in the blood. Kidney function tests, however, have a limited ability to detect early or less severe renal involvement, which can be picked up by urinalysis or individual chemistry procedures.

The more common kidney function studies are screening tests to determine the extent and nature of renal dysfunction, follow its clinical course, and evaluate the kidneys' response to treatment. However, these tests give little indication of the cause of the dysfunction. Depressed renal function may result from numerous organic kidney diseases, as well as severe anemia, poorly compensated congestive heart failure, shock, severe dehydration, or any other condition in which the renal blood supply is altered.

As with any other laboratory procedure, the results of kidney function studies must be interpreted in conjunction with direct observation and evaluation of the patient. Health history factors, such as age (renal function normally decreases with age), severe muscle exercise, and marked reduction in dietary protein, deserve consideration when interpreting these tests as an index of overall renal performance.

A specific kidney function test is available to measure the kidney's filtration, reabsorption, and secretion abilities. The **creatinine clearance test** reflects glomerular filtration; the **urine concentration test** indicates the efficiency of tubular reabsorption; and the **phenolsulfonphthalein test** (PSP) measures renal plasma flow and tubular secretion.

Creatinine Clearance Test

Creatinine is a nonprotein nitrogenous substance excreted by the kidney in amounts close to the glomerular filtration rate. An adult normally excretes 1.2–1.7 g of creatinine in 24 hours. Creatinine also is secreted to a slight extent by the renal tubules, and therefore the amount of creatinine in the urine is not due entirely to glomerular filtration. If glomerular filtration decreases during renal disease, the rate of creatinine clearance falls, causing serum creatinine concentrations to rise. (Serum creatinine levels are discussed in Chapter 4.)

    Creatinine clearance appears to be the most practical and effective test available for the clinical evaluation of kidney function. Clearance refers to the volume of blood that can be completely cleared of a substance in 1 minute. Three factors are considered in determining the creatinine clearance: the level of creatinine in the blood, creatinine level in the urine, and volume of urine excreted in a unit of time.

Clinical Significance

Creatinine clearance is a measure of the glomerular filtration rate (GFR), which is inferred from the rate at which any substance leaves the bloodstream and enters the glomerular filtrate to be excreted with the urine. Individuals with advanced renal disease usually have a decreased creatinine clearance rate; however, additional factors, such as tubular secretion, may interfere with the meaningful comparison of the creatinine clearance rate in these individuals. Therefore, in most instances sequential clearance tests should be used to monitor changes in kidney function. Creatinine clearance is also a sensitive indicator of renal allograft rejection.

    Clearance values for women are routinely lower than those for men because women normally have a lower muscle mass (the source of circulating creatinine). Some laboratories request the age, weight, and height of the patient to report and interpret their findings more accurately. Laboratory determinations of creatinine clearance rate are used mainly to follow the progress of renal insufficiency.

Normal Values

The normal values for creatinine clearance are:

Females	87–132 mL/min
Males	107–141 mL/min

Variations

Although an elevation in the creatinine clearance rate usually is not significant, a **decrease in the creatinine clearance rate** may be associated with:

- Acute tubular necrosis
- Congestive heart failure
- Decreased renal blood flow caused by shock, renal artery atherosclerosis, or dehydration
- Drugs such as anabolic steroids, androgens, and thiazide diuretics
- Glomerulonephritis
- Polycystic kidney disease
- Renal tuberculosis
- Tumors of the kidney

Methodology

A 24-hour urine specimen usually is preferred for the creatinine clearance study, although shorter periods, such as 2, 6, or 12 hours, also may be used. Whatever the time span, the most important points concerning test validity are accurate timing and complete specimen collection. A serum creatinine concentration must be measured along with the urine to calculate and interpret the significance of urine levels. The blood sample for a creatinine determination may be drawn at any time during the test period because serum creatinine levels for an individual remain fairly constant during a 24-hour period.

Ascorbic acid, L-dopa, methyldopa, nitrofurans, and PSP dye interfere with the test procedure and produce falsely increased urine creatinine test results. In addition, falsely low urine creatinine clearance test values will result if the urine specimen is not refrigerated or if a bacterial inhibitor such as thymol is not added to the specimen container.

▶▶ Nursing Responsibilities and Implications

1. Determine if the patient is taking any medications, such as furosemide, phenacetin, gentamicin, or thiazide diuretics, that might influence the test results.

2. Inform the patient that, although a regular diet can be eaten, excessive intake of meat should be avoided before and during the test period.

3. The nurse usually is responsible for collecting and preserving the urine specimen. The procedure follows:
   a. Encourage the patient to drink enough water during the test period to ensure adequate urine flow.
   b. Ask the patient to empty the bladder completely at the beginning of the test period and discard this urine.
   c. Instruct the patient to save all urine.
   d. Save the urine, using appropriate preservative measures (ice, refrigeration, preservatives).
   e. Include the exact starting and completion times of the test period on the specimen label.
   f. Collect or notify the laboratory technician to draw the blood specimen for serum creatinine determinations before the end or at the beginning of the test period.
   g. Send the entire 24-hour collection specimen to the laboratory.

Concentration Test

The **concentration test** measures the ability of the kidneys to conserve water when the intake of water is limited. If the kidneys are capable of reabsorbing water, they also are assumed to be capable of reabsorbing vital substances from the glomerular filtrate. After an individual is deprived of water for 14–16 hours, the urine will reflect the greatest concentrating capability of the kidneys.

Clinical Significance

One of the earliest kidney functions lost in renal disease is tubular reabsorption or the ability to reclaim water and solutes that were filtered out of the blood along with the wastes. When the kidneys fail to concentrate urine, it normally signifies renal damage, with a reduction in the number of nephrons capable of reabsorbing water from their tubules. Normally, the amount of water and essential solutes conserved by the kidneys varies according to the diet and body requirements. Failure of the renal tubules to perform this function quickly leads to a serious depletion of the body's fluid and electrolyte reserves.

Therefore, tubular reabsorption helps to maintain the volume, osmolality, and electrolyte content of body fluids within normal limits.

Abnormal concentration test results frequently indicate subtle kidney damage or unsuspected infection before an increase in the levels of nitrogenous waste products (urea nitrogen, creatinine, and others) occurs in the serum. This is true in such conditions as polycystic kidney disease, pyelonephritis, and hydronephritis because these conditions damage the renal medulla, which contains the renal tubules, before they damage the cortex, where filtration occurs. However, major renal disease does not always result in loss of concentrating ability. Many patients with active kidney disease excrete urine with a specific gravity of 1.025 or greater.

Patients on low-protein or low-salt diets often fail to excrete urine with an increased specific gravity because of the lack of sufficient urinary solids. Test results are also unreliable and inconclusive in the presence of any severe water or electrolyte imbalance, pregnancy, chronic liver disease, formation or excretion of edema fluid, and adrenocortical insufficiency.

Normal Values

The normal values for urine concentrating ability are:

14–16 hours without fluid   Specific gravity of 1.025–1.035

Variations
Decreased urine concentrating ability (specific gravity of less than 1.025) may be found in:

Chronic pyelonephritis	Patients receiving diuretics
Congestive heart failure	Polycystic kidney disease
Fanconi's syndrome	Protein deficiency
Hydronephrosis	Reduced antidiuretic hormone (ADH) production
Hypercalcemia	
Hypokalemia	Renal insensitivity to ADH
Nephritis	Sickle cell trait

Methodology
Concentrating ability normally is determined by measuring specific gravity with a refractometer or urinometer or by ascertaining the osmolality of urine. (Osmolality is discussed in Chapter 5.)

▶▶ **Nursing Responsibilities and Implications**

1. Discontinue diuretics at least 2 days prior to the testing period.

2. Discontinue all medications for the duration of the test.

3. Provide the appropriate diet:
   a. Provide a diet adequate in protein and fluids for several days prior to the test.
   b. Provide the patient with a high-protein diet limited to 200 mL of fluid at 6 PM the evening before the test.
   c. Restrict food or fluid thereafter until the test is completed.

4. Instruct the patient to empty the bladder before retiring and discard this urine; urine voided during the night should be sent to the laboratory as a separate specimen.

5. Instruct the patient to empty the bladder completely at 7, 8, and 9 AM.

6. Collect each specimen in its entirety and label with the appropriate time.

7. Send the specimens to the laboratory.

Phenolsulfonphthalein Test

The **phenolsulfonphthalein (PSP) test** measures a slightly different facet of kidney function. Together with the creatinine clearance test it provides a more exact diagnosis of renal dysfunction. A normal kidney quickly removes an intravenous test dose of the PSP dye from the blood and excretes it in the urine. This test indicates both tubular secretion and renal blood flow by measuring the amount of dye excreted in various urine specimens collected at precisely timed intervals. The more severe the renal disease, the less PSP dye excreted. Although the test has little ability to measure minimal renal impairment, it is more sensitive in detecting abnormalities than a blood urea nitrogen (BUN) determination or a creatinine clearance test.

Almost all of the intravenous PSP binds reversibly with the albumin in the plasma, although a minute amount remains unbound in the blood. A normal kidney separates the dye from the albumin and actively secretes it through the tubular epithelium into the urine. At the same time the kidney filters the unbound portion through the glomerulus. Thus, virtually all of the dye is removed by the normal kidney.

Clinical Significance

The amount of dye excreted, as measured in urine specimens collected 15, 30, 60, and 120 minutes after the injection, is a fairly accurate guide to the severity of any renal impairment. Test results correlate rather well with the rate of renal blood flow. The 15-minute specimen is the most significant because later specimens are influenced by additional factors that cause difficulties in interpretation. Phenolsulfonphthalein excretion varies directly with urine volume, especially in patients with marked renal damage.

Conditions such as acute renal insufficiency or diminished renal function, as indicated by an increased BUN level, definitely contraindicate the PSP test because rapid hydration could be dangerous. Interpretation of the PSP test is difficult in individuals with cardiac and vascular problems because these conditions alter circulation. Inaccurate test results also occur in patients with edema or urinary retention (as in prostatic hypertrophy).

Normal Values

The normal values for the excretion of the PSP test dose are:

Time	Total Excretion
15-minute specimen	25%–35%
30-minute specimen	40%–60%
60-minute specimen	50%–75%
120-minute specimen	75%–80%

Variations
Increased PSP excretion may be associated with hypoproteinemia and a low albumin concentration.

Decreased PSP excretion may be associated with:

Advanced essential hypertension	Edema
Amyloidosis	Lower nephron nephrosis
Chronic nephritis	Nephrosclerosis
Cirrhosis with normal kidneys	Prostatic obstruction
Congenital polycystic kidney disease	Pyelonephritis
Congestive heart failure	Renal vascular disease
Cystitis	

▶▶ **Nursing Responsibilities and Implications**
Proper patient preparation before the PSP test is as important as the test period itself. The nurse should proceed as follows:

1. Restrict medications and other substances for the 24 hours preceding the test because they may interfere with the test results. For example, probenecid, sulfinpyrazone, and injected contrast media inhibit PSP excretion; chlorthiazide, penicillin G, salicylates, BSP dye, and sulfonamides compete with PSP for tubular secretion; and drugs such as phenazopyridine give a marked color to the urine.

2. Obtain a detailed history of any allergies, especially those related to shellfish. Report positive findings to the physician.

3. Encourage the patient to drink four to five glasses of water during the 30 minutes before the test and a glass of water every 20 minutes during the test to ensure an adequate urine flow. This increases the validity of the test results.

4. Instruct the patient to empty the bladder completely and discard the urine at the start of the test period.

5. Make certain an anaphylaxis tray is available before the dye is administered.

6. Record the exact time the PSP dye is administered intravenously by the physician. (The dye should not be administered subcutaneously or intramuscularly because it is absorbed into the blood at variable rates, altering the test results. This variable absorption causes the dye to enter the kidneys gradually, and the excretion rate will not accurately indicate secretion capabilities.)

7. Observe the patient for any adverse reactions to the dye.

8. Collect and carefully label urine specimens at the exact times specified: 15, 30, 60, and 120 minutes after the administration of the dye. The bladder must be emptied completely at each collection time because large amounts of residual urine invalidate the test results.

9. Use a catheter if the patient is unable to void; if an indwelling catheter is in place, clamp it between specimen collections.

RENAL CALCULI

Renal calculi (kidney stones) are deposits of organic material and mineral salts that have precipitated from the urine. Renal stones consist of an organic core, such as a mucoid carbohydrate-protein complex, blood clots, epithelial or pus cells, or bacteria, that becomes the matrix for the crystallization of minerals and other urine components. Calculi may appear in various sizes described as sand, gravel, and stone; large, round stones characteristically are found in the bladder. Laboratory determination of kidney stone composition helps to identify the disease or condition responsible and prevent further stone development.

Clinical Significance
A number of factors can contribute to kidney stone formation, including renal tubule cell injury (neoplasm, ulceration), pH changes, increased excretion of mineral salts, and vitamin deficiency. Calculi formation also is stimulated by urinary stasis from infections, spinal cord injury, foreign bodies (sutures, catheters), and pathologic changes from urethral strictures, prostatic hyperplasia, or bladder diverticuli. The reduced volume and increased concentration of urine accompanying excessive perspiration and dehydration predispose many individuals to kidney stones. Thus, kidney stones are more common in patients living in areas that are hot and dry during the summer than in individuals living in cold, wet areas.

The passage of kidney stones through the ureters is accompanied by renal colic and causes severe back pain that radiates to the groin. The movement of stones from the bladder through the urethra is also extremely painful. When calculi are too large to pass through the ureter, they obstruct the renal pelvis and passage of urine, causing hydronephrosis and pyelonephrosis. These clinical symptoms of renal calculi commonly are accompanied by hematuria.

Normal Values
Normally, there is an equilibrium between the precipitation and dissolution of urinary crystalloid substances that prevents the formation of renal calculi.

Variations
Renal calculi formation may result from:

Alkali excess	Endocrine disorders	Oxaluria
Avitaminosis A	Cushing's disease	Polycythemia
Berylliosis	Diabetes mellitus	Prolonged immobility
Carcinoma	Hyperparathyroidism	Purine drug excess
Chemotherapy	Fixed urinary pH	Randall's plaques
Cystinuria	Gout	Urinary obstruction
Dehydration	Infection with urea-	
Dietary deficiency	splitting organisms	

Calcium-Containing Stones. There are two major types of calcium-containing stones: calcium oxalate calculi and calcium phosphate calculi. Patients with a normal diet who excrete more than 250 mg of calcium per day in the urine (**hypercalciuria**) have the potential to form calcium-containing stones. **Hypercalciuria and calcium-containing stone formation** may be associated with:

Alkali excess	Osteoporosis	Renal tubular acidosis
Excessive intake of milk	Paget's disease	Sarcoidosis
Hyperparathyroidism	Prolonged immobilization	Vitamin D excess
Idiopathic hypercalciuria		

Calcium oxalate, the most common constituent of calculi in conditions associated with calcium-containing stones, is precipitated when stasis occurs in any part of the urinary tract. Oxalates are formed in the body during the metabolism of carbohydrates, proteins, and fats. Oxalates also are ingested with common foods such as apples, asparagus, cabbage, grapes, lettuce, rhubarb, spinach, and tomatoes and are excreted unchanged in the urine. In addition to the conditions previously listed that promote the formation of calcium-containing stones, calcium oxalate calculi occur in patients who excrete more than 47 mg of oxalate per day in the urine (**oxalosis**). Calcium oxalate stones are very hard, with tiny, sharp surface edges, are often a dark color, and occur in persistently acid urine. **Oxalosis and calcium oxalate stone formation** may be associated with:

Acetazolamide inhibition of carbonic anhydrase	Fractures causing immobilization
	Liver disease
Diabetes mellitus	Poliomyelitis
Excess glycogen breakdown	Spinal cord injuries

Calcium phosphate, a precipitate composed of tricalcium phosphate, calcium hydrogen phosphate dihydrogen, and apatite (calcium-phosphate complex with carbonate), appears as light-colored stones that crumble easily. The carbonate-apatite complex often is found in persistently alkaline urine during urinary tract infections caused by urea-splitting organisms. It is also a principal constituent of stones in the lacrimal duct, prostate gland, and bronchi and the calcified plaques of arteriosclerosis. Ammonium and magnesium also may combine with phosphate in alkaline urine to form triple-phosphate stones.

Uric Acid Stones. Uric acid calculi, yellow to brown-red, moderately hard stones, occur mainly in middle-aged and elderly patients with persistently acid urine. These stones frequently result from hyperuricemia as a complication of gout but also may form without evidence of high serum uric acid levels. **Uric acid stones** may be associated with:

Chemotherapy for leukemia	Liver disease	Rapid protein catabolism
	Lymphoma	Theophylline
Chronic diarrhea	Polycythemia	Thiazide diuretics
Ileostomy		

Cystine Stones. Cystine stones appear smooth and waxy and are formed when more than 300 mg of cystine per day is excreted in the urine (**cystinuria**). They occur most frequently in patients with congenital cystinuria and usually are accompanied by increased excretion of other amino acids, including ornithine, lysine, and arginine. **Cystine stones** also occur in patients with:

Heavy metal nephrotoxicity

Pyelonephritis—acute phases

Renal tubular acidosis (Fanconi's syndrome, Lowe's syndrome)

Wilson's disease

Xanthine Stones. Xanthine stones are uncommon and usually occur in children who have a genetic disorder in which the production of the liver enzyme xanthine oxidase is decreased. These stones appear primarily in persistently acid urine and may occur in renal disease that results in excessive xanthine clearance from the blood. Excretion of more than 25 mg of xanthine per day in the urine (**xanthinuria**) is excessive.

Methodology

Stones are placed in a clean beaker, covered with several thicknesses of gauze held in place with rubber bands, and carefully washed free of blood and mucus under gently running, cold tapwater. Tiny stones and renal sand are rinsed with water from a squeeze bottle instead of tapwater to prevent breaking delicate formations. At this time, the composition of the stone is determined.

▶▶ Nursing Responsibilities and Implications

1. Instruct the patient to collect all urine in a bedpan and strain the urine through several thicknesses of gauze.

2. Examine the gauze carefully in bright light to determine the presence of minute sand stones.

3. Chart the presence and characteristics of the stones.

4. Place the stones in a clean, dry container, label it, and send it to the laboratory.

5. When necessary, provide medication for pain as ordered.

6. Provide a minimum of 3000 mL of fluid daily to flush precipitates through the urinary system and assist the passage of formed calculi.

7. Instruct the patient regarding a proper diet once the composition of the calculi is identified:
   a. Calcium oxalate and calcium phosphate calculi—low-calcium, low-phosphorus, and low-oxalate diet.
   b. Uric acid calculi—low-purine diet.
   c. Cystine calculi—low-protein diet.

AMINOACIDURIA

Amino acids, the chief components of proteins, are organic substances that are essential to human metabolism and nutrition as well as nitrogen equilibrium in adults. The amino acids most vital to human metabolism are isoleucine, leucine, lysine, methionine, phenylalanine, threonine, tryptophan, and valine; an additional amino acid, histidine, is vital to infants. Other essential amino acids include alanine, arginine, asparagine, aspartic acid, cystine, glutamic acid, glutamine, glycine, ornithine, proline, serine, taurine, thyroxine, and tyrosine.

Amino acids appear in the urine (**aminoaciduria**) during kidney disease when renal dysfunction prevents adequate reabsorption of the normal glomerular filtrate. Aminoaciduria also results when abnormal amino acid metabolism causes an abnormal metabolite or a larger than normal amount of a normal metabolite to be excreted in the urine. Examples of this latter type of aminoaciduria include alkaptonuria, phenylketonuria, tyrosinosis, maple syrup urine disease, and the generalized aminoaciduria of liver disease. Most of these disorders result from inborn errors of metabolism and are associated with mental deficiency or retardation, degeneration of the nervous system, and failure to thrive.

Homogentisic Acid

The excretion of homogentisic acid, which is associated with alkaptonuria, results from the defective metabolism of phenylalanine and tyrosine. Normally, phenylalanine and tyrosine are metabolized to the intermediary product homogentisic acid, which is then oxidized to maleyl acetoacetic acid by the enzyme homogentisic acid oxidase. Patients with a hereditary deficiency of this enzyme are unable to metabolize homogentisic acid, causing it to accumulate in the blood and large amounts to appear in the urine. Laboratory screening tests for urinary homogentisic acid help to diagnose alkaptonuria.

Clinical Significance
Homogentisic acid appears in the urine of patients with alkaptonuria shortly after birth and remains throughout life. It also may be deposited in the cartilage and connective tissue, where it is oxidized slowly to a dark blue-black pigment and produces the pathologic condition known as ochronosis. Alkaptonuria frequently is not suspected or diagnosed until arthritis develops or symptoms of connective tissue and joint degeneration appear late in adult life.

Normal Values

Normally, homogentisic acid is completely oxidized to maleyl acetoacetic acid and is not present in the urine.

Methodology
Laboratory determinations of homogentisic acid require a fresh, random urine specimen collected without preservatives. Specimens containing homogentisic acid darken at the surface through oxidation and gradually turn black when allowed to stand exposed to the air. This darkening process occurs more quickly in alkaline urine specimens because acid urine or the presence of ascorbic acid inhibits oxidation. Certain screening procedures for homogentisic acid, such as Benedict's test, give false-positive results when the urine contains glucose or other reducing substances.

▶▶ *Nursing Responsibilities and Implications*

1. Inform the patient that there are no food or fluid restrictions.
2. Indicate on the laboratory slip if the patient has diabetes mellitus or is spilling glucose in the urine.

Phenylpyruvic Acid

Increased amounts of **phenylpyruvic acid** are found in the urine of individuals with **phenylketonuria** (PKU), a hereditary disease caused by the defective metabolism of phenylalanine. Normally, most phenylalanine is converted to tyrosine by the liver enzyme phenylalanine hydroxylase. Patients with PKU have a deficiency of this enzyme that causes phenylalanine and its metabolites to accumulate in the blood and appear in the urine in abnormal amounts.

Laboratory screening tests for increased urinary phenylpyruvic acid levels are required for all newborns in many states to aid in the early detection of PKU. Screening tests for serum phenylalanine (Guthrie's test) also may be used to detect the possible presence of this disorder. Positive PKU screening tests must be followed by quantitative determinations of serum phenylalanine and tyrosine levels to confirm the diagnosis.

Clinical Significance

Infants with PKU usually have normal phenylalanine levels at birth because the mother metabolizes this amino acid for the fetus during pregnancy. However, once feeding begins, phenylalanine from milk or formula accumulates in the blood and tissues of these infants and hinders the normal development of central nervous system cells. Increased blood levels of phenylalanine also appear in unaffected premature infants weighing less than 11 kg without PKU because development of the appropriate liver enzyme activity is delayed.

Phenylalanine levels of 10 mg/dL or greater in the blood during the first few weeks of life cause brain damage and neurologic manifestations (hyperkinesia, epilepsy, microcephaly, and severe mental retardation). Phenylalanine appears in the blood of children with PKU 4 days after their first milk feeding; phenylpyruvic acid can be detected in their urine 2–8 weeks later. If PKU is detected before the infant is 4 months old, dietary restriction of foods containing phenylalanine will prevent the accumulation of toxic compounds until alternative metabolic pathways can be developed.

Normal Values
Normally, only minute amounts of phenylpyruvic acid and phenylalanine occur in the urine.

Methodology

Reagent strip screening tests for urine phenylpyruvic acid (Phenistix) require a small amount of fresh urine or a urine-soaked diaper. The reagent-impregnated portion of the strip is dipped into the urine specimen or pressed against the wet diaper and compared with the color chart after 30 seconds. Specimens containing salicylates, phenothiazine derivatives, or high concentrations of bilirubin interfere with color reactions but do not cause false-positive or false-negative test results.

Ferric chloride screening tests require 5 mL of fresh urine or a urine-soaked diaper. This test is nonspecific for phenylpyruvic acid, giving positive results in several other amino acid disorders, including alkaptonuria, histidinemia, tyrosinosis, oasthouse urine disease, and maple syrup urine disease. Substances such as ketones, bilirubin, phosphate, salicylates, phenothiazines, and L-dopa in the urine interfere with accurate color development in this test method.

▶▶ *Nursing Responsibilities and Implications*

The nurse usually performs the reagent strip screening test (Phenistix) at the 6-week well-baby visit or if a baby over 2 weeks of age is admitted to the hospital. The nurse should proceed as follows:

1. Use a urine-impregnated diaper or collect urine by using a plastic collection bag.

2. If a reagent strip is used with collected urine, see the guidelines for reagent strip use under Routine Urinalysis—Nursing Responsibilities and Implications.

3. If a reagent strip is used with a wet diaper, press the strip on the diaper to saturate it with urine.

4. Compare the results with the color chart provided by the manufacturer in 30 seconds.

5. If the test is positive, refer the mother for dietary counseling and emphasize the importance of adhering to a low-phenylalanine diet.

OTHER URINE STUDIES

A number of other studies are routinely performed on urine. These studies, which are discussed in other chapters, include:

Electrolyte studies
  Chloride (Chapter 5)
  Magnesium (Chapter 5)
  Osmolality (Chapter 5)
  Phosphorus (Chapter 5)
  Potassium (Chapter 5)
  Sodium (Chapter 5)
Endocrine studies
  Aldosterone (Chapter 6)
  Catecholamines (Chapter 6)
  Cortisol (Chapter 6)
  Estradiol (Chapter 6)
  Estriol (Chapter 6)
  Estrogen (Chapter 6)
  Estrone (Chapter 6)
  Follicle-stimulating hormone (FSH) (Chapter 6)
  17-Hydroxycorticosteroids (17-OHCS) (Chapter 6)
  5-Hydroxyindoleacetic acid (5-HIAA) (Chapter 6)
  17-Ketosteroids (17-KS) (Chapter 6)

17-Ketogenic steroids (17-KGS) (Chapter 6)
Luteinizing hormone (LH) (Chapter 6)
Metanephrines (Chapter 6)
Pregnanediol (Chapter 6)
Vanillylmandelic acid (VMA) (Chapter 6)
Miscellaneous studies
  Amylase (Chapter 4)
  Ascorbic acid (Chapter 4)
  Copper (Chapter 4)
  Creatine (Chapter 4)
  Creatinine (Chapter 4)
  Culture (Chapter 10)
  Delta-aminolevulinic acid (ALA) (Chapter 3)
  Hemosiderin (Chapter 3)
  Protein electrophoresis (Chapter 4)
  Urea nitrogen (Chapter 4)
  Uric acid (Chapter 4)
  Zinc (Chapter 4)

Toxicology studies
  Alcohol (Chapter 7)
  Arsenic (Chapter 7)
  Barbiturates (Chapter 7)

Drug screen (Chapter 7)
Lead (Chapter 7)
Phenothiazines (Chapter 7)
Salicylates (Chapter 7)

REFERENCES

Ames Company. 1978. *N-Multistix reagent strips for urinalysis product profile.* Elkhart, Ind.: Miles Laboratories.

Bauer, J. D. 1982. *Clinical laboratory medicine.* 9th ed. St. Louis: The C. V. Mosby Co.

Bologna, C. V. 1971. *Understanding laboratory medicine.* St. Louis: The C. V. Mosby Co.

Cannon, D. C. 1979. The identification and pathogenesis of urine casts. *Lab. Med.* 10(1): 8–11.

Collins, R. D. 1975. *Illustrated manual of laboratory diagnosis.* 2nd ed. Philadelphia: J. B. Lippincott Co.

Dienhart, M. 1979. *Basic human anatomy and physiology.* 3rd ed. Philadelphia: W. B. Saunders Co.

Doucet, L. P. 1981. *Medical technology review.* Philadelphia: J. B. Lippincott Co.

Frankel, S., Reitman, S., and Sonnenwirth, A. C., editors. 1980. *Gradwohl's clinical laboratory methods and diagnosis.* 8th ed. St. Louis: The C. V. Mosby Co.

Free, A. H., and Free, H. M. 1978. Rapid convenience urine tests: their use and misuse. *Lab. Med.* 9(12):9–17.

Freeman, J. A., and Beehler, M. F. 1983. *Laboratory medicine—clinical microscopy.* 2nd ed. Philadelphia: Lea & Febiger.

French, R. M. 1980. *Guide to diagnostic procedures.* 5th ed. New York: McGraw-Hill Book Co.

Henry, J. B. 1984. *Clinical diagnosis and management by laboratory methods.* 17th ed. Philadelphia: W. B. Saunders Co.

Kark, R. M., et al. 1964. *A primer of urinalysis.* 2nd ed. Hagerstown, Md.: Harper & Row, Publishers, Inc.

Lancaster, R. G. 1975. *Listen, look and learn—urinalysis.* Bethesda, Md.: National Committee for Careers in Medical Laboratory.

Marsh, M. M. *Basic urine analysis.* Chicago: American Society of Clinical Pathologists.

Miale, J. B. 1982. *Laboratory medicine—hematology.* 6th ed. St. Louis: The C. V. Mosby Co.

O'Connor, L. J. June, 1981. Acute intermittent porphyria. *Am. J. Nurs.* 1184–1186.

Race, G. J., and White, M. G. 1979. *Basic urinalysis.* Hagerstown, Md.: Harper & Row, Publishers, Inc.

Strand, M. M., and Elmer, L. A. 1983. *Clinical laboratory tests.* 3rd ed. St. Louis: The C. V. Mosby Co.

Tilkian, S. M., Conover, M. H., and Tilkian, A. G. 1983. *Clinical implications of laboratory tests.* 3rd ed. St. Louis: The C. V. Mosby Co.

White, W. L., Erikson, M. M., and Stevens, S. C. 1976. *Chemistry for the medical laboratory.* 4th ed. St. Louis: The C. V. Mosby Co.

Widmann, F. K. 1983. *Clinical interpretation of laboratory tests.* 9th ed. Philadelphia: F. A. Davis Co.

2

Hematology

SPECIMEN COLLECTION AND HANDLING   63
Capillary Blood   ·   Venipuncture

COMPLETE BLOOD COUNT   65
Hemoglobin   ·   Hematocrit   ·   Erythrocyte Count   ·   Leukocyte Count   ·   Differential White Blood Cell Count   ·   Stained Red Blood Cell Examination

ERYTHROCYTE INDICES   89

ERYTHROCYTE SEDIMENTATION RATE   93

RETICULOCYTE COUNT   96

ERYTHROCYTE OSMOTIC FRAGILITY TEST   98

PLATELET COUNT   100

EOSINOPHIL COUNT AND THORN TEST   102

LUPUS ERYTHEMATOSUS CELL TEST   104

LEUKOCYTE ALKALINE PHOSPHATASE STAIN   106

GLUCOSE-6-PHOSPHATE DEHYDROGENASE DEFICIENCY TEST   108

HEMOGLOBIN ELECTROPHORESIS   109

SICKLE CELL TEST   113

ALKALI DENATURATION TEST FOR FETAL HEMOGLOBIN   114

BONE MARROW EXAMINATION   116

OTHER TESTS OF HEMOGLOBIN METABOLISM   120

Clinical hematology, which literally means the study of blood, is the branch of laboratory medicine concerned with the cellular elements of peripheral blood, namely erythrocytes, leukocytes, and platelets. A constant balance generally exists between the rate of formation and destruction of each of these cells, with each type of cell performing its own specialized function. Any disturbance in this critical balance due either to a change in the nature or rate of formation or an increase in cell utilization or destruction usually causes problems.

Hematology procedures provide significant information regarding the number of blood cells present, the relative distribution of each cell type, and any structural or biochemical abnormalities that may cause disease. A thorough hematology evaluation routinely includes a complete blood count, stained blood smear examination, erythrocyte sedimentation rate, reticulocyte count, and calculation of the red blood cell indices. Additional hematology procedures, such as the erythrocyte osmotic fragility test, hemoglobin electrophoresis, and special staining techniques, are also available to determine the cellular structure, internal composition, and histochemical properties of blood cells. Accurate hematology determinations are helpful in the diagnosis and evaluation of many diseases but are most valuable to patient care when they are correlated with the entire clinical picture.

SPECIMEN COLLECTION AND HANDLING

Capillary Blood

Although most hematology procedures require venous blood specimens, many tests, such as hemoglobin, hematocrit, and stained blood cell examinations, also may be performed on capillary blood obtained from a skin puncture. However, red and white blood cell counts, as well as the enumeration of platelets and reticulocytes, should not be performed on capillary blood because variations in capillary blood flow cause poor test precision.

The appropriate skin puncture site depends on the age and physical status of the patient. The plantar surface of the heel or great toe in infants and an earlobe or palmar fingertip surface in adults are the most commonly used sites. Finger punctures are recommended for small children and patients with poor veins and are generally more convenient for bedridden patients because the fingertip is more accessible than the earlobe. In other situations puncturing the free margin of the earlobe is preferable because it is a less sensitive area; this site is useful for patients in shock, those with extensive burns, and those with edematous extremities.

Because the finger is difficult to cleanse adequately, patients with lowered resistance to infection are more likely to get an infection from a fingerstick puncture than from venipuncture. Thus, the alcohol swab should remain in contact with the puncture site for 7–10 minutes before capillary blood is collected from patients with leukemia, agranulocytosis, diabetes, uremia, and immune deficiency diseases.

Precautions
To ensure accurate results when testing capillary blood, the following precautions should be observed:

1. Do not use an edematous or congested site because free blood flow is essential to obtain test results that are comparable to those of venous blood. Poor blood flow can

produce test results that are significantly different from those of venous blood because of hemoconcentration from stasis or dilution with tissue fluid from squeezing.

2. Do not use a cold or cyanotic area for the puncture site. Poor circulation causes falsely elevated hemoglobin results and cell counts.

3. Do not squeeze the puncture site because this will alter the composition of the blood specimen. Tightly squeezing the puncture site causes interstitial tissue fluids to be expelled along with the blood and produces inaccurate test results.

▶▶ **Nursing Responsibilities and Implications**

1. Select one of the usual puncture sites—earlobe or finger in adults and children and heel or great toe in infants. Make certain the site is pink and warm to ensure a dilated skin vessel and free blood flow. Circulation may be improved by rubbing the earlobe with a piece of cotton or by immersing the hand or heel in warm water for 5 minutes and drying it briskly with a towel.

2. Wash the site using a gauze pad saturated with 70% alcohol or another suitable skin disinfectant to remove dirt and epithelial debris. This action also increases the amount of blood in the area. Allow the skin to dry before puncturing to prevent hemolysis from mixture of the blood with moisture.

3. Puncture the skin with a sterile lancet or a No. 11 scalpel blade to a depth of 2–3 mm. The puncture should be made with a firm, quick stab, controlling both the site and depth. A deep puncture causes no more pain than a superficial one and makes repeating the procedure unnecessary.

4. Wipe away the first drop of blood with a sterile gauze because it contains tissue fluids that will dilute the blood and may cause inaccurate test results. Collect the subsequent drops for examination, allowing them to well up naturally without squeezing or applying more than gentle pressure to the area immediately adjacent to the puncture site. If the blood is difficult to obtain, warm the hand or allow it to remain in a dependent position for several minutes.

5. Collect the blood quickly into microhematocrit tubes or micropipettes and expel it into tubes containing the necessary diluents. Wipe excess blood from the sides of pipettes before inserting them into the diluent tubes, making sure to adjust the blood level in the pipette with a fingertip. Carefully prepare several thin blood smears with feathered edges on clean, new microscopic slides. A thin blood film is needed for reliable microscopic examination.

6. Apply slight pressure to the puncture site with a sterile gauze pad until the bleeding has stopped.

Venipuncture

Venipuncture is the most convenient means of collecting sufficient blood for a number of hematology procedures, and the amount of available blood makes it possible to repeat a test in case of accident, error, or doubtful results. Venipuncture techniques also significantly reduce the collection variables, such as dilution with tissue fluid or vasoconstriction from cold and emotion, that frequently are associated with skin puncture. (Venipuncture techniques and precautions are discussed in Chapter 4.)

Anticoagulants Used in Hematology

Four anticoagulants are currently used for various hematology tests because no single anticoagulant is all-purpose and not all are equally satisfactory for every procedure.

EDTA (Sequestrene, Versene). EDTA (ethylenediaminotetraacetate) is the preferred anticoagulant for most hematology procedures in a concentration of 1–2 mg/mL of blood. EDTA preserves cellular morphology and only occasionally causes artifact formation, even after prolonged standing, making it useful for blood smears. EDTA also prevents platelet agglutination and is excellent for preserving cells for all blood cell counts.

Balanced Oxalate. Oxalates may be used to perform cell counts as well as hemoglobin and hematocrit determinations in a concentration of 2 mg/mL of blood. When combined in the proportion of six parts of ammonium oxalate to four parts of potassium oxalate, the mixture prevents significant cellular distortion and does not affect the mean corpuscular volume. However, double oxalate is unsuitable for making blood films because it causes the rapid development of crenation, platelet clumping, nuclear artifacts, cytoplasmic vacuoles, and other malformations or changes.

Heparin. Heparin is the best anticoagulant when it is extremely important to maintain red blood cell size and prevent hemolysis, and it is used in a concentration of 0.1–0.2 mg/mL of blood. Heparin is used in tests for blood pigments, osmotic fragility, and erythrocyte sedimentation rate but is not satisfactory for leukocyte counts or stained blood films. Blood smears prepared with heparinized blood exhibit poor cellular integrity and develop a blue background when stained with Wright's stain.

Sodium Citrate. Citrate is used mainly for blood coagulation studies and as an anticoagulant for blood transfusions in a mixture of one part of 3.8 aqueous solution and nine parts of blood. Sodium citrate also may be used as the anticoagulant for obtaining erythrocyte sedimentation rates.

Precautions

To ensure accurate test results, the following precautions should be observed when using venipuncture to collect specimens:

1. Completely fill the specimen collection tubes to ensure the proper proportion of blood and anticoagulant and prevent erythrocyte distortion.

2. Prepare blood films immediately.

3. Perform the tests within 2–3 hours after the blood is drawn unless the specimen is refrigerated (Table 2-1). Certain hematology test errors may occur in anticoagulated blood that is left at room temperature following venipuncture because of changes in erythrocyte morphology. The erythrocyte swelling that normally occurs after 6 hours at room temperature causes a falsely elevated hematocrit and mean corpuscular volume (MCV) along with a falsely decreased mean corpuscular hemoglobin concentration (MCHC) and erythrocyte sedimentation rate.

COMPLETE BLOOD COUNT

The **complete blood count** (CBC) is a series of screening tests that are an important part of most physical examinations and every hospital admission workup. The CBC consists of hemoglobin and hematocrit measurements to detect the presence of anemia, red and white blood cell counts to enumerate the cells in a cubic millimeter of whole blood,

TABLE 2-1 Approximate Keeping Time of Oxalated or Sequestrinized Blood

Test	Keeping Time	
	Room Temperature	Refrigerated
Differential white blood cell count	1 hour	—
Stained red blood cell examination	1 hour	—
Reticulocyte count	1 hour	24 hours
Platelet count	1 hour	24 hours
Malaria smears	1 hour	—
Erythrocyte sedimentation rate	2 hours	12 hours
Eosinophil count	2 hours	—
Abnormal hemoglobins	2 hours	—
Mean corpuscular values	3 hours	24 hours
Hematocrit determination	3 hours	24 hours
Hemoglobin determination	24 hours	24 hours
Red blood cell count	24 hours	24 hours
White blood cell count	24 hours	24 hours

and a differential white blood cell count and red blood cell examination to assess cellular morphology and evaluate cell distribution.

Test values for CBC procedures are closely interrelated and significant when considered collectively and interpreted as part of an entire hematology examination. The CBC provides a fairly complete evaluation of all the formed elements in blood. It can supply a great deal of the information necessary to diagnose a hematologic disorder, help to identify disease states not directly related to the hematopoietic system, and help to evaluate the stages and prognosis of certain diseases.

Hemoglobin

Hemoglobin (Hgb), the main component of red blood cells, is the essential protein that combines with and transports oxygen to the body cells for nourishment. Hemoglobin also collects carbon dioxide, the end product of cellular metabolism. The carbon dioxide is later released by the lungs, acting as a buffer to help maintain pH equilibrium. Any condition that reduces the number of circulating red blood cells or decreases the concentration of hemoglobin in the peripheral blood lowers the oxygen-combining capacity of the blood and results in anemia.

Hemoglobin values and red blood cell counts do not always rise and fall equally because some red blood cells contain more hemoglobin than others. This is an important factor in the differential diagnosis of anemia because the oxygen-combining capacity of blood and the degree of anemia are directly related to the hemoglobin concentration rather than to blood volume or the number of red blood cells present. Laboratory measurements of hemoglobin are a simple means of establishing the presence of anemia and are useful in evaluating the effectiveness of therapy.

Clinical Significance

Hemoglobin concentrations below 12 g/dL in men and 10.2 g/dL in women indicate an anemic condition and produce symptoms progressing from weakness, tachycardia, and dizziness to dyspnea at rest, cardiac failure, and coma. Symptoms of anemia range from mild to severe and depend on the degree of the hemoglobin deficit, extent of physiologic adaptation, and intensity of physical exertion. Thus, a moderately severe anemia of acute onset (hemorrhage) may produce severe symptoms, whereas the same degree of anemia developing gradually can be asymptomatic because of compensatory changes.

Hemoglobin values also may be affected by other disease states, as well as non-pathologic conditions such as age, sex, altitude, and the degree of fluid retention or dehydration. Newborn infants normally exhibit hemoglobin concentrations that are higher than those of adults to sustain them until active erythropoiesis begins. After puberty, male and female hemoglobin values differ because men have a greater body mass and higher oxygen requirements than women.

Normal Values
The normal values for hemoglobin determinations are:

Children

Neonates	18–27 g/dL
3 months	10.6–16.5 g/dL
1 year	9.0–14.6 g/dL
3 years	9.4–15.5 g/dL
10 years	10.7–15.5 g/dL

Adults

Males	14–18 g/dL
Females, nongravid	12–16 g/dL
Pregnant females	
3 months	11.4–15.0 g/dL
6 months	10.0–14.3 g/dL
9 months	10.2–14.4 g/dL
Postpartum females	10.4–15.0 g/dL

Variations
Elevated hemoglobin levels may occur with:

Dehydration (prolonged vomiting, severe diarrhea)

Hemoconcentration (shock, following hemorrhage)

High altitude

Polycythemia or erythrocytosis

Severe burns

Decreased hemoglobin levels may occur with:

Anemia from increased blood destruction or decreased blood production

Cirrhosis

Hemorrhage (trauma, childbirth)

Hydremia of pregnancy or fluid retention

Hypothyroidism

Idiopathic steatorrhea

Intravenous overload

Leukemia

Many chronic diseases

Methodology

Hemoglobin determinations require at least 1 mL of venous blood collected with EDTA anticoagulant (lavender-stoppered tube) that must not be kept at room temperature for more than 24 hours. Capillary blood from a finger puncture also may be used for hemoglobin measurements when the blood is collected in the appropriate pipette and diluted immediately in Drabkin's solution.

Precautions

To ensure accurate test results, the following precautions should be observed when collecting specimens for hemoglobin determinations:

1. Do not draw the blood specimen from the same arm or hand being used for the administration of intravenous solutions because the extra fluid may cause falsely decreased hemoglobin values.

2. Do not leave the tourniquet on for longer than 1 minute during specimen collection because elevated hemoglobin values may result from prolonged hemostasis due to vasoconstriction.

▶▶ *Nursing Responsibilities and Implications*

1. Inform the patient that there are no food or fluid restrictions.

2. Determine whether the patient is taking any medications or has any illness that might alter the test results.

3. Observe the patient for signs of dehydration and, if present, encourage fluid intake.

4. Monitor the hematocrit level if the hemoglobin level is decreased.

5. If the hemoglobin level is decreased, encourage the patient to rest; observe the patient for signs of anemia.

Hematocrit

The **hematocrit** (Hct), or packed cell volume, measures the percentage of a given volume of whole blood that is occupied by erythrocytes. Thus, a hematocrit value of 45% indicates that 45 mL of each deciliter of peripheral blood is composed of red blood cells. Hematocrit determinations aid in the diagnosis and evaluation of anemia and also may be used to calculate erythrocyte indices, total erythrocyte mass, and blood volume.

Clinical Significance

Hematocrit values generally parallel both the hemoglobin level and erythrocyte count directly because any variation of one value produces an equal change in the other values when red blood cells are a normal size. Hemoglobin and erythrocyte counts may be estimated from the microhematocrit reading of normal blood according to the following formulas:

1 hematocrit point = 0.34 g of hemoglobin per deciliter of blood

1 hematocrit point = 107,000 erythrocytes per microliter of blood

The accuracy of the hemoglobin and hematocrit relationship on laboratory reports also may be checked easily according to the following formula:

$$\text{Hematocrit reading} = \text{Hemoglobin value} \times 3 \pm 3\%$$

For example, a hemoglobin value of 13.0 g/dL should be accompanied by a hematocrit value between 36% and 42% (13.0 × 3 = 39% ± 3% = 36%–42%). Any consistent deviation of laboratory results from this relationship indicates the presence of many red blood cells of abnormal size or hemoglobin content.

The normal relationship between hematocrit and hemoglobin or erythrocyte count does not exist in certain pathologic conditions in which the red blood cells are larger or smaller than normal. Thus, patients with macrocytic red blood cells, which usually contain a larger amount of hemoglobin than normal, demonstrate a hematocrit value higher than the corresponding erythrocyte count would indicate. Conversely, microcytic red blood cells, which generally contain less hemoglobin than normal, produce a decreased hematocrit in spite of a normal erythrocyte count because smaller cells pack into a smaller volume.

Normal Values

The normal values for hematocrit determinations are:

Children	
Neonates	42%–68%
3 months	29%–54%
1 year	29%–41%
3 years	31%–44%
10 years	34%–45%

Adults	
Males	40%–54%
Females, nongravid	37%–47%
Pregnant females	
3 months	35%–46%
6 months	30%–42%
9 months	32%–44%
Postpartum females	34%–44%

Variations

Elevated hematocrit levels may occur with:

Dehydration (prolonged vomiting, severe diarrhea)

Hemoconcentration (shock, surgery, hemorrhage)

Polycythemia vera

Severe burns

Decreased hematocrit levels may occur with:

Anemia (decreased blood production, increased blood destruction)

Cardiac decompensation

Excessive fluid administration

Hemorrhage or prolonged blood loss

Hydremia of pregnancy

Hypothyroidism

Idiopathic steatorrhea

Leukemia

Methodology

Hematocrit determinations require approximately 3 mL of venous blood collected with EDTA anticoagulant (lavender-stoppered tube); the tube should be filled entirely so that the proper proportion of blood to anticoagulant is obtained to preserve cellular morphology. This test also may be done on a capillary blood specimen collected directly from a fingertip or earlobe puncture into microhematocrit tubes.

Precautions

To ensure accurate hematocrit test results, the following precautions should be observed:

1. Do not draw the blood specimen from the same arm or hand being used for the administration of intravenous solutions because the extra fluid may cause falsely decreased hematocrit values.

2. Do not leave the tourniquet on for longer than 1 minute during specimen collection because hematocrit values may be falsely elevated as much as 2%–5% by prolonged stasis due to vasoconstriction.

▶▶ Nursing Responsibilities and Implications

1. Quiet or comfort the patient, especially the young child, before the blood for the hematocrit is drawn because agitation causes a temporary rise in hemotocrit values.

2. Inform the patient that there are no food or fluid restrictions.

3. Obtain the blood specimen before the bath, shower, or morning care because cold water and massage cause a temporary rise in hematocrit values.

4. Encourage adequate fluid intake if the patient's hematocrit level is increased.

5. Assess the patient for anemia if the hematocrit is decreased.

6. Determine if the patient is taking any medications or has any illness that might alter the test results.

Erythrocyte Count

The **red blood cell count** (RBC) is a determination of the number of circulating erythrocytes present in 1 μL or 1 mm^3 of whole blood. The level of circulating erythrocytes is regulated by erythropoiesis in the bone marrow. Erythropoiesis is affected by **erythropoietin**, a renal hormone, and controlled by the oxygen demands of the body.

The rate of red blood cell production generally remains stable within certain limits during normal body functioning but may be altered by erythropoietic dysfunction or physiologic and environmental conditions. Thus, any increase in the level of circulating red blood cells inhibits erythropoiesis, whereas hypoxia caused either by altitude variations or anemia stimulates erythropoiesis. Laboratory determinations of red blood cell counts are occasionally useful in the diagnosis of various anemias and are necessary to calculate the red blood cell indices.

Clinical Significance

Red blood cell levels below 4.2 million/μL in men and 3.6 million/μL in women commonly characterize an anemic condition. Significant variations in the red blood cell count also may result from several physiologic factors such as posture, extreme physical exercise, excitement, age, sex, severe dehydration, and altitude. Red blood cell counts may be decreased by as much as 5% when blood specimens are drawn with the patient recumbent rather than upright. The normal erythrocyte count of infants is highest immediately following birth to fulfill the newborn's oxygen requirements until active erythropoiesis begins. After puberty, red blood cell levels are routinely lower in women than in men because of a smaller body mass, lesser oxygen requirements, and repeated menstrual blood loss.

Strong emotions such as fear, anger, or excitement, as well as abdominal massage and cold showers, may cause a temporary increase in the red blood cell count. Blood counts obtained under conditions of extreme excitement may be of doubtful clinical significance, especially in children, in whom this factor exhibits its greatest effect. Erythropoiesis actually increases at high altitude because of the lower oxygen tension and stimulating effect of hypoxia. Thus, a moderate but significant difference in erythrocyte levels will exist between individuals residing at an altitude greater than 750 m and those living closer to sea level.

Normal Values
The normal values for the red blood cell count are:

Children

Neonates	4.8−7.0 million/μL
3 months	3.8−5.5 million/μL
1 year	3.6−5.5 million/μL
3 years	3.8−5.4 million/μL
10 years	3.9−5.2 million/μL

Adults

Males	4.5−6.2 million/μL
Females, nongravid	4.0−5.5 million/μL
Pregnant females	
3 months	4.0−5.0 million/μL
6 months	3.2−4.5 million/μL
9 months	3.0−4.9 million/μL
Postpartum females	3.2−5.0 million/μL

Variations

Elevated red blood cell counts (erythrocytosis) may occur with:

Anoxia

Cardiovascular disease

Cushing's disease

Hemoconcentration (shock, trauma, surgery, hemorrhage)

High altitude

Polycythemia vera (erythremia)

Profound dehydration

Severe burns

Decreased red blood cell counts may occur with:

Acute blood loss due to hemorrhage

Addison's disease

Anemia resulting from abnormal blood destruction or diminished blood production

Chronic infections

Excessive intravenous fluids

Gaucher's disease

Hodgkin's disease

Hydremia of pregnancy

Hypothyroidism

Idiopathic steatorrhea

Leukemia

Lupus erythematosus

Recovery phase following hemo-concentration (shock or trauma)

Methodology

Red blood cell counts require approximately 3 mL of venous blood collected with EDTA anticoagulant (lavender-stoppered tubes) and kept at room temperature for no more than 24 hours.

Precautions

To ensure accurate red blood cell counts, the following precautions should be observed:

1. Do not draw blood specimens for red blood cell determinations from the same extremity being used for intravenous infusions because the additional fluid may dilute the blood and produce falsely decreased test values.

2. Do not leave the tourniquet in place for more than 1 minute because red blood cell counts may be falsely elevated by hemoconcentration from stasis due to vasoconstriction.

▶▶ *Nursing Responsibilities and Implications*

1. Inform the patient that there are no food or fluid restrictions.

2. Determine if the patient is taking any medications or has any illness that might alter the test results.

3. Encourage rest if the patient's red blood cell count is reduced.

4. Encourage the patient to eat foods high in iron, such as organ meats and green leafy vegetables, which promote red blood cell production, if the red blood cell count is decreased.

Leukocyte Count

The **white blood cell count** (WBC) is a determination of the number of circulating leukocytes present in 1 μL or 1 mm^3 of whole blood. White blood cells are produced in the bone marrow and lymphatic tissues and enter the bloodstream for transportation to the extravascular location where they function. Leukocytes leave the blood when they reach their destination and enter body tissues to help defend against invading microorganisms through phagocytosis and antibody formation.

Five types of normal white blood cells are routinely recognized in the bloodstream, namely the neutrophils, eosinophils, and basophils, known as granulocytes, and the lymphocytes and monocytes. Each cell type has its own unique function in defending the body against foreign threats, and the cells assume certain recognizable distribution patterns in response to different types of disease. However, the total leukocyte count does not distinguish these different cell types, which is the purpose of the differential count, but only indicates the leukocyte response to various conditions. Laboratory determination of the total white blood cell count, accompanied by a differential count of cell distribution and morphology, is a vital aid to the diagnosis and evaluation of many pathologic disorders.

Clinical Significance

Significant changes in the number and distribution of white blood cells in the peripheral blood are extremely valuable indicators of the presence and cause of disease. Any rise above normal leukocyte values results from stimulation of the bone marrow by bacteria or invading organisms, whereas decreased white blood cell levels follow bone marrow depression caused by viruses or toxic chemicals. Minor variations from normal values are not significant when accompanied by normal differential smears, although this situation does not rule out some early infections or myeloproliferative disorders.

Pathologic leukocyte values can be defined only after assessing the effect of physiologic factors such as age, stress, exercise, and other deviations from basal conditions. Physiologic factors, including bathing, eating, and physical or emotional activity, may cause slightly increased leukocyte counts, but the level of maximum elevation usually does not exceed twice the normal minimum level. Physiologic leukocyte elevations generally subside to normal levels within several hours; therefore, white blood cell counts should be repeated under more relaxed circumstances if the elevation is of doubtful significance. Leukocyte values for men and women are affected equally by a diurnal rhythm that increases white blood cell levels as much as 2000/μL between morning and evening, independent of food intake.

Normal Values

The normal values for the leukocyte count are:

Children

Neonates	9000–30,000/μL
3 months	5700–18,000/μL
1 year	6000–17,500/μL
3 years	5700–16,300/μL
10 years	4500–13,500/μL

(continued)

Adults	
Males	4500–11,000/μL
Females, nongravid	4500–11,000/μL
Pregnant females	
3 months	6600–14,100/μL
6 months	6900–17,100/μL
9 months	5900–14,700/μL
During labor	9800–17,800/μL
Postpartum females	
1 week	9700–25,700/μL
1–2 months	6400–11,800/μL

Interpretation

The significance of the total leukocyte count may be interpreted as follows:

Mildly decreased	<3000/μL
Moderately decreased	1500–3000/μL
Severely decreased	<1500/μL
Slightly elevated	<20,000/μL
Moderately elevated	30,000–40,000/μL
Markedly elevated	>50,000/μL

Variations

Elevated leukocyte counts (leukocytosis) may occur in physiologic conditions such as:

Adrenaline injections	Exposure to cold	Strenuous exercise or work
Anesthesia	Immediately following trauma or hemorrhage	
Anorexia		Ultraviolet irradiation or sunlight
Anoxia	Menstruation	
Convulsive seizures	Paroxysmal tachycardia	
Emotional stress (pain, fear, anger, excitement)	Pregnancy and childbirth	

Elevated leukocyte counts also may occur in pathologic conditions such as:

Abscess	Cushing's disease	Leukemoid reactions accompanying severe sepsis or miliary tuberculosis
Anemia	Diphtheria	
Appendicitis	Erythroblastosis fetalis	
Bacterial infections, acute and chronic	Infectious mononucleosis	Meningitis
Chickenpox	Leukemia	Parasitic infestations

Peritonitis	Rheumatic fever	Transfusion reaction
Pneumonia	Smallpox	Ulcers
Polycythemia vera	Tonsillitis	Uremia

Decreased leukocyte counts (leukopenia) may occur with:

Agranulocytosis	Hypersplenism	Protein therapy
Anemia	Infectious hepatitis and cirrhosis	Psittacosis
Bacterial infections, overwhelming	Influenza	Radiation therapy
Brucellosis	Leukemia (some forms)	Rheumatic fever
Drug and chemical toxicity	Lupus erythematosus	Typhoid fever and para-typhoid fever
Gaucher's disease	Measles	Viral infections
	Myxedema	

Methodology

White blood cell counts require 3 mL of venous blood collected in EDTA anticoagulant (lavender-stoppered tube) because these specimens permit repeat testing and produce accurate results for up to 24 hours.

Differential White Blood Cell Count

The **differential white blood cell count** (Diff) enumerates individual leukocyte distribution on a stained slide of peripheral blood. A differential cell count is performed by microscopically identifying 100 or more white blood cells, classifying them according to morphology, and calculating the relative percentage of each cell type present. Reliable white blood cell classifications help to direct attention toward particular diseases because characteristic abnormal cell distribution patterns are generally consistent with certain disorders.

Differential cell counts routinely report leukocyte morphology, including immature or abnormal cells and cellular inclusions, which helps to identify the stage and severity of some specific diseases. An accurate differential report, combined with a hemoglobin determination, provides as much as 90% of the significant diagnostic information available through hematologic procedures. Laboratory determinations of white blood cell distribution are helpful in diagnosis and can be used to monitor patient progress as well as to indicate the effects of chemotherapy or radiotherapy.

Clinical Significance

A differential white blood cell count classifies leukocytes according to three morphologic categories: monocytes, lymphocytes, and the granulocytes, which are identified as neutrophils, eosinophils, and basophils (Figure 2-1). The cells routinely identified during a differential cell count are mature cells with normal morphology and no cytoplasmic inclusions. Each cell fulfills a definite need and performs a unique specific function in the defense and protection of the body.

Neutrophils, the most numerous circulating white blood cells in normal adults, form the primary line of defense against infections and other trauma. Neutrophilic granu-

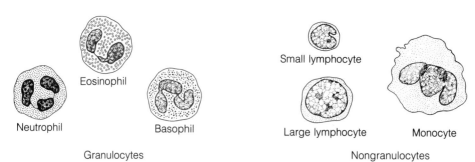

Figure 2-1   Major leukocyte types.

locytes seek out bacteria or necrotic tissue at the site of injury and destroy them through the engulfment process known as **phagocytosis**. Segmented neutrophils actively ingest the invading organism as well as the debris of dead tissue cells and liberate certain enzymes to digest local tissues in preparation for future healing. Neutrophils must be present at a site of injury before lymphocytes, monocytes, or other cells can be attracted to continue the healing process.

A constant level of circulating neutrophils is maintained normally in healthy individuals, but larger numbers of cells are demanded and released from the bone marrow when bacteria invade the body. A prolonged demand for high neutrophil levels causes the bone marrow to release cells that are not completely developed, resulting in an increased number of immature band neutrophils. Any significant increase in the number of circulating neutrophils is almost always accompanied by a rise in the total leukocyte count, indicating that the body is fighting the infection. However, a decreased total leukocyte count with an increased number of immature band neutrophils during an overwhelming infection is an ominous indication that the body is losing its fight.

Lymphocytes, the second line of defense against foreign organisms, are produced in the thymus, lymph nodes, and bone marrow and protect the body through antibody formation and immune reactions. Lymphocytes identify invading substances, including viruses, bacteria, incompatible erythrocytes, tissue grafts or transplants, and neoplasms, respond to their structure chemically, and produce a specific antibody against each particular organism. An individual's own cells and secretions also can stimulate antibody production and evoke hypersensitivity reactions if the body recognizes these substances as foreign.

Two types of lymphocytes are currently recognized—T-lymphocytes and B-lymphocytes—each having their own distinct life cycle and specific function. T cells (formed in the thymus) comprise 80%–90% of circulating lymphocytes (65%–75% of the total lymphocytes) and have a life span ranging from many months to 30 years. They are responsible for initiating cellular immunity in delayed hypersensitivity reactions such as skin rashes, tissue allograft rejection, and graft versus host reactions. They also attack intracellular bacterial and rickettsial pathogens, fungi, and many viruses. B cells (from the bone marrow) have a short life span and produce antibodies to neutralize viruses, interfere with absorption of foreign proteins, and detoxify other toxic proteins. Their primary functions, however, are the defense against virulent, encapsulated bacterial pathogens, synthesis of immunoglobulin and specific antibodies, and production of plasma cells. (T-lymphocytes and B-lymphocytes also are discussed in Chapter 11.)

B-lymphocytes have the additional ability to transform themselves into plasma cells, which rapidly secrete antibodies for short periods of time to help combat invading organisms. Plasma cells seldom appear in the bloodstream, but increased numbers may accompany severe infections, especially in children, to reinforce immunity when sufficient antibodies are unavailable.

Children and young adolescents exhibit a physiologic increase of circulating lymphocytes as the developing immune system struggles to meet the ongoing need for new antibodies. A nonphysiologic lymphocytosis may result from an actual stimulation of lymphocyte production in response to greater antibody requirements. This response is sufficient to produce an increase in the total leukocyte count. An apparent lymphocytosis also can be an illusion created by a concurrent decrease of some other cell or cells, generally the neutrophil.

Monocytes, the all-purpose cleanup cells, are produced by the bone marrow and transported in the bloodstream to the tissues, where they perform their phagocytic function. Monocytes complement the phagocytic activity of neutrophils and prepare tissues for healing by removing pus and dead cellular debris after an abscess or acute inflammatory reaction subsides. However, unlike neutrophils, whose activities are directed primarily against bacteria, monocytes also ingest larger protozoa, such as fungi and parasites, that the neutrophils are not equipped to remove.

Monocytes function as scavenger cells to dispose of noninfectious foreign substances, including crystals of altered hemoglobin remaining in the tissues from previous bleeding. Additional substances, such as particles inhaled into the lungs, products of tissue breakdown, and particles of any foreign material thrust into traumatized tissues, also are removed from the body by monocyte ingestion. Recently, monocytes have been suspected of supplying a factor necessary to stimulate granulocyte growth and therefore may be involved in regulating neutrophil production.

Eosinophils, phagocytic and bactericidal cells arising from the bone marrow, are segmented granulocytes that respond to immune complexes and limit chronic inflammatory reactions. Eosinophils are closely associated with allergic and parasitic conditions, although their exact role in the etiology and manifestation of allergic reactions is unclear. Circulating eosinophils are attracted to sites of foreign antigen by tissue histamine late in the course of inflammatory processes and respond by breaking down protein material and ingesting antigen-antibody complexes.

Eosinophils generally exhibit a diurnal variation, with circulating levels declining during the morning until about noon and rising throughout the afternoon, reaching a maximum level between midnight and 3 AM. However, this normal rhythm is reversed in asthmatics and night workers, who exhibit a maximum peak between 9 AM and noon. Eosinophils also accumulate in skin, lungs, and tissues within the gastrointestinal tract in numbers 100 times greater than in blood.

Basophils, a third variety of segmented granulocytes originating in the bone marrow, are the most poorly understood cells found in the blood. Basophils carry about one-half of the blood histamine, which is released in response to IgE-stimulated antigen-antibody reactions. They play an active role in allergic reactions and anaphylactoid states. Basophils also contain heparin and hydroxytryptamine, which causes these cells to be closely associated with fibrinolysis, the prevention of stasis and coagulation, and lipid metabolism.

The differential count also may identify immature or abnormal white blood cells and cellular anomalies or inclusion bodies, which can be classified as follows:

Immature white blood cells, predominantly of the neutrophilic series, indicate that the bone marrow is responding to a heavy demand by rapidly producing and releasing

Normal Values

The normal values for the differential white blood cell count are:

	Neutrophils	Band Neutrophils	Lymphocytes	Monocytes	Eosinophils	Basophils
Neonates	6000–26,000/μL 61%	1600/μL 9%	2000–11,000/μL 31%	400–3100/μL 6%	20–850/μL 2%	0–640/μL 0.6%
3 months	1000–9000/μL 34%	470/μL 4%	3300–15,000/μL 59%	150–1600/μL 5%	70–800/μL 3%	0–200/μL 0.5%
1 year	1500–8500/μL 31%	350/μL 3%	4000–10,500/μL 61%	50–1100/μL 5%	50–700/μL 3%	0–200/μL 0.4%
3 years	1500–8500/μL 38%	300/μL 3%	2500–8700/μL 54%	25–900/μL 5%	30–650/μL 3%	0–200/μL 0.5%
10 years	1800–8000/μL 54%	240/μL 3%	1500–6500/μL 38%	0–800/μL 4%	0–600/μL 2%	0–200/μL 0.5%
Adults (males and nongravid females)	1800–7700/μL 54%–75%	220/μL 3%–8%	1000–4800/μL 25%–40%	0–800/μL 2%–8%	0–450/μL 1%–4%	0–200/μL 0%–1%
Pregnant females						
3 months	3750–10,700/μL 57%–76%		1100–4650/μL 17%–33%	60–1100/μL 1%–8%	30–700/μL 1%–5%	
6 months	4700–13,600/μL 67%–81%		700–3900/μL 10%–23%	0–1350/μL 0%–8%	20–500/μL 0.3%–3%	
9 months	4100–11,900/μL 68%–81%		700–3500/μL 12%–24%	0–1150/μL 0%–8%	0–320/μL 0%–2%	
During labor	7500–15,600/μL 72%–88%		780–3500/μL 8%–20%	0–1400/μL 0%–8%	0–100/μL 0%–0.6%	
Postpartum females						
1 week	6800–24,100/μL 70%–94%		450–7700/μL 5%–30%	200–500/μL 2%	0–380/μL 0%–1.5%	
1–2 months	3300–9300/μL 52%–79%		1050–5200/μL 17%–44%	250–470/μL 4%	60–800/μL 1%–7%	

unsegmented young cells. Neutrophils normally mature in the bone marrow, progressing from myeloblasts (most immature cells) to promyelocytes, myelocytes, and metamyelocytes, before entering the peripheral circulation as bands and segmented neutrophils (mature cells). The appearance of immature neutrophils in the peripheral blood is known as a **shift to the left** because neutrophil maturation is usually illustrated from left to right (the youngest cells on the left). Immature neutrophils appear in the bloodstream during such conditions as granulocytic leukemia, acute infections, neutrophilic leukemoid reactions, toxemia, and hemorrhage.

The degree of shift to the left, together with the accompanying total leukocyte level, indicates the severity of infection and the extent of an individual's resistance. Thus, a low total white blood cell count with a marked increase of young cells indicates bone marrow depression and a block in the maturation process known as a **degenerative shift**. On the other hand, a high total white blood cell count with numerous immature cells reflects bone marrow response to increased stimulation and is known as a **regenerative shift**. The term **shift to the right** implies hypersegmented neutrophils that have more than the usual number of nuclear segments. These cells develop in individuals with liver disease, Down's syndrome, or megaloblastic anemias, including pernicious anemia.

Toxic granulation refers to dark-staining particles present in the cytoplasm of neutrophils during inflammatory or toxic states. The degree of granulation reflects the severity of conditions such as acute infections, toxemia of pregnancy, chemical poisoning, liver disease, x-ray irradiation, and agranulocytosis.

Atypical lymphocytes, also known as virocytes or reactive lymphocytes, are B cells that differ from normal lymphocytes in morphology and staining characteristics; this occurs as a reaction to antigen stimulation. The presence of atypical lymphocytes on a differential report generally indicates a reaction to viral infections such as infectious mononucleosis, acute viral hepatitis, viral pneumonia, cytomegalovirus, chickenpox, mumps, or rubella. Reactive lymphocytes may accompany such nonviral conditions as tuberculosis, rickettsialpox, syphilis, diphtheria, malaria, scarlet fever, and typhus, along with drug reactions to para-aminosalicylic acid (PAS), phenytoin, mephenytoin, barbiturates, and phenylbutazone. Reactive lymphocytes also occur with serum sickness, agranulocytosis, acute myocardial infarction, ulcerative colitis, and Addison's disease and following open-heart surgery, irradiation, or massive blood transfusions.

Interpretation (See Normal Values on facing page)

Differential white blood cell reports occasionally include an estimated total leukocyte count as a check on electronic white blood cell count results. White blood cell count test results frequently appear lower than actual circulating levels because many leukocytes, particularly leukemic cells, are fragile and disintegrate easily in the electronic counter. The total white blood cell count can be estimated microscopically in a high-power field as follows:

Average Number of White Blood Cells per High-Power Field	Estimated Total Leukocyte Count per Microliter
1–4	2000–8000
4–6	8000–12,000
6–10	12,000–20,000
10–20	20,000–40,000

Differential white blood cell counts must be evaluated carefully to obtain the maximum diagnostic information from reports that express only the relative proportion of cells. Relative values can be misleading because an increased percentage of any cell type may reflect an actual rise in the number of that particular cell or a decrease in one or more cells of another type. Accurate analysis of patient status requires a knowledge of the actual circulating level of each type of cell to provide absolute values that are not subject to misinterpretation.

The absolute value for each cell may be calculated by multiplying the total leukocyte count by the relative percentage each particular cell occupies in the blood:

$$\begin{array}{c} \text{Total leukocyte} \\ \text{count (WBCs/}\mu L) \end{array} \times \begin{array}{c} \text{Relative value} \\ (\%) \end{array} = \begin{array}{c} \text{Absolute value} \\ (\text{cells/}\mu L) \end{array}$$

For example, a total leukocyte count of 8000/μL with a differential report of 30% lymphocytes indicates that the absolute or actual number of lymphocytes in circulation is 2400/μL, which is a normal level (8000 × 30% = 2400).

Relative and absolute leukocyte values are significant because they allow a determination of the problem in an abnormal blood picture. The following examples demonstrate the usefulness of absolute values in diagnosis:

$$\begin{array}{c} \textit{Total WBC} \\ \textit{9500/}\mu L \end{array} \times \begin{array}{c} \textit{Differential} \\ \textit{Count (\%)} \end{array} = \begin{array}{c} \textit{Absolute} \\ \textit{Values} \\ \textit{(cells/}\mu L) \end{array}$$

	Differential Count (%)	Absolute Values (cells/μL)
Neutrophils	60	5700
Band neutrophils	20	1900
Lymphocytes	12	1400
Monocytes	4	380
Eosinophils	3	285
Basophils	1	95

Interpretation: Relative and absolute increase in neutrophils (**neutrophilia**), along with a relative and absolute decrease in lymphocytes (**lymphopenia**).

$$\begin{array}{c} \textit{Total WBC} \\ \textit{25,000/}\mu L \end{array} \times \begin{array}{c} \textit{Differential} \\ \textit{Count (\%)} \end{array} = \begin{array}{c} \textit{Absolute} \\ \textit{Values} \\ \textit{(cells/}\mu L) \end{array}$$

	Differential Count (%)	Absolute Values (cells/μL)
Neutrophils	65	16,250
Band neutrophils	15	3750
Lymphocytes	16	4000
Monocytes	2	500
Eosinophils	1.5	375
Basophils	0.5	125

Interpretation: Although this differential report appears much the same as example 1, this patient exhibits a relative and absolute neutrophilia but only a relative lymphopenia.

$$\frac{Total\ WBC}{3000/\mu L} \times \frac{Differential}{Count\ (\%)} = \frac{Absolute}{Values}$$
$$(cells/\mu L)$$

Neutrophils	20	600
Band neutrophils	0	0
Lymphocytes	72	2160
Monocytes	5	150
Eosinophils	2	60
Basophils	1	30

Interpretation: Relative increase in lymphocytes but no actual increase in their absolute number; relative and absolute decrease in neutrophils.

Variations
Elevated neutrophil levels (neutrophilia) may occur with:

Acute infections with pyogenic bacteria and other organisms

  Abscesses and boils

  Anthrax

  Appendicitis

  Chickenpox

  Cholecystitis

  Cholera

  Diphtheria

  Empyema

  Endocarditis

  Osteomyelitis

  Otitis media

  Peritonitis

  Pneumonia

  Purulent meningitis

  Pyelonephritis

  Pyemia

  Rheumatic fever

  Salpingitis

  Scarlet fever

  Septicemia

  Smallpox

  Tonsillitis

  Typhus

Noninfective tissue damage

  Burns

  Carcinoma and tumors

  Coronary thrombosis

  Crushing injury

  Drugs (epinephrine, ACTH, digitalis, benzene, ethylene glycol, potassium chlorate, corticosteroids)

  Gangrene

  Myocardial infarction

  Poisoning (carbon monoxide, lead, mercury, arsenic, turpentine)

  Pulmonary infarction

Metabolic disorders

  Cushing's disease

  Diabetic acidosis

  Eclampsia

  Gout

  Thyroiditis

  Uremia

Myeloproliferative disorders

  Acute myeloblastic leukemia

  Chronic myelocytic leukemia

  Di Guglielmo disease

  Lymphoma

  Myelophthisic anemias

  Neutrophilic leukemoid reaction

  Polycythemia vera

Stress conditions

  Allergies

  Anger

  Anoxia

  Anxiety

  Electric shock and electroconvulsive therapy

  Extreme heat or cold

  Fear

  Hemorrhage

  Labor and delivery

Panic	Hemolysis	Chronic hemolytic anemia crisis
Strenuous exercise	Acute hemolytic anemia	
Surgery		Hemolytic transfusion reaction

Decreased neutrophil levels (neutropenia) may occur with:

Infections, bacterial, viral, protozoal

  Bacterial infections, overwhelming

  Brucellosis

  Infectious hepatitis

  Infectious mononucleosis

  Influenza

  Kala-azar

  Malaria

  Measles

  Miliary tuberculosis

  Mumps

  Paratyphoid fever

  Primary atypical pneumonia

  Psittacosis

  Relapsing fever

  Rubella

  Rubeola

  Septicemia

  Tularemia

  Typhoid fever

Hematopoietic disorders

  Agranulocytosis

  Aleukemic leukemia

  Aplastic anemia

Felty's syndrome

Gaucher's disease

Hypersplenism

Myelofibrosis

Pernicious anemia

Cachexia and inanition

  Anorexia nervosa

  Carcinoma

  Folic acid deficiency

  Myeloma

  Sarcoma

  Starvation

  Vitamin B_{12} deficiency

Hormone diseases

  Acromegaly

  Addison's disease

  Thyrotoxicosis

Toxic agents

  Antimetabolites

  Benzene

  Nitrogen mustard

  X-ray irradiation and radiation therapy

Chemical agents

  Acute alcohol ingestion

Analgesics (antipyrine, aminopyrine, phenylbutazone, phenacetin)

Antibiotics (penicillin, chloramphenicol, streptomycin)

Anticonvulsants (phenytoin, mephenytoin, phenacemide)

Antihistamines (tripelennamine hydrochloride, methaphenilene hydrochloride)

Hematopoietic depressants (6-mercaptopurines, phenylhydrazines, urethan)

Miscellaneous (phenindione, aminophylline, quinine, chlorpromazine, barbiturates, arsenic compounds, dinitrophenol, cinchophen)

Sulfonamides

Other causes

  Anaphylactoid shock

  Disseminated lupus erythematosus

Elevated lymphocyte levels (lymphocytosis) may occur with:

Acute and chronic infections, bacterial or viral

  Brucellosis

  Chickenpox

  Cytomegalovirus

Infectious lymphocytosis

Infectious mononucleosis

Influenza

Measles or German measles

Mumps

Paratyphoid fever

Pertussis

Syphilis

Tuberculosis

Tularemia

Typhoid fever

Typhus

Viral hepatitis

Viral pneumonia

Hematopoietic disorders

Agranulocytosis

Aplastic anemia

Banti's disease

Felty's syndrome

Leukosarcoma

Lymphocytic leukemia

Multiple myeloma

Non-Hodgkin lymphomas

Miscellaneous

Active antibody for-mation in young children

Addison's disease

Carcinoma

Hyperthyroidism, thyrotoxicosis

Malnutrition

Rickets

Scurvy in later childhood

Waldenström's macroglobulinemia

Decreased lymphocyte levels (lymphopenia) may occur with:

Aplastic anemia

Cardiac failure

Cushing's disease

Di Guglielmo disease

Epinephrine, cortisone, or ACTH administration

Hodgkin's disease

Immunoglobulin defi-ciencies (Wiskott-

Aldrich syndrome, dysgammaglobulinemia)

Leukemias (chronic granulocytic, monocytic)

Lymphosarcoma

Nitrogen mustard

Radiation of lymphatics

Stress reactions follow-ing burns or trauma

Systemic lupus erythematosus

Terminal carcinoma

Thymic hypoplasia in children

Uremia

Elevated plasma cell levels (plasmacytosis) may occur with:

Carcinoma

Chickenpox

Gaucher's disease

Infections during childhood

Infectious mononucleosis

Lymphocytosis

Measles

Multiple myeloma

Plasma cell leukemia

Postirradiation damage

Scarlet fever

Serum sickness

Skin diseases

Elevated monocyte levels (monocytosis) may occur with:

Agranulocytosis

Amebic dysentery

Bacterial infections, especially during the recovery phase

Banti's disease

Brucellosis

Chickenpox

Chronic tuberculosis

Cirrhosis

Collagen disease

Gaucher's disease

Hodgkin's disease

Infectious mononucleosis

Kala-azar

Leishmaniasis

Malaria

Malignant tumors

Monocytic leukemia

Mumps

Myeloma

Non-Hodgkin lymphomas

Normal newborns

Overexposure to x-rays

Paratyphoid fever

Polycythemia vera

Regional enteritis

Rickettsial infections such as Rocky Mountain spotted fever

Sarcoidosis

Subacute bacterial endocarditis

Trypanosomiasis

Typhoid fever

Typhus

Ulcerative colitis

Weil's disease

Elevated eosinophil levels (eosinophilia) may occur with:

Allergic conditions
  Allergic eczema
  Angioneurotic edema
  Bronchial asthma
  Drug sensitivity
  Gastrointestinal allergy to foods
  Hay fever
  Löffler's syndrome
  Periarteritis nodosa
  Serum sickness
  Urticaria
Chronic skin diseases
  Eczema
  Erythema multiforme
  Exfoliative dermatitis
  Ichthyosis
  Leprosy
  Pruritus of jaundice
  Psoriasis
Drug therapy
  Allopurinol

Digitalis
Heparin
Penicillin
Phenothiazine
Procainamide
Propranolol
Quinidine
Streptomycin
Parasitic infestations
  Ancylostoma
  Ascaris
  Filaria
  Hookworm
  Malaria
  Schistosoma
  Strongyloides
  Toxoplasma
  Trichinosis
Hematopoietic disorders
  Chronic granulocytic leukemia
  Eosinophilic leukemia

Eosinophilic leukemoid reaction
Hodgkin's disease
Pernicious anemia
Polycythemia vera
Postsplenectomy
Sarcoidosis
Sickle cell anemia
Miscellaneous
  Addison's disease
  Brucellosis
  Chorea
  Chronic bacterial infections
  Metastatic carcinoma
  Postirradiation therapy
  Scarlet fever
  Subacute infections
  Tuberculosis
  Ulcerative colitis

Decreased eosinophil levels (eosinopenia) may occur with:

Acromegaly

Adrenaline, epi-nephrine, ACTH administration

Cushing's disease

Disseminated lupus erythematosus

Increased adrenocortical activity

Intermenstrual period

Stress situations (trauma, burns, surgery,

electroconvulsive therapy, strenuous exercise)

Thyroxine administration

Elevated basophil levels (basophilia) may occur with:

Chronic myelogenous leukemia

Erythroderma

Hemolytic anemias

Hodgkin's disease

Hypothyroidism or myxedema

Infections, especially during the recovery phase	Irradiation	Splenectomy
	Myelofibrosis	Ulcerative colitis
	Polycythemia vera	Urticaria

Decreased basophil levels (basopenia) may occur with:

Acute allergic reactions

Anaphylactoid reactions

Hyperthyroidism, thyrotoxicosis

Steroid therapy or increased corticosteroid production

Stress reactions

Methodology

Differential white blood cell counts require two air-dried peripheral blood smears made on new microscope slides. The most significant test results are obtained from fresh capillary or EDTA-anticoagulated venous blood films that cover approximately two-thirds of the slide and have a well-formed, feathered edge. Well-made blood smears may be prepared by a number of recently designed automated devices as well as the conventional coverslip and slide-wedge procedures. When stained with Wright's stain, these blood films allow the morphologic examination of red blood cells and platelets along with white blood cell differentiation.

▶▶ Nursing Responsibilities and Implications

1. Inform the patient that there are no food or fluid restrictions.

2. Record the time the blood sample is drawn because the counts vary depending on the time of day.

3. List any drugs the patient has been or is taking because many drugs decrease the white blood cell count (agranulocytosis, leukopenia, and neutropenia); identify any illnesses that might alter the test results.

4. Protect the patient from infection if the white blood cell count is decreased.

Stained Red Blood Cell Examination

A thorough inspection of red blood cell morphology is conducted routinely on a stained smear of peripheral blood at the same time as the differential white blood cell count. Laboratory identification of abnormal or immature red blood cells is an important means of distinguishing various anemias and blood dyscrasias and may indicate the need for additional diagnostic procedures.

Clinical Significance

Normal-sized and shaped erythrocytes are referred to as **normocytes**. That the majority of red blood cells fall within the normal size range does not necessarily exclude the diagnosis of anemia. Normal shape enables the red blood cells to withstand severe distortion and pass undamaged through small capillaries. The depth of red blood cell color and stain on a blood film provides a rough guide to the amount of hemoglobin in each cell. Erythrocytes that contain a normal hemoglobin concentration are known as **normochromic cells**.

Red blood cell morphologic variations include changes in size, shape, color, maturation, and content, all of which are reported according to the type and degree of abnormality. The degree of variation may be classified as occasional, slight, moderate, marked, or very marked, depending on the number and severity of the abnormal forms identified. A more uniform grading system for evaluating changes in morphology also may be employed to help standardize subjective impressions among various examiners, as follows:

Abnormal RBCs/hpf	Score	Interpretation
3–6	1+	Slight
7–10	2+	Moderate
11–20	3+	Marked
Over 20	4+	Very marked

Normal Values

Normal red blood cell morphologic features are:

Size	6.7–7.7 μm (average is 7.2 μm)
Shape	Biconcave disk with a thin central area that resembles a donut
Color	Well-filled, uniformly stained, buff-orange disk with central pallor
Contents	No nucleus, nuclear remnants, or cellular inclusions

---

Variations

Size. **Anisocytosis** refers to a pathologic variation from normal cell size, either increased or decreased, a nonspecific feature seen in many disorders. Variations from normal cell dimensions generally reflect changes in bone marrow function and red blood cell development, frequently resulting from deficiencies of such raw materials as iron, vitamin B_{12}, and folic acid. Anisocytosis is common in newborns and may be recorded in individuals with leukemia and many anemias, including pernicious anemia and iron deficiency anemia. The most severe anemias are accompanied by the most marked size variations.

Microcytes are mature red blood cells with a smaller than normal diameter of 6.0 μm or less that frequently contain an insufficient amount of hemoglobin. The abundance of microcytic cells may be caused by hemoglobin abnormalities or a deficiency of the hematopoietic materials required to produce hemoglobin. Microcytosis can occur in such hemoglobinopathies as thalassemia and hereditary spherocytosis, as well as iron deficiency anemia and anemia secondary to chronic hemorrhage.

Macrocytes are red blood cells that are larger than normal, with an average diameter of 8.0 μm or greater. The abundance of macrocytic cells usually is associated with disorders characterized by a deficiency of such erythropoietic factors as vitamin B_{12} and folic acid. Macrocytosis generally occurs in newborns, as well as individuals with pernicious anemia, thalassemia, reticulocytosis, liver disease, hypothyroidism, and idiopathic steatorrhea.

Shape. **Poikilocytosis** refers to any variation from the normal red blood cell shape and may result from a number of pathologic conditions. Abnormally shaped erythrocytes can range from mildly irregular, oval, or spherical shapes to such peculiar distortions as tear drops, pear-shaped, and dumbbell-like forms. Significant poikilocytosis usually indicates faulty erythropoiesis caused by defective formation and maturation within the bone marrow or red blood cell fragmentation due to stress within the bloodstream. Increased poikilocytes are characteristic of myelofibrosis and also may occur with many types of anemias, including iron deficiency and megaloblastic anemias.

Elliptocytes, also known as ovalocytes, are mature erythrocytes that assume an elliptic or oval shape and compose up to 1% of the red blood cells in normal blood. The presence of numerous elliptocytes is characteristic of hereditary elliptocytosis, a dominantly inherited condition that seldom produces any symptoms. A form of symptomatic elliptocytosis accompanies blood dyscrasias affecting the red blood cell membrane such as thalassemia, iron deficiency anemia, sickle cell anemia, and pernicious anemia.

Spherocytes are small, globelike red blood cells that are thicker than normal cells and lack the usual central pallor on a stained blood smear. Significant spherocytosis is characteristic of congenital hemolytic anemia, a familial condition, also known as hereditary spherocytosis, that results from a dominant autosomal trait. Spherocytic cells usually are found in individuals with acquired hemolytic anemia and infants with ABO hemolytic disease of the newborn, as well as following blood transfusions or thermal injury in which the normal red blood cell membrane is damaged.

Target cells, also known as leptocytes and Mexican hat cells, are thin erythrocytes with a dark central area surrounded by a lighter ring that resemble a bull's-eye on a stained smear. The presence of a significant number of target cells may be due to inherited hemoglobin abnormalities such as thalassemia, hemoglobin C disease, and sickle cell anemia. Target cells also may occur during iron deficiency anemia, following splenectomy, or in individuals with liver disorders such as hepatitis, obstructive jaundice, and cirrhosis.

Acanthocytes are abnormally crenated erythrocytes that have a thorny appearance on a stained blood smear because of a defect in their cell membrane. Acanthocytes result from a metabolic defect, either congenital or acquired, associated with dysfunction of lipid absorption from the small intestine. Acanthocytosis is characteristic of β-lipoproteinemia but also may occur in individuals with retinitis pigmentosa, alcoholic cirrhosis, hemolytic anemia due to pyruvate kinase deficiency, and following splenectomy or heparin administration.

Burr cells are erythrocytes with abnormal blunt cytoplasmic projections that closely resemble acanthocytes on a stained blood smear. Although the exact mechanism responsible for producing this peculiar formation is not known, the cells have little diagnostic significance. Burr cells may be recorded in individuals with bleeding gastric ulcers, carcinoma of the stomach, renal failure and uremia, extensive burns, pyruvate kinase deficiency, thrombotic thrombocytopenic purpura, disseminated intravascular coagulation (DIC), and microangiopathic hemolytic anemia.

Schistocytes are fragments of damaged red blood cells that appear as distorted and irregularly shaped particles on a stained blood smear. The presence of a significant number of schistocytes indicates a hemoglobinopathy and hemolysis or mechanical fragmentation involving the clothesline effect of a fibrin strand on a passing red blood cell. Schistocytes may occur in individuals with DIC, microangiopathic hemolytic anemia, untreated valvular stenosis, prosthetic heart valves, severe burns, uremia, pyruvate kinase deficiency, and the acute phase of hemolytic anemia.

Color. **Anisochromia** refers to an inequality or variation in the staining intensity of erythrocytes and reflects the distribution of hemoglobin among the cells. Anisochromia may occur following a blood transfusion during iron deficiency anemia, indicating several distinct red blood cell populations that do not contain a uniform amount of hemoglobin.

Hypochromic cells are erythrocytes that have less than the normal amount of color on a stained blood smear, indicating a lower than normal concentration of hemoglobin in each cell. Hemoglobin deficiency produces cells with a large area of central pallor; in some severe conditions, cells appear as nothing more than a pale rim of hemoglobin. Hypochromia may occur during conditions associated with abnormal or decreased hemoglobin production, including leukemia, iron deficiency anemia, thalassemia, chronic posthemorrhagic anemia, and numerous other anemias.

Hyperchromic cells are erythrocytes that stain more deeply than normal on a stained blood smear and have a smaller than normal or nonexistent area of central pallor. Hyperchromia usually is not related to an oversaturation of hemoglobin in the red blood cells because a natural physiologic upper limit regulates the amount of hemoglobin a cell can contain. Hyperchromic cells may occur during very severe prolonged dehydration or during conditions associated with spherocytes in which the average cell thickness is increased.

Polychromatophilia refers to normal erythrocytes that exhibit a bluish tinge on a stained blood smear because a small amount of basophilic nuclear substance remains in the cytoplasm. Polychromatophilic cells are slightly larger than normal, which helps to identify them as recently released reticulocytes that can be seen without the supervital stain that is required for their identification. Significant polychromatophilia reflects increased erythropoietic activity and may occur following acute blood loss from hemorrhage or hemolysis and during therapy for pernicious or iron deficiency anemia.

Structure and Content. **Nucleated red blood cells**, also known as normoblasts, are immature, developing erythrocytes normally present in the peripheral blood of the fetus and very young infant. Red blood cells containing a nucleus usually are confined to the bone marrow of healthy adults, whereas only more mature, non-nucleated erythrocytes are released into the bloodstream. Normoblasts enter the bloodstream prematurely in response to an increased physiologic demand for erythrocytes that the bone marrow is unable to fulfill with mature cells. The number of nucleated cells in the bloodstream reflects the extent of bone marrow reaction to the red blood cell deficiency rather than the degree or severity of the condition.

Nucleated red blood cells are identified and enumerated on a stained blood smear during the differential white blood cell count, with the number encountered reported as NRBC/100 WBC. A significant number of nucleated red blood cells may reflect a disturbance of erythrocyte maturation, particularly untreated megaloblastic anemia, but usually appears during hemolytic conditions, including thalassemia, sickle cell crises, erythroblastosis fetalis, or transfusion reactions. Nucleated erythrocytes also accompany severe anoxia resulting from congestive heart failure or pulmonary disease, as well as space-occupying bone marrow lesions such as leukemia, metastatic carcinoma, multiple myeloma, and myelofibrosis.

Basophilic stippling is an aggregation of coarse dark granules seen in some red blood cells on a stained blood smear, which indicates the presence of underdeveloped erythrocytes. Basophilic stippling is normal in approximately 1 red blood cell per 10,000 erythrocytes but occurs in much higher concentrations with heavy metal intoxication, particularly involving lead, silver, bismuth, and mercury. The appearance of basophilic stippling aids in diagnosis when the symptoms or occupation of the patient suggest the possibility of lead poisoning. Counts of 30 or more stippled cells per 10,000 erythrocytes provide strong evidence of lead poisoning. Basophilic stippling also may be recorded in patients with leukemia, gastrointestinal hemorrhage, and most types of severe anemia, including sickle cell anemia and thalassemia.

Cabot rings are light bluish-purple, fine ringlike or figure 8-shaped structures that may be found in red blood cells on a stained blood smear. Cabot rings are believed to be nuclear remnants, although their presence may be merely artifactual because these peculiar inclusion bodies have been produced artificially. Cabot rings frequently accompany severe anemias, particularly pernicious anemia, but they also occur in individuals with lead poisoning and myelofibrosis with myeloid metaplasia.

Howell-Jolly bodies are small, round, deeply staining remnants of nuclear material that may be seen in mature erythrocytes on a stained blood smear. These cellular inclusions measure less than 1 μm in diameter and normally are removed from the red blood cell as it passes through the sinusoids of the spleen. Thus, Howell-Jolly bodies frequently accompany splenectomy and may be found in individuals with splenic atrophy or congenital absence of the spleen. Howell-Jolly bodies also have been identified in some individuals with leukemia, various hemolytic anemias, and anemias resulting from abnormal erythropoiesis, including megaloblastic anemia.

Siderotic granules are particles of nonhemoglobin iron that appear on a stained blood smear as purple-blue specks aggregated around the periphery of mature erythrocytes known as siderocytes. These free-iron granules commonly occur in the developing normoblasts and reticulocytes of premature or normal newborn infants during hemoglobin formation but occasionally are seen in adults. A high siderocyte count, up to 100%, may reflect impaired hemoglobin synthesis, resulting in such chronic hemolytic anemias as thalassemia and congenital spherocytic anemia. A significant number of siderotic granules also may occur following splenectomy or in individuals with severe burns, pernicious anemia, lead poisoning, infections, and hemochromatosis.

Heinz bodies are small, round, oval, or irregular particles of denatured hemoglobin within mature erythrocytes that are clinically significant indicators of potential red blood cell instability. Heinz bodies are invisible on the Wright-stained preparations generally used for red blood cell examination but appear as blue-black granules of 1−2 μm on smears stained with cresyl blue. The number of Heinz bodies per cell varies from 1 to 20 and may occasionally indicate an unsuspected hemolytic anemia resulting from defective erythrocytes or certain hemoglobinopathies such as glucose-6-phosphate dehydrogenase (G-6-PD) deficiency or thalassemia. Heinz bodies also may be associated with drug-induced erythrocyte injury produced by toxic agents, including resorcinol, pyridine, chlorates, acetanilid, sulfapyridine, phenothiazine, phenacetin, and aniline.

ERYTHROCYTE INDICES

The **erythrocyte indices**, also known as the corpuscular constants, are measurements that indicate the size, weight, and hemoglobin content of an average red blood cell. Red blood cell corpuscular values are the most effective means of describing the red blood cell changes that occur in anemias and various other diseases. Laboratory determinations of erythrocyte indices are used to identify changes in red blood cell size and shape, classify characteristic morphologic patterns, and diagnose certain types of anemias.

The three distinct erythrocyte values that describe red blood cell morphology are the mean corpuscular volume (MCV), mean corpuscular hemoglobin (MCH), and mean corpuscular hemoglobin concentration (MCHC). The MCV expresses the average volume and size of individual erythrocytes in cubic microns, microcubic millimeters, or femtoliters (fL). The MCH expresses the average amount and weight of hemoglobin contained in a single erythrocyte in micrograms or picograms (pg). The MCHC expresses the average hemoglobin concentration or proportion of each red blood cell occupied by hemoglobin as a percentage.

Clinical Significance

A **mean corpuscular volume** (MCV) within the normal range classifies red blood cells as normocytic, whereas increased values indicate large, or macrocytic, cells and decreased results reflect small, or microcytic, cells. Mean corpuscular volume results must be evaluated by carefully inspecting erythrocytes on a stained blood smear because values reflect only the average volume of many cells. Red blood cells may exhibit anisocytosis, varying widely in size from microcytic to macrocytic, and still produce a MCV within the normal range. Microcytes and a decreased MCV commonly are associated with iron deficiency anemia and thalassemia. Macrocytes and an increased MCV generally are reported during megaloblastic anemias resulting from a vitamin B_{12} or folic acid deficiency, chronic emphysema, Down's syndrome, or the reticulocytosis found in newborn infants and during active erythrocyte regeneration.

Mean corpuscular hemoglobin (MCH) usually fluctuates directly with the MCV because larger cells can accommodate more hemoglobin than smaller cells. Thus, MCH values are higher than normal in newborn infants and patients with macrocytic anemia, whereas lower than normal values accompany microcytosis, particularly when it results from iron deficiency anemia. Although the MCH expresses the average weight of individual erythrocytes, it provides less clinical information than the MCHC combined with an evaluation of erythrocyte appearance on a stained blood smear.

A **mean corpuscular hemoglobin concentration** (MCHC) below the normal range indicates the presence of red blood cells deficient in hemoglobin, which are classified as hypochromic. Decreased MCHC values generally accompany iron deficiency anemia, thalassemia, sideroblastic anemia, and overhydration or water intoxication. Increased MCHC values, indicating an elevated hemoglobin concentration or hyperchromic cells, are not possible because normal erythrocytes already contain the maximum amount of hemoglobin. However, MCHC values may genuinely rise above the normal range in individuals with hereditary spherocytosis, extensive burns, or severe prolonged dehydration. Red blood cells that contain the proper amount of hemoglobin for their size have a normal MCHC and are classified as normochromic. Both microcytic and macrocytic cells may have normal MCHC values if their hemoglobin content increases or decreases in proportion to the volume of the cell.

Interpretation (See Normal Values on facing page)

The erythrocyte indices, evaluated in conjunction with red blood cell appearance on a stained blood smear, provide an accurate picture of erythrocyte morphology. Morphologic classification of red blood cell characteristics furnishes valuable clinical information concerning the etiology of various anemias and helps to classify them into several broad categories. Anemias may be identified roughly as normocytic, microcytic, or macrocytic depending on the MCV and as normochromic or hypochromic depending on the MCH and MCHC.

Normal Values

The normal values for the erythrocyte indices are:

	Mean Corpuscular Volume	Mean Corpuscular Hemoglobin	Mean Corpuscular Hemoglobin Concentration
Newborns	106 fL (average)	38 pg (average)	38% (average)
3 months	82 fL	28 pg	34%
1 year	77 fL	25 pg	34%
3 years	79 fL	26 pg	33%
10 years	80 fL	27 pg	33%
Adults	82–98 fL	26–34 pg	31%–38%

The classification of various anemias is based on their morphologic characteristics, as follows:

Anemia	Mean Corpuscular Volume	Mean Corpuscular Hemoglobin Concentration
Normocytic, normochromic	82–98 fL	31%–38%
Microcytic, hypochromic	60–76 fL	20%–30%
Microcytic, normochromic	60–76 fL	30%–38%
Macrocytic, normochromic	100–160 fL	30%–38%

Variations

Normocytic, normochromic anemia is associated with:

Acute blood loss following hemorrhage or hemolysis

Aplastic and hypoplastic anemias caused by:

    Chemical agents, drugs

    Myasthenia gravis

    Myelophthisic anemia

    Irradiation

    Thymic tumors

Chronic disease

Endocrine disorders

    Addison's disease

    Myxedema

    Panhypopituitarism

Hemolytic anemias, including:

    Acquired hemolytic anemias

    Anemias induced by conditions such as infections, burns, insertion of an intracardiac prosthesis causing a mechanical hemolysis, and hypersplenism

    Drug- or toxin-induced anemia

    Hemoglobinopathies

    Hereditary spherocytosis

    Paroxysmal nocturnal hemoglobinuria

    Renal failure

    Sideroblastic anemia

Microcytic, hypochromic anemia is associated with:

Iron deficiency caused by:

Excessive iron loss resulting from hemorrhage or parasitic infestation

Inadequate iron absorption resulting from chronic diarrhea or gastro-intestinal resection

Increased iron demand due to pregnancy, growth spurts, or blood regeneration

Sideroachrestic (sideroblastic) anemias caused by:

Alcoholism

Drugs

Hemoglobinopathies such as thalassemia, sickle cell anemia, or hemoglobin C disease

Infection

Lead poisoning

Rheumatoid arthritis

Transferrin deficiency

Microcytic, normochromic anemia is associated with:

Chemicals, drugs	Lead poisoning	Irradiation
Infection	Liver disease	Rheumatoid arthritis
Kidney disease	Malignancy	

Macrocytic, normochromic anemia is associated with:

Acute blood loss

Administration of anti-convulsants or antimetabolites

Aplastic anemia

Chronic liver disease

Folic acid deficiency resulting from:

Pregnancy

Some acute leukemias

Sprue or celiac disease

Hemolytic anemia

Myxedema, hypothyroidism

Pernicious anemia

Reticulocytosis

Vitamin B_{12} deficiency resulting from:

Gastric resection or gastric carcinoma

Kwashiorkor

Pregnancy

Sprue or celiac disease

Methodology

The erythrocyte indices are rarely ordered as a separate study but are routinely computed and reported with complete blood counts performed on electronic counters. Erythrocyte values always must be supplemented by a peripheral blood smear because they represent only a homogeneous cell population and may not convey the true red blood cell picture. For example, patients with sideroblastic anemia exhibit a mixed cell population containing enough normocytic, normochromic cells with the characteristic microcytic, hypochromic erythrocytes to produce an unrepresentative picture.

Erythrocyte indices also may be calculated from accurate red blood cell, hemoglobin, and hematocrit test results. The various indices are calculated according to the following formulas:

Mean corpuscular volume (MCV) represents the relationship between the packed cell volume, or hematocrit, and the red blood cell count.

$$MCV = \frac{Hematocrit \times 10}{RBC \ count}$$

Mean corpuscular hemoglobin (MCH) reflects the relationship between hemoglobin values and the red blood cell count.

$$MCH = \frac{Hemoglobin \times 10}{RBC\ count}$$

Mean corpuscular hemoglobin concentration (MCHC) represents the relationship between the amount of hemoglobin present in each cell and the volume of the cell containing it.

$$MCHC = \frac{Hemoglobin \times 100}{Hematocrit}$$

▶▶ *Nursing Responsibilities and Implications*

1. Inform the patient that there are no food or fluid restrictions.

2. Observe the patient for signs of dehydration or overhydration because these conditions will influence the test results.

3. Note if the patient is receiving anticonvulsants or antimetabolites because these drugs elevate the MCV; determine whether the patient is taking any other medications or has any illnesses that might alter the test results.

4. Note if the patient is receiving radiation therapy because it will decrease the MCV.

5. If erythrocyte indices are decreased, encourage the patient to eat foods high in iron such as red meats, liver, and green leafy vegetables, which will promote red blood cell production.

6. If the erythrocyte indices are decreased, encourage rest to counter the accompanying fatigue.

ERYTHROCYTE SEDIMENTATION RATE

The **erythrocyte sedimentation rate** (ESR), more commonly referred to as the sedimentation rate, is a measure of the speed with which red blood cells in anticoagulated whole blood settle to the bottom of a calibrated tube. The test measures the distance the upper part of a red blood cell column descends in a specified amount of time and usually is reported in millimeters per hour. Sedimentation normally takes place slowly, but the rate is increased in numerous conditions involving an inflammatory process or tissue necrosis, frequently in proportion to the severity of the disease.

The ESR is a nonspecific indicator of the physiologic responses associated with connective tissue diseases, dysproteinemia, malignancy, and infectious diseases, although it is not directed at any particular organ or disorder. When used as a general screening test, a normal ESR significantly reduces the probability of unsuspected disease processes, whereas elevated results indicate the need for further testing. A gradually increasing ESR is indicative of continuing or increasing problems, whereas a gradually diminishing ESR reflects clinical improvement and is a favorable sign of an abating inflammatory condition. Laboratory determinations of the ESR may be used to detect occult organic disease and follow the course of inflammatory conditions such as rheumatic fever, tuberculosis, rheumatoid arthritis, and myocardial infarction.

Clinical Significance

The ESR is of greatest value when used to indicate an active, although obscure, disease process and to differentiate between certain conditions with similar clinical findings and symptoms. For example, the ESR rises in myocardial infarction but remains normal in angina pectoris; increases during rheumatic fever, rheumatoid arthritis, and pyogenic arthritis but not osteoarthritis; and is elevated with hepatic carcinoma but is generally normal with cirrhosis. The ESR also helps to differentiate advanced cancer of the stomach from peptic ulcer because sedimentation is usually rapid when metastases and tumor inflammation are present.

The speed of red blood cell settling is affected by many factors, including the concentration of various plasma protein fractions, mainly fibrinogen and globulin, as well as the size, shape, and number of erythrocytes. The ESR is accelerated by the increased quantities of fibrinogen associated with tissue necrosis, infection, pregnancy, and the abnormal globulins or globulin fractions seen in multiple myeloma and other gammopathies. Active antibody formation, along with the loss of albumin caused by kidney disease, enteritis, or faulty synthesis, also alters the ESR by increasing the ratio of globulins to albumin.

Significant variations from the normal range for the erythrocyte count have a predictable effect on sedimentation velocity, with low counts (anemia) accelerating the ESR and high counts (polycythemia) retarding it. A newer test, the zeta sedimentation rate, is unaffected by anemia, provides test results in 3–5 minutes, and has the same normal range in men and women.

Normal Values

The normal values for the erythrocyte sedimentation rate vary according to the particular method used, as follows:

Method	Men (mm/hr)	Women (mm/hr)	Children (mm/hr)
Wintrobe			
<70 years	0–9	0–20	0–15
>70 years	0–50	0–50	—
Westergren			
<17 years	—	—	0–20
17–50 years	1–7	3–9	—
51–60 years	3–9	4–14	—
>60 years	2–10	5–15	—
Landau			
<2 years	—	—	1–6
2–14 years	—	—	1–9
>14 years	0–6	0–9	—

Zeta sedimentation rate: 40–51 mL/dL

Variations
An **elevated erythrocyte sedimentation rate** may occur with:

Marked elevation (>100 mm/hr)
  Acute severe bacterial infection
  Carcinoma
  Collagen diseases
  Leukemia
  Malignant lymphoma
  Multiple myeloma
  Portal or biliary cirrhosis
  Sarcoma
  Severe anemia
  Severe renal disease
  Ulcerative colitis
  Viral pneumonia
  Waldenström's macroglobulinemia
Moderate elevation (>40 mm/hr)
  Acute and chronic infectious diseases
  Acute glomerulonephritis
  Acute localized infections
  Acute viral hepatitis
  Advanced age
  Agranulocytosis
  Anaphylactoid purpura
  Coronary thrombosis
  Cryoglobulinemia

Drug therapy
  Methyldopa
  Methysergide
  Penicillamine
  Theophylline
  Trifluperidol
  Vitamin A
Ectopic pregnancy
Hyperthyroidism, hypothyroidism
Internal hemorrhage
Intravenous dextran administration
Lead and arsenic intoxication
Malignant tumors with necrosis
Menstruation
Myocardial infarction
Nephritis, nephrosis
Normal pregnancy after first trimester
Oral contraceptives
Postcommissurotomy syndrome
Rheumatic fever
Rheumatoid arthritis
Syphilis
Systemic lupus erythematosus
Tuberculosis

A **normal erythrocyte sedimentation rate** may occur with benign neoplasms, infectious mononucleosis, localized infection, or uncomplicated viral infections.

A **decreased (zero) erythrocyte sedimentation rate** may occur with:

Cryoglobulinemia	Salicylates	Hyperviscosity syndrome
Drug therapy	Steroids	Polycythemia vera
Quinine	Hemoglobin C disease	Sickle cell anemia

Methodology
The ESR requires 3 mL of blood collected in EDTA anticoagulant (lavender-stoppered tube) and delivered promptly to the laboratory. Erythrocytes tend to become spherical after prolonged standing, making them less inclined to stack or settle normally and thus retarding the ESR. Therefore, when the specimen is kept at room temperature, the ESR must be performed within 3 hours. Testing may be delayed for up to 12 hours when the specimen is refrigerated.

▶▶ *Nursing Responsibilities and Implications*

1. Inform the patient that there are no food or fluid restrictions.

2. Note if the patient has been taking oral contraceptives for a prolonged period because they may increase the ESR.

3. Determine if the patient is taking any other medications or has any illnesses that might alter the test results.

4. Handle the specimen gently to prevent hemolysis and take the specimen to the laboratory immediately.

5. Observe the patient for signs of infection or inflammation if the ESR is elevated.

RETICULOCYTE COUNT

Reticulocytes are immature, non-nucleated erythrocytes that retain a portion of their basophilic nuclear material in the form of a filamented reticulum during their maturation period. The meshlike network of RNA may be abundant or sparse, depending on the stage of erythrocyte development, but is visible only when stained with a supravital dye. The reticulocyte count provides a valuable index of bone marrow function, with an elevated count reflecting accelerated erythropoietic activity and decreased levels resulting from erythrocyte hypoplasia. Laboratory determinations of the reticulocyte count aid in the diagnosis of several types of anemia and in evaluating the patient's response to therapy.

Clinical Significance
The reticulocyte count is affected by several factors, including the rate of erythrocyte production and release from the bone marrow, along with the rate of red blood cell destruction or blood loss. An increased number of circulating reticulocytes indicates bone marrow hyperactivity, which occurs following hemorrhage or hemolysis as well as during treatment of and recovery from anemia. Discovery of an increased reticulocyte count may lead to the recognition of occult or unsuspected conditions such as chronic hemorrhage or undiagnosed hemolysis. The degree of reticulocytosis is roughly proportional to the initial severity of the anemia or condition, to bone marrow reactivity, and to the utilization of available hematopoietic substances. Conversely, a persistently low reticulocyte count, particularly in the presence of anemia, suggests markedly defective erythropoiesis resulting from bone marrow hypofunction or depression.

Normal Values
The normal values for the reticulocyte count are:

Neonates	2.5%–6.0% (falls to adult range within 2 weeks)
Adults	0.5%–2.0%
	25,000–75,000 reticulocytes/μL (slightly higher in women)

Interpretation

Reticulocyte values are most significant when an absolute count expressing the number of reticulocytes present in 1 mm^3 or 1 μL of blood is reported with the red blood cell percentage. The absolute number of reticulocytes may be calculated according to the following formula:

$$RBCs/\mu L \times Reticulocyte/100 \; (\%) = Reticulocyte \; count/\mu L$$

For example, a reticulocyte report of 2% with a total erythrocyte count of 6 million/μL reflects an absolute reticulocyte count of 120,000/μL, which is above the normal range despite the normal percentage (6,000,000/μL $\times$ 2/100 = 120,000 reticulocytes/μL).

Variations

An **elevated reticulocyte count (reticulocytosis)** may occur with:

Acquired autoimmune hemolytic anemia	Hereditary spherocytosis
	Paroxysmal nocturnal hemoglobinuria
Acute posthemorrhagic anemia	Sickle cell anemia
Chronic erythremic myelosis	Thalassemia major
Chronic hemorrhage	Treatment of iron deficiency anemia
Di Guglielmo disease	Treatment of vitamin B$_{12}$ and folic acid
Erythroblastosis fetalis	deficiencies

A **decreased reticulocyte count (reticulocytopenia)** may occur with:

Aplastic anemia

Aplastic crisis of hemolytic anemia

Untreated iron deficiency anemia

Untreated megaloblastic anemia

Methodology

Reticulocyte counts require 3 mL of freshly drawn venous blood collected in EDTA anticoagulant (lavender-stoppered tube). Reticulocyte counts also may be performed on a fresh drop of capillary blood drawn into a white blood cell pipette and mixed with an equal volume of new methylene blue solution.

The percentage of reticulocytes present is determined by recording the number of reticulocytes encountered while examining 1000 erythrocytes microscopically on a thin blood film and dividing the number counted by 10.

Precautions

To ensure accurate test results, the following precautions should be observed when collecting specimens for the reticulocyte count:

1. Do not draw the blood specimen from the same arm or hand being used for the administration of intravenous solutions because the extra fluid may cause hemodilution.

2. Do not leave the tourniquet on for longer than 1 minute during the specimen collection because alterations in the reticulocyte count may result from prolonged hemostasis due to vasoconstriction.

▶▶ *Nursing Responsibilities and Implications*

1. Inform the patient that there are no food or fluid restrictions.
2. Note any drugs that the patient has been or is taking such as cytotoxic or sulfa drugs or any illness that might alter the reticulocyte count.

ERYTHROCYTE OSMOTIC FRAGILITY TEST

The **erythrocyte osmotic fragility test** indicates any significant change from the normal biconcave disk shape of the red blood cells by measuring their ability to resist hemolysis in a hypotonic solution. This test is based on the fact that erythrocytes are surrounded by a semipermeable membrane that permits the exchange of water and electrolytes and allows cells to change their volume in response to ionic variations of the extracellular fluid. Therefore, erythrocytes suspended in a solution with the same ionic concentration as serum retain their original volume and shape because of a balanced electrolyte exchange between the cells and their surrounding environment. Erythrocytes placed in hypotonic saline strive to establish osmotic equilibrium with their external environment by drawing in water; the cells then swell, become spherical, and eventually burst.

The osmotic fragility test is performed by suspending erythrocytes in decreasing concentrations of saline (increasing hypotonicity) to determine at which concentration hemolysis begins and at what point all cells are hemolyzed. Cells that hemolyze in relatively high concentrations of saline (barely hypotonic) have an increased osmotic fragility, whereas those requiring lower saline concentrations (greatly hypotonic) for hemolysis exhibit decreased osmotic fragility. Incubation of blood for 24 hours before testing accentuates increased osmotic fragility and may reveal abnormal fragility not detectable using the standard method. Laboratory determinations of osmotic fragility are a sensitive index to the presence and extent of spherical erythrocytes and are most useful in diagnosing hereditary spherocytosis.

Clinical Significance

Erythrocytes have the ability to withstand a certain amount of fluid intake without bursting, the amount depending on the initial ratio of the cell volume to its surface area. Thus, spherical cells rupture more easily than thin, flat cells, which can accept a greater amount of fluid and swell to a greater degree before hemolyzing. Although the test is governed by the osmosis of fluids, actual cell rupture is caused by a diminished resistance to osmotic pressure resulting from an abnormal erythrocyte membrane. Red blood cell resistance to hemolysis also is influenced by the age of the erythrocyte, with older cells lysing first in barely hypotonic saline concentrations, whereas younger cells are more resistant.

Normal Values
The normal values for erythrocyte osmotic fragility are:

Screening test	Initial hemolysis 0.40%−0.46% saline	Complete hemolysis 0.30%−0.35% saline

Quantitative test	Saline solution (%)	Hemolysis (%)
	0.30	97−100
	0.35	90−99
	0.40	50−95
	0.45	5−45
	0.50	0−5
	0.55	0

Incubated test	Saline solution (%)	Hemolysis (%)
	0.20	95−100
	0.30	85−100
	0.35	75−100
	0.40	65−100
	0.45	55−95
	0.50	40−85
	0.55	5−70
	0.60	0−40
	0.65	0−19
	0.70	0−9
	0.75	0
	0.85	0

Variations
Increased osmotic fragility (spherical cells) may occur with:

Acquired hemolytic anemia

Burns

Chemical poisoning or drugs

Hemolytic disease due to ABO incompatibility

Hemolytic disease due to Rh incompatibility

Hereditary spherocytic anemia or congenital hemolytic anemia

Pernicious anemia

Symptomatic hemolytic anemia associated with:

Cirrhosis

Hodgkin's disease

Leukemia

Myelosclerosis

Pneumonia

Syphilis

Tuberculosis

Decreased osmotic fragility (flat cells) may occur with:

Hemoglobin C disease

Iron deficiency anemia

Liver disease

Obstructive jaundice

Polycythemia vera (erythremia)

Sickle cell anemia

Splenectomy

Thalassemia major

Methodology

The osmotic fragility test is most accurate when performed within 3 hours after the collection of 5 mL of venous blood drawn into a tube containing EDTA or heparin anticoagulant (lavender- or green-stoppered tube). Erythrocyte osmotic fragility is greatly affected by the pH, temperature, and glucose concentration of the blood, as well as by the age of the erythrocyte and time interval between blood collection and testing.

Precautions

To ensure accurate results, the following precautions should be observed when collecting specimens for erythrocyte osmotic fragility tests:

1. Do not leave the tourniquet on for longer than 1 minute during specimen collection because erythrocytes are fragile and easily damaged.

2. Mix and handle the specimen gently to prevent hemolysis.

▶▶ ### Nursing Responsibilities and Implications

1. Inform the patient that there are no food or fluid restrictions.

2. Send the specimen to the laboratory immediately because osmotic fragility increases as the specimen ages.

3. Assess the patient for signs and symptoms of anemia if the results are outside the normal range.

4. Determine if the patient is taking any medications or has any illnesses that might alter the test results.

PLATELET COUNT

The **platelet count** is an actual enumeration of the thrombocytes (tiny fragments of cytoplasm originating in the bone marrow) that are present in 1 mm^3 or 1 μL of whole blood. Because platelets accelerate the coagulation mechanism and promote overall hemostasis, any change in the platelet count alters the clotting process and reflects bone marrow response to various diseases and physiologic or chemical stimuli. Laboratory determinations of the platelet count are vital to the diagnosis and treatment of hemorrhagic diseases and frequently are used to monitor patients receiving chemotherapy or radiation therapy.

Clinical Significance

An adequate number of normal platelets is necessary to maintain hemostasis through functions that include:

- Agglutination to form a mechanical plug for sealing blood vessels
- Release of serotonin to cause local vasoconstriction and reduce bleeding after an injury
- Release of accessory factors to accelerate the coagulation process
- Release of factors to promote retraction of the newly formed clot

Platelet counts usually below 75–100,000/μL reflect a tendency toward spontaneous bleeding and can affect other coagulation studies at even higher levels. Abnormal platelet counts may result from normal conditions or activities as well as a number of blood dyscrasias and diseases. (Platelets and platelet counts are also discussed in Chapter 10.)

Normal Values
The normal values for the platelet count are:

Newborns	100,000–300,000/μL
3 months	260,000/μL (average)
1 year	250,000/μL
3 years	250,000/μL
10 years	250,000/μL
Adults	150,000–400,000/μL

Interpretation
Total platelet counts usually are supplemented in the laboratory by a careful examination of the stained blood smear to confirm the number of cells counted and evaluate their morphologic characteristics. The presence of 3–8 platelets per 100 red blood cells on the stained smear or 8–20 platelets per oil-immersion field indicates a count within the normal range. In general, the total platelet count is roughly equal to the number of platelets counted in ten oil-immersion fields multiplied by 2000. For example, observation of 15 platelets in each of ten oil-immersion fields reflects a total platelet count of 300,000/μL ($15 \times 10 \times 2000 = 300,000$ platelets/μL).

Variations
An **elevated platelet count** (**thrombocytosis**) may occur with:

Acute blood loss	Myeloproliferative disorders
Asphyxia	Polycythemia vera
Chronic granulocytic leukemia	Reticulocytosis
Epinephrine injections	Strenuous exercise, excitement
High altitudes	Splenectomy
Idiopathic thrombocythemia	Trauma (fractures, surgery)
Iron deficiency anemia	Tuberculosis
Metastatic carcinoma	

A **decreased platelet count** (**thrombocytopenia**) may occur with:

Acute granulocytic leukemia	Bone marrow depressant drugs:
Acute lymphocytic leukemia	Amidopyrine
Acute rheumatic fever	Nitrogen mustard
Aplastic anemia	Quinidine

Quinine	Incompatible blood transfusion
Salicylates	Monocytic leukemia
Streptomycin	Multiple myeloma
Sulfonamides	Pernicious anemia
Chronic lymphocytic leukemia	Premenstruation
Diphtheria	Septicemia
Gaucher's disease	Severe burns
Hemolytic disease of newborns	Typhoid fever
Hypersplenism	X-ray irradiation
Idiopathic thrombocytopenic purpura	

Methodology

Platelet count procedures produce accurate results when performed within 1 hour on a 5 mL blood specimen collected in EDTA anticoagulant (lavender-stoppered tube) and maintained at room temperature.

Precautions

To ensure accurate results, the following precautions should be observed when collecting specimens for platelet counts:

1. Do not leave the tourniquet on for longer than 1 minute during specimen collection because platelets are fragile and easily damaged.

2. Avoid trauma when performing venipuncture to avoid injury to platelets and prevent hematoma formation.

3. Mix and handle the specimen gently to prevent hemolysis.

▶▶ Nursing Responsibilities and Implications

1. Inform the patient that there are no food or fluid restrictions.

2. Note if the patient is receiving chemotherapy or radiation therapy because these treatments might decrease the platelet count; determine if the patient is taking any other medications or has any illnesses that might alter the test results.

3. Carefully observe the venipuncture site for prolonged bleeding; apply pressure as necessary.

4. Observe the patient for signs of bleeding (petechiae, purpura, hematuria, melena, and hematemesis) if the platelet count is decreased.

5. Teach the patient with a decreased platelet count how to avoid injury; handle the patient gently.

EOSINOPHIL COUNT AND THORN TEST

The total or absolute **eosinophil count** is an enumeration of the actual number of eosinophils present in 1 mm^3 or 1 μL of blood. The eosinophil count uses a special stain to permit the direct counting of this particular type of leukocyte, and this method is preferred to estimations calculated from total white blood cell and relative eosinophil values. Direct eosinophil counts generally are performed when circulating levels are persistently low or when eosinophils are entirely absent from differential reports. Laboratory determination of the eosinophil count mainly is used to assess the degree of eosinopenia, evaluate eosinophil response to ACTH or epinephrine administration, and monitor treatment of eosinophilic conditions.

Clinical Significance

Total eosinophil response to ACTH or epinephrine injections forms the basis of a screening procedure for adrenal cortex function known as the Thorn test. Administration of ACTH or epinephrine stimulates adrenocortical activity and increases hormone production. This action in turn produces an absolute decrease in the number of circulating eosinophils. Individuals with normal adrenal cortex function respond to ACTH stimulation with a 50% or greater decrease in the total eosinophil count from baseline values 4 hours following the ACTH injection.

Patients with primary adrenal insufficiency (Addison's disease) fail to react normally to ACTH stimulation and exhibit an absolute eosinophil decrease of 20% or less from preinjection values. However, individuals with adrenal insufficiency secondary to pituitary disease respond to ACTH injection with a normal eosinophil decrease. In these individuals epinephrine administration does not change the eosinophil count significantly.

Normal Values

The normal values for the absolute eosinophil count are:

Random	50–450/μL
Following ACTH administration (Thorn test)	≥50% decrease in baseline values after 4 hours

---

Variations

Elevated eosinophil counts (eosinophilia) may occur with:

Allergies	Parasitic infestations
Brucellosis	Scarlet fever
Chronic granulocytic leukemia	Skin diseases
Copper poisoning	Splenectomy
Digitalis administration	Tuberculosis
Hodgkin's disease	

Decreased eosinophil counts (eosinopenia) may occur with:

Administration of ACTH, epinephrine, adrenocortical hormones, or insulin

Eclampsia

Excessive exercise

Hyperadrenalism (Cushing's disease)

Stress situations (trauma, burns, major surgery, shock, severe infections)

Methodology

Direct eosinophil counts require 5 mL of venous blood collected in a tube with EDTA anticoagulant (lavender-stoppered tube). When performed as part of the Thorn test to evaluate adrenocortical stimulation, a total eosinophil count is measured immediately before and 4 hours after a test injection of ACTH.

▶▶ **Nursing Responsibilities and Implications**

1. Inform the patient that there are no food or fluid restrictions when a random eosinophil count is to be done.

2. Note if the patient has any infections or allergies.

3. Record the time the specimen for the eosinophil count is drawn because counts are lower in the morning, higher in the late afternoon, and peak after midnight.

4. Note if the patient is receiving ACTH, epinephrine, adrenocortical hormones, or insulin because these drugs can decrease the eosinophil count; determine if the patient is taking any other medications or has any illnesses that might alter the test results.

5. When a Thorn test is to be done:
   a. Inform the patient that both food and fluid are totally restricted for 12 hours prior to and 4 hours after the injection of ACTH.
   b. Obtain a venous blood specimen and send it to the laboratory for a baseline eosinophil count.
   c. Administer 25 mg of ACTH intramuscularly; note the time of administration.
   d. Obtain a venous blood specimen exactly 4 hours after the ACTH injection and send it to the laboratory for an eosinophil count.

LUPUS ERYTHEMATOSUS CELL TEST

The **lupus erythematosus (LE) cell test** is used to detect the presence of the **LE plasma factor**, an autoimmune antinuclear antibody that reacts with components of cell nuclei. The LE cell consists of a structureless globular mass of modified nuclear protein engulfed by a mature segmented leukocyte, generally a neutrophil. The LE cell phenomenon does not occur in the bloodstream but can be demonstrated in the laboratory by incubating blood or body fluids containing the LE factor with a supply of nuclear material. Laboratory identification of LE cells is most helpful in the diagnosis of systemic lupus erythematosus (SLE) and may appear in 50%–75% of the patients with the active form of this disease.

Clinical Significance

The LE cell test is a moderately sensitive and specific indicator of the presence of the LE factor, although both false-positive and false-negative test results may occur. Unfortunately, negative test reports do not eliminate a diagnosis of SLE because these cells are not formed during spontaneous remission of the disease or with the administration of corticosteroid and immunosuppressive drugs. Typical LE cells also have been observed with other diseases, although many of these conditions may either be part of the syndrome or precede the development of the typical syndrome. The number of LE cells present does not necessarily reflect the stage or clinical severity of the disease, but identification of two or three cells does help confirm the diagnosis of SLE.

LE test reports occasionally include the observation of **LE rosettes**, which are clusters of neutrophils surrounding but not engulfing a central mass of transformed nuclear material. This phenomenon also is found in specimens from patients with SLE, but positive test results may be recorded only when typical LE cells are identified. A sensitive and accurate antinuclear antibody (ANA) screening procedure also is available for the diagnosis of SLE, although it lacks specificity and may produce positive results with other autoimmune or collagen diseases. However, a negative ANA virtually eliminates a diagnosis of SLE. (The ANA test also is discussed in Chapter 11.)

Normal Values

The normal values for the LE cell test are:

Screening test   No LE cells seen

Antinuclear antibody test for the   Negative
LE factor

Variations

The **presence of typical LE cells** is diagnostic of SLE but also may occur with:

Chronic discoid lupus erythematosus   Reserpine

Dermatomyositis   Streptomycin

Drug reactions to: Sulfonamides

   Anticonvulsant drugs (phenytoin,   Tetracycline
   mephenytoin, trimethadione,
   primidone)   Glomerulonephritis

   Hydralazine hydrochloride   Hemolytic anemia

   Isoniazid   Lupoid hepatitis

   Methyldopa   Polyarteritis nodosa

   Oral contraceptives   Rheumatoid arthritis

   Penicillin   Serum sickness

   Procainamide hydrochloride   Sjögren's syndrome

                                    Systemic sclerosis

Methodology

The LE cell test requires 10 mL of blood collected without anticoagulants (red-stoppered tube) or 5 mL of blood mixed with heparin (green-stoppered tube). Specimen collection requirements vary with different laboratory techniques and must be followed to demonstrate the LE cell phenomenon and ensure accurate test results.

Precautions

To ensure accurate test results, the following precautions should be observed when collecting specimens for the LE cell test:

1. Avoid mixing the specimen with large amounts of heparin; use a red- or green-stoppered tube.

2. Mix and handle the specimen gently to prevent hemolysis.

▶▶ *Nursing Responsibilities and Implications*

1. Note if the patient is receiving adrenocorticoid therapy or has a low white blood cell count; determine if the patient is taking any other medications or has any illnesses that might alter the test results.

2. Inform the patient that there are no food or fluid restrictions.

3. Keep the venipuncture site covered for at least 24 hours; protect the patient from infection because individuals with SLE have depressed immune systems.

LEUKOCYTE ALKALINE PHOSPHATASE STAIN

The **leukocyte alkaline phosphatase stain** is a cytochemical procedure performed on blood smears to estimate alkaline phosphatase enzyme activity in neutrophilic granulocytes. This stain reflects the rate of intercellular metabolism within neutrophils but has little relationship to serum alkaline phosphatase levels. The specific granules present in leukocytes of the myeloid series generally exhibit a strong reaction but show minimal enzyme activity when leukemia and certain other diseases are present. Laboratory evaluation of leukocyte alkaline phosphatase stain is most useful in differentiating chronic granulocytic leukemia from neutrophilic leukemoid reactions and polycythemia vera from secondary erythrocytosis.

Clinical Significance
The leukocyte alkaline phosphatase stain is determined by incubating blood with a specific substrate to react with the granules of neutrophilic granulocytes according to their enzyme content and activity. Cells are evaluated on an arbitrary scale ranging from 0 to 4, depending on the degree of phosphatase staining, which may vary from colorless to dark, coarse granulation. A semiquantitative estimation of alkaline phosphatase activity is obtained by examining 100 neutrophils under the microscope and scoring them individually to achieve a total value for a given blood smear.

Normal Values
The normal values for the leukocyte alkaline phosphatase stain are:

Neonates (up to 2 weeks)	≥200
Adults	15–100 (average is 60)

Variations
Elevated leukocyte alkaline phosphatase activity (over 100) may be found in:

ACTH administration

Cushing's disease

Down's syndrome

Leukocytosis (15,000–50,000/μL) associated with a variety of infections

Lymphoproliferative disorders (acute lymphocytic leukemia, malignant lymphoma)

Multiple myeloma

Neutrophilic leukemoid reactions
(50,000–170,000/μL)

Diphtheria

Eclampsia

Hemolytic anemia

Hemorrhage

Hodgkin's disease

Lobar pneumonia

Malaria

Meningitis

Mercury poisoning

Myeloid metaplasia

Severe burns

Syphilis

Tuberculosis

Tumors

Oral contraceptives

Polycythemia vera

Postoperative period, immediate

Pregnancy

Stress situations

Tissue necrosis

Trauma

Normal leukocyte alkaline phosphatase activity may be found in:

Chronic lymphocytic leukemia

Acute and chronic myelomonocytic leukemia

Kwashiorkor

Lymphosarcoma

Secondary polycythemia, erythrocytosis

Viral infection

Decreased leukocyte alkaline phosphatase activity (under 20) may be found in:

Acute and chronic myelocytic leukemia

Acute monocytic leukemia

Aplastic anemia

Collagen diseases

Di Guglielmo disease

Hereditary hypophosphatasia

Infectious mononucleosis during the acute phase

Idiopathic thrombocytopenic purpura

Myelosclerosis

Paroxysmal nocturnal hemoglobinuria

Pernicious anemia, especially during relapse

Methodology

Leukocyte alkaline phosphatase stain may be performed on fresh blood smears prepared from either capillary or venous blood specimens. However, capillary blood is preferred to avoid the effects of the anticoagulant and should be used whenever possible. Blood smears must be prepared as soon as possible after collection from venous blood specimens drawn into tubes containing heparin. Specimens drawn into tubes with EDTA anticoagulant are not suitable for a leukocyte alkaline phosphatase stain because EDTA inhibits the activity of the enzyme.

▶▶ Nursing Responsibilities and Implications

1. Note if the patient is taking oral contraceptives or is pregnant.

2. Note if the patient is receiving adrenocorticoid therapy; determine if the patient is taking any other medications or has any illnesses that might alter the test results.

3. Inform the patient that there are no food or fluid restrictions.

GLUCOSE-6-PHOSPHATE DEHYDROGENASE DEFICIENCY TEST

Glucose-6-phosphate dehydrogenase (G-6-PD) is an enzyme present in erythrocytes that preserves the normal balance of oxidation and reduction reactions and protects red blood cells from injury. A deficiency of G-6-PD is an inherited, sex-linked red blood cell defect that makes the affected individual exceptionally susceptible to drug-induced non-spherocytic hemolytic anemia. Variants of G-6-PD enzyme appear in most races and populations, and G-6-PD deficiency is the most common of the numerous red blood cell enzyme defects associated with hemolytic anemia. Laboratory determination of G-6-PD deficiency is most useful in diagnosing hemolytic anemia caused by oxidant drugs and also may be helpful in genetic counseling.

Clinical Significance

Individuals with a moderate G-6-PD deficiency generally possess sufficient enzyme to maintain red blood cells under normal conditions and have no readily detectable abnormality except for a slightly shortened erythrocyte survival time. However, the administration of therapeutic doses of a variety of nontoxic drugs or their metabolites produces an oxidizing action within the erythrocytes that results in hemoglobin degradation and hemolysis. The severity of hemolysis in G-6-PD deficiency and the frequency of hemolytic episodes depend on the dose and nature of the inducing drug, as well as the particular G-6-PD variant involved.

Clinical evidence of hemolysis appears 2–3 days after an affected individual is exposed to an offending drug, with the hemolytic crisis becoming more pronounced during the next 7–10 days. The effect of drug exposure is more severe if the patient is already ill because infections and metabolic disorders can precipitate hemolytic episodes or accentuate drug-induced hemolysis. Renal damage and hepatic disease cause severe hemolysis and dramatically intensify the effects of small doses of oxidant drugs as a result of the reduced ability to eliminate the offending compound.

Normal Values

The normal G-6-PD test values may vary depending on the particular laboratory method used but generally are:

Screening test	Negative
Quantitative test	4.5–10.8 U/g of hemoglobin

Variations

Hemolytic anemia due to **G-6-PD deficiency** may occur with:

Diabetic acidosis	Antipyrine	Naphthalene
Exposure to certain drugs:	Ascorbic acid	Nitrofurantoin
	Aspirin	Nitrofuran
Acetanilid	Chloramphenicol	Pentaquine
Acetylphenylhydrazine	Nalidixic acid	Phenacetin

Phenylhydrazine	Quinidine	Ingestion of fava beans
Primaquine	Quinine	Septicemia
Probenecid	Sulfonamides	Viral and bacterial infections
Quinacrine	Vitamin K	

Methodology

Glucose-6-phosphate dehydrogenase deficiency tests require 2 mL of venous blood collected in acid citrate dextrose (ACD), heparin, or EDTA anticoagulant (blue-, green-, or lavender-stoppered tube), depending on the type of specimen indicated by the individual laboratory. Specimen collection procedures requested by each laboratory for the various test methods should be followed to ensure accurate results.

▶▶ ### Nursing Responsibilities and Implications

1. Inform the patient that there are no food or fluid restrictions.

2. Determine if the patient is taking any medications or has any illnesses that might alter the test results.

3. Monitor the patient's urinary output for decreases because prolonged hemolysis can cause renal impairment.

4. Observe the patient for clinical signs of hemolysis such as jaundice.

HEMOGLOBIN ELECTROPHORESIS

Hemoglobin electrophoresis is a specialized screening procedure used to distinguish the different types of hemoglobin most commonly present in red blood cells and determine the relative percentage of each. Hemoglobin electrophoresis separates various hemoglobins according to their molecular composition, electrical charge, and speed of migration to identify the characteristic mobility pattern associated with each particular variant. The types of hemoglobin most commonly identified by electrophoresis are the normal hemoglobins A_1, A_2, and F, as well as the abnormal hemoglobins S, G, C, E, O, and D. Laboratory evaluation of hemoglobin by electrophoresis helps to detect abnormal concentrations of normal hemoglobins, as well as establish the presence of and identify an abnormal hemoglobin variant.

Clinical Significance

More than 400 types of abnormal hemoglobin have been identified, most differing from normal hemoglobin by the variation of a single amino acid in the globin molecule. Abnormal hemoglobins frequently are associated with hemolytic anemias, in varying degrees from mild to severe, although not all variants cause disease. The abnormal hemoglobins of diagnostic significance are those responsible for recognizable clinical symptoms and the so-called hemoglobin diseases or hemoglobinopathies.

Several of these hemoglobin variants have nearly identical electrophoretic mobility patterns, which prevents their adequate separation by electrophoresis when more than one variant is present. These variants must be differentiated and measured by additional methods such as the sickling tests for hemoglobin S or the alkali denaturation test for hemoglobin F. Because routine electrophoretic techniques are insensitive to most unstable hemoglobins, many abnormal and variant hemoglobin types must be identified by special citrate agar or globin chain fractionation procedures.

Normal Values

The normal values for the important types of hemoglobin that can be identified by electrophoresis are:

Hemoglobin A$_1$ (major component of adult blood)	
Infants	10%–30%
Children and adults (>1 year)	95%–98%
Hemoglobin A$_2$ (minor component of adult blood)	2%–3%
Hemoglobin F (predominant hemo-globin molecule during fetal life)	
Neonates	70%–80%
1 month	70%
2 months	50%
3 months	25%
6 months–1 year	3%
2 years	2%
3 years	1%
Adults	0.8%

Variations

The more commonly encountered abnormal hemoglobin variants that are identified by electrophoresis include Hemoglobin S, C, H, D, and E (Table 2-2).

Hemoglobin S, the most common and widely distributed hemoglobin variant, occurs in approximately 10% of American blacks. Hemoglobin S exhibits greatly decreased solubility characteristics at reduced oxygen tensions. Erythrocytes containing Hb S become grossly distorted and assume a crescent or sickle shape when the available supply of oxygen in the blood is reduced locally or generally. Erythrocyte sickling can occur with serious consequences at high altitudes and during deep anesthesia, strenuous exercise, or flying.

The sickling phenomenon and the speed with which it develops are influenced by the concentration of Hb S and the presence of other hemoglobins in the red blood cell. Hemoglobin S can occur in the homozygous state (S/S), producing sickle cell anemia, and in the heterozygous state (A/S), producing the sickle cell trait with no demonstrable clinical symptoms. Hemoglobin S also can be found in combination with Hb C and Hb D (S/C and S/D) to produce red blood cells that sickle more rapidly than A/S cells with a similar amount of Hb S.

Several laboratory tests, such as Sickledex and the older sickle cell preparation, frequently are used to screen individuals for the presence of Hb S. However, these tests give

TABLE 2-2 Qualitative Distribution of Hemoglobins by Electrophoresis

Hemoglobin Variants	Percent Distribution of Hemoglobins
Normal adult blood	
Hb A_1	95%–98%
Hb A_2	2%–3% (not visible on electrophoretogram)
Hb F	0.8% (not visible on electrophoretogram)
Sickle cell disease	
Hb S	80%–100%
Hb A_1	Absent
Hb A_2	2%–3%
Hb F	Over 2% (visible on electrophoretogram)
Sickle cell trait	
Hb S	20%–40%
Hb A_1	60%–80%
Hb A_2	2%–3%
Hb F	2% (not visible on electrophoretogram)
Hb C disease	
Hb C	90%–100%
Hb A_1	Absent
Hb A_2	2%–3%
Hb F	2% or slightly higher
Hb C trait	
Hb C	45%
Hb A_1	55%
Hb S-thalassemia major	
Hb A_1	Absent
Hb S	70%–80%
Hb F	15%–25%
Hb S-thalassemia minor	
Hb A_1	30%
Hb A_2	2%–3%
Hb S	60%
Hb F	Over 2% (not visible on electrophoretogram)
Thalassemia major	
Hb A_1	5%–20%
Hb A_2	2%–3%
Hb F	65%–100%
Thalassemia minor	
Hb A_1	50%–85%
Hb A_2	4%–6%
Hb F	5%–20%

positive results regardless of whether the affected red blood cells contain predominantly Hb S or Hb S combined with a normal or another abnormal hemoglobin. Therefore, positive and doubtful screening test results must be confirmed by hemoglobin electrophoresis to distinguish between homozygous and heterozygous Hb S and to document the presence of other abnormal hemoglobins. False-positive screening test results are seldom encountered, although false-negative reports are not uncommon.

Hemoglobin C occurs in 2%–3% of American blacks and produces red blood cells with a reduced osmotic fragility that may sickle under certain circumstances. Hemoglobin C can occur in the homozygous state (C/C) to produce Hb C disease with a mild hemolytic anemia and in the heterozygous state (A/C) to produce the Hb C trait, which is asymptomatic. Hemoglobin C also can be found in combination with Hb S to produce a moderate to severe condition known as Hb S/C disease. Individuals affected by Hb S/C disease exhibit an intermediate type of hemolytic anemia quite similar to sickle cell anemia, the severity of which is proportional to the amount of Hb S present.

Hemoglobin H is an unstable hemoglobin that may precipitate quite easily to form numerous inclusion bodies within the red blood cells. Hemoglobin H has an abnormally high affinity for oxygen, binding with rather than releasing it to the tissues and interfering with normal oxygen transport. It often is found in association with a mild variety of thalassemia minor, producing Hb H disease. Red blood cells containing Hb H have a diminished life span of approximately 40 days because the cell membrane is damaged by the numerous inclusion bodies formed by the precipitated hemoglobin and the cell is removed prematurely by the spleen.

Hemoglobin D and hemoglobin E are abnormal variants that are rarely encountered in the United States but can occur in the homozygous state (D/D and E/E) to produce a mild hemolytic anemia or in the heterozygous state (A/D and A/E), in which they are asymptomatic. The combination of these abnormal hemoglobins with Hb S (sickle cell-Hb D disease) or thalassemia (Hb D-thalassemia and Hb E-thalassemia) causes severe disease. Because Hb D migrates like Hb S, routine electrophoresis may result in the misdiagnosis of the Hb D trait as the sickle cell trait. However, red blood cells containing Hb D do not sickle.

Methodology

Hemoglobin electrophoresis requires 5 mL of freshly drawn venous blood collected in heparin, EDTA, or oxalate anticoagulant (green-, lavender-, or black-stoppered tube). Prompt processing of the specimen helps to ensure reliable test results because prolonged storage of whole blood, particularly at warm temperatures, may produce artifacts that stimulate the production of abnormal hemoglobin variants. When the presence of an unstable hemoglobin is suspected, it is essential to avoid any delay between obtaining the specimen and performing the test.

Precautions

To ensure accurate test results, the following precautions should be observed when collecting a specimen for hemoglobin electrophoresis:

1. Wait at least 3–4 months after transfusion therapy before performing hemoglobin electrophoresis because mobility patterns can be obscured by the presence of donor red blood cells following blood transfusions.

2. Deliver the blood specimen to the laboratory without delay because abnormal hemoglobin is unstable.

▶▶ *Nursing Responsibilities and Implications*

1. Inform the patient that there are no food or fluid restrictions.
2. Note if the patient has received a transfusion in the past 3–4 months.
3. Observe the patient for signs of anemia such as fatigue and dyspnea.
4. Promote adequate rest.
5. Encourage the patient to wear a medical alert tag or card if genetic or chronic anemia is present.
6. Inform the patient and family of the availability of genetic counseling if appropriate.

SICKLE CELL TEST

The **sickle cell test** is a screening procedure used to demonstrate the presence of hemoglobin S, an abnormal hemoglobin variant that causes red blood cells to sickle. Red blood cells containing Hb S retain their proper shape under conditions of normal oxygen tension but assume a distorted crescent or sickle shape when the oxygen supply is reduced. Erythrocytes containing other types of abnormal hemoglobin also have been found to sickle under appropriate reducing conditions and can produce test results similar to those associated with Hb S. Laboratory procedures based on the low solubility of Hb S help to confirm the presence of a hemoglobinopathy and are useful in the diagnosis of sickle cell anemia and the sickle cell trait.

Clinical Significance

The sickling phenomenon and the speed with which it occurs are influenced by the concentration of Hb S and the presence of other hemoglobins in the red blood cell. Thus, erythrocytes sickle and give positive test results regardless of whether they contain predominantly Hb S or a combination of Hb S and the normal Hb A. However, screening procedures cannot reliably differentiate the homozygous state responsible for sickle cell anemia from the heterozygous sickle cell trait.

Erythrocytes may not exhibit the sickling reaction during testing if the Hb S concentration is less than 25%, the minimum required for sickling to occur. Unreliable sickling reactions and test results may occur when the total hemoglobin concentration is extremely low, as in severe anemia, or abnormally high, as in polycythemia. False-positive results also are encountered in patients with high protein levels, such as occurs in lupus erythematosus or multiple myeloma, in which the globulin is precipitated instead of the sickling hemoglobin. Hemoglobin electrophoresis is required to completely identify hemoglobin patterns and accurately diagnose the various hemoglobinopathies involved in the sickling disorders.

Normal Values

The normal values for hemoglobin S and the sickling phenomenon are:

Screening test	Negative No sickled red blood cells seen
Hemoglobin S	0%

Variations

Erythrocytes may exhibit the sickling reaction under appropriate conditions if they contain the following hemoglobin variants:

Hb I	Hb C Harlem
Hb I-thalassemia	Hb Alexandria
Hb Bart	Hb Memphis/S
Hb C Georgetown	

Methodology

The sickle cell test requires 5 mL of freshly drawn venous blood collected in EDTA anticoagulant (lavender-stoppered tube).

Precautions

To ensure accurate test results, the following precautions should be observed when collecting a specimen for the sickle cell test:

1. Wait 3–4 months after transfusion therapy before performing the sickle cell test because results may be altered by the presence of donor red blood cells.

2. Deliver the blood specimen to the laboratory without delay because abnormal hemoglobin is unstable.

▶▶ **Nursing Responsibilities and Implications**

1. Inform the patient that there are no food or fluid restrictions.

2. Note if the patient has received a transfusion in the past 3–4 months.

3. Determine if the patient is receiving phenothiazine drugs because concentrations higher than 128 μg/mL may inhibit or reverse the sickling reaction.

4. Observe the patient for clinical symptoms of sickle cell anemia such as fatigue, dyspnea, bone pain, swollen joints, or chest pain.

5. Promote rest.

6. Teach the patient to avoid situations that promote hypoxia such as high altitudes, strenuous activity, or extreme cold.

7. Instruct the patient to avoid infections.

8. Inform the patient and family of the availability of genetic counseling.

ALKALI DENATURATION TEST FOR FETAL HEMOGLOBIN

The **alkali denaturation test** is a simple method for measuring fetal hemoglobin (Hb F) levels when thalassemia is suspected or when increased concentrations of this hemoglobin type are detected during routine hemoglobin electrophoresis. Because the electrophoretic mobility pattern of Hb F is close to that of adult hemoglobin (Hb A) in many electrophoretic techniques, measurement of Hb F by molecular separation and densitometry is inaccurate. The alkali denaturation test isolates Hb F by denaturing Hb A with strong alkali (Hb F resists alkali denaturation but Hb A does not), precipitating the denatured hemoglobin, and measuring the residual alkali-resistant Hb F.

Clinical Significance

The amount of Hb F measured by alkali denaturation helps to determine the severity of thalassemia and other hemoglobinopathies by differentiating the homozygous and heterozygous forms. For example, Hb F usually comprises 30%–100% of the total hemoglobin in homozygous β-thalassemia (thalassemia major) but only 2%–5% in the heterozygous form (thalassemia minor). Likewise, the homozygous condition of hereditary persistence of fetal hemoglobin (HPFH) is accompanied by 100% of Hb F, whereas the heterozygous form contains 40% or less of Hb F. Patients with sickle cell anemia and β-thalassemia have Hb F values up to 20%; Hb F levels in individuals with the sickle cell trait are normal.

Normal Values

The normal values for hemoglobin F are:

Alkali denaturation test	<2%
Infants	
Newborns	60%–90%
6 months	<5%
1 year	<2%
Adults (reached by 2 years of age)	0.9%

Variations

Increased concentrations of fetal hemoglobin (more than 2%) occur with:

Aplastic anemia	Paroxysmal nocturnal hemoglobinuria
Erythroleukemia	Pernicious anemia
Hereditary persistence of fetal hemoglobin (HPFH)	Pregnancy
	Refractory anemia
Leakage of fetal hemoglobin into the maternal bloodstream	Sickle cell anemia
	Spherocytic anemia
Leukemia	Thalassemia
Megaloblastic anemia	Thyrotoxicosis
Metastatic disease with bone marrow involvement	Trisomy D syndrome
Myelofibrosis	

Methodology

Alkali denaturation tests require 5 mL of venous blood collected in a tube containing EDTA anticoagulant (lavender-stoppered tube) or heparin (green-stoppered tube). Specimens for Hb F determinations remain stable for 4 days at room temperature.

▶▶ *Nursing Responsibilities and Implications*

1. Inform the patient that there are no food or fluid restrictions.

2. Determine if the patient has any illness that might alter the test results by increasing the presence of fetal hemoglobin.

BONE MARROW EXAMINATION

Bone marrow, the major site of erythrocyte, leukocyte, and thrombocyte formation, can provide revealing information about cell production when abnormal or defective hematopoiesis is suspected. The hematopoietic process is best studied by obtaining a marrow sample by aspiration or biopsy and evaluating the cells for characteristic abnormalities that may indicate disease. Active hematopoiesis in adults occurs almost entirely in the red marrow of such membranous bones as the vertebral spinous processes, ribs, sternum, and iliac crest. The last two sites are the most readily accessible regions for marrow puncture and aspiration.

Unlike peripheral blood studies, which yield limited information about the pathogenesis of an abnormal condition, bone marrow examinations can confirm a diagnosis suggested by other clinical or laboratory findings. Diagnosis of blood disorders through bone marrow examination usually is based on an evaluation of the balance between the rate and quality of hematopoietic activity and the rate of cell release and survival. Bone marrow studies should be performed only when it is necessary to obtain additional information concerning a specific disease or to follow the progress of therapy for leukemia and anemia.

Clinical Significance

Bone marrow studies are of particular interest in the diagnosis and treatment of a variety of disorders, including anemia, leukemia, multiple myeloma, thrombocytopenic purpura, splenomegaly, lymph node enlargement, and metastatic carcinoma. Thorough evaluation of marrow histopathology is essential to the correct diagnosis of aplastic anemia, myelofibrosis, and granulomas and can help exclude the diagnosis of leukemia and other primary blood dyscrasias. However, bone marrow examinations are contraindicated in patients with hemophilia and other major disturbances of hemostasis or coagulation.

Test reports should include a description of the general marrow cellularity and type of erythropoiesis observed, as well as a reference to the maturity of erythropoietic and leukopoietic cells. Marrow cellularity normally varies with the age of the individual and the site of examination and reflects the ratio of fat content to the total content of hematopoietic cells. A differential count is useful in selected cases to record the relative proportion of different cell types but does not indicate the total number of cells present in the marrow.

The estimated ratio of total myeloid cells to nucleated erythroid cells is expressed as the myeloid-erythroid, or M:E, ratio. A high M:E ratio with a low fat content suggests hyperplastic marrow, whereas a low M:E ratio and high fat content indicates hypoplasia, at least of the particular marrow area sampled. A normal M:E ratio does not necessarily guarantee a normal marrow or exclude the existence of a disease process.

Normal Values

The normal values for the bone marrow differential cell count are:

Hemocytoblast	0.1%–1.0%
Myeloblasts	0.1%–5.0%
Promyelocytes	0.5%–8.0%
Myelocytes	
Neutrophilic	5.0%–20%
Eosinophilic	0.1%–3.0%
Basophilic	0%–0.5%
Metamyelocytes	
Neutrophilic	10%–32%
Eosinophilic	0.3%–3.7%
Basophilic	0%–0.3%
Band cells	
Neutrophilic	10%–35%
Eosinophilic	0.2%–2.0%
Basophilic	0%–0.3%
Segmented cells	
Neutrophilic	7.0%–30%
Eosinophilic	0.2%–4.0%
Basophilic	0%–0.7%
Lymphocytes (all stages)	2.7%–24%
Monocytes (all stages)	0%–2.7%
Plasmacytes	0.1%–1.5%
Megakaryocytes	0.03%–0.5%
Pronormoblasts	0.2%–4.0%
Basophilic normoblasts	1.5%–5.8%
Polychromatophilic normoblasts	5.0%–26.4%
Orthochromic normoblasts	1.6%–21%
Reticulum cells	0.1%–2.0%
M:E ratio	
Birth	1.85:1
2 weeks	11:1
1–2 months	5.5:1
1–20 years	2.95:1
Adult	4:1 (range of 6:1–2:1)

Variations

An **elevated M : E ratio** (7 : 1 or more) may occur with:

Erythroid hypoplasia

Infections

Leukemoid reaction

Myeloid leukemia

A **normal M : E ratio** may occur with aplastic anemia, myeloma, and myelosclerosis.
A **decreased M : E ratio** (2 : 1 or less) may occur with:

Depressed myeloid formation
(agranulocytosis)

Increased erythroid activity:

  Iron deficiency anemia

  Liver disease

Pernicious anemia

Polycythemia vera

Posthemolytic anemia

Posthemorrhagic anemia

Generalized bone marrow hyperplasia may occur with myeloproliferative syndromes and a reaction to pancytopenia.
Generalized bone marrow hypoplasia may be idiopathic or occur with:

Myelofibrosis

Myelosclerosis

Myelotoxic agents (chemicals, drugs,
ionizing radiation)

Advancing age

Osteopetrosis

Tumor, cellular infiltrations

Viral infections (rubella, dengue fever)

Elevated bone marrow lymphocytes may occur with:

Aplastic anemia

Decreases in other cell types

Infectious lymphocytosis

Infectious mononucleosis

Lymphatic leukemoid reaction

Lymphocytic leukemia

Lymphoma

Macroglobulinemia

Myelofibrosis

Viral infections

Elevated bone marrow granulocytes may occur with:

Decreases in other cell types

Infections

Myelocytic leukemia

Myelocytic leukemoid reaction, myeloproliferative syndrome

Decreased bone marrow granulocytes may occur with agranulocytosis, increases
in other cell types, and ionizing radiation.
Elevated bone marrow plasma cells may occur with:

Acute rheumatic fever

Agranulocytosis

Amyloidosis

Aplastic anemia

Hepatic cirrhosis

Hodgkin's disease

Hypersensitivity states

Irradiation

Macroglobulinemia

Malignant tumors or carcinomatosis

Multiple myeloma

Rheumatoid arthritis

Serum sickness

Syphilis

Ulcerative colitis

Elevated bone marrow normoblasts may occur with:

Chronic blood loss

Decreases in other cell types

Erythemia

Erythroid-type myeloproliferative disorders

Hemolytic anemias

Iron deficiency anemia

Megaloblastic anemias that have been treated

Elevated bone marrow megakaryocytes may occur with:

Acute hemorrhage

Chronic myeloid leukemia

Infections, especially pneumonia

Megakaryocytic myelosis

Myelofibrosis

Polycythemia vera

Secondary hypersplenism associated with Gaucher's disease, systemic lupus erythematosus, or Felty's syndrome

Thrombocytopenia (secondary to peripheral destruction or sequestration of platelets)

Decreased bone marrow megakaryocytes may occur with:

Aplastic anemia

Cirrhosis

Excessive irradiation

Marrow overgrowth with carci-nomatous or leukemic deposits

Pernicious anemia

Thrombocytopenic purpura (some cases)

Toxic substances (benzene, cytotoxic drugs, chlorothiazides)

Methodology

Bone marrow studies are performed on specimens aspirated or collected under a local anesthetic by a qualified physician with the assistance of a specially trained technologist or nurse. Marrow smears should be obtained for examination before the patient receives any iron, liver, vitamin B_{12}, folic acid, or cytotoxic agents that might alter the cells. The interpretation of bone marrow smears also may be difficult if the patient has received a blood transfusion within the preceding few weeks.

▶▶ Nursing Responsibilities and Implications

1. Make certain the patient has signed an informed consent form.

2. Inform the patient that a local anesthetic will be used but that some pain and pressure will be experienced during the procedure.

3. Prepare the area and shave it if necessary; the sternum or iliac crest are the most fre-quently used sites in adults. The iliac crest is the most frequently used site in children over 1½ years of age; the tibia is the most commonly used site in infants under 1½ years of age.

4. Obtain baseline vital signs before the procedure begins.

5. Position the patient—supine for sternal or tibial punctures and side lying or prone for punctures of the iliac crest.

6. Assist the patient to maintain this position and remain still during the procedure.

7. Apply direct pressure to the puncture site to limit bleeding; maintain bedrest for 30−60 minutes.

8. Send the specimen to the laboratory immediately; note if the patient has had a recent blood transfusion or is receiving iron, liver, vitamin B_{12}, folic acid, or cytotoxic agents.

9. Monitor the patient's vital signs. The immediate concern is shock caused by hemorrhage; infection is a later concern.

OTHER TESTS OF HEMOGLOBIN METABOLISM

A number of other tests pertaining to hemoglobin metabolism are discussed in other chapters, including:

Delta-aminolevulinic acid (ALA) (Chapter 3)

Bilirubin (Chapter 3)

Ferritin (Chapter 3)

Folate (Chapter 3)

Haptoglobin (Chapter 3)

Plasma hemoglobin (Chapter 3)

Porphyrins (Chapter 3)

Serum iron (Chapter 3)

Total iron-binding capacity (Chapter 3)

Transferrin (Chapter 3)

Urobilinogen (Chapter 3)

Vitamin B_{12} (Chapter 3)

REFERENCES

Bauer, J. D. 1982. *Clinical laboratory medicine*. 9th ed. St. Louis: The C. V. Mosby Co.

Bologna, C. V. 1971. *Understanding laboratory medicine*. St. Louis: The C. V. Mosby Co.

Collins, R. D. 1975. *Illustrated manual of laboratory diagnosis*. 2nd ed. Philadelphia: J. B. Lippincott Co.

Dougherty, W. M. 1976. *Introduction to hematology*. 2nd ed. St. Louis: The C. V. Mosby Co.

Eastham, R. D. 1970. *Clinical hematology*. 3rd ed. Baltimore: The Williams & Wilkins Co.

French, R. M. 1980. *Guide to diagnostic procedures*. 5th ed. New York: McGraw-Hill Book Co.

Garb, S. 1976. *Laboratory tests in common use*. 6th ed. New York: Springer Publishing Co.

Gerarde, H. W., and Anderson, E. 1972. *Hematology laboratory procedures using the Unopette disposable diluting pipette*. Rutherford, N.J.: Becton-Dickinson and Co.

Henry, J. B. 1984. *Clinical diagnosis and management by laboratory methods*. 17th ed. Philadelphia: W. B. Saunders Co.

Hammond, K. B. 1980. Blood specimen collection from infants by skin puncture. *Lab. Med.* 11(1):9−12.

Marchand, A. 1980. Restoring energy to a tired anemia diagnosis. *Diagn. Med.* 3(5): 23−24.

Maslow, W. C., et al. 1980. *Hematologic disease.* Boston: Houghton Mifflin Co.

Miale, J. B. 1982. *Laboratory medicine—hematology.* 6th ed. St. Louis: The C. V. Mosby Co.

Raphael, S. S., et al. 1983. *Medical laboratory technology.* 4th ed. Philadelphia: W. B. Saunders Co.

Seivard, C. 1983. *Hematology for medical technologists.* 5th ed. Philadelphia: Lea & Febiger.

Strand, M. M., and Elmer, L. A. 1983. *Clinical laboratory tests.* 3rd ed. St. Louis: The C. V. Mosby Co.

Tilkian, S. M., Conover, M. H., and Tilkian, A. G. 1983. *Clinical implications of laboratory tests.* 3rd ed. St. Louis: The C. V. Mosby Co.

Widmann, F. K. 1983. *Clinical interpretation of laboratory tests.* 9th ed. Philadelphia: F. A. Davis Co.

3

Chemistry: Tests of Hemoglobin Metabolism

HEMOGLOBIN SYNTHESIS AND BREAKDOWN   123
Hemoglobin Synthesis · Hemoglobin Breakdown

TESTS OF HEMOGLOBIN SYNTHESIS   125
Vitamin B_{12} · Folic Acid · Porphyrins and Their Precursors · Serum Iron · Transferrin, Total Iron-Binding Capacity, and Percent Saturation · Serum Ferritin

TESTS OF HEMOGLOBIN BREAKDOWN   139
Plasma Hemoglobin · Haptoglobin · Bilirubin · Urobilinogen

OTHER HEMOGLOBIN STUDIES   149

HEMOGLOBIN SYNTHESIS AND BREAKDOWN

Hemoglobin Synthesis

Hemoglobin synthesis (Figure 3-1) involves two main constituents, heme and globin, which must be present in adequate amounts to allow optimal formation and function of this respiratory pigment. **Heme** is a complex substance composed of protoporphyrin and iron; **globin** is a normal plasma protein (see Proteins, Chapter 4). Heme synthesis begins when succinyl coenzyme A (coA) and glycine, produced with the aid of vitamin B_{12} and folate, combine to form a substance that becomes delta-aminolevulinic acid (ALA), the first porphyrin precursor. Subsequent steps in heme metabolism include: (1) the combination of ALA molecules to form porphobilinogen; (2) conversion of porphobilinogen to uroporphyrin; and (3) synthesis of coproporphyrin and protoporphyrin from uroporphyrin. Protoporphyrin is then coupled with the iron ions bound by transferrin or ferritin to form heme.

Iron is absorbed from the diet in the small intestine and bound in the bloodstream to **transferrin**, a plasma protein that serves as its principal transport agent. Transferrin plays a crucial role in delivering iron to the bone marrow and storage organs such as the liver, along with facilitating the entry of iron into hemoglobin-producing erythropoietic cells. Iron that is not bound to transferrin is conserved by storing the surplus within **ferritin**, a highly specialized intracellular protein present in the bone marrow, spleen, and liver.

The body also stores excess iron in hemosiderin granules that are believed to be derived from ferritin, although iron in this form is less readily available than the iron in ferritin. **Hemosiderin granules** are insoluble iron-loaded particles that accumulate in reticuloendothelial cells and connective tissue when abnormal red blood cell destruction releases large amounts of iron to be placed in storage. Hemosiderin frequently is excreted in the urine during hemochromatosis, siderosis of the kidneys following chronic hemolytic anemia, or multiple transfusions when iron stores become excessive.

Hemoglobin Breakdown

Normal destruction of red blood cells by the reticuloendothelial cells of the spleen releases heme, globin, and iron as the byproducts of hemoglobin degradation (see Figure 3-1). Iron is processed by reticuloendothelial cells and either bound to transferrin to be returned to the bone marrow for the synthesis of new red blood cells or stored as ferritin and hemosiderin. Globin chains are broken down into their constituent amino acids to be available for further protein synthesis.

Heme is first degraded to biliverdin, which is reduced by the reticuloendothelial system to bilirubin and transported to the liver for excretion (see Bilirubin later in this chapter). Bilirubin traveling to the liver is insoluble in water, but when the bilirubin reaches the liver, it combines with glucuronic acid to form a water-soluble compound that passes freely into the bile. As conjugated bilirubin descends through the biliary system and intestinal tract, it is degraded into a series of compounds that are excreted in the feces as urobilinogen, urobilin, and stercobilinogen. Minimal amounts of the soluble urobilinogen are reabsorbed from the colon into the bloodstream and are carried to the liver by the portal circulation for excretion in the bile and finally the urine (see Urobilinogen later in this chapter).

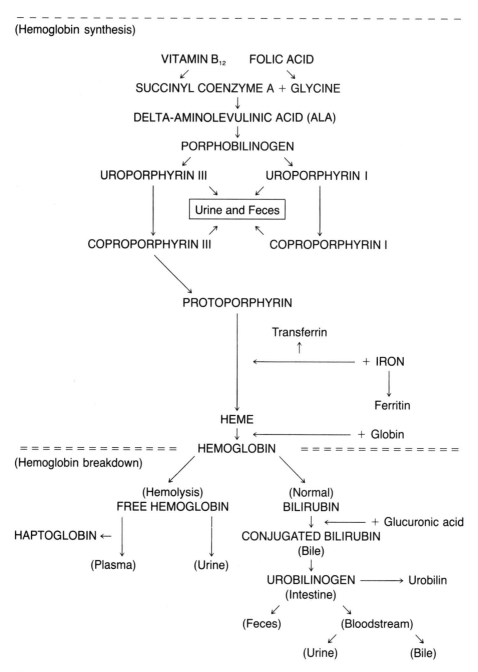

Figure 3-1 Hemoglobin synthesis and breakdown.

Destruction of red blood cells within the bloodstream during intravascular hemolysis releases free hemoglobin into the circulation, where it combines with the α_2-globulin, haptoglobin. This hemoglobin-haptoglobin complex is metabolized directly by the reticuloendothelial system, which returns hemoglobin constituents to the body storage pool. Saturation of the hemoglobin-binding capacity of circulating haptoglobin by pathologic red blood cell destruction causes free hemoglobin to remain in the bloodstream and to cross the glomerular filter into the urine.

Free hemoglobin remaining in the plasma that is not excreted by the kidneys after saturation of the haptoglobin-binding capacity is oxidized into heme molecules and firmly bound to hemopexin. **Hemopexin** is a normal plasma globulin that conserves iron by binding the free or loosely bound heme released into the bloodstream by dissociated hemoglobin proteins after the haptoglobin-binding capacity has been exceeded. In contrast to the hemoglobin-haptoglobin complexes, which are cleared by reticuloendothelial cells, heme-hemopexin complexes are rapidly degraded by hepatic parenchymal cells.

TESTS OF HEMOGLOBIN SYNTHESIS

Vitamin B$_{12}$

Vitamin B$_{12}$, a complex organic compound also known as cyanocobalamin, is synthesized by certain microorganisms and required for normal hematopoiesis as well as many biochemical reactions. It is essential for the conversion of methylmalonate to succinyl CoA, a substance necessary for hemoglobin synthesis (see Figure 3-1), and is also required for normal folic acid metabolism and DNA synthesis. A normal diet containing foods such as liver, meat, fish, eggs, and dairy products supplies an excess of the minimum daily requirement of vitamin B$_{12}$, but an intrinsic factor is needed in the gastric juice for absorption. Thus, the average adult stores sufficient vitamin B$_{12}$ to withstand at least 3 years of zero intake unless rapid growth periods occur or cell turnover increases.

Deficiencies of vitamin B$_{12}$ most frequently develop therefore only in strict vegetarians or individuals who completely lack gastric secretion of the intrinsic factor. Significant vitamin B$_{12}$ deficiency produces morphologic changes in all body cells, particularly red blood cell precursors, which are manifested by the development of pernicious anemia. However, because megaloblastic anemia also results from folate deficiency, folic acid level evaluations frequently accompany vitamin B$_{12}$ determinations to differentiate these disorders and allow correct therapy (see Folic Acid later in this chapter). Laboratory measurement of vitamin B$_{12}$ is valuable in diagnosing pernicious anemia, establishing the cause of megaloblastic anemia, and distinguishing vitamin B$_{12}$ deficiency from folic acid deficiency.

Clinical Significance

Vitamin B$_{12}$ deficiency caused by a lack of the intrinsic factor causes the megaloblastic disease known as **pernicious anemia**, which is characterized by large, oval, red blood cells and hypersegmented neutrophils. Thus, decreased vitamin B$_{12}$ test results must be interpreted along with red blood cell indices and stained red blood cell examinations to help distinguish pernicious anemia from other vitamin B$_{12}$ deficiencies. On the other hand, misleadingly high vitamin B$_{12}$ levels may result from the overproduction of B$_{12}$-binding proteins in patients with myeloproliferative disorders and hepatocellular damage.

Because protein production in these conditions raises serum concentrations of vitamin B_{12}, body cells are deprived of the vitamin. This causes B_{12} tissue deficiency to coexist with normal serum levels.

Vitamin B_{12} and folic acid each have specific biochemical functions but are also interrelated and overlap in their physiologic response patterns to a deficiency of either substance. For example, patients with vitamin B_{12} deficiency frequently develop higher than normal serum folate levels, which drop sharply when vitamin B_{12} is administered therapeutically. Thus, although vitamin B_{12} and folic acid are capable of stimulating normoblastic red blood cell growth in megaloblastic bone marrow, each cannot by itself fully correct a deficiency of the other.

Normal Values

The clinically significant values for vitamin B_{12} are:

Normal range	330–900 pg/mL
Borderline	270–330 pg/mL
Low	<270 pg/mL
High	>1000 pg/mL

Variations

Increased vitamin B_{12} may occur with:

Cirrhosis

Hepatitis, infectious

Hyperproteinemia

Myeloproliferative disorders (1000–10,000 pg/mL)

Myelocytic leukemia, acute and chronic

Myelosclerosis

Polycythemia vera

Vitamin B_{12} deficiency (<100 pg/mL) may occur with:

Blind loop syndrome

Celiac disease

Cirrhosis

Dietary deficiency

Diverticulosis

Diphyllobothrium latum infection (fish tapeworm)

Enteritis, regional

Gastrectomy

Gastric carcinoma

Hepatitis

Ileal resection, extensive (bypass procedure)

Kwashiorkor

Malabsorption, drug-induced

Pancreatic dysfunction

Pernicious anemia (intrinsic factor deficiency)

Sprue

Vegetarian diets

Methodology

Vitamin B_{12} determinations require 5 mL of blood collected without anticoagulants (red-stoppered tube) from a fasting individual. Specimens must not be collected using ascorbic acid or high concentrations of fluoride as preservatives because these two agents destroy vitamin B_{12}.

Folic Acid

Folic acid (pteroylglutamic acid) is the vitaminlike precursor of several organic substances, collectively known as the folates, that are involved in DNA synthesis and essential for normal hematopoiesis. Folates are present in many foods of plant and animal origin, including eggs, liver, milk, fruit, cereal, yeast, nuts, and leafy vegetables, and are stored in the liver. However, because the body can store only limited amounts of folic acid, serum folate levels are easily influenced by dietary factors and increase or decrease abruptly in response to dietary changes.

Folic acid stores are adequate to withstand 4–6 months of decreased intake, but this supply may be rapidly depleted by abnormal intestinal absorption or increased utilization. A diet severely deficient in folate therefore can cause persistently low serum folate levels, impair DNA synthesis, and produce a megaloblastic anemia similar to that resulting from vitamin B_{12} deficiency. An index of total folic acid status is provided by red blood cell folate levels, which reflect tissue folate stores more accurately than serum folate values. Laboratory measurement of serum and red blood cell folate concentrations helps in the diagnosis of folic acid deficiency and should be performed on every patient with megaloblastic anemia to ensure proper therapy.

Clinical Significance

Slightly decreased serum folate levels usually accompany the appearance of the enlarged red blood cells and hypersegmented neutrophils characteristically associated with megaloblastic anemia but also may occur before these hematologic abnormalities develop. In patients with borderline values who exhibit little or no hematologic changes, red blood cell folate levels should be measured to help assess the presence and severity of folate deficiency. Subnormal red blood cell folate levels, together with decreased serum folate values, indicate a severe depletion of hematopoietic and liver stores, the proper treatment of which is folic acid administration. However, low red blood cell folate values also can mean that the patient has a primary vitamin B_{12} deficiency that is blocking the ability of cells to take up folate (see the previous section on vitamin B_{12}). In this case the proper therapy would be vitamin B_{12} rather than folic acid because neurologic damage may result if treatment with folate is used when the problem is vitamin B_{12} deficiency.

It is impossible therefore to determine the cause of megaloblastosis by therapeutic trials alone because the administration of vitamin B_{12} can correct the hematologic abnormalities of folate deficiency. Conversely, folate administration corrects the hematologic abnormalities of B_{12} deficiency while allowing the underlying disease to progress unhindered in other organs. Because folate and vitamin B_{12} values in these two deficiencies frequently overlap, differentiation of the cause of megaloblastic anemia requires serum and red blood cell folate measurements plus vitamin B_{12} level determinations. Thus, all three values should be determined simultaneously to differentiate these overlapping areas, obtain a more accurate clinical assessment, and ensure proper therapy for megaloblastosis.

Normal Values

The normal values for folic acid are:

Serum folate	3–20 ng/mL of serum
Red blood cell folate	160–600 ng/mL of red blood cells

Variations

Decreased serum folate levels (<3ng/mL) may occur with:

Alcoholism	Phenytoin	Leukemia, acute
Celiac disease	Pyrimethamine	myelomonocytic
Dermatitis herpetiformis	Triamterene	Malabsorption syndromes
Dietary deficiency	Trimethoprim	Malnutrition
Drug therapy	Hemolytic anemia	Myelosclerosis
Glutethimide	Hyperthyroidism	Neoplastic diseases
Isoniazid	Infants	Pregnancy
Methotrexate	Iron and folate deficiency	Sickle cell anemia
Oral contraceptives	combined	Sprue

Increased serum folate levels may occur with:

Blind loop syndrome	Liver disease
Folic acid administration, oral	Vitamin B_{12} deficiency
Kidney failure	

Decreased red blood cell folate levels (<125 ng/mL) may occur with folic acid deficiency or a primary vitamin B_{12} deficiency.

Methodology

Serum folate determinations require 5 mL of blood collected without trauma in a tube with no anticoagulants (red-stoppered tube). Specimens must not be hemolyzed because inadvertent hemolysis before the serum is separated from the clot causes test results to be falsely elevated.

Measurement of red blood cell folate levels also requires 5 mL of serum (the same specimen collected for the serum folate level determination can be used) along with 5 mL of blood collected in EDTA (ethylenediaminotetraacetate) (lavender-stoppered tube). Red blood cell folate levels are calculated from the amount of folate measured in serum and hemolysate. Specimens for both determinations must be collected from fasting individuals because recent food intake increases folic acid levels appreciably.

Porphyrins and Their Precursors

The **porphyrins** are biochemical compounds produced in all tissues, especially bone marrow and liver cells, that are involved in heme synthesis during the early stages of hemoglobin metabolism. The first porphyrin precursor and the earliest substance in heme synthesis is delta-aminolevulinic acid (ALA), a chemical building block of porphobilinogen. Subsequent conversion of porphobilinogen to uroporphyrin by enzymatic action within normoblasts of the bone marrow is followed by further transformation to coproporphyrin and protoporphyrin. The addition of iron to protoporphyrin results in the final formation of heme (see Figure 3-1).

Metabolism of these substances and their precursors usually is evaluated by measuring porphyrin concentrations in the urine, blood, and feces. The predominant porphyrin in urine is coproporphyrin, although small amounts of ALA and porphobilinogen are also normal. Protoporphyrin normally is the predominant porphyrin in red blood cells, although much larger amounts of coproporphyrin and uroporphyrin also may be found in abnormal conditions. Feces normally contain uroporphyrin, coproporphyrin, and protoporphyrin (the bacterial breakdown products of hemoglobin breakdown) derived from meat ingestion or intestinal hemorrhage.

Laboratory determination of porphyrin concentrations in urine, blood, and feces helps to identify abnormal porphyrin metabolism, verify the diagnosis of porphyria, and evaluate other disturbances of heme synthesis. Measurement of porphyrin concentrations in erythrocytes aids in the detection of subacute lead poisoning and also can be used to differentiate iron deficiency anemia from the thalassemias. If the increase in total erythrocyte porphyrins is not sufficient for diagnostic purposes, additional tests can be performed to aid in distinguishing between abnormal amounts of coproporphyrins and uroporphyrins.

Clinical Significance

Overaction of the various enzymes involved in heme synthesis interferes with porphyrin metabolism, increasing the excretion of these substances and their precursors in blood, urine, and feces, a disorder known as **porphyria** (see Porphobilinogen and Porphyrins in Chapter 1). For example, ALA excretion is increased in individuals during acute porphyric attacks, as well as in asymptomatic carriers in whom porphobilinogen values are normal. Total urine porphyrin levels are greatly increased in all forms of clinically active porphyria except erythropoietic protoporphyria and erythropoietic coproporphyria, and range from normal to moderately increased in latent porphyria. Analysis of blood for free erythrocyte porphyrins aids in the evaluation of erythropoietic protoporphyria and is required in patients under observation for cutaneous porphyria if the test for urinary porphyrin is normal. Likewise, fecal porphyrins are often, but not regularly, elevated in variegate porphyria, porphyria cutanea tarda, and erythropoietic porphyria.

Porphyrin analysis for the evaluation of diseases other than the porphyrias is limited to the diagnosis of lead poisoning, although increased erythrocyte protoporphyrin levels also occur in individuals with iron deficiency. Because lead poisoning interferes with heme synthesis, increased concentrations of ALA in urine and protoporphyrin in erythrocytes are the most sensitive laboratory indicators of subclinical lead intoxication. Thus, measurement of these substances is particularly useful in the early recognition of low-level lead toxicity in children from high-risk areas and prevention of the more severe neurologic sequelae.

Normal Values

The normal values for the porphyrins and their precursors are:

Erythrocytes

ALA	<1 mg/dL
Coproporphyrin	$0.5-2.3$ μg/dL
Protoporphyrin	$4-52$ μg/dL
Uroporphyrin	Trace

(continued)

Normal Values *(Continued)*

Feces

    Coproporphyrin   400−1200 μg/24 hours

    Protoporphyrin   <1800 μg/24 hours

    Uroporphyrin   10−40 μg/24 hours

Free erythrocyte porphyrin   20−75 μg/dL

Urine

    ALA   1.3−7.5 mg/24 hours

    Coproporphyrin   50−160 μg/24 hours

    Porphobilinogen   <2.0 mg/24 hours

    Uroporphyrin   <30 μg/24 hours

Variations

Increased ALA levels may occur with:

Alcoholic cirrhosis	Porphyrias, congenital and acquired
Lead poisoning	Toxic chemical poisoning

Increased coproporphyrin levels may occur with:

Alcoholic cirrhosis	Hemolytic anemia
Erythroid hyperplasia	Hodgkin's disease
Erythropoietic porphyria, congenital (>90 μg/dL)	Lead poisoning
	Leukemia
Erythropoietic protoporphyria (>140 μg/dL)	Myocardial infarction, acute
	Pernicious anemia
Erythropoietic coproporphyria	Poliomyelitis, acute
Exercise, strenuous	Sideroachrestic anemia
Fever	Thyrotoxicosis
Hemochromatosis	Vitamin deficiency

Increased porphobilinogen levels may occur with acute intermittent porphyria.

Increased protoporphyrin levels may occur with:

Erythropoiesis, increased	Iron deficiency (>200 μg/dL)
Erythropoietic protoporphyria (>2200 μg/dL)	Lead poisoning (>200 μg/dL)
	Sideroachrestic anemia, acquired (>50 μg/dL)
Hemolytic anemia (>50 μg/dL)	
Infection (>50 μg/dL)	Thalassemia

Decreased protoporphyrin levels may occur with megaloblastic anemia (< 30 μg/dL).

Increased uroporphyrin levels may occur with:

Cirrhosis

Erythropoietic porphyria, congenital
($>$300 μg/dL)

Lead intoxication

Porphyria, acute, intermittent

Methodology

Determination of the porphyrins and their precursors in urine requires a 24-hour urine specimen that has been protected from exposure to light and refrigerated during the collection period. Test procedures require only a 50 mL aliquot of urine, but the total volume of urine collected during the 24-hour period should be indicated on the laboratory request slip. Although the 24-hour collection method is preferred, measurement of total porphyrin values in the first-morning urine specimen provides the same clinical information more rapidly and without the inevitable errors associated with the longer test period.

Evaluation of erythrocyte porphyrin concentrations requires 3 mL of whole blood collected without hemolysis in heparin, EDTA, or oxalate anticoagulant (green-, lavender-, or black-stoppered tube, respectively).

Measurement of fecal porphyrin levels requires about 10 g of a 48- to 72-hour stool specimen that has been mixed well and weighed.

Precautions

To ensure accurate results when testing for porphyrins and their precursors, the following precautions should be observed:

1. Collect the specimen in a dark bottle (to protect it from light because the porphyrins decompose when exposed to light) with 5 grams sodium carbonate.

2. Test the specimen immediately because porphobilinogen in acid urine is converted to uroporphyrin, causing erroneous test results.

3. False-positive results with urine screening tests for porphobilinogen may occur in patients receiving large doses of such drugs as acriflavin, antipyretics, barbiturates, ethoxazene, phenazopyridine, phenothiazines, phenylhydrazine, procaine, sulfamethoxazole, sulfonamides, and tetracycline.

▶▶ Nursing Responsibilities and Implications

1. Obtain a single morning urine specimen or 24-hour urine specimen as ordered.

2. Protect the specimen from light and send it to the laboratory immediately; refrigerate the specimen during the 24-hour collection period.

3. Obtain a stool specimen; total stool specimens for 48–72 hours may be ordered.

4. Obtain a 3 mL venous specimen of whole blood in a green-, lavender-, or black-stoppered tube.

5. Note on the laboratory slip any medications such as phenothiazines, barbiturates, antibiotics, sulfonamides, diethylstilbestrol, and griseofulvin that might interfere with the test results.

6. If the test results are positive, teach the patient to avoid strong sunlight because the patient may be photosensitive and develop dermatitis as a result of exposure to sunlight.

Serum Iron

Iron, an inorganic element widely distributed in foods such as meat, eggs, legumes, and leafy vegetables, is essential to the formation of hemoglobin and various cellular enzymes. It is absorbed into the bloodstream from the small intestine, bound to the protein transferrin, and carried to the bone marrow for hemoglobin synthesis and red blood cell formation (see Figure 3-1). Although most of the body's total iron is contained in red blood cells, serum iron levels indicate the amount bound to transferrin that is available for hemoglobin formation. Serum iron determinations measure the amount of iron in transit at any specific moment as a result of such processes as iron absorption, hemoglobin breakdown, and iron release from body stores.

Absorption of approximately 2 mg of iron per day is usually sufficient to replace the minimal amounts routinely excreted in perspiration, feces, and urine. However, the typical American diet frequently is inadequate to replace the larger amounts of iron lost in women during menstruation, pregnancy, and childbirth and may contribute to the development of iron deficiency. Iron intake also may be inadequate in infants because the low iron content of milk will not supplement body stores, which are not sufficient to meet the infant's needs beyond 6 months of age. Laboratory measurement of the relatively small amount of iron remaining in serum helps to diagnose certain disorders and identify disturbances in iron absorption, storage, and utilization.

Clinical Significance

Serum iron levels are generally high when excessive iron is released from body stores, when red blood cell destruction is excessive, or when red blood cells are produced more slowly than normal. Decreased serum iron levels generally are the result of impaired release of iron from body stores, increased body requirements, or dietary deficiency. A single serum iron measurement is usually not enough to diagnose abnormal iron levels accurately, and diagnosis usually requires the additional measurement of total iron-binding capacity and a calculation of percent saturation.

Serum iron concentrations fluctuate widely during the day, with the highest levels occurring between 7 and 10 AM and decreasing steadily as the day progresses. Normal variations of 20%–30% (40–100 μg/dL) between morning and evening levels prevent the satisfactory comparison of random serum specimens. This diurnal variation disappears in individuals with hematologic disorders and is directly reversed in individuals who work at night and sleep during the day. Thus, when monitoring the course of disease or the results of therapy, comparison of serum iron levels should be based on specimens collected at the same time each day.

Normal Values

The normal serum iron values are:

Men	80–200 μg/dL
Women	60–130 μg/dL
Children	55–185 μg/dL
<2 years	<100 μg/dL
>2 years	Rises until adolescence
Elderly	60–80 μg/dL

Variations
Increased serum iron levels may occur with:

Aplastic anemia	Iron therapy	Pyridoxine deficiency
Blood transfusion	Lead poisoning	Sideroblastic anemia
Hemochromatosis	Oral contraceptives	Thalassemia
Hemolytic anemia	Pernicious anemia	Transfusion siderosis
Hepatitis, acute	Polycythemia	

Decreased serum iron levels may occur with:

Blood loss, chronic	Hemorrhage	Nephrotic syndrome
Burns, extensive	Infections, chronic	Postoperative period
Dietary iron deficiency	Iron deficiency anemia	Pregnancy
Erythropoiesis, increased	Kwashiorkor	Renal disease, chronic
Gastrectomy	Malabsorption syndromes	Rheumatoid arthritis
Genitourinary neoplasms, stones, inflammation	Malignancy	Uremia
	Menstrual bleeding, excessive	

Methodology
Serum iron determinations require 5 mL of blood collected without hemolysis in a tube with no anticoagulants (red-stoppered tube) or a special iron-free tube with a Parafilm cover. Specimens containing visible hemolysis are not acceptable for serum iron determinations because ruptured erythrocytes release their high iron content and can falsely elevate test values by 10 μg/dL or more. Although traces of hemolysis will not significantly affect the validity of serum iron determinations, specimens containing visible hemolysis should be disregarded because iron levels increase in proportion to the degree of hemolysis.

Precautions
To ensure accurate results when testing for serum iron levels, the following precautions should be observed:

1. Discontinue, as ordered, any medications that might interfere with the test results or note that the patient is receiving them on the laboratory slip; decreased results may occur with adrenocorticotropic hormone (ACTH), folic acid, vitamin B$_{12}$, and EDTA derivatives; increased results may occur with parenteral iron compounds, estrogens, chloramphenicol, and oral contraceptives.

2. Obtain a blood sample at the same time of day for each specimen to avoid variations caused by diurnal influences.

▶▶ Nursing Responsibilities and Implications

1. Inform the patient that there are no food or fluid restrictions; occasionally, the laboratory or physician may request that the patient fast for 8 hours prior to the test.

2. Obtain the blood specimen in the morning when serum iron levels are at their peak; note the time the specimen was obtained on the laboratory slip.

3. Note any signs of iron deficiency anemia such as fatigue, pallor, tachycardia, and exertional dyspnea.

4. If serum iron levels are low, encourage the patient to eat foods high in iron such as organ meats, eggs, and dried fruit.

5. If serum iron levels are low, encourage the patient to avoid activity that precipitates dyspnea; encourage rest periods.

Transferrin, Total Iron-Binding Capacity, and Percent Saturation

Total iron-binding capacity (TIBC) measures the amount of iron-transporting protein (**transferrin**) available in the blood to bind with and carry iron throughout the body. The amount of available transferrin is determined by measuring serum iron levels after completely saturating transferrin with iron in the laboratory. However, the binding sites of transferrin normally are only about one-third saturated with iron and actually could transport much more iron than is contained in the serum. Thus, the total transferrin pool acts as a cushion to buffer large amounts of absorbed or released iron that would otherwise produce toxic effects.

Total iron-binding capacity values represent the actual iron content of the serum plus the amount of additional iron that transferrin could absorb and carry if it were completely saturated. The ratio between serum iron and the transferrin available to bind with it is called the **percent saturation** and is the most widely recognized measurement of iron status. The percent of transferrin saturation is calculated from values for TIBC and serum iron content according to the following formula:

$$\text{Percent saturation} = (\text{serum iron}/\text{TIBC}) \times 100$$

Laboratory determinations of TIBC and percent saturation are useful in establishing the cause of abnormal serum iron concentrations and in diagnosing disorders of iron metabolism.

Clinical Significance

The combined analysis of TIBC, percent saturation, and serum iron, rather than any one value alone, provides the most clinically significant information for evaluating suspected disorders of iron metabolism (see Table 3-1). In general, TIBC levels are decreased in debilitating diseases characterized by protein loss or poor protein synthesis, iron overload, and decompensated chronic hemolytic anemia. Values for percent saturation remain normal when iron stores are adequate but fall when these stores become depleted. Total iron-building capacity and percent saturation levels follow the same diurnal variation pattern as serum iron, with the highest levels occurring in the morning and the lowest levels occurring in the late afternoon and early evening.

Normal Values
The normal values for TIBC and percent saturation are:

Transferrin	155–400 mg/dL
TIBC	
Adults	250–420 μg/dL
Newborn	225 μg/dL (average)
Percent saturation	
Men	35%–50%
Women	20%–35%

Variations

Elevated transferrin levels may occur with:

Blood loss	Iron deficiency	Oral contraceptives
Hemolysis	Malabsorption syndromes	Pregnancy

Decreased transferrin levels may occur with:

Cirrhosis	Liver disease	Protein deficiency
Iron therapy	Nephrotic syndrome	

Elevated total iron-binding capacity may occur with:

Blood loss, acute and chronic	Mestranol	Iron deficiency
Drug therapy	Oral contraceptives	Muscular exercise (immediate and several hours after)
Estrogens	Hepatitis	
Iron salts	Infancy	Pregnancy

Decreased total iron-binding capacity may occur with:

Blood transfusion-induced iron overload	Infections, acute and chronic
Collagen-vascular disease	Inflammations, acute and chronic
Drug therapy	Kwashiorkor
Asparaginase	Liver disease, chronic
Chloramphenicol	Malignancy
Corticotropin	Nephrosis
Cortisone	Newborns
Dextran	Pernicious anemia
Testosterone	Renal disease, chronic
Hemochromatosis	Sideroblastic anemia
Hemosiderosis	Starvation
	Thalassemia

Elevated percent saturation may occur with:

Blood loss, acute	Kwashiorkor	Pyrixodine deficiency
Hemochromatosis	Lead poisoning	Sideroblastic anemia
Hemosiderosis	Liver disease	Starvation
Iron overload	Nephrosis	Thalassemia

Decreased percent saturation (under 15%) may occur with:

Infections, acute and chronic	Malignancy
Inflammations, acute and chronic	Pregnancy, late
Iron deficiency anemia	

Table 3-1 summarizes the changes in serum iron, iron-binding capacity, and percent saturation in various clinical disorders.

TABLE 3-1   Serum Iron, Iron-Binding Capacity, and Percent Saturation in Selected Conditions

Clinical Condition	Serum Iron	Total Iron-Binding Capacity	Percent Saturation
Aplastic anemia	Increased	Decreased	Increased
Cirrhosis	No change	Decreased	Increased
Iron intake, excess	Increased	Decreased	Increased
Hemochromatosis	Increased	No change or decreased	Increased
Hemolytic anemia	Increased	No change or decreased	Increased
Hepatitis, acute	Increased	Increased	No change or increased
Hypothyroidism	No change	Decreased	Decreased
Infections, chronic	Decreased	Decreased	Decreased
Iron deficiency anemia	Decreased	Increased	Decreased
Kwashiorkor	Decreased	Decreased	Increased
Menstruation	Decreased	No change	Decreased
Neoplastic disease	Decreased	Decreased	Decreased
Nephrosis	Decreased	Decreased	Increased
Oral contraceptives	No change or increased	Increased	No change
Pernicious anemia	Increased	Decreased	Increased
Pregnancy, late	Decreased	Increased	Decreased
Pyridoxine deficiency	Increased	No change	Increased
Renal disease	Decreased	Increased or decreased	Decreased
Thalassemia	Increased	Decreased	Increased
Uremia	Decreased	Decreased	No change

Methodology

Determination of transferrin, TIBC, and percent saturation requires 7 mL of blood collected without anticoagulants (red-stoppered tube) or with special iron-free tubes and needles. Because iron-containing medications can affect test results, specimens should be collected at least 24 hours or more after therapy with such medications has been discontinued. Specimens for TIBC and percent saturation determinations should be collected in the morning after the patient has fasted for at least 8 hours. Because tests for TIBC and percent saturation frequently accompany serum iron analysis, blood samples are collected most conveniently in the same serum tube at a definite time each morning (see Serum Iron earlier in this chapter).

Precautions

To ensure accurate results when testing for TIBC, transferrin, and percent saturation, the following precautions should be observed:

1. Handle the specimen gently to avoid hemolysis and the release of iron into the serum.
2. Send the specimen to the laboratory immediately.
3. Discontinue, as ordered, any medications that might interfere with test results or note that the patient is receiving them on the laboratory slip; decreased results may occur with ACTH and steroids; increased results may occur with preparations containing iron, oral contraceptives, and chloramphenical.

▶▶ Nursing Responsibilities and Implications

1. Inform the patient that no food or fluid will be permitted for 8 hours prior to the test.
2. Note any signs of iron deficiency anemia such as fatigue, pallor, tachycardia, and exertional dyspnea.
3. If the test results are decreased, encourage the patient to eat foods high in iron such as organ meats, eggs, and dried fruit.
4. If the test results are decreased, encourage the patient to avoid activity that precipitates dyspnea and encourage rest periods.

Serum Ferritin

Ferritin, a highly specialized iron-storage protein, is the body's primary means of conserving surplus iron, with 1 ng of ferritin representing about 8 mg of stored iron. Ferritin is produced in direct proportion to the amount of iron stored in body tissues; iron reserves exceeding body requirements stimulate ferritin synthesis, whereas depleted iron supplies depress ferritin synthesis. Normally, ferritin is produced in the liver, spleen, and bone marrow, but it also is released by inflamed tissues and proliferating tumor cells. Ferritin mobilizes stored iron from the body's tissue reserves when metabolic requirements exceed dietary supply. It also stores excess serum iron to help prevent the damaging effects of iron overload when quantities exceed body requirements.

Decreased ferritin levels reflect a depletion of the total iron reserves available for hemoglobin synthesis. Increased ferritin values frequently accompany neoplastic activity, and a return to normal concentrations usually indicates successful therapy. Laboratory determinations of serum ferritin levels supplement the investigation of iron metabolism disorders, help to monitor therapy during the treatment of iron deficiency or overload, and provide an index of liver damage. They also can help in diagnosing certain malignancies, evaluating the prognosis of patients with breast cancer, and detecting persistent or recurrent tumors following mastectomy before the appearance of clinical symptoms.

Clinical Significance

Ferritin values reflect iron status more reliably than determinations of serum iron or percent of transferrin saturation, with levels below 10 ng/mL corresponding to a transferrin saturation of less than 16% (see the previous section on Transferrin, Total Iron-Binding Capacity, and Percent Saturation). Serum ferritin levels become depressed before iron stores are depleted and can be used to detect iron deficiency states that previously went undetected until iron stores were totally depleted. Thus, they can either provide an early warning of potential incipient iron deficiency anemia or confirm that the condition already exists. Ferritin values therefore help to distinguish uncomplicated iron deficiency from the anemias associated with chronic disease that mimic iron deficiency. These anemias result from the impaired release or utilization of iron stores.

Normal ferritin levels, however, do not eliminate the possibility of iron deficiency. Diseases that produce a concomitant increase in ferritin concentrations also may be present simultaneously and mask an underlying deficiency state. Ferritin test results may be within the normal range in individuals with hematopoietic malignancies, liver disease, and rheumatoid arthritis while iron stores are actually depleted. Therefore, serum ferritin determinations frequently are combined with serum iron and TIBC measurements to provide a more accurate assessment of the patient's entire iron status.

Normal Values

The normal values for serum ferritin are:

Adults

Men (18−45 years)	35−255 ng/mL
Men (>45 years)	40−300 ng/mL
Women (18−45 years)	12−100 ng/mL
Women (>45 years)	25−155 ng/mL
Newborns	101 ng/mL (average)

Infants

First month	350 ng/mL (average)
6 months	30 ng/mL (average)
Children (6 months−15 years)	10−140 ng/mL

Variations
Increased serum ferritin levels may occur with:

Carcinomas, general

Hematopoietic disorders

    Anemia associated with chronic disease

    Hemolytic anemia

    Pernicious anemia

    Polycythemia

    Leukemia

Hemochromatosis, idiopathic (>1000 ng/mL)

Hepatic diseases (approximately 500 ng/mL)

    Cirrhosis

    Hepatic necrosis (drug- or viral-induced)

Hepatitis, infectious (>1000 ng/mL)

Hepatoma, primary

Metastatic carcinoma

Obstructive jaundice, surgical

Hodgkin's disease

Inflammation, chronic

Iron overload (>10,000 ng/mL)

    Refractory anemia, primary

    Transfusion therapy

Multiple myeloma

Rheumatoid arthritis

Siderosis, nutritional

Thalassemia

Tissue damage

Decreased serum ferritin levels may occur with:

Gastric surgery

Hemodialysis

Inflammatory bowel disease

Iron deficiency (<10 mg/mL)

Pregnancy

Methodology
Measurement of serum ferritin requires 5 mL of blood collected without hemolysis in a tube containing no anticoagulants (red-stoppered tube), although plasma specimens collected in a heparinized tube (black-stoppered tube) also may be used.

▶▶ *Nursing Responsibilities and Implications*

1. Inform the patient that there are no food or fluid restrictions.

2. Note on the laboratory slip if the patient is receiving any medications that contain iron because they might interfere with the test results.

TESTS OF HEMOGLOBIN BREAKDOWN

Plasma Hemoglobin

Plasma hemoglobin is the free hemoglobin that escapes during intravascular hemolysis and remains in the bloodstream after the saturation of haptoglobin (see the following section on Haptoglobin). Plasma normally contains minute amounts of free hemoglobin from physiologic red blood cell breakdown, but massive hemolysis raises this level several hundred times and causes the plasma to appear pink (**hemoglobinemia**). In contrast, the golden yellow-orange coloration of plasma that results from increased bilirubin production after extravascular red blood cell destruction does not reflect elevated plasma hemoglobin levels (see Bilirubin later in this chapter). Laboratory evaluation of plasma hemoglobin concentration provides a supplement to haptoglobin determinations and helps to identify the origin of plasma pigmentation in the differential diagnosis of intravascular and extravascular hemolysis.

Normal Values
The normal and clinically significant values for plasma hemoglobin are:

Normal	0.5–5.0 mg/dL
Hemoglobinemia (orange plasma)	>10 mg/dL
Intravascular hemolysis (pink plasma)	>30 mg/dL
Hemoglobinuria	>150 mg/dL
Cherry-red plasma	>200 mg/dL

Variations
Increased plasma hemoglobin levels may occur with:

Autoimmune hemolytic anemia (idiopathic, drug-induced)	Malaria (*Plasmodium falciparum*)
	Paroxysmal nocturnal hemoglobinuria
Cold hemagglutinins	Prosthetic heart valve
Disseminated intravascular coagulation (DIC)	Septicemia
	Thrombotic thrombocytopenic purpura
Exercise, strenuous	Transfusion reaction
Intravascular hemolysis	Traumatic hemolytic anemia
Lupus erythematosus	

Methodology
Plasma hemoglobin determinations require 5 mL of blood collected without trauma in a tube containing heparin or EDTA (green- or lavender-stoppered tube) to prevent the mechanical hemolysis of red blood cells during clotting. Specimen collection is a critical part of plasma hemoglobin determinations because any damage to red blood cells during venipuncture or the separation of plasma and cells produces erroneously high test results.

Precautions
To ensure accurate results when testing for plasma hemoglobin, the following precautions should be observed:

1. Do not draw the blood specimen from the same arm or hand being used for the administration of intravenous solutions because the extra fluid may cause falsely decreased hemoglobin values.

2. Do not leave the tourniquet on for longer than 1 minute during specimen collection

because elevated hemoglobin values may result from prolonged hemostasis due to vasoconstriction.

▶▶ *Nursing Responsibilities and Implications*

1. Inform the patient that there are no food or fluid restrictions.

2. Deliver the specimen to the laboratory immediately because plasma must be separated from cells within 1–2 hours after collection of the specimen.

3. Note any signs of anemia such as pallor, exertional dyspnea, tachycardia, or fatigue.

4. If plasma hemoglobin levels are increased, encourage the patient to avoid activities that precipitate dyspnea; encourage periods of rest because the amount of usable hemoglobin is decreased.

Haptoglobin

Haptoglobin is an α_2-globulin that combines with free hemoglobin to form a complex which is removed by the reticuloendothelial system rather than by urinary excretion. This complex can bind up to 200 mg of free hemoglobin to prevent significant loss of iron and other cellular constituents in the urine. However, haptoglobin reserves are rapidly diminished by any condition that destroys red blood cells and are almost completely saturated by even small amounts of intravascular hemolysis. Thus, lysis of 10 mL of red blood cells reduces haptoglobin supplies by about 100 mg/dL and can depress the entire haptoglobin reserve to zero.

Decreased or absent haptoglobin levels therefore imply haptoglobin saturation resulting from increased red blood cell destruction or decreased haptoglobin synthesis due to genetic factors. Not until this hemoglobin-binding capacity of haptoglobin has been exceeded can free hemoglobin remain in the bloodstream or appear in the urine. The lowest haptoglobin levels occur 8–12 hours after a hemolytic episode and remain depressed, even when no further hemolysis occurs, until hepatic synthesis restores haptoglobin concentrations to prehemolytic values.

Haptoglobin is also an acute-phase reactant that increases to five to eight times the normal value during conditions such as malignancy, tissue necrosis, inflammation, and pregnancy. However, increased haptoglobin concentrations may accompany increased hemoglobin binding and actually mask a haptoglobin deficiency caused by hemolysis. Thus, normal or slightly elevated haptoglobin values in patients with such conditions do not rule out hemolysis and may interfere with the accurate interpretation of test results. Laboratory determination of haptoglobin provides a valuable index to the presence of hemolysis and, because myoglobin is not bound by haptoglobin, also may be used to differentiate hemoglobinemia from myoglobinemia.

Clinical Significance

Totally absent haptoglobin values frequently occur in athletes because the normal process of hemolysis may be exaggerated by blows to any part of the body during contact sports. Zero haptoglobin values also occur in musicians who use their hands vigorously or patients with seizure disorders whose violent muscular contractions result in low-level mechanical red blood cell breakdown. In addition, decreased haptoglobin values are not uncommon in pediatric patients who must be restrained when blood specimens are obtained.

Haptoglobin levels are normally low or totally absent in newborns, particularly premature infants, but appear in the blood of normal full-term infants within a few days after birth. However, neonates suffering from infections acquired in utero can have haptoglobin values as high as 100 mg/dL. Thus, caution must be exercised in interpreting low haptoglobin test results in children.

Normal Values

The normal and clinically significant values for haptoglobin are:

Normal range

Adults	40−245 mg/dL
Neonates	0−40 mg/dL
Hemolysis	<25 mg/dL
Inflammation	>200 mg/dL

Variations

Decreased or absent haptoglobin levels may occur with:

Ahaptoglobinemia, congenital

Artificial heart valve implantation

Haptoglobin variant, congenital

Hemolysis, intravascular or extravascular

Hemolytic anemia

Hepatocellular disease, acute and chronic

Infectious mononucleosis

Liver failure

Megaloblastic anemia

Tissue hemorrhage

Transfusion reaction, hemolytic

Increased haptoglobin levels may occur with:

Abscess

Androgen administration

Burns

Hypernephroma

Infection

Inflammation

Malignancies

Myocardial infarction

Oral contraceptives

Pneumonia

Pregnancy

Rheumatoid arthritis

Steroid therapy

Subacute bacterial endocarditis

Surgery

Tissue necrosis

Tuberculosis

Ulcerative colitis

Methodology

Serum haptoglobin determinations require 5 mL of blood collected with no anticoagulants (red-stoppered tube) and without trauma to avoid hemolysis. Specimens should be delivered to the laboratory immediately for prompt analysis to prevent red blood cells and serum from remaining in contact for a prolonged period.

Precautions

To ensure accurate results when testing for serum haptoglobin, the following precautions should be observed:

1. Obtain the specimen without trauma and handle it gently to prevent red blood cell lysis because this will result in falsely decreased values.

2. Deliver the specimen to the laboratory immediately.

3. Do not permit the serum specimen to come in contact with peroxidase or other oxidants because these substances may cause falsely elevated test results.

▶▶ ### Nursing Responsibilities and Implications

1. Inform the patient that there are no food or fluid restrictions.

2. Deliver the specimen to the laboratory immediately.

3. Note any signs of anemia; assess the patient's vital signs, particularly the pulse and respirations, for increases.

4. If the test results are elevated, assess the patient for possible inflammation or infection.

Bilirubin

Bilirubin, the waste product of hemoglobin breakdown, is produced in the reticuloendothelial cells of the liver, spleen, and bone marrow from hemoglobin released by old or damaged red blood cells. Low concentrations of free bilirubin normally circulate in the bloodstream; the kidneys excrete small amounts of bilirubin in urine, and the liver processes the remainder to form conjugated bilirubin. Most of this water-soluble, conjugated bilirubin is excreted into the duodenum as a constituent of bile, but a very small amount returns to the general circulation (see Figure 3-1).

Once in the gastrointestinal tract, conjugated bilirubin is reduced by bacterial action in the colon to urobilinogen and urobilin, the substances that give feces its characteristic brown color. Most of the urobilinogen is excreted in feces, although some is reabsorbed from the colon into the bloodstream, returned to the liver, and excreted in bile. A very small amount of the urobilinogen reabsorbed into the bloodstream is excreted by the kidneys in urine.

Free and conjugated bilirubin fractions are differentiated during laboratory measurement of bilirubin concentrations according to their reaction with test reagents. Conjugated bilirubin, which requires only one reagent and can be measured immediately, is known as **direct bilirubin**, whereas an additional reagent is needed to measure free bilirubin, which also is called **indirect bilirubin**. Alternative laboratory procedures measure only total and direct bilirubin concentrations rather than direct and indirect bilirubin levels on the assumption that the difference between these values represents the indirect fraction.

Accumulation of increased bilirubin concentrations in the bloodstream and tissues is associated with jaundice and may result from a number of disorders. Laboratory measurement of the total bilirubin level is useful in assessing the severity and progress of jaundice, detecting hemolysis, and diagnosing the presence of liver disease. Determination of direct and indirect bilirubin levels, together with an evaluation of urine bilirubin, urine urobilinogen, and fecal urobilinogen levels, provides a valuable guide to the differential diagnosis of jaundice.

Clinical Significance

Serum bilirubin concentrations rise significantly and produce jaundice when red blood cell destruction becomes excessive and when the liver is unable to conjugate or properly excrete the quantities of bilirubin presented to it. Because overt jaundice appears with bilirubin concentrations above 2 mg/dL, it is advantageous to recognize rising serum levels before jaundice occurs. However, the sudden onset of jaundice occasionally may be the first indication of hemolytic anemia, acute or chronic liver disease, or other disease processes.

There are three general types of jaundice that may be distinguished according to the nature of bilirubin formation and excretion (Table 3-2).

Hemolytic Jaundice. Hemolytic jaundice occurs when an increased rate of red blood cell destruction produces more bilirubin and bile pigments than the liver can cope with. Even when liver function is relatively normal, if the increased rate of hemolysis exceeds the liver's conjugating capacity, bilirubin accumulates and increases total and free (indirect) bilirubin concentrations. Hemolytic jaundice may accompany hemolytic anemias, transfusion reactions, and massive heart or lung infarcts.

Hepatic Jaundice. Hepatic jaundice occurs when toxic, infectious, or mechanical damage to the liver parenchymal cells interferes with efficient bilirubin metabolism and excretion. A damaged liver is unable to excrete bilirubin in normal amounts, thus greatly decreasing the output of bile and increasing serum concentrations of total, free (indirect), and conjugated (direct) bilirubin. Hepatic jaundice may accompany cirrhosis, infectious hepatitis, toxic hepatitis resulting from poison ingestion or drug abuse, liver necrosis, and damage from a trauma or wound. Hepatic jaundice also may accompany liver damage caused by the prolonged administration of many drugs such as some antiarthritic preparations, antibiotics, diuretics, and tranquilizers.

Obstructive Jaundice. Obstructive jaundice occurs when a blockage of the excretory ducts of the liver prevents the flow of bile into the duodenum, causing it to back up into the bloodstream. In the presence of an obstructed biliary tract, normal bilirubin conjugation and bile excretion by the liver result in an increased serum concentration of both total and conjugated (direct) bilirubin. Obstructive jaundice may result from stones, tumors, or scar tissue in either the excretory ducts of the liver or the common bile duct.

TABLE 3-2 Differentiation of Jaundice by Bilirubin Metabolism

| | Type of Jaundice | | |
	Hemolytic	Hepatic	Obstructive
Serum bilirubin (total)	Moderate increase	Marked increase	Marked increase
Serum bilirubin (direct)	Normal	Moderate increase	Moderate increase
Serum bilirubin (indirect)	Moderate increase	Moderate increase	Normal
Urine bilirubin	Negative	Increased	Increased
Urine urobilinogen	Marked increase	Increased	Decreased
Fecal urobilinogen	Marked increase	Normal	Decreased

Normal Values

The normal values for serum bilirubin are:

Total bilirubin

Adults	0.3−1.4 mg/dL
Children	0.2−0.8 mg/dL
Newborns	1.0−12.0 mg/dL
Direct bilirubin	0.1−0.4 mg/dL
Indirect bilirubin	0.2−0.8 mg/dL

Interpretation

A differential diagnosis of the various types of jaundice is not always possible from serum bilirubin measurements alone. Accurate interpretation of serum bilirubin test results and a thorough clinical assessment frequently require the additional measurement of urine bilirubin and urobilinogen values and fecal urobilinogen levels (see Table 3-2) (see Bilirubin and Urobilinogen in Chapter 1 and Urobilinogen in Chapter 8).

Hemolytic Jaundice. Hemolytic jaundice is characterized by a moderately increased total bilirubin level and a direct bilirubin level that is less than 20% of the total. The indirect bilirubin level is increased because the liver cannot adequately conjugate the large amounts of bilirubin that result from excessive hemolysis. Urine bilirubin is absent because the large quantities of indirect bilirubin are not water-soluble and cannot be cleared from the blood by the kidneys. Urine and fecal urobilinogen levels are increased because of the presence of large amounts of bilirubin that must be converted to urobilinogen.

Hepatic Jaundice. Hepatic jaundice is characterized by a moderate to marked increase in the total bilirubin level and a direct bilirubin level that is 20%−50% of the total. The indirect bilirubin level is also greatly increased because inefficient liver function prevents bilirubin excretion in the bile. The urine bilirubin level is increased because of elevated concentrations of water-soluble conjugated bilirubin, which is excreted by the kidneys. The urine urobilinogen level may or may not be increased, whereas the fecal urobilinogen level is normal to slightly decreased because less bile reaches the colon to be converted to urobilinogen.

Obstructive Jaundice. Obstructive jaundice is characterized by a markedly increased total bilirubin level and a direct bilirubin level that is greater than 50% of the total. The indirect bilirubin level is normal because it already has been conjugated by the normally functioning liver and little remains in the blood. The urine bilirubin level is increased because of the elevated concentration of water-soluble direct bilirubin that is excreted by the kidneys. Both urine and fecal urobilinogen levels are decreased because, depending on the extent of bile obstruction, the bilirubin-containing bile never reaches the intestine to be converted to urobilinogen. However, very low fecal urobilinogen levels are not diagnostic of obstructive jaundice because broad-spectrum antibiotics, which suppress the intestinal bacteria, also interrupt the conversion of bilirubin to urobilinogen.

Variations

Elevated total serum bilirubin levels (**hyperbilirubinemia**) may occur with:

Drug therapy (Table 3-3)

Hemolytic jaundice

    Erythroblastosis fetalis

    Hereditary spherocytosis

    Myocardial infarction

    Sickle cell anemia

    Transfusion reactions

Hepatic jaundice

    Cirrhosis

    Hepatitis (infectious, viral, or toxic)

Obstructive jaundice

    Carcinoma of the head of the pancreas

    Impaired excretory function of the liver (caused by stones or scar tissue)

Elevated direct bilirubin levels may occur with:

Alcoholic hepatitis, acute

Biliary obstruction

    Calculi

    Iproniazid therapy

    Methyltestosterone therapy

    Oral contraceptive therapy

    Scar tissue

Thorazine therapy

Tumor

Carcinoma of the head of the pancreas

Cirrhosis

Drug therapy (Table 3-3)

Dubin-Johnson syndrome

Hepatitis (infectious, viral, or toxic)

Elevated indirect bilirubin levels may occur with:

Alcoholic cirrhosis, acute

Autoimmune hemolysis

Cirrhosis

Crigler-Najjar syndrome

Drug therapy (Table 3-3)

Erythroblastosis fetalis

Gilbert's disease

Hemorrhage into body cavities and soft tissues

Hereditary spherocytosis

Hepatitis (infectious, viral, or toxic)

Malaria

Myocardial infarction

Pernicious anemia

Septicemia

Sickle cell disease

Transfusion reaction (hemolytic)

Methodology

Serum bilirubin determinations require 5 mL of blood collected without anticoagulants (red-stoppered tube). Serum specimens for bilirubin determinations remain stable for up to 1 week when stored in the dark at refrigerator temperatures and for 3 months when frozen.

Precautions

To ensure accurate results when testing for serum bilirubin, the following precautions should be observed:

1.   Determine whether the patient has received an injection of radiopaque contrast media for radiographic studies within the past 24 hours because these substances inter-

TABLE 3-3 Commonly Used Drugs That Affect Bilirubin Tests

Increased Value	Decreased Value
Antimalarials	Barbiturates
Aspirin	Corticosteroids
Cholinergics	Sulfonamides
Coumarin	Thioridazine
Ethoxazene	
Morphine	
Oral contraceptives	
Penicillin	
Phenylbutazone	
Primaquine	
Procainamide	
Quinidine	
Quinine	
Rifampin	
Streptomycin	
Sulfa drugs	
Tetracycline	
Thiazides	

fere with the color reaction of the test; if this is the case, serum bilirubin determinations should be delayed for 24 hours.

2. Obtain the blood specimen without trauma and handle it gently because liberated hemoglobin caused by red blood cell lysis can produce falsely decreased results.

3. Protect the specimen from strong sunlight because bilirubin concentrations may drop as much as 50% within 1 hour if the serum is allowed to stand in a well-lighted area.

4. Determine whether the patient is receiving any drugs that give the serum a yellow or orange color because they can falsely elevate the bilirubin level. Elevated bilirubin values also may result from the prolonged administration of drugs that temporarily modify liver function and are considered hepatotoxic. Drugs that cause falsely elevated serum bilirubin values include:

Acetazolamide	Isoniazid	Radiopaque contrast media, certain
Androgens	Methanol	Salicylates
Chlordiazepoxide	Nitrofurantoin	Sulfonylureas
Chlorpromazine	Oxacillin	Sulfonamides
Erythromycin	Phenothiazines	Vitamin A
Indomethacin	Phenylbutazone	
Iproniazid	Pyrazinamide	

▶▶ *Nursing Responsibilities and Implications*

1. Instruct the patient to avoid orange and yellow foods, such as carrots and yams, several days prior to the test because they give the serum a yellow to orange color.

2. Instruct the patient to avoid food and fluid for the 4 hours prior to the test; substances that cause a high lipid content in the blood will interfere with the test reaction and produce a falsely low bilirubin level.

3. Protect the specimen from direct light and deliver it to the laboratory immediately.

4. If the physician orders a serum bilirubin measurement and a test employing a dye, schedule the serum bilirubin determination first because contrast media will affect the test results.

Urobilinogen

Urobilinogen, the end product of hemoglobin breakdown, is formed by the bacterial degradation of conjugated bilirubin excreted in the bile. The quantity of urobilinogen produced depends on the amount of bilirubin contained in the bile pigments that reach the intestine. About half the urobilinogen formed is absorbed into the bloodstream and carried to the kidneys, where it readily enters the urine; the remainder is excreted in the feces (see Figure 3-1). Urobilinogen levels in urine and feces are influenced by the degree of red blood cell destruction, amount of bilirubin produced, and rate of bile flow from the liver.

Any condition that increases the rate of bilirubin degradation and stimulates the production or accumulation of abnormal quantities of bile and urobilinogen in the intestine increases urinary and fecal urobilinogen excretion. Conversely, interruption or obstruction of the flow of bile into the intestinal tract decreases urobilinogen production and lowers the amount excreted in the urine and feces. Laboratory determination of urobilinogen concentrations helps in evaluating bilirubin metabolism and aids in the differential diagnosis of jaundice (see Table 3-2). (See Bilirubin in this chapter and Urobilinogen in Chapters 1 and 8.)

Clinical Significance
Urobilinogen levels in urine and feces are increased in individuals with conditions characterized by excessive red blood cell destruction and bile excretion. However, excretion is diminished in proportion to the decrease of bile flow, with a total absence of urobilinogen indicating complete obstruction. Urobilinogen levels also are used in the management of hepatic disorders because increased values are the first indication of incipient liver disease and provide a sensitive gauge of liver damage. Urine urobilinogen levels are more widely used as a chemical indicator of hemolysis and hemoglobin turnover than fecal urobilinogen determinations because they are much easier to measure.

Normal Values
The normal values for urine and fecal urobilinogen are:

Fecal urobilinogen	
Qualitative	Positive
Quantitative	40−250 mg/24 hours
	75−350 mg/100 g of stool
Urine urobilinogen	0.5−4.0 Ehrlich units/24 hours
	0.05−2.5 mg/24 hours

Variations
Increased fecal urobilinogen levels may occur with:

Hemolytic anemia

   Sickle cell anemia

   Hereditary spherocytosis

Thalassemia

Hemolytic jaundice

Decreased fecal urobilinogen levels may occur with:

Antibiotic administration

Aplastic anemia

Bile duct obstruction

Obstructive jaundice

Increased urine urobilinogen levels may occur with:

Erythropoietic porphyria

Hemolytic disorders

Intestinal obstruction

Parenchymal liver disease

Cirrhosis

Hepatitis (infectious or toxic)

Infectious mononucleosis

Decreased urine urobilinogen levels may occur with:

Absence of intestinal bacteria

Antibiotic administration, broad-spectrum

Carcinoma of the head of the pancreas

Hepatitis with cholestasis

Obstruction of the common bile duct

Rapid intestinal transit time

Starvation

Methodology
Specimen collection procedures for urobilinogen determinations are discussed under Urobilinogen in Chapters 1 and 8.

Precautions
Precautions to observe during urobilinogen determinations are discussed under Urobilinogen in Chapters 1 and 8.

▶▶ *Nursing Responsibilities and Implications*
Nursing responsibilities for urobilinogen determinations are discussed under Urobilinogen in Chapters 1 and 8.

OTHER HEMOGLOBIN STUDIES

A number of additional tests pertaining to hemoglobin are discussed in other chapters, including:

Alkali denaturation test for fetal hemoglobin (Chapter 2)

Hemoglobin (Chapter 2)

Hemoglobin electrophoresis (Chapter 2)

Sickle cell test (Chapter 2)

REFERENCES

Bauer, J. D. 1982. *Clinical laboratory methods.* 9th ed. St. Louis: The C. V. Mosby Co.

Becton-Dickinson Immunodiagnostics. 1980. *Iron-binding capacity RIA kit protocol.* Orangeburg, N.Y.: Becton-Dickinson Immunodiagnostics.

———. 1981. *Vitamin B$_{12}$/folate RIA kit protocol.* Orangeburg, N.Y.: Becton-Dickinson Immunodiagnostics.

Bio-Science Laboratories. 1982. *The Bio-Science handbook.* 13th ed. Van Nuys, Calif.: Bio-Science Laboratories.

Clinical Assays, Inc. 1980. *Ferritin RIA test kit protocol.* Cambridge, Mass.: Clinical Assays, Inc.

Collins, R. D. 1975. *Illustrated manual of laboratory diagnosis.* 2nd ed. Philadelphia: J. B. Lippincott Co.

French, R. M. 1980. *Guide to diagnostic procedures.* 5th ed. New York: McGraw-Hill Book Co.

Garb, S. 1975. *Laboratory tests in common use.* 6th ed. New York: Springer Publishing Co.

Henry, J. B. 1984. *Clinical diagnosis and management by laboratory methods.* 17th ed. Philadelphia: W. B. Saunders Co.

Krause, J. R. 1981. Serum ferritin test and its relationship to iron deficiency. *Lab. Med.* 12(9):536–540.

Larson, F. C. 1983. *Clinical significance of tests available on DuPont Automated Clinical Analyzer.* Wilmington, Del.: DuPont Industries.

Maslow, W. C., et al. 1980. *Hematologic disease.* Boston: Houghton Mifflin Co.

Miale, J. B. 1982. *Laboratory medicine—hematology.* 6th ed. St. Louis: The C. V. Mosby Co.

Raphael, S. S., et al. 1983. *Medical laboratory technology.* 4th ed. Philadelphia: W. B. Saunders Co.

RIA Products, Inc. 1977. *Clinical radioimmunoassay of serum ferritin.* Waltham, Mass.: RIA Products, Inc.

———. 1979. *In vitro measurement of serum ferritin by radioimmunoassay.* Waltham, Mass.: RIA Products, Inc.

Strand, M. M., and Elmer, L. A. 1983. *Clinical laboratory tests.* 3rd ed. St. Louis: The C. V. Mosby Co.

Tilkian, S. M., Conover, M. B., and Tilkian, A. G. 1983. *Clinical implications of laboratory tests.* 3rd ed. St. Louis: The C. V. Mosby Co.

White, W. L., Erickson, M. M., and Stevens, S. C. 1976. *Chemistry for the clinical laboratory.* 4th ed. St. Louis: The C. V. Mosby Co.

Widmann, F. K. 1983. *Clinical interpretation of laboratory tests.* 9th ed. Philadelphia: F. A. Davis Co.

With, T. K. 1980. Diagnostic tests for porphyrins. *Lab. Med.* 11(7):446–454.

4

Chemistry: Routine Studies

SPECIMEN COLLECTION AND HANDLING   152
Specimen Types   ·   Anticoagulants Used to Prevent Clotting   ·   Collection Times   ·   Collection Tubes   ·   Order of Specimen Draw   ·   Performing a Venipuncture   ·   Preserving and Processing Blood Specimens

AUTOMATION IN THE CHEMISTRY LABORATORY   157

CARBOHYDRATES   157
Fasting Blood Glucose   ·   Two-Hour Postprandial Blood Glucose   ·   Glucose Tolerance Test   ·   Glycohemoglobin Test   ·   D-Xylose Absorption Test   ·   Lactose Tolerance Test

ENZYMES   172
Amylase   ·   Lipase   ·   Acid Phosphatase   ·   Alkaline Phosphatase   ·   Cholinesterase and Pseudocholinesterase   ·   Aldolase   ·   Creatine Phosphokinase (Creatine Kinase)   ·   Lactic Dehydrogenase   ·   Hydroxybutyric Dehydrogenase   ·   Aspartate Aminotransferase   ·   Alanine Aminotransferase   ·   Gamma-Glutamyl Transferase   ·   5′-Nucleotidase

LIPIDS   201
Cholesterol   ·   Triglycerides   ·   Lipoproteins   ·   Free Fatty Acids, Phospholipids, and Total Lipids

LIVER FUNCTION TESTS   213

MISCELLANEOUS TESTS   214
Ascorbic Acid   ·   Carotene and Vitamin A   ·   Copper   ·   Zinc

NONPROTEIN NITROGEN COMPOUNDS   219
Blood Ammonia   ·   Blood Urea Nitrogen   ·   Creatinine   ·   Blood Urea Nitrogen/Creatinine Ratio   ·   Uric Acid

SERUM PROTEINS   230
Total Protein, Albumin, and Globulins   ·   Immunoglobulins   ·   Serum Protein Electrophoresis and Immunoelectrophoresis

TUMOR MARKERS   241
α-Fetoprotein   ·   Carcinoembryonic Antigen

Accurate chemical analysis of blood and urine composition is a valuable tool in recognizing certain changes caused by disease. Because blood and other body fluid components must remain within rather narrow limits for the body to function properly, variations can indicate many pathologic or physiologic conditions. The normal balance of electrolytes, enzymes, hormones, proteins, carbohydrates, and other constituents may easily be disturbed during disease by many factors that influence their rate of formation and their utilization or removal. Any change in the structure or function of organs such as the lungs, liver, or kidneys may alter the concentration of the chemical constituents of blood and urine.

SPECIMEN COLLECTION AND HANDLING

Specimen Types

Urine is used as a specimen in certain chemistry procedures, especially those concerned with the measurement of kidney function and hormone metabolites. (The procedure for collecting urine specimens is discussed in Chapter 1.)

Plasma, the liquid portion of anticoagulated blood, is an ideal specimen for most chemistry procedures, especially when heparin is used as the anticoagulant. **Serum**, the liquid portion of clotted blood, is also ideal for many chemical analyses because it avoids the potential interference that may result from the addition of various anticoagulants. Most procedures are equally accurate with either plasma or serum specimens, although serum must be used for a few determinations such as serum enzyme measurements or serum electrophoresis.

Whole blood has been practically eliminated as a specimen for chemistry procedures because the distribution of many blood constituents varies significantly between red blood cells and serum or plasma. This factor adds an unnecessary variable to laboratory determinations due to the inconsistent number of red blood cells in each specimen.

Anticoagulants Used to Prevent Clotting

An anticoagulant must be added to prevent clotting during specimen collection for laboratory tests that require plasma or whole blood. Several anticoagulants are available, but not all of them are equally satisfactory for every test because some may interfere with chemical reactions or alter morphologic characteristics of the formed elements. The following are the four most popular types of anticoagulants.

Oxalates include the single salts of sodium, potassium, or lithium and the double oxalate mixture of ammonium and potassium salts. Oxalates are used extensively in chemical determinations, although the double oxalate mixture may not be used for potassium or urea nitrogen determinations because it will cause erroneous test results. However, the double oxalate mixture frequently is used for a number of hematology procedures such as the mean corpuscular value, erythrocyte sedimentation rate, hematocrit, and red blood cell count which require that red blood cell size and shape be retained. Sodium oxalate often is used to prevent clotting in specimens for prothrombin time and other coagulation studies. All oxalates are toxic and must not be added to prevent clotting in blood that is to be used for transfusion therapy.

Heparin is available as a sodium, lithium, or ammonium salt. The form of heparin used for various laboratory determinations is governed by specific test requirements. Heparin is the best anticoagulant for preventing hemolysis and commonly is added to specimens for special hematology tests such as osmotic fragility, blood pigments, and the lupus erythematosus (LE) cell preparation because hemolyzed blood interferes with these results. Heparin is nontoxic and may be added to blood for transfusion therapy when multiple units of blood are required.

EDTA is available as sodium or potassium salts of ethylenediaminetetraacetic acid. EDTA is the preferred anticoagulant for all hematology procedures because it does not distort cellular morphology or produce cellular artifacts and vacuoles. EDTA is used for all red and white blood cell studies, as well as platelet counts and blood smears. EDTA is also nontoxic and may be added to blood for transfusion therapy.

Sodium citrate is the principal anticoagulant added to blood for transfusion therapy. Sodium citrate frequently is used to prevent clotting of blood for coagulation studies because it eliminates many of the problems caused by the other anticoagulants.

Collection Times

Most chemical components of blood are not changed significantly after a standard breakfast; therefore, it usually is not essential that the patient fast before blood specimens are collected. For example, an average breakfast has no significant effect on sodium, potassium, chloride, carbon dioxide, urea nitrogen, creatinine, total protein, albumin, cholesterol, cholesterol esters, calcium, and uric acid levels.

Chief exceptions to this rule are glucose, inorganic phosphorus, and triglyceride levels, which demonstrate significant variations when specimens are drawn following a meal. In addition, the plasma or serum turbidity produced by lipemia following a meal containing fat may interfere with the color reaction or accurate reading of many chemical determinations. Thus, it is good routine practice whenever possible, but especially for lipid determinations, to collect all blood specimens following a 12- to 14-hour overnight fast, although a 4- to 6-hour fast is usually sufficient.

It is also important that specimens for timed tests be obtained precisely at the specified intervals to overcome the effects of certain medications or physiologic variations. Tests for corticosteroids, serum iron, and glucose tolerance require timed specimens because diurnal or other metabolic effects may be anticipated. Likewise, specimens for therapy-monitoring tests such as the prothrombin time, activated partial thromboplastin time, and salicylate and digoxin levels must be collected at a specified time that is related to the dose of the medication administered.

Collection Tubes

All blood specimens should be collected in syringes or tubes that are chemically clean and free from organic and inorganic contaminants that may alter the results of a chemical analysis. Venipuncture is performed using either the syringe method, with the correct test tube immediately available to receive the blood, or the evacuated tube method, in which a needle is attached to a vacuum tube. Tubes are selected with or without the premeasured anticoagulant or other additive, depending on the test to be performed. A general listing of the type of tube and additives required for the collection of blood for many laboratory tests is presented in Appendix B, although a more thorough discussion is included whenever necessary under the specific tests.

Order of Specimen Draw

When multiple blood samples are drawn from the same patient in a single venipuncture, special attention must be given to the order in which the tubes are filled.

- **First draw**—blood culture tubes and sterile tubes to prevent possible contamination with nonsterile tube stoppers.
- **Second draw**—tubes with no additives to allow the specimens to clot undisturbed while the other specimens are being drawn.
- **Third draw**—tubes for coagulation studies.
- **Last draw**—tubes with additives to allow the specimens to mix with anticoagulants or preservatives immediately.

Performing a Venipuncture

The venous blood required for most laboratory procedures usually is collected from the veins of the forearm, wrist, or hand. The median cubital vein of the forearm is chosen most frequently in adults because it is larger, closer to the surface, easier to enter, and least painful for the patient. Veins located in the ankle or foot are also satisfactory for venipuncture but should not be used in patients with diabetes or cardiovascular or circulatory problems. However, the collection of blood specimens from routine venipuncture sites may not be possible in individuals with problematic veins such as extremely obese patients, infants and children, cardiac patients, and oncology or leukemia patients who require frequent blood testing.

Venipuncture should be performed in a calm, quiet, reassuring manner with the patient lying relaxed in bed or seated comfortably alongside a table. The patient must remain still with the arm extended and resting flat on the bed or supported firmly on the tabletop.

Precautions

Several common difficulties may interfere with the venipuncture procedure or cause blood specimens to become hemolyzed, which can invalidate laboratory results. To perform a successful venipuncture and prevent hemolysis, the nurse or venipuncture technician should observe the following precautions:

1. Do not use a healed burn site with extensive scarring for venipuncture because circulation may be impaired.
2. Do not collect blood specimens from the same side on which a mastectomy has been performed because lymphostasis may interfere with truly representative specimens.
3. Do not perform a venipuncture in an area adjacent to a hematoma because poor circulation in this region may cause erroneous test results. However, if another venipuncture site is not available, the specimen may be collected distal to the hematoma.
4. Avoid prolonged use of the tourniquet because excessive venous stasis can falsely elevate the concentration of red blood cells, plasma protein, and plasma-bound constitu-

ents such as calcium and hormones. Hemoconcentration also can increase the plasma concentration of such intracellular contents as potassium and lactic acid.

5. Collect all blood specimens from the arm opposite an intravenous infusion site because blood drawn above an intravenous site will be diluted by the fluid being administered. Various constituents in the intravenous fluid may cause local concentrations that are not an accurate indication of amounts circulating in the rest of the body. However, if intravenous lines are running in both arms and no other venipuncture site can be found, satisfactory samples may be drawn below the intravenous site if the following procedures are followed:

    a. Ask the primary nurse to temporarily slow the intravenous infusion to a minimal drip rate that will maintain patency (nursing personnel must be aware that the administration of fluid has been interrupted).

    b. Wait 2 minutes and then apply the tourniquet below the intravenous site; select a vein other than the one with the intravenous line.

    c. Perform the venipuncture; withdraw 5 mL of blood and discard.

    d. Draw the blood sample for the test; apply a firm, but not tight, bandage after withdrawing the needle.

    e. Ask the primary nurse to readjust the rate of flow of the intravenous infusion.

    f. Note on the laboratory request slip that the sample was drawn below an intravenous site.

6. Prevent moisture in or contamination of needles, syringes, or blood containers.

7. Do not use excessive traction on the syringe plunger, especially with a small-lumen needle. A 20-gauge needle with minimum suction should be used for trauma-free blood collection.

8. Avoid leakage of air into the tube or syringe during specimen collection because this can produce foaming and cause cells to hemolyze.

9. Do not expel blood through the needle from the syringe into another container because forcing the blood out of the syringe vigorously causes hemolysis. Instead, remove the needle from the syringe and allow the blood to flow gently into the containers.

10. Do not shake the blood vigorously in the container to mix it with the anticoagulant. Mix the blood by gently inverting the tube or container six to eight times.

11. Do not agitate a tube of blood that does not contain an anticoagulant.

▶▶ *Nursing Responsibilities and Implications*

1. Identify the patient to ensure that the blood specimen is drawn from the individual designated on the request form.

2. Select the appropriate evacuated tube or the correct syringe and test tube, depending on the test to be performed.

3. Select either a 20- or 21-gauge needle for veins of the forearm and a 25-gauge needle for veins of the wrist, hand, or ankle (remember, the larger the needle gauge number, the smaller the needle bore).

4. Apply the tourniquet or blood pressure cuff just above the bend in the arm to enlarge the veins and make them more prominent. Instruct the patient to make a fist and

maintain it as the vein to be used is located. However, vigorously pumping the fist before and during venipuncture may increase the concentration of certain blood constituents and falsely alter certain test results.

5. Select the site for venipuncture by palpating the area below the tourniquet. This step should be performed as quickly as possible because prolonged use of the tourniquet can cause venous stasis and falsely elevate the concentration of many blood constituents.

6. Cleanse the venipuncture site with 70% alcohol or any other disinfectant such as povidone-iodine (Betadine) and allow the site to dry. Once the area has been cleansed, do not palpate the vein again.

7. Enter the skin and vein in a single motion with the needle held bevel side up and pointing in exactly the same direction as the path of the vein. Hold the syringe or evacuated tube in the vein so that it makes a 15-degree angle with the patient's arm. A proper angle of entry is important because the needle will slide along the top of the vein if the angle is too shallow and will go through the vein if the angle is too great. It is much easier to enter the vein cleanly if the vein is stabilized by placing the thumb below the proposed point of entry and applying downward pressure.

8. Remove the tourniquet once the blood begins to flow freely into the tube or syringe. Prolonged application of the tourniquet, even for 60 seconds, produces hemoconcentration, which measurably increases blood test values.

9. Instruct the patient to open the fist as the needle is removed. Immediately apply gentle pressure to the venipuncture site with a sterile pad to stop the bleeding and prevent hematoma formation.

10. Remove the needle from the syringe and immediately transfer the blood into the proper tube. Immediately cover and gently mix the tube if an anticoagulant is being used to prevent clotting.

11. Carefully label all tubes with the patient's name and room number and deliver them to the laboratory as soon as possible.

Preserving and Processing Blood Specimens

All chemical analyses ideally should be performed within 1 hour after the blood is collected because the concentrations of many blood constituents change rapidly if the specimen is allowed to stand at room temperature for an extended period of time. Prolonged contact of serum or plasma with the red blood cells results in glycolysis and the continued metabolism of blood glucose, as well as a shift of intracellular constituents into the serum or plasma.

Precautions
When a blood specimen cannot be transported to the laboratory shortly after collection or prompt laboratory testing is not possible, the following precautions should be observed:

1. Separate serum or plasma from cells and refrigerate as soon as possible. If serum or plasma specimens must be retained for an extended period of time, they should be frozen because freezing preserves nearly all chemical constituents.

2. DO NOT FREEZE whole blood because this causes red blood cells to rupture.

3. Chill blood immediately in an ice bath when the specimen must be retained for several hours and it is not possible to separate serum or plasma from the cells. Refrigeration also is helpful in slowing down glycolysis and other enzymatic or bacteriologic processes. However, cooling may proceed very slowly, especially if several tubes are placed together in a small container, which allows significant chemical changes to occur.

4. DO NOT CHILL freshly collected blood until it has clotted.

5. Add thymol or fluoride to preserve the blood specimen when glucose analysis will be delayed or specimen will be sent to a commercial laboratory. Fluoride inhibits glycolysis as well as all other enzyme action; therefore, these specimens cannot be used for enzyme determinations. Fluoride, however, does not prevent glycolysis in bacterially contaminated specimens.

AUTOMATION IN THE CHEMISTRY LABORATORY

Advances in automation and technology have made it possible to perform many chemistry tests simultaneously from very small specimen samples and more quickly than with other methods. Some automated systems have become so well known that the combination of tests performed from a single specimen has become synonymous with a laboratory test. One example is Technicon's SMA 12/60 (Sequential Multiple Analyzer), which performs 12 different chemistry studies on each specimen at a rate of 60 specimens per hour. The SMAC (SMA with computer) is another type of analyzer that offers an even wider variety of tests and performs 20 chemical determinations on 150 specimens within 1 hour. These groups of tests include several from each of the screening panels so that most organs or body systems are represented in a single procedure. Several variable selection analyzers perform as many or more procedures than the SMA and give added flexibility to laboratory testing. These discrete sampling systems offer the option of running the complete battery of tests in one system or performing any combination of tests on each specimen. (See Appendix A for a complete discussion of organ panels.)

CARBOHYDRATES

Carbohydrates, which exist mainly in the form of glucose circulating in the bloodstream from dietary starch and sugars, are the primary source of energy for all body functions. Most carbohydrates are ingested in the form of starch from grains, vegetables, or legumes, including rice, wheat, corn, and potatoes. The other important dietary source of carbohydrates is sugar, including fructose and pentoses (contained in fruits), lactose (found in milk and milk products), and sucrose (contributed by sugar cane and sugar beets).

These various forms of carbohydrates are interconverted to glucose by several intestinal enzymes during digestion; glucose is then made available to all body tissues by insulin from the pancreas. Adequate amounts of insulin are necessary from the beta cells of the islets of Langerhans in the pancreas to make circulating glucose available to body tissues to fuel metabolism. Insufficient or ineffective insulin supplies deprive cells of their energy source, which results in an increased level of circulating glucose.

Additional causes of elevated blood glucose levels include increased secretion of other hormones such as epinephrine, hydrocortisone, glucagon, thyroxine, and the growth hormone. Thus, abnormal blood glucose levels frequently are good indicators of hormone imbalance. Glucose metabolism also is controlled by the liver, which stores excess glucose in the form of glycogen for use as a reserve energy source. When the glucose supply is insufficient to meet energy demands, the body compensates by synthesizing glucose from amino acids and fatty acid fragments.

The detection of disorders involving glucose metabolism, particularly diabetes mellitus, rests mainly on the measurement of glucose either in the fasting state or following the controlled ingestion of glucose. The diagnosis of diabetes mellitus is based on laboratory procedures to identify and classify patients with carbohydrate metabolic disorders and accurate interpretation of test results to determine the stage of disease. However, the blood glucose levels of many healthy individuals also may be affected by several physiologic factors that are not related to any disease process, including:

Age—blood glucose levels tend to rise in older individuals.

Emotional state—fear and anxiety cause blood glucose levels to rise.

Dietary pattern—a low-carbohydrate diet several days before testing tends to dull the insulin response to a recent glucose load and can elevate blood glucose above its normal fasting level.

Exercise—normal exercise immediately before testing tends to decrease the blood glucose level slightly. However, if the exercise is accompanied by excitement, glucose levels may rise.

Fasting—a 48-hour fast before the test reduces blood glucose levels significantly below normal fasting levels.

Laboratory determination of glucose levels can be divided into two categories: enzymatic tests, which are most specific for glucose, and chemical tests, which depend on the reducing properties of glucose. Because most automated laboratory procedures in current use involve enzymatic reactions, test results normally reflect true glucose values. However, many older chemical test methods are nonspecific for glucose because they measure all reducing substances present in the blood that react in the same manner as glucose. Newer dipstick tests for blood glucose have glucose oxidase reagent imbedded in the pad to greatly reduce the incidence of false positive results.

The fasting blood glucose determination, the most frequently ordered test of carbohydrate metabolism, and the 2-hour postprandial glucose determination are effective screening tests for diabetes mellitus. Individuals who exhibit abnormal values with either test should be evaluated further with a glucose tolerance test. (Urine tests for glucose are discussed in Chapter 1.) A newer study, the glycosylated hemoglobin test, provides an index of long-term glucose control by reflecting the time-averaged glucose level in diabetic patients during the preceding 3−8 weeks.

Fasting Blood Glucose

The **fasting blood glucose**, also known as the fasting blood sugar (FBS), is the most specific but least sensitive method for diagnosing diabetes mellitus. A fasting blood glucose should be the first test used as part of a routine screening procedure to detect diabetes mellitus when symptoms are present. Fasting blood glucose test values also are used to evaluate the current status of diabetics.

Clinical Significance
Glucose test results are classified as hyperglycemic or hypoglycemic. Both definitions, however, are arbitrary, and there is no clear-cut distinction between normal and abnormal. Although normal test results rule out significant diabetic problems, they do not completely exclude the possibility of diabetes because only 30%−40% of individuals with diabetes can be diagnosed by a fasting blood glucose. For example, most individuals with prediabetes or mild, latent, or adult-onset diabetes show fasting blood glucose values within the normal range, although they are diabetic by definition. In addition, fasting blood glucose results alone are inadequate to detect some hypoglycemic conditions.

Normal Values
The normal and clinically significant values for fasting blood glucose are:

50−110 mg/dL	Normal following an overnight fast
110−120 mg/dL	Significant; should be monitored regularly
120−140 mg/dL	Borderline; indicates possibility of diabetes mellitus
>140 mg/dL	Diagnostic for diabetes mellitus

Variations
Elevated fasting blood glucose levels (mild hyperglycemia; 120−150 mg/dL) may be caused by:

Eclampsia

Endocrine disorders (hyperthyroidism, hyperpituitarism, hyperadrenalism):

  Acromegaly

  Adrenal pheochromocytoma

  Cushing's disease

  Infections, acute and chronic

  Injury, acute

  Myocardial infarction

Pancreatic carcinoma, pancreatitis, pancreatic insufficiency

Shock

Steroid drugs

Stress, emotional

Trauma

Hypertension

Obesity

Pregnancy

Thiazide diuretics

Moderate hyperglycemia (200–500 mg/dL) may be caused by:

Anesthesia

Carbon monoxide poisoning

Infectious diseases

Intracranial diseases, cerebral lesions (convulsions, cerebrovascular accident, encephalitis, meningitis, hemorrhage, skull fracture, tumors)

Marked hyperglycemia (>500 mg/dL) is always associated with diabetes mellitus. **Decreased fasting blood glucose levels (hypoglycemia**; <65 mg/dL) may be caused by:

Cold, exposure to severe

Exercise, strenuous

Fever, prolonged

Liver disease, extensive (advanced cirrhosis)

Hyperinsulinemia (insulin overdose, pancreatic lesion [beta-cell adenoma])

Hypoadrenalism (Addison's disease)

Hypopituitarism (Simmonds' disease)

Hypothyroidism (cretinism, myxedema)

Malnutrition, starvation

Vomiting, severe

von Gierke's disease (glycogen storage disease)

Methodology

Fasting blood glucose determinations require 5 mL of blood collected without anti-coagulants (red-stoppered tube) after an overnight fast. Specimens collected following a 12- to 14-hour fast show less variation than specimens collected at other times during the day. When blood cannot be processed within 1 hour after collection, 2 mg of sodium fluoride should be added for each milliliter of blood and the specimen refrigerated to prevent glycolysis for 48 hours.

Precautions

To ensure an adequate specimen for a fasting blood glucose test, the following precautions should be observed:

1. Delay specimen collection for glucose determination, whenever possible, if the patient has taken any medication within the previous 24 hours that might affect glucose physiologically or interfere chemically with certain test procedures. **Falsely increased** glucose test values may be caused by:

Acetaminophen

ACTH (corticosteroids)

Ascorbic acid

Dextran

Epinephrine

Ethacrynic acid

Furosemide

Hydralazine

Isoproterenol

L-dopa

Mercaptopurine

Methimazole

Methyldopa

Nalidixic acid

Oxazepam

Para-aminosalicylic acid

Phenytoin

Propylthiouracil

Tetracycline

Thiazide diuretics

Tolbutamide

Falsely decreased glucose values may be caused by:

Ascorbic acid	Isoniazid	Phenazopyridine
Chlorpropamide	Nitrazepam	Phenformin
Hydralazine	Para-aminosalicylic acid	Propranolol
Isocarboxazid	Phenacetin	

2. Deliver the specimens to the laboratory for prompt analysis because continued metabolism of red and white blood cells may decrease glucose values 5%−7% per hour when blood stands at room temperature.

▶▶ *Nursing Responsibilities and Implications*

1. Withhold all foods and fluids (except water) after midnight until the blood specimen is collected.
2. Withhold the patient's insulin injection until the specimen is drawn.
3. Deliver the blood specimen to the laboratory within 30 minutes after collection so that serum can be separated promptly from the red blood cells. Once the cells have been removed, glucose levels remain stable in unhemolyzed serum for 8 hours at room temperature and 72 hours at 4 C.
4. If the procedure is for screening purposes, inform the patient that additional tests probably will be done if the glucose level is elevated.

Two-Hour Postprandial Glucose

The **2-hour postprandial blood glucose**, the most sensitive screening test of carbohydrate metabolism, is more reliable in detecting diabetes mellitus than the fasting blood glucose. Once glucose is absorbed into the bloodstream, glucose concentrations normally rise to peak values of 120−150 mg/dL within 60−90 minutes after a meal and return to fasting levels within 2 hours. Conversely, glucose concentrations in individuals with diabetes mellitus approach fasting levels only after an extended period of time, and significantly increased 2-hour postprandial glucose test values are found in diabetics.

Laboratory measurement of 2-hour postprandial glucose levels frequently is used to screen for diabetes, diagnose diabetes mellitus, and monitor glucose control. In addition, repeatedly normal 2-hour postprandial glucose values may rule out the diagnosis of diabetes mellitus. However, this procedure is not useful in diagnosing hypoglycemia.

Clinical Significance

The significance of 2-hour postprandial glucose levels is limited by the absence of rigidly controlled conditions, including the amount of carbohydrate ingested, the patient's age, and any intercurrent infections. For example, test interpretation occasionally may be difficult because of variations in the number of calories ingested in addition to abnormally rapid or slow rates of carbohydrate absorption. The interpretation of test results also must take into account such factors as previous diet, drugs, or hormonal disease, as well as the patient's age (glucose levels may be slightly higher in older individuals). Therefore, the diagnostic value of the 2-hour postprandial glucose test is debatable, and elevated or borderline results warrant a glucose tolerance test.

Normal Values
The normal and clinically significant values for a 2-hour postprandial glucose test are:

Diagnosis of diabetes mellitus

<140 mg/dL	Normal
>140 mg/dL	Requires further evaluation
<160 mg/dL	Normal in individuals over 60 years of age
>160 mg/dL	Suggests diabetes mellitus or a hormone imbalance
>200 mg/dL	Diagnostic of diabetes mellitus

Monitoring glucose control

<130 mg/dL	Good control
>150 mg/dL	Poor control

Variations
Increased 2-hour postprandial glucose levels (>160 mg/dL) may occur in:

Acromegaly	Diabetes mellitus	Pancreatitis, chronic
Cirrhosis, advanced	Hyperthyroidism	Pheochromocytoma
Cushing's disease	Malnutrition	

Decreased 2-hour postprandial glucose levels (<65 mg/dL) may occur in:

Addison's disease

Hyperinsulinism (islet-cell adenoma)

Pituitary insufficiency, anterior

Steatorrhea, idiopathic

von Gierke's disease (glycogen storage disease)

Methodology
Measurement of 2-hour postprandial glucose values requires 5 mL of blood collected in a tube without anticoagulants (red-stoppered tube) exactly 2 hours after the patient has ingested a standardized glucose load. Specimens must be delivered to the laboratory promptly to prevent a decrease in test values due to glycolysis.

Precautions
To ensure accurate 2-hour postprandial glucose test results, the following precautions should be observed:

1. Make certain that all pretest dietary regulations are followed as ordered.

2. Deliver the specimens to the laboratory promptly because continued metabolism by red and white blood cells may decrease glucose values 5%–7% per hour when blood stands at room temperature.

▶▶ *Nursing Responsibilities and Implications*

1. Provide the patient with a high-carbohydrate diet for 2−3 days prior to the test.

2. Withhold food and fluids (except water) for 8 hours before testing.

3. Give the patient a 50−100 g glucose load or a high-carbohydrate meal (containing 75−100 g of carbohydrate) on the day of the test. A breakfast of orange juice, cereal with sugar, toast with butter, and milk supplies sufficient calories and carbohydrates for proper test interpretation. However, the 2-hour postprandial glucose test produces higher, more sensitive results following a glucose load than tests performed after a high-carbohydrate meal or a mixed carbohydrate and protein meal.

4. Collect a single blood specimen for glucose determination exactly 2 hours after the meal or glucose load.

5. Understand that this test also may be performed after a high-carbohydrate lunch or noontime glucose load.

Glucose Tolerance Test

The **glucose tolerance test** (GTT) is a sensitive test designed to measure carbohydrate metabolism by evaluating insulin response to a glucose load. This procedure is based on the fact that in nondiabetics a test load of glucose will be removed from the bloodstream faster than it will in diabetics. During glucose absorption, the blood glucose level normally peaks at 160−180 mg/dL within 30 minutes to 1 hour after glucose ingestion, triggering the release of insulin, and returns to fasting levels or below within 2−3 hours. In diabetics, however, blood glucose values peak at much higher levels and are slower to return to fasting levels because of an inadequate insulin response to the glucose.

The glucose tolerance test is therefore a valuable diagnostic tool in diabetes mellitus because it gives a more complete picture of glucose metabolism than either the 2-hour postprandial glucose test or the fasting blood glucose test. The fasting, 1-, and 2-hour samples provide the most relevant information for routine use. Specimens must be obtained at 3, 4, 5, and 6 hours if postprandial hypoglycemia or the malabsorption syndrome is suspected. Glucose tolerance tests, on the other hand, are usually contraindicated for diagnostic purposes in patients with a fasting blood glucose level above 140 mg/dL or a 2-hour postprandial glucose level above 180 mg/dL.

Clinical Significance

The standard **oral glucose tolerance test** is the most widely used, sensitive, and practical test for the diagnosis of latent or asymptomatic diabetes mellitus. However, the significance of test findings may be reduced by pregnancy, endocrine disorders, prolonged physical inactivity, infectious diseases, surgical or other trauma, acute illness, and pyrexia. In addition, there is no consensus as to what constitutes an abnormal glucose response because the test outcome may be influenced by diet as well as other test variables.

An **intravenous glucose tolerance test** should be used to diagnose diabetes mellitus in patients who are unable to ingest an oral glucose load. In addition, the intravenous procedure eliminates the variable glucose utilization that accompanies impaired or erratic absorption from the gastrointestinal tract, which influences insulin response. Thus, the intravenous glucose tolerance test should be used in patients with conditions that produce virtually flat oral glucose tolerance curves such as sprue, celiac disease, gastric resection, Addison's disease, hypopituitarism, or hypothyroidism. This method is also advantageous in individuals with thyrotoxicosis, a condition in which a hyperglycemic curve is produced as a result of accelerated absorption, and organic or functional hyperin-sulinism, in which the full glucose dose enters the system.

The **cortisone glucose tolerance test**, a special procedure that is rarely used, may accentuate carbohydrate intolerance and be helpful in detecting latent or subclinical diabetes because cortisone promotes gluconeogenesis. It is performed the same way as the standard glucose tolerance test, except that two doses of cortisone are added prior to the orally administered glucose dose. The cortisone induces a chemical stress that affects glucose tolerance similar to the effect that occurs during pregnancy and produces blood glucose levels that are somewhat higher than those that occur with the standard glucose tolerance test. However, the prognostic implications of this test are uncertain.

Normal Values

The normal and clinically significant values for the glucose tolerance test are:

Oral Glucose Tolerance Test

Normal

Fasting blood glucose	80 mg/dL
½-hour blood glucose	155 mg/dL
1-hour blood glucose	165 mg/dL
1½-hour blood glucose	150 mg/dL
2-hour blood glucose	120 mg/dL
3-hour blood glucose	80 mg/dL
Urine glucose	Negative

Suggestive of diabetes mellitus

1-hour blood glucose	>185 mg/dL
1½-hour blood glucose	>160 mg/dL
2-hour blood glucose	>140 mg/dL
Urine glucose	Positive

Intravenous Glucose Tolerance Test

Normal

Fasting blood glucose	80 mg/dL
5-minute blood glucose	250 mg/dL
½-hour blood glucose	150 mg/dL
1-hour blood glucose	80 mg/dL

Suggestive of diabetes mellitus

2-hour blood glucose	>80 mg/dL

Cortisone Glucose Tolerance Test

Normal

2-hour blood glucose	<140 mg/dL

Suggestive of diabetes mellitus

2-hour blood glucose	>140 mg/dL

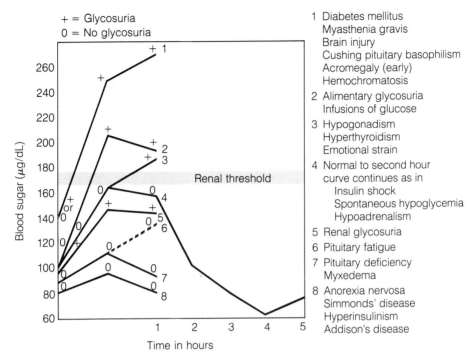

Figure 4-1 Glucose tolerance curves. (From Bauer, J., 1982. CLINICAL LABORATORY METHODS. 9th ed. St. Louis: The C. V. Mosby Co.)

Interpretation

Several systems for interpreting glucose tolerance test results take into account not only the highest blood glucose level attained during testing but also the pattern of test values after the peak. A correction factor for older individuals is recommended to prevent the false diagnosis of mild diabetes in persons whose blood glucose levels are actually normal for their age. Normal test values should be increased by 10–15 mg/dL for individuals in their 60s and by 20–30 mg/dL for those in their 70s.

In general, patients with diabetes mellitus demonstrate:

1. Elevated fasting blood glucose levels along with glycosuria in the fasting urine specimen.

2. Glucose peak values higher than the peak values of a healthy person.

3. Glucose peak values that persist for longer than normal—frequently as long as 4 hours.

4. Urine specimens that exhibit glycosuria in degrees that parallel blood glucose values.

Abnormal glucose curves usually are diagnostic of diabetes mellitus, although various other curves indicate the presence of additional diseases (Figure 4-1). Healthy individuals on a low-carbohydrate, quick weight-loss diet may exhibit a diabetic-type response (abnormal increase in the blood glucose level and delayed decrease) because the pancreas has been unaccustomed to coping with a high-carbohydrate load. Conversely, a patient whose diet contains an extremely high carbohydrate concentration will have an abnormally low blood glucose curve (small increase in the blood glucose level and small decrease).

Methodology

The glucose tolerance test requires 5 mL of blood collected in a tube without anti-coagulants (red-stoppered tube) immediately before glucose administration and at carefully timed intervals thereafter. Blood samples should be delivered to the laboratory within 30 minutes after collection to allow prompt separation of serum from the red blood cells and prevent glycolysis. When blood will be retained in the laboratory for the simultaneous analysis of all samples, specimens may be collected in a tube containing a glycolytic inhibitor (gray-stoppered tube) or 2 mg of sodium fluoride per milliliter of blood. A urine specimen must be obtained at the same time as the fasting and 30, 60, 120, and 180 minute blood samples.

The glucose tolerance test must be performed under rigidly controlled conditions for meaningful test values to be obtained. For example, to obtain a true test response, the patient must consume a regular diet containing adequate amounts of carbohydrate for several days prior to testing. Therefore, the presence of anorexia or other conditions that prevent adequate food intake, such as severe weight-loss diets, automatically invalidate the test.

In addition, the patient must avoid alcohol, tea, and coffee during the 12 hours prior to testing and must not smoke or exercise, even mildly, during testing. The patient also should discontinue the use of many drugs for at least 3 days prior to testing; oral contraceptives should be omitted for at least one complete cycle before this procedure is performed. The glucose tolerance test should be performed only on ambulatory patients because prolonged inactivity, such as extended bedrest, may reduce glucose tolerance and produce inaccurate test results. In addition, the test should not be performed on patients who have had an infectious disease, surgery, or other trauma during the 2 weeks prior to testing.

Precautions

A number of drugs are known to interfere with the glucose tolerance test and must be considered when patients receiving them are evaluated for hyperglycemia or hypoglycemia. Because the methods of glucose determination and the types of drugs in common clinical use keep changing, it is often difficult to state the effects of a particular compound on a given method or the physiology of the patient. However, an abnormal glucose tolerance curve may occur with the following drugs:

Acetazolamide	Estrogens	Phenytoin
Alcohol	Nicotinic acid	Reserpine
Ascorbic acid	Oral contraceptives	Salicylates
Corticosteroids	Phenylbutazone	Thiazide diuretics
Diazoxide		

▶▶ Nursing Responsibilities and Implications

To ensure accurate oral glucose tolerance test results, the nurse should proceed as follows:

1. Discontinue drugs such as oral contraceptives, large doses of salicylates, thiazide diuretics, and steroids for at least 3 days before the test.

2. Make sure the patient has eaten a regular diet containing at least 150 g of carbohydrate per day for at least 3 days before the test.

3. Discontinue hypoglycemic drugs (insulin or sulfonylureas) at least on the day of the test. When these drugs must be administered on the day of testing, their effect must be considered in the interpretation of the test results.

4. Make sure the patient did not consume any alcohol the evening before the test.

5. Make sure the patient has not eaten any food since midnight and continues to fast during the entire test period. Remind the patient that drinking tea and coffee is considered breaking the fast, although water should be encouraged to produce urine specimens as required.

6. Obtain a fasting blood sample for glucose determination in a tube containing sodium fluoride and thymol for anticoagulation and preservation. This is important because frequently all blood samples are retained until the end of the test period to allow simultaneous testing of specimens.

7. Obtain a fasting urine specimen for glucose and acetone determinations.

8. Make certain the patient's fasting glucose level is determined before the test because fasting hyperglycemia contraindicates a large test load of glucose. Notify the physician if fasting hyperglycemia is present.

9. Make certain the test begins between 7 and 9 AM after the patient has been fasting for at least 8 hours and not more than 16 hours.

10. Caution the patient to remain in the room during the test period to assure availability at the proper times and to minimize exercise, which could affect the glucose level. Outpatients should remain in quiet, comfortable surroundings during the test period.

11. Caution the patient not to smoke during the test period because smoking produces physiologic stimulation, which may alter the test results.

12. Give the patient the glucose test dose at the rate of 40 g/m^2 of body surface area as calculated by a nomogram based on height and weight. A test dose based on 1.75 g of glucose per kilogram of body weight or a standard adult dose of 100 g of glucose is also satisfactory. Encourage the patient to consume the entire amount within 5 minutes and note the exact time of administration because all specimen collections are based on the time of glucose intake.

13. Make certain that blood and urine specimens are collected 30, 60, 120, and 180 minutes after glucose intake, although some procedures require a 90-minute specimen or a 4- and 5-hour specimen. Record the actual time of each voiding on the specimen slip because the patient may not always be able to void at the scheduled time. A few milliliters of urine for each timed collection is sufficient for laboratory testing. Results of urine testing do not affect the diagnosis but give information about the renal threshold, which is necessary for planning successful patient therapy.

14. Observe the patient for any signs of impending hypoglycemic shock or coma such as headache, irrational speech or behavior, fainting, or profuse sweating, especially during the 5-hour glucose tolerance test. Report any unfavorable patient reaction, such as excessive nausea, vomiting, weakness, fainting, giddiness, or undue sweating, and terminate the procedure immediately. These symptoms require immediate remedial action from the nurse or medical staff.

Nursing responsibilities for patient preparation and the test procedure for the intravenous glucose tolerance test are similar to those for the oral method, with the following exceptions:

1. Make sure that the patient has eaten a regular diet containing 300 g of carbohydrate daily for 3 days prior to the test.

2. Administer an intravenous infusion of 0.5 g of 50% glucose solution per kilogram of body weight over 2−4 minutes. A standard dose of 50 mL of 50% glucose solution is also satisfactory. The nurse should begin timing the test exactly halfway through the injection.

3. Obtain blood and urine specimens for glucose determinations immediately after completing the glucose injection.

4. Collect additional blood and urine specimens 1, 2, 5, 10, 20, 30, 60, 90, and 120 minutes after the end of the infusion.

Glycohemoglobin Test

Glycohemoglobin, also known as glycosylated hemoglobin, is a compound composed of glucose bound irreversibly to hemoglobin A that accumulates within circulating erythrocytes and remains throughout their life span. The amount of glycohemoglobin formed and stored in the red blood cells depends on the concentration of glucose present in the plasma during the life span of the erythrocyte. Glycohemoglobin values therefore are very revealing of the true degree of hyperglycemia because they represent the average of many glucose determinations taken at frequent intervals over the preceding 120 days. Thus, diabetics with a higher than normal glucose concentration will also have an increased concentration of glycohemoglobin in their red blood cells.

Laboratory determination of glycohemoglobin provides a reliable index of glucose control and helps to evaluate the effectiveness of long-term dietary or insulin therapy in diabetics. However, because glycohemoglobin values do not reflect recent glucose changes, the test is less useful than plasma glucose values in monitoring acute changes in glycemic control such as diabetic ketoacidosis. In addition, glycohemoglobin test values do not appear to be any more useful in the diagnosis of diabetes mellitus than the fasting blood glucose and oral glucose tolerance tests.

Clinical Significance

Glycohemoglobin concentrations do not fluctuate with acute variations in glucose concentration because they are unaffected by the recent ingestion of sugar-containing substances, exercise, or antidiabetic drugs on the day of testing. Thus, individuals with diabetes may have normal glucose values after temporarily decreasing their glucose intake or increasing their exercise prior to the test, which could lead to the false assumption that the patient's condition is under control at home. Normal glycohemoglobin levels, however, indicate good control over a prolonged period of time, whereas elevated values show that poor control has existed for many weeks prior to testing.

Glycohemoglobin determinations are most significant when performed at 2- to 3-month intervals because the test values of diabetics with poorly controlled disease will approach the normal range within 5−8 weeks when treatment is carefully controlled.

Newly diagnosed diabetics and those with poorly controlled disease frequently exhibit glycohemoglobin values that are two to three times the normal test levels; the higher the percentage, the greater the severity of the disease. Elevated glycohemoglobin concentrations also indicate the pathogenesis of many diabetic complications, including neuropathy, cataracts, microangiopathy, leukocyte and platelet dysfunction, skin lesions, myopathy, and cardiocerebrovascular disease.

Normal Values

The normal and clinically significant glycohemoglobin values are:

Percentage of total hemoglobin

5.5%–8.5%	Normal, nondiabetic
8.5%–12%	Transitional, unknown significance
>9.5%	Poor glucose control
12%–20%	Uncontrolled diabetes
14.3%–20%	Ketoacidosis

Variations

Falsely increased glycohemoglobin levels may occur with a number of conditions that result in elevated hemoglobin F concentrations, including:

Fetal-maternal transfusion during pregnancy

Hereditary persistence of fetal hemoglobin (HPFH)

Neonatal period

Pregnancy, last trimester

Renal dialysis

Falsely decreased glycohemoglobin levels may occur with:

Hemolytic anemias	Renal failure, chronic
Pernicious anemia	Sickle cell anemia
Post splenectomy	Thalassemias

Methodology

Glycohemoglobin determinations require 5 mL of blood collected in a tube containing EDTA, heparin, or oxalate anticoagulant (lavender-, green-, or gray-stoppered tube). Specimens must be delivered to the laboratory promptly so that red blood cells can be separated from the plasma without delay. Red blood cell specimens remain stable for glycohemoglobin studies for 6 days when frozen.

▶▶ Nursing Responsibilities and Implications

1. Inform the patient that there are no food or fluid restrictions.

2. Collect the blood specimen with a minimum of hemostasis or hemolysis and deliver the tube to the laboratory as soon as possible.

D-Xylose Absorption Test

The **D-xylose absorption test**, a procedure used to diagnose malabsorption states, is helpful in differentiating between intestinal and pancreatic causes of steatorrhea. During the test, a standard test dose of D-xylose, which is not present in the blood, is administered orally and the amount excreted in the urine is measured. When D-xylose is administered to a normal individual, it is rapidly absorbed into the bloodstream from the intestine, a small amount is metabolized, and most is excreted in the urine. However, if there is a defect in the intestinal absorption process, D-xylose will not be absorbed into the blood-stream, and very little will be excreted in the urine. Intestinal absorption and urinary excre-tion of D-xylose proceed normally if the malabsorption and steatorrhea are the result of pancreatic malfunction because pancreatic enzymes are not needed for D-xylose absorption.

Clinical Significance

The D-xylose absorption test is most significant when blood D-xylose concentrations and urinary excretion levels are interpreted together to eliminate most of the false-positive and false-negative results. Few patients with disease of the small intestines demonstrate normal test results for both of these specimens, whereas few individuals without gastro-intestinal disorders have abnormal findings in both specimens.

Normal Values

The normal values for the D-xylose absorption test are:

Blood

1 hour	21−57 mg/dL
2 hours	32−58 mg/dL
3 hours	19−42 mg/dL
4 hours	11−29 mg/dL
5 hours	6−18 mg/dL

Urine

Normal	4−9 g/5 hours

Variations

False-positive D-xylose absorption may result from bacterial overgrowth in the intes-tines and a decreased rate of urinary excretion caused by impaired renal function. For example, a combination of low urinary xylose excretion and high blood levels may be caused by renal disease.

False-negative D-xylose absorption may occur in patients with celiac disease.

Methodology

The rate of D-xylose absorption is determined by measuring the concentration of D-xylose in blood and urine specimens collected for 5 hours after administering a 25 g test dose to a fasting patient. Measurement of D-xylose absorption requires 5 mL of blood collected in a tube containing oxalate anticoagulant (gray-stoppered tube) exactly 1 hour after ingestion of the test dose and after each additional hour of testing. Determination of D-xylose excretion requires a 25–100 mL aliquot of the total urine specimen collected during the 5-hour test period.

▶▶ **Nursing Responsibilities and Implications**

1. Instruct the patient to void immediately before the test period begins and to discard the urine.

2. Administer an oral test dose of 25 g of D-xylose in 500 mL of water after the patient has been fasting for 12 hours and note the exact time. (A test dose of 5 g of D-xylose may be substituted if the 25 g dose causes nausea or vomiting.)

3. Collect a blood specimen exactly 1, 2, 3, 4, and 5 hours after the administration of the D-xylose test dose.

4. Collect and refrigerate all urine voided during the 5-hour test period and write the total 5-hour volume on the laboratory request slip.

5. Send the entire urine specimen to the laboratory immediately after the test period ends.

Lactose Tolerance Test

The **lactose tolerance test** is a procedure designed to detect a deficiency of the digestive enzyme lactase in the small intestinal mucosa of individuals who exhibit an intolerance to milk and milk products. When lactase activity is adequate, lactose is converted to glucose and galactose for absorption into the bloodstream. However, inadequate lactase activity causes lactose intolerance, which is manifested by gastrointestinal discomfort and diarrhea following the ingestion of milk and relieved by eliminating milk from the diet.

Clinical Significance

An oral glucose tolerance test is performed to provide a baseline for comparison, and a lactose tolerance test is performed the next day. In the lactase tolerance procedure, an equal amount of lactose is substituted for the glucose, and blood samples are collected periodically to be analyzed for glucose concentration. If lactase activity and absorption are normal, digestion of the lactose will be reflected by an elevation of the blood glucose level, and similar glucose tolerance curves will be observed on both days. Conversely, if a patient has a lactase deficiency, the lactose tolerance curve will be flat and there will be an insignificant increase in the blood glucose level over the fasting glucose concentration.

Normal Values

The normal and clinically significant values for the lactose tolerance test are:

<20 mg/dL rise over the fasting glucose level	Lactase deficiency
20–50 mg/dL rise over the fasting glucose level	Normal, lactose tolerance

---

Variations

False-positive lactose tolerance test results may occur in patients whose blood glucose levels fail to rise 20 mg/dL within 1 hour because of slow gastric emptying.

Methodology

Lactose tolerance tests require 5 mL of blood collected in a tube containing an oxalate anticoagulant (gray-stoppered tube). This procedure requires a total of four blood specimens; one collected before testing begins and then ½ hour, 1 hour, and 2 hours after administration of the lactose test dose. It is important to conduct the test in an area with a bathroom nearby because some patients experience sudden and severe intestinal discomfort.

▶▶ Nursing Responsibilities and Implications

1. Follow the procedures for performing an oral glucose tolerance test to establish baseline values for the comparison of lactose tolerance test results. (See Glucose Tolerance Test—Nursing Responsibilities and Implications.)

2. On the following day, collect a fasting blood specimen from the patient (after a 12-hour fast).

3. Administer a test dose of lactose, using an amount of lactose that is equal to the test dose of glucose given the preceding day.

4. Collect blood specimens for glucose analysis exactly ½, 1, and 2 hours later.

5. Ensure easy access to a bathroom or bedpan during the test.

ENZYMES

Enzymes are complex proteins found in all body tissues that act as catalysts to speed the rate of many metabolic reactions. Each organ or structure contains its own characteristic enzymes that appear in the blood in increased concentrations when tissue cells are damaged or destroyed by trauma, infection, or infarction. The presence of significant quantities of these enzymes in the blood indicates the probable site of tissue damage because changes in enzyme concentrations reflect parallel changes in a specific organ or tissue.

Laboratory determinations of enzyme levels provide evidence of a disease process, indicate the location of the abnormality, evaluate the extent and severity of the illness, and identify the probable cause of the condition. Once a diagnosis has been established, enzyme values also help to monitor and control treatment and, whenever possible, substantiate clinical recovery. Abnormal enzyme values readily distinguish certain diseases from other clinically similar states in which abnormal enzyme levels do not occur. For example, enzyme concentrations distinguish myocardial infarction from other causes of chest pain, identify the recurrence of infarction, or aid in identifying additional complications during recovery. Enzyme determinations also aid in the differential diagnosis of hepatobiliary and muscle diseases, the diagnosis of pancreatitis, and the recognition of metastases to the liver or bones. Enzyme activity in various conditions is summarized in Table 4-1.

A simultaneous study of several enzymes frequently is necessary to localize the source of pathologic conditions because many enzymes are common to more than one type of tissue and most tissues contain more than one type of enzyme. Many enzymes are found in two or more slightly different forms known as **isoenzymes** that catalyze the same reaction but have unique chemical, structural, and physical properties. Identification of a specific isoenzyme provides diagnostic information about the organ responsible for the increased enzymatic activity because different proportions of various isoenzymes are found in each type of tissue.

Enzyme determinations have an advantage over most other clinical chemistry values in that they closely reflect intracellular processes rather than just the result of biochemical reactions. Enzyme levels commonly are expressed in units of activity rather than in milligrams or milliequivalents because actual concentrations are so low that the usual measurements are impractical. However, because standardized units to report enzyme concentration have not yet been established, a variety of units are still used for each enzyme.

Serum enzymes are easily destroyed by changes in pH or elevated temperature and remain stable outside the body for a limited time. Most enzymes remain stable when specimens are kept at room temperature for several hours or refrigerated for 24 hours, but the specimens must be frozen when laboratory analysis cannot be performed promptly. A more thorough discussion of specimen handling requirements is included whenever necessary with the individual tests.

Amylase

Amylase is a digestive enzyme produced by the pancreas and salivary glands that splits dietary starch into its component sugars, maltose and glucose. Certain types of pancreatic disease allow increased amounts of amylase to escape into surrounding tissues, where it is picked up by the blood and excreted in the urine. Laboratory determinations of amylase frequently are requested on an emergency basis for patients with severe abdominal pain to assist in distinguishing acute pancreatitis from other conditions requiring immediate surgery. Serum amylase studies also are frequently performed during the first few days following abdominal surgery to detect any inadvertent damage to the pancreas.

Clinical Significance
Serum amylase levels rise rapidly in acute pancreatitis and reach at least twice the normal value within 4–12 hours after the onset of symptoms, although levels remain high for only a short time. Serum amylase values also fall rapidly, returning to normal levels within 48–72 hours, even though active inflammation persists. On the other hand, urine amylase levels rise within several hours of a serum increase but remain elevated for about 1 week after an acute pancreatic episode. Therefore, urine amylase determinations provide a retrospective diagnosis of acute pancreatitis even after serum values have already declined. Patients with severe renal disease may have impaired excretion of amylase and retain it in the serum, causing serum amylase levels to remain elevated for a prolonged time.

Normal Values
The normal values for serum and urine amylase are:

Serum	60–180 Somogyi units/dL
	80–330 IU/L
	4–25 U/mL
Urine	35–260 Somogyi units/hr
	100–1600 IU/L

TABLE 4-1 Enzyme Activity in Specific Conditions

	Creatinine Phospho-kinase	Lactic Dehydro-genase	Hydroxy-butyric Dehydrogenase	Aspartate Aminotrans-ferase*	Alanine Aminotrans-ferase[†]
Liver					
Hepatitis	—	Increase	Increase	Very marked increase	Very marked increase
Infectious mono-nucleosis	—	Marked increase	Increase	Marked increase	Marked increase
Cirrhosis	—	Increase	Variable	Increase	Increase
Jaundice	—	Increase	Variable	Increase	Increase
Carcinoma	—	Marked increase	Increase	Increase	Increase
Heart					
Myocardial infarction (early)	Very marked increase	Increase	Increase	Increase	—
Myocardial in-farction (late)	Increase	Marked increase	Very marked increase	Marked increase	Variable
Muscle					
Dystrophy	Very marked increase	Marked increase	Variable	Marked increase	Marked increase
Bone	—	—	—	—	—
Pancreas	—	—	—	—	—
Prostate	—	—	—	—	—

*Formerly glutamic-oxaloacetic transaminase (GOT).
[†]Formerly glutamic-pyruvic transaminase (GPT).

Variations
Elevated serum amylase levels may occur with:

Diabetic ketoacidosis

Ectopic pregnancy, ruptured

Empyema of the gallbladder

Ethanol intoxication, acute

Gastroduodenal ulcers, perforated

Hyperthyroidism

Macroamylasemia

Narcotic analgesics

Obstruction, intestinal or pancreatic duct

Pancreatitis, acute

Pancreatic carcinoma

Pancreatic trauma

Peritonitis

Renal disease, severe

Salivary gland disease (i.e., mumps)

Splenic trauma, acute

Gamma-Glutamyl Transferase	Pseudo-cholin-esterase	Alkaline Phosphatase	Amylase	Lipase	Acid Phosphatase
Increase	Decrease	Increase	—	—	—
—	Decrease	Marked increase	—	—	—
Increase	Decrease	Increase	—	—	—
Marked increase	Variable	Very marked increase	—	—	—
Very marked increase	—	Marked increase	—	—	—
—	—	—	—	—	—
Marked increase	—	—	—	—	—
—	—	—	—	—	—
—	—	Marked increase	—	—	—
—	—	—	Marked increase	Marked increase	—
—	—	—	—	—	Marked increase

Decreased serum amylase levels may occur with:

Alcoholism, acute

Cirrhosis

Glucose administration

Hepatic carcinoma

Hepatitis

Liver disease (abscess, alcohol, carcinoma, cirrhosis, hepatitis)

Pancreatitis, chronic

Toxemia of pregnancy

Methodology

Serum amylase determinations require 5 mL of blood collected in a tube without anti-coagulants (red-stoppered tube). Amylase remains stable in serum specimens at room temperature for approximately 1 week and for several months when the specimens are refrigerated or frozen immediately after collection.

Urinary amylase measurements require an accurately timed urine specimen collected without preservatives during a 2-, 12-, or 24-hour period. Urinary amylase remains stable when specimens are refrigerated or stored on ice until they are sent to the laboratory.

Precautions

To ensure accurate serum and urinary amylase determinations, the following precautions should be observed:

1. Do not contaminate the specimen with saliva by coughing or sneezing near an open specimen container because saliva contains high amylase concentrations that can cause falsely elevated test results.

2. Delay the collection of blood and urine specimens if the patient has received any of the following drugs within the previous 24 hours:

Bethanechol	Ethanol	Morphine
Cholinergics	Indomethacin	Oral contraceptives
Codeine	Meperidine	Pentazocine
Diatrizoate sodium	Methacholine	Thiazide diuretics

▶▶ Nursing Responsibilities and Implications

1. Collect a blood specimen 2 hours after the patient has eaten and before any diagnostic measures using dyes or medications have been started.

2. Collect an accurately timed urine specimen as directed by the laboratory.
   a. Instruct the patient to empty the bladder and discard the urine at the beginning of the collection period.
   b. Save all subsequent urine voided, including urine obtained at the end of the collection period.
   c. Keep the specimen refrigerated or on ice until it can be sent to the laboratory.

3. Indicate on the laboratory request slip any drugs or intravenous glucose administered to the patient within 24 hours of testing.

Lipase

Lipase is a digestive enzyme produced by the pancreas that hydrolyzes or splits dietary fats and triglycerides into fatty acids and glycerol. Like amylase, lipase appears in the bloodstream following damage to pancreatic cells; serum levels rise 12–24 hours after the onset of symptoms. Thus, elevations of serum lipase usually parallel changes in serum amylase. Laboratory determination of serum lipase frequently is used in the diagnosis of acute pancreatitis or other pancreatic disorders.

Clinical Significance

Although serum levels of both amylase and lipase rise at approximately the same rate in pancreatic diseases, elevations in lipase concentration persist for as long as 10 days. Therefore, lipase values frequently are useful in the diagnosis and follow-up of acute pancreatitis when too much time has elapsed for amylase levels to remain elevated or after clinical symptoms have subsided.

Normal Values
The normal values for serum lipase, depending on the laboratory method used, are:

<1.5 units

30−125 IU

20−180 IU/L

Variations
Elevated serum lipase levels may occur with:

Cholecystitis, acute

Cirrhosis

Duodenal ulcers, perforated

Obstruction, pancreatic duct or high intestinal

Pancreatic carcinoma

Pancreatitis, acute

Renal disease with impaired excretion

Methodology
Serum lipase determinations require 5 mL of blood collected without trauma in a tube with no anticoagulants (red-stoppered tube). Lipase remains stable in serum specimens for 1 week at room temperature and for up to 6 weeks when refrigerated or frozen immediately after collection.

Precautions
To ensure accurate serum lipase determinations, the following precautions should be observed:

1. Prevent hemolysis of red blood cells during specimen collection because hemoglobin inhibits lipase activity and will cause inaccurate test results.

2. Delay the collection of blood specimens if the patient has received any of the following drugs within 24 hours:

Bethanechol

Cholinergics

Codeine

Meperidine

Methacholine

Morphine

Narcotics

Protamine

▶▶ Nursing Responsibilities and Implications

1. Collect the blood specimen after an overnight fast before the patient has eaten breakfast as a precaution because it has not been determined whether food interferes with lipase test results.

2. Indicate on the laboratory request slip any opiates or other narcotic drugs administered to the patient within 24 hours of testing.

Acid Phosphatase

Acid phosphatase, an enzyme found mainly in the prostate but also in the kidneys, spleen, liver, and erythrocytes, catalyzes the split of certain phosphate esters during several important body reactions. Small amounts of acid phosphatase occur normally in the blood, whereas prostatic tissue has a concentration 1000 times greater than other tissues. Elevated serum acid phosphatase levels therefore are a useful marker for the presence of advanced metastatic carcinoma of the prostate in which the tumor extends beyond the capsule surrounding the prostate gland.

Laboratory determinations of acid phosphatase concentrations usually are performed on men to establish or confirm a diagnosis of metastatic prostatic carcinoma and to assess the extent of known prostatic adenocarcinoma. The test also is useful in monitoring tumor regression or progression in response to treatment. Acid phosphatase determinations also may be performed on vaginal aspirates as part of the examination for alleged rape because seminal fluid receives high acid phosphatase concentrations from the prostate gland.

Clinical Significance

Significantly elevated serum acid phosphatase concentrations nearly always indicate prostatic cancer that has metastasized to bone, although concentrations also may be elevated with prostatic tumors that have not metastasized. Unfortunately, test values are of little help in detecting prostatic carcinoma in its early stages. Acid phosphatase levels decrease following a course of estrogen therapy, which generally indicates a favorable response; any subsequent increase in the serum acid phosphatase level usually heralds renewed metastatic activity.

Although the routine measurement of acid phosphatase isoenzymes has not proved clinically significant, a specific procedure that detects the prostatic acid phosphatase isoenzyme has recently gained acceptance. A slightly different form of acid phosphatase also has been found in women with cancer of the breast that has metastasized to bone.

Normal Values

The normal values for serum acid phosphatase, depending on the laboratory method used, are:

Total	2.5–11.7 IU/L, men
	0.3–9 IU/L, women
Prostatic Acid	
Enzymatic	<0.3 IU/L
	0.2–3.5 IU/L, men
	0–0.8 IU/L, women
Radioimmunoassay	<4.0 ng/mL

Variations
Elevated total acid phosphatase levels may occur with:

Bone fractures	Myelogenous leukemia, acute
Carcinoma of the breast with bone metastases	Osteogenesis imperfecta
	Paget's disease
Embolism, arterial or pulmonary	Prostatic carcinoma with metastases
Gaucher's disease	Renal disease, acute
Hepatitis, viral	Renal insufficiency
Hyperparathyroidism	Sickle cell crisis
Liver damage	Thrombocythemia, thrombocytosis
Multiple myeloma	Thrombophlebitis

Elevated prostatic acid phosphatase levels occur only with prostatic carcinoma that has metastasized.

Methodology
Acid phosphatase determinations require 5 mL of blood collected without anticoagulants (red-stoppered tube) and delivered to the laboratory immediately for prompt testing. Serum specimens for acid phosphatase determinations deteriorate rapidly at room temperature but remain stable for up to 1 week when refrigerated or frozen with 0.01 mL of 20% acetic acid per milliliter of serum.

Precautions
To ensure accurate acid phosphatase test results, the following precautions should be observed:

1. Do not collect the blood specimen if the patient has received clofibrate in the previous 24 hours.
2. Do not collect the blood specimen if the patient has had a transurethral resection (TUR), prostatic massage, or extensive palpation of the prostate in the previous 24 hours.
3. Prevent hemolysis of the blood specimen because test results may be falsely elevated by large concentrations of acid phosphatase released from hemolyzed red blood cells.
4. Prevent contamination of the blood specimen with fluoride, oxalate, or phosphate, all of which produce falsely decreased test results.

▶▶ Nursing Responsibilities and Implications

1. Collect the serum specimen carefully and without trauma, taking care to prevent hemolysis during venipuncture.
2. Deliver the specimen to the laboratory immediately because prostatic acid phosphatase may lose up to 50% of its activity within 1 hour at room temperature. If the acid phosphatase determination cannot be performed immediately, the serum must be separated from the cells, acetic acid added to the serum, and the specimen refrigerated or kept on ice.

Alkaline Phosphatase

Alkaline phosphatase, found in the bone, liver, intestine, and sometimes the placenta, is a nonspecific enzyme that becomes active mainly during the formation of new bone matrix. Alkaline phosphatase activity in the blood represents a total of five isoenzyme types derived from the various tissues, each having different characteristics that aid in identification. Specific laboratory tests to separate the various isoenzymes are now available to identify the exact source of alkaline phosphatase when total serum levels are elevated.

Small amounts of alkaline phosphatase appear normally in blood, but levels rise during active bone formation and liver or biliary tract disorders in proportion to the severity of the condition. Laboratory determination of total alkaline phosphatase activity is therefore useful in the differential diagnosis of metabolic bone diseases, including tumors. It is also helpful in evaluating calcium or phosphate metabolism and space-occupying hepatic lesions with impaired excretion and in identifying the degree of biliary tract blockage.

Clinical Significance

Elevated alkaline phosphatase concentrations generally direct immediate attention to bone or liver diseases, although physiologic elevations must be considered in women and children. Elevated concentrations associated with liver disease are related to bile duct obstruction, which impedes phosphatase excretion and closely correlates with clinical findings such as jaundice. Increased alkaline phosphatase levels without evidence of liver disorders may signal bone disease in which the formation of osseous tissue is increased such as bone tumors. High serum alkaline phosphatase levels also occur during the last trimester of pregnancy, reflecting placental activity, and are useful in evaluating the status of the pregnancy.

Elevated alkaline phosphatase levels routinely occur in infants and children during periods of active bone growth when a natural increase in osteoblastic activity occurs. Although alkaline phosphatase levels vary markedly from child to child depending on the rate of bone growth, activity normally peaks during the first year after birth and at puberty. A rapid increase in alkaline phosphatase activity parallels adolescent growth spurts and is more pronounced (but occurs several years later) in boys than in girls.

Normal Values

The normal values for alkaline phosphatase, depending on the test method used, are:

Total	30–105 IU/L, adults
	50–350 IU/L, children
Isoenzymes	
Bone	20–120 U/L
Liver	20–130 U/L
Intestines	0–18 U/L

Variations
Elevated alkaline phosphatase levels may occur with:

Bone disease (osteoblastic activity)
  Bone malignancy
  Familial hyperphosphatasemia
  Fibrous dysplasia
  Fractures, extensive
  Growth hormone, excess production
  Hyperparathyroidism
  Myositis ossificans
  Osteoblastic metastases
  Osteomalacia
  Osteogenic sarcoma
  Paget's disease
  Rickets
  Vitamin D deficiency
Liver disease
  Biliary cirrhosis
  Hepatic carcinoma
  Hepatitis, infectious or viral
  Hepatotoxic drug therapy
  Infectious mononucleosis
  Liver abscess

Obstruction, pancreatic duct
Obstructive jaundice
Miscellaneous
  Carbohydrate ingestion, large amounts
  Diabetes mellitus
  Fat ingestion
  Gaucher's disease
  Gastrointestinal disease
  Graves' disease
  Human albumin, massive infusion
  Hyperalimentation
  Idiopathic steatorrhea
  Kidney tissue rejection
  Leukemia
  Lymphoma
  Phosphate depletion
  Renal infarct
  Rheumatoid disease
  Sickle cell crisis
  Ulcer, perforated

Decreased alkaline phosphatase levels may occur with:

Celiac disease
Cretinism
Hypophosphatasia
Malnutrition
Nephritis, chronic
Osteolytic sarcoma

Pernicious anemia
Protein malnutrition
Scurvy
Transfusion therapy, massive
Vitamin D intoxication
Zinc depletion

Drugs that produce **falsely increased alkaline phosphatase levels** include:

Acetohexamide
Allopurinol
Chlorpropamide
Colchicine
Erythromycin
Indomethacin

Lincomycin
Methyldopa
n-Hydroxyacetamide
Oral contraceptives, some
Oxacillin

Penicillamine
Procainamide
Thiothixene
Tolazamide
Tolbutamide

Methodology

Alkaline phosphatase determinations require 3 mL of blood collected in a tube without anticoagulants (red-stoppered tube). Alkaline phosphatase remains stable in serum specimens for at least 8 hours at room temperature, 1 week if refrigerated, and about 1 month when frozen. Alkaline phosphatase activity increases at room temperature, however, because of a change in the pH of the specimen.

Precautions

To ensure accurate results, the following precautions should be observed when collecting specimens for alkaline phosphatase tests:

1. Do not collect the blood specimen if the patient has received any hepatotoxic drugs within the past 12 hours.

2. Do not schedule the test if the patient has had a recent intravenous infusion of albumin because alkaline phosphatase values will be significantly increased.

▶▶ Nursing Responsibilities and Implications

1. Withhold the patient's food and medications for 12 hours before collecting the blood specimen because alkaline phosphatase activity may rise 25% or more depending on the type of food and the time interval since the meal.

2. Deliver the specimen to the laboratory immediately. When alkaline phosphatase determinations cannot be performed shortly after specimen collection, the serum must be separated from the cells and refrigerated as soon as possible.

Cholinesterase and Pseudocholinesterase

Cholinesterase, an enzyme existing in the body in two forms, hydrolyzes choline esters such as acetylcholine, which is produced at nerve endings and helps to transmit nerve cell impulses. The first form, **true cholinesterase**, is found in nerve tissue, skeletal muscle, and red blood cells; the second form, **pseudocholinesterase** (PCHE), is distributed throughout the body and plasma. Pseudocholinesterase hydrolyzes the muscle relaxant succinylcholine, and its activity is inhibited by organic phosphorous insecticides, which can interrupt nerve impulses, causing death. Laboratory determinations of pseudocholinesterase concentrations most frequently are used to assess patient susceptibility to succinylcholine and indicate the degree of exposure to phosphorus insecticides.

Clinical Significance

Pseudocholinesterase determinations frequently are included in the screening of patients for major surgery or electroconvulsive therapy in which succinylcholine will be used. Individuals with normal enzyme levels readily inactivate succinylcholine, but those with low activity, whether from heredity or acquired disease, are slow to metabolize the relaxant. Thus, patients with low pseudocholinesterase levels sustain the exaggerated effects of succinylcholine for several hours and experience dyspnea or apnea and a prolonged period of muscle relaxation.

Normal Values

The normal values for serum cholinesterase, depending on the test method used, are:

Pseudocholinesterase	3.0−8.0 U/mL
	8−18 IU/L
	0.5−1.3 pH units
	204−532 IU/dL
True cholinesterase	3−5 IU/mL

Variations

Elevated pseudocholinesterase levels may occur with diabetes mellitus, hyperthyroidism, and nephrotic syndrome.

Decreased pseudocholinesterase levels may occur with:

Anemia, severe	Insecticide exposure (Parathion, Sevin)
Carcinomatosis	Malnutrition
Cirrhosis	Muscular dystrophy
Hepatic carcinoma, metastatic	Shock
Hepatitis, infectious	Succinylcholine hypersensitivity
Hypoproteinemia	Tuberculosis
Infections, acute	Uremia
Infectious mononucleosis	

Methodology

Pseudocholinesterase determinations require 5 mL of blood collected in a tube without anticoagulants (red-stoppered tube). Tests for true cholinesterase require 5 mL of blood collected in a tube containing heparin anticoagulant (green-stoppered tube). Cholinesterase and pseudocholinesterase remain stable in serum or plasma specimens for up to 1 week at room temperature, 2 weeks if refrigerated, and for up to 3 months when frozen.

Precautions

To ensure accurate pseudocholinesterase results, the blood specimen should be collected with as little trauma as possible to prevent hemolysis, which can cause falsely elevated test values by releasing true cholinesterase from red blood cells.

Aldolase

Aldolase, an enzyme found in all body cells, occurs in highest concentrations in skeletal muscles. Aldolase levels usually rise before any overt clinical manifestations of muscle disease in patients destined to develop progressive muscular dystrophy and decrease with progression of the disease as muscle mass diminishes. The chief clinical application of aldolase determinations is in the investigation of progressive muscular dystrophy, in which levels may increase up to six times the upper limit of normal.

Laboratory determinations of aldolase activity are most useful in monitoring skeletal muscle disorders, including primary myopathy, severe traumatic injury, and inflammatory skeletal muscle diseases such as dermatomyositis and trichinosis. Aldolase determinations also provide a sensitive measure of neoplastic and hepatic diseases such as acute infectious hepatitis, in which concentrations may be as much as 20 times the average normal level. However, because CPK determinations are more senstive and specific for these disorders, aldolase levels may be infrequently ordered.

Normal Values
The normal values for aldolase, depending on the test method used, are:

Adults	1.0−7.5 U/L
	0−7 units
	1.3−8.2 U/dL
Men	8.5−20 U/L
	3.1−7.5 IU/L
Women	7−14 U/L
	2.7−5.3 IU/L
Children	Two times adult levels
Neonates	Four times adult levels

Variations
Elevated aldolase levels may occur with:

Anemia, megaloblastic or hemolytic

Cirrhosis

Crushing injuries

Dermatomyositis

Erythroblastosis fetalis

Heart failure

Hepatic necrosis

Hepatitis

Hepatoma

Infectious mononucleosis

Injections, intramuscular

Jaundice, obstructive

Lead intoxication

Leukemia, chronic granulocytic

Lymphoma

Metastatic carcinoma

Muscular dystrophy, progressive

Myocardial infarction

Pancreatitis, acute

Pericarditis, hemorrhagic

Polycythemia vera

Prostatic carcinoma, advanced

Pulmonary infarct, large

Skeletal muscle disease

Surgery

Trauma, muscle

Trichinosis

Methodology
Aldolase determinations require 5 mL of blood collected without trauma in a tube with no anticoagulants (red-stoppered tube). Aldolase remains stable in serum specimens for 6 days at room temperature.

Precautions

To ensure accurate aldolase determinations, the following precautions should be observed:

1. Do not collect specimens if the patient has received ACTH or cortisone within the previous 24 hours because these medications falsely elevate aldolase values up to five times the normal level.

2. Do not submit hemolyzed specimens to the laboratory because erythrocytes contain an abundance of aldolase, which can produce falsely elevated test values.

Creatine Phosphokinase (Creatine Kinase)

Creatine phosphokinase (CPK), also known as **creatine kinase** (CK), is an enzyme found in cardiac muscle, skeletal muscle, and brain tissue that helps to control the amount of energy available to the body. Creatine phosphokinase may be separated by isoenzyme electrophoresis into three individual molecular species: CPK_3 (MM), found primarily in skeletal muscle, CPK_2 (MB), found mostly in cardiac muscle, and CPK_1 (BB), found mainly in brain and nervous tissue. The relative amounts of each CPK isoenzyme present frequently are determined to help distinguish conditions causing total CPK values to be elevated.

Normal isoenzyme patterns show moderate concentrations of the CPK_3 (MM) fraction, which generally is responsible for most of the total CPK activity in serum. Thus, individuals with an unusually large muscle mass, such as athletes, frequently have higher CPK levels than most of the population. Total CPK activity is increased by acute pulmonary and myocardial infarction as well as by any condition that destroys muscle tissue, including muscle disease, injury, and strenuous exercise. Laboratory determinations of CPK and its isoenzymes are used to diagnose Duchenne's muscular dystrophy and for the early differential diagnosis of myocardial infarction. Creatine phosphokinase levels also may be used to indicate active tissue damage, monitor reinfarction, and screen patients at risk of developing malignant hyperpyrexia or hyperthermia.

Clinical Significance

The most striking increase in CPK activity occurs in the early stages of Duchenne's muscular dystrophy, in which levels may reach 300−400 times normal. These markedly elevated CPK concentrations, caused primarily by increased CPK_3 (MM) activity, frequently precede any definite clinical symptoms and remain elevated during the course of the disease. Creatine phosphokinase levels fall slowly as the disease progresses, reflecting the decreased muscle mass and limited physical activity of the patient. Elevated CPK and CPK_3 (MM) levels of up to three times normal also may occur following strenuous exercise, although these elevations disappear within 24−36 hours.

Creatine phosphokinase activity begins to rise 2−6 hours after myocardial infarction, reaches peak concentrations within 18−36 hours, and returns to normal levels within 3−6 days (see Table 4-3). Increased concentrations of the CPK_2 (MB) isoenzyme appear approximately 4−8 hours after the onset of chest pain following myocardial infarction, reach peak activity within 18−24 hours, and remain elevated for another 2 days. Maximum values may reach ten or more times the upper limit of normal, although values three to six times the normal level are more common. However, the level of the CPK_3 (MM) isoenzyme also increases during myocardial infarction and remains elevated for 4−5 days, longer than CPK_2 (MB) is elevated. Thus, CPK isoenzyme testing 4 days after myocardial infarction may reveal only CPK₃ (MM) activity, but there is no way to determine if this isoenzyme came from the heart or skeletal muscle. Therefore, although CPK determinations are most valuable in detecting cardiac necrosis within the first 36 hours following myocardial infarction, beyond that time serum aspartate aminotransferase (AST, formerly known as glutamic-oxaloacetic transaminase, or GOT) and lactic dehydrogenase (LDH) values are more significant diagnostically.

Normal Values

The normal values for creatine phosphokinase and its isoenzymes, depending on the test method used, are:

Total creatine phosphokinase	45–235 IU/L
Men	5–35 U/mL
	20–170 U/L
	5–55 mU/mL
Women	5–25 U/mL
	10–135 U/L
	5–35 mU/mL
Children (<1 year)	40–350 U/L
Following strenuous exercise	60–500 U/L
CPK₃ (MM)	90%–100% of total creatine phosphokinase
CPK₂ (MB)	0%–5% of total creatine phosphokinase
CPK₁ (BB)	0%–3% of total creatine phosphokinase

Variations

Creatine phosphokinase isoenzyme patterns in various conditions are summarized in Table 4-2.

Elevated creatine phosphokinase levels may occur with:

Heart disorders
  Cardiac surgery
  Myocardial infarction, acute
  Myocarditis
  Rejection of heart transplant
  Tachycardia
Miscellaneous
  Bowel injury, surgery, infarction
  Hepatic coma

Intoxication, severe alcohol or salicylate
Pregnancy
Prostate injury, surgery, infarction
Pulmonary infarction
Thyrotoxicosis
Neurologic disorders
  Brain tumor
  Cerebral accident

TABLE 4-2   Creatine Phosphokinase Isoenzyme Patterns

Condition	CPK$_3$ (MM)	CPK$_2$ (MB)	CPK$_1$ (BB)
Normal pattern	Normal to moderate increase	—	—
Acute myocardial damage	Slight to very marked increase	Trace to marked increase	—
Active skeletal muscle damage	Moderate to very marked increase	Normal to slight increase	—
Brain injury	Normal to moderate increase	Normal to trace	Normal to slight increase
Malignant tumors with metastases	Slight to moderate increase	Normal to trace	Normal to moderate increase
Severe shock	Slight to very marked increase	Normal to slight increase	Normal to trace
Chronic renal failure	Slight to very marked increase	Normal to slight increase	Normal to slight increase
Malignant hyperthermia	Slight to very marked increase	Normal to slight increase	Normal to slight increase

Cerebral infarction

Convulsions

Hyperthermia, malignant (20,000–100,000 U/L)

Head injury

Meningoencephalitis

Psychosis, acute

Subarachnoid hemorrhage

Skeletal muscle disorders

Crushing injury

Delirium tremens

Electrocautery

Exercise, strenuous

Hypothyroidism

Injections, intramuscular

Muscular dystrophy

Polymyositis

Surgery

Normal creatine phosphokinase levels may occur with hemolytic anemia, acute hepatitis, and obstructive jaundice.

Elevated CPK$_3$ (MM) levels may occur with:

Cardiac catheterization

Coronary arteriography

Electrical countershock to correct cardiac arrhythmia

Injections, intramuscular

Muscle trauma

Myocardial infarction

Shock

Surgery

Elevated CPK$_2$ (MB) levels may occur with:

Angina pectoris (uncommon)

Lung carcinoma

Anoxia, severe	Myocardial infarction, acute
Carbon monoxide poisoning	Myocarditis
Congestive heart failure (uncommon)	Pulmonary embolism
Coronary angiography (uncommon)	Surgery, open-heart
Coronary insufficiency (uncommon)	Trauma, cardiac

Elevated CPK$_1$ (BB) levels may occur with:

Bowel infarction	Oat cell carcinoma
Breast malignancy	Renal dialysis
Carcinoma, gastrointestinal or prostatic	Renal failure
Hemorrhagic strokes	Reye's syndrome
Hyperpyrexia, malignant	Shock
Hypothermia	Surgery, central nervous system
Labor	

Drugs that produce falsely increased test results include:

Clofibrate	Furosemide	Lithium carbonate
Codeine	Glutethimide	Meperidine
Dexamethasone	Halothane anesthesia	Morphine
Digoxin	Heroin	Phenobarbital
Ethanol	Imipramine	

Methodology

Creatine phosphokinase determinations require 5 mL of blood collected in a tube without anticoagulants or containing heparin (red- or green-stoppered tube). Creatine phospho-kinase concentrations remain stable in serum and plasma specimens for up to 4 days at room temperature and for up to 11 days when refrigerated.

Precautions

To ensure accurate CPK determinations, the following precautions should be observed:

1. Collect blood samples for CPK determinations as soon as possible after the patient is admitted to the hospital as well as 12 and 24 hours after the onset of symptoms of myocardial infarction so that the increased CPK$_2$ (MB) concentrations will not be missed.

2. Whenever possible, do not collect specimens for CPK determinations if the patient has received any of the drugs that produce falsely increased test results within the past 24 hours (see Variations).

▶▶ Nursing Responsibilities and Implications

1. Notify the laboratory if the specimen was collected less than 24–48 hours after sur-gery because this amount of time is required to clear CPK released by tissue trauma.

2. Notify the laboratory if the patient has received any medications within the previous 24 hours because a number of compounds can affect the test results.

3. If myocardial infarction is suspected, collect subsequent blood specimens at 24-hour intervals to evaluate changes in lactic dehydrogenase and its isoenzymes, which become elevated after CPK.

Lactic Dehydrogenase

Lactic dehydrogenase (LDH), an enzyme found in nearly all body cells undergoing metabolism, occurs in high concentrations in the heart, liver, brain, skeletal muscles, kidneys, and red blood cells. Elevated LDH activity is a nonspecific indicator of disease because tissue damage resulting from many pathologic conditions releases the enzyme into the bloodstream, increasing LDH concentrations. Lactic dehydrogenase may be separated by isoenzyme electrophoresis into five distinct molecular forms, labeled LDH_1 through LDH_5, that occur in varying proportions and concentrations in every tissue and organ. High concentrations of LDH isoenzymes appear in various tissues as follows:

LDH_1—heart, red blood cells, brain

LDH_2—heart, red blood cells, brain

LDH_3—lungs, spleen, pancreas, thyroid, adrenals, kidneys

LDH_4—liver, skeletal muscle, kidneys, brain

LDH_5—liver, skeletal muscle, kidneys

When tissue cells are damaged, they release a characteristic LDH isoenzyme pattern that forms a mirror image of the damaged tissue, giving more specific diagnostic information than total LDH measurements alone. For example, myocardial tissue contains high concentrations of LDH_1 and LDH_2 but very small amounts of LDH_4 and LDH_5; thus, a corresponding isoenzyme pattern is highly suggestive of myocardial infarction. Elevated concentrations of LDH_3 occur in patients with pulmonary infarction, but the characteristic pattern may be somewhat confused by the interference of additional isoenzymes caused by associated health problems. Hepatic tissue, on the other hand, contains high concentrations of LDH_4 and LDH_5 but only trace amounts of LDH_1 and LDH_2; therefore, this isoenzyme pattern is characteristic of liver disease.

Abnormal isoenzyme concentrations cannot always be detected by serum LDH values alone because marked changes in the isoenzymes may affect only their relative distribution and cause little variation in the total level of LDH. Laboratory determination of total LDH and LDH isoenzyme activity aids in the differential diagnosis of myocardial infarction, pulmonary infarction, and liver disease and helps in monitoring the course of cancer chemotherapy. A favorable response to therapy frequently is accompanied by a fall in LDH concentrations, whereas a recurrence of the tumor generally is signaled by a rise in total LDH and its isoenzymes.

Clinical Significance

High LDH activity (two- to fortyfold elevations) occurs in individuals with megaloblastic anemia, extensive carcinomatosis, severe shock, and hypoxia, whereas relatively slight

TABLE 4-3 Serum Enzyme Activity after Myocardial Infarction

Enzyme	Rise Begins (Hours)	Peak Activity (Hours)	Return to Normal (Days)
Creatine phosphokinase	2–6	18–36	3–6
Lactic dehydrogenase	6–12	48–72	6–14
Hydroxybutyric dehydrogenase	8–10	48–96	16–18
Aspartate aminotransferase*	6–10	24–48	4–7

*Formerly glutamic-oxaloacetic transaminase (GOT).

elevations develop in hepatic disorders such as hepatitis, obstructive jaundice, and cirrhosis. Marked elevation of hepatic isoenzymes frequently occurs before clinical jaundice appears and returns to normal concentrations during convalescence even though jaundice persists. Variations of LDH_4 and LDH_5 activity also may be used to monitor the effect of drugs such as chlorpromazine and toxic materials such as carbon tetrachloride on the liver.

Moderately elevated LDH values (two- to fourfold), composed mainly of LDH_1 and LDH_2, most often occur in patients with myocardial infarction (see Table 4-3). Enzyme activity rises perceptibly 24–48 hours following myocardial necrosis and reaches peak concentrations of two to ten times normal within 3–6 days, which closely parallels the extent of cardiac damage. The normal isoenzyme ratio of LDH_1/LDH_2 assumes a "flipped" profile, in which LDH_1 is greater than LDH_2, approximately 12–24 hours after acute myocardial infarction and remains elevated for up to 7 days. Elevated LDH levels usually return to normal in 6–14 days, later than CPK or AST, making LDH values most valuable in the delayed diagnosis of myocardial infarction.

Normal Values

The normal values for lactic dehydrogenase and its isoenzymes, depending on the test method used, are:

Total lactic dehydrogenase	80–120 Wacker units
	150–450 Wroblewski units
	70–250 U/L
LDH_1	16%–33% of total LDH
LDH_2	28%–40% of total LDH
LDH_3	16%–30% of total LDH
LDH_4	5%–16% of total LDH
LDH_5	2%–20% of total LDH
LDH_1/LDH_2 ratio	<1

Variations

Abnormal LDH isoenzyme patterns are summarized in Table 4-4.

Elevated lactic dehydrogenase levels may occur with:

Anoxia

Arrhythmias, ventricular

Carcinoma, metastatic (>800 U/L)

Cerebrovascular accident

Cirrhosis (>800 U/L)

Delirium tremens (>450 U/L)

Heart failure, acute congestive

Hemolytic anemia (>450 U/L)

Hepatic neoplasm (>800 U/L)

Hepatitis, acute and toxic (>800 U/L)

Infectious mononucleosis (>450 U/L)

Jaundice, obstructive

Leukemia, untreated acute (>800 U/L)

Lymphoma, malignant

Megaloblastic anemia (>800 U/L)

Muscular dystrophy (>450 U/L)

Myocardial infarction (>450 U/L)

Pernicious anemia

Pneumonia

Pulmonary embolism

Pulmonary infarction (>450 U/L)

Renal infarct, infection, or malignancy

Sickle cell anemia

Shock

Trauma

TABLE 4-4 Abnormal Lactic Dehydrogenase Isoenzyme Patterns

Condition	LDH_1	LDH_2	LDH_3	LDH_4	LDH_5
Myocardial infarction	Increased	Increased	—	—	—
Myocardial infarction with liver congestion	Increased	Increased	—	—	Increased
Pulmonary infarct	—	Increased	Increased	—	—
Shock	Increased	Increased	Increased	Increased	Increased
Hepatitis	—	—	—	Increased	Increased
Active cirrhosis	—	—	—	Increased	Increased
Infectious mononucleosis	—	—	Increased	Increased	Increased
Pernicious anemia	Increased	Increased	—	—	—
Sickle cell anemia	Increased	Increased	—	—	—
Dermatomyositis	—	—	—	—	Increased
Muscular dystrophy	—	—	Increased	Increased	Increased
Acute pancreatitis	—	—	Increased	Increased	Increased
Cerebrovascular accident	Increased	Increased	—	Increased	—
Acute glomerulonephritis	—	—	—	Increased	Increased
Renal necrosis	Increased	Increased	Increased	Increased	Increased

Methodology

Lactic dehydrogenase determinations require 5 mL of blood collected without trauma in a tube containing heparin (green-stoppered tube) or no anticoagulants (red-stoppered tube) and delivered to the laboratory immediately. Specimens for total LDH determination remain stable for about 4 days at room temperature and for 1 week at refrigerator temperatures. However, LDH isoenzymes are unstable and should be processed as soon as possible after blood collection to ensure an accurate isoenzyme pattern.

Precautions

To ensure an accurate LDH determination, the following precautions should be observed:

1. Do not submit hemolyzed blood to the laboratory because falsely elevated values may be obtained if the test is performed on specimens in which hemolysis is apparent or the serum hemoglobin level is above 0.1 g/dL.

2. Prevent contamination of the specimen with any oxalate compounds, such as ammonium or potassium oxalate anticoagulants, which can produce falsely decreased test values.

3. If possible, do not collect blood specimens for LDH determinations if the patient has received any anesthetic agents, clofibrate, codeine, dicumarol, morphine, or theophylline in the previous 24 hours because these drugs produce physiologic effects or chemical interferences and affect the test results.

▶▶ ## Nursing Responsibilities and Implications

1. Collect the blood specimen in heparin or without anticoagulants because contact with oxalate or EDTA causes falsely decreased test results.

2. Prevent hemolysis of the blood specimen because the release of LDH from red blood cells into the serum produces falsely elevated test results.

3. Collect blood specimens for LDH analysis every 24 hours for 2 or 3 days after the acute episode in patients with myocardial infarction to detect the reversed, or "flipped," LDH_1/LDH_2 ratio.

4. Note on the laboratory slip any medications the patient is receiving that might affect the test results.

5. Deliver the specimen to the laboratory immediately because LDH isoenzymes are unstable and the test is most accurate when performed shortly after blood collection.

Hydroxybutyric Dehydrogenase

Hydroxybutyric dehydrogenase (HBDH), an enzyme found in highest concentrations in heart muscle, kidneys, brain, and red blood cells, has a clinical significance similar to LDH_1 and LDH_2. Thus, HBDH determinations provide the same information concerning myocardial damage as interpretation of the electrophoretic isoenzyme patterns for LDH_1 and LDH_2. However, HBDH values are not entirely specific for LDH_1 activity because elevated levels also can occur in individuals with hepatocellular disorders and skeletal muscle damage. Laboratory determinations of HBDH are not as specific or sensitive as LDH, but may be used to aid in the diagnosis of myocardial infarction when total LDH levels are not sufficiently significant or when the complete LDH isoenzyme pattern is unavailable.

Clinical Significance

Hydroxybutyric dehydrogenase levels begin to rise 8–10 hours following myocardial infarction, reach peak concentrations within 48–96 hours, and return to normal 16–18 days after cardiac necrosis (see Table 4-3). Hydroxybutyric dehydrogenase determinations are considered superior to CPK, AST, and total LDH measurements for the confirmation of myocardial infarction because elevated values are specific for this condition and remain at abnormal levels longer.

The relationship of HBDH values to LDH levels has recently been calculated in an attempt to interpret HBDH assays, although this ratio may be misleading. For example, myocardial infarction complicated by cardiogenic shock or hepatic congestion may produce elevations in heart and liver/muscle isoenzyme fractions, resulting in a normal HBDH/LDH ratio as one increase balances the other.

Normal Values

The normal and clinically significant hydroxybutyric dehydrogenase values, depending on the test method used, are:

Hydroxybutyric dehydrogenase	140–350 IU/L
	56–125 IU/L
	82–163 mU/mL
HBDH/LDH ratio	
Normal	0.5
Cardiac disorders	>0.5
Liver or skeletal muscle disorders	<0.5

Variations

Elevated hydroxybutyric dehydrogenase levels may occur with:

Anemia, hemolytic or megaloblastic	Muscular dystrophy
Leukemia	Myocardial infarction
Lymphomas	Nephrotic syndrome
Malignant melanomas	Orthopedic hip surgery

Methodology

Hydroxybutyric dehydrogenase determinations require 5 mL of blood collected without anticoagulants (red-stoppered tube) or hemolysis. Hydroxybutyric dehydrogenase is stable at room temperature for 5 days and may be stored as long as 10 days if refrigerated. Specimens are not suitable for HBDH analysis after freezing because enzyme activity is lost during thawing.

▶▶ Nursing Responsibilities and Implications

The blood specimen must be collected without incurring trauma or hemolysis, which releases HBDH from the red blood cells and produces falsely elevated test results.

Aspartate Aminotransferase

Aspartate aminotransferase (AST), formerly known as glutamic-oxaloacetic transaminase (GOT), is an enzyme found in high concentrations in cardiac, hepatic, skeletal muscle, brain, spleen, pancreas, lung, and kidney tissue. Aspartate aminotransferase activity in blood is generally relatively low, but during certain diseases the enzyme leaks into the bloodstream from dead or damaged cells and is found in much higher concentrations. The amount of enzyme liberated is a reliable indicator of the extent and severity of tissue destruction because serum levels rise in proportion to the degree of tissue damage.

Although AST levels are sensitive indicators of tissue necrosis, they cannot pinpoint the exact site of disease because many organs contain high transaminase concentrations. Thus, the greatest amount of diagnostic information is obtained when AST is measured simultaneously with other enzymes, particularly alanine aminotransferase (formerly called glutamic-pyruvic transaminase), CPK, LDH, and alkaline phosphatase. Laboratory determinations of AST are used primarily to investigate the progress and prognosis of patients with myocardial infarction and liver disease (Table 4-5).

Clinical Significance

Extremely elevated AST levels, up to 100 times normal, accompany massive destruction of liver tissue and severe hepatic necrosis such as occurs in the acute stages of fulminating hepatitis. These enzyme changes occur early in the disease, often before the appearance of clinical jaundice, and remain elevated longer than other liver function tests. A sudden AST elevation superimposed on a pattern of declining levels or persistently high levels when test values should be falling suggest the development of complications, postnecrotic cirrhosis, or a recurrence of the original problem.

The ratio of LDH to AST helps to distinguish liver metastases from other liver diseases and may be used to evaluate the prognosis of patients with liver metastases and non-metastatic hepatocellular disease. The relationship of these enzymes is more specific

TABLE 4-5 Aspartate Aminotransferase* and Alanine Aminotransferase[†] Elevations in Heart and Liver Disease

Disease	Aspartate Aminotransferase (AST)	Alanine Aminotransferase (ALT)
Infectious hepatitis	Marked increase	Very marked increase
Obstructive jaundice	Marked increase	Moderate increase
Cholangiolitic hepatitis	Moderate increase	Marked increase
Laennec's cirrhosis	Moderate increase	Slight increase
Postnecrotic cirrhosis	Marked increase	Moderate increase
Toxic hepatitis	Marked increase	Very marked increase
Infectious mononucleosis	Marked increase	Very marked increase
Myocardial infarction	Marked increase	Slight increase

*Formerly glutamic-oxaloacetic transaminase (GOT).
[†]Formerly glutamic-pyruvic transaminase (GPT).

for the detection of metastases than the interpretation of alkaline phosphatase, 5'-nucleotidase, gamma-glutamyl transferase, LDH, or AST levels obtained separately. This LDH/AST ratio is not specific for liver metastases, however, because it also is increased by hemolysis, leukemia, renal infarction, hemolytic anemia, pulmonary embolism, and congestive heart failure.

Significant increases of AST levels occur within 6–12 hours following a myocardial infarction and reach peak concentrations of four to ten times the normal range after 24–48 hours. Aspartate aminotransferase activity usually falls to normal levels in 4–7 days, making this procedure more useful than CPK determinations in the delayed diagnosis of myocardial infarction (see Table 4-3). Recurrent AST elevations in the absence of liver damage indicate additional areas of myocardial necrosis resulting from coronary insufficiency or congestive heart failure. However, the availability of total CPK and LDH determinations, along with their isoenzyme patterns, has made AST analysis redundant and caused it to be largely discontinued as a cardiac enzyme determination.

Normal Values
The normal values for aspartate aminotransferase, depending on the test method used, are:

Adults	1–70 IU/L
	12–30 U/L
	8–40 U/mL
	13–55 units
Infants	Four times adult levels

Variations
Elevated aspartate aminotransferase levels may occur with:

Marked elevations (>300 U/L)
  Hepatitis, infectious or toxic
  Myocardial infarction, acute
Slight to moderate elevations
(>60 U/L)
  Amebic infections
  Bile duct obstruction
  Cardiac arrhythmias
  Cardiac catheterization
  Cerebral infarction
  Cirrhosis
  Congestive heart failure
  Crushing injuries
  Dermatomyositis
  Delirium tremens

Hepatic carcinoma, metastatic
Infectious mononucleosis
Jaundice, cholangiolitic or obstructive
Liver abscess
Muscular dystrophy, progressive
Muscle injury
Pancreatitis, acute interstitial
Pericarditis
Pulmonary infarction
Renal disease
Shock, prolonged
Skeletal muscle disease
Toxemia of pregnancy
Trauma, extensive

Decreased aspartate aminotransferase levels may occur with pregnancy and renal dialysis.

Falsely elevated aspartate aminotransferase levels may be caused by:

Ascorbic acid	Ethyl biscoumacetate	Narcotics
Ampicillin	Guanethidine	Oxacillin
Azaserine	Hydralazine	Para-aminosalicylic acid
Carbenicillin	Isoniazid	Pyrazinamide
Carbon tetrachloride	Lead (even without evi-dent poisoning)	Pyridoxine
Cholinergics		Salicylates
Chlorpromazine	Meperidine	Sulfamethoxypyridazine
Codeine	Methyldopa	Tolbutamide
Dicumarol	Morphine	Vitamin B$_6$
Erythromycin		

Methodology

Aspartate aminotransferase determinations require 5 mL of blood collected without anti-coagulants (red-stoppered tube). Aspartate aminotransferase remains stable in serum specimens for 3 days at room temperature and for 1 week if refrigerated but is unstable when frozen because enzyme activity is altered during thawing.

Precautions

To ensure an accurate AST determination, the following precautions should be observed:

1. Do not submit hemolyzed blood specimens to the laboratory because this can produce inaccurate test results.

2. Do not collect blood specimens for AST analysis if the patient has received any medi-cations within the previous 12 hours. Falsely elevated AST levels may be caused by a number of drugs and chemicals (see Variations), although it is not certain whether these elevations are artifactual or caused by slight drug-induced liver damage.

▶▶ Nursing Responsibilities and Implications

1. Stop all medications 12 hours before collecting the blood specimen because many drugs and chemicals can produce falsely elevated test results; if the medication can-not be withheld, list it on the laboratory slip.

2. Note the time the blood is collected and keep the specimen refrigerated after a clot has formed until it can be sent to the laboratory; AST remains stable for 4 days when refrigerated.

3. Collect the blood specimen without causing trauma or hemolysis, which can inter-fere with accurate test results.

Alanine Aminotransferase

Alanine aminotransferase (ALT), formerly called glutamic-pyruvic transaminase (GPT), is an enzyme found primarily in the liver; smaller amounts also occur in the kidneys, heart, and skeletal muscles. In liver disease elevated amounts of ALT are released into the bloodstream by damaged or destroyed hepatic tissue in concentrations that directly parallel the degree of liver necrosis. Laboratory determinations of ALT are used mainly in the diagnosis of liver disease and frequently are measured along with AST to help distinguish between cardiac and hepatic tissue damage (see Table 4-5).

Clinical Significance

Transaminase activity increases early in the course of liver disease, often several days before jaundice appears, and returns to normal in about 2–3 months unless complications occur. However, ALT levels remain increased longer than AST levels and reach greater elevations (often as high as 4000 units) in individuals with hepatitis or hepatic necrosis caused by drugs and chemicals. Thus, measurement of ALT levels aids in the diagnosis of liver disease in the absence of jaundice because levels considerably higher than 300 units are common in hepatic disorders, whereas levels under 300 units usually result from extrahepatic conditions.

The AST/ALT ratio increases the diagnostic value of both transaminase enzymes and is most helpful when activity is two to ten times the upper limit of normal. The ratio is of little value, however, when the enyzme activities are very high (>500 units), at which point the diagnosis is usually obvious. A ratio of greater than 2 indicates the possibility of alcoholic hepatitis or cirrhosis, whereas a ratio of less than 2 is unusual in other types of cirrhosis and acute or chronic hepatitis. Although the reason for the increased ratio is unknown, ALT activity is lower in patients with alcoholic liver disease than it is in normal patients and those with acute viral hepatitis.

Comparison of AST and ALT levels also yields valuable information in individuals with suspected myocardial infarction because AST activity always increases following myocardial infarction, whereas ALT levels may not rise proportionally. Thus, an elevated AST concentration accompanied by normal ALT values confirms a diagnosis of cardiac disease rather than hepatic necrosis.

Normal Values

The normal values for alanine aminotransferase, depending on the test method used, are:

Alanine aminotransferase	5–30 U/L
	1–36 U/mL
	6–53 units
	1–70 IU/L
AST/ALT ratio	1

Variations

Elevated alanine aminotransferase levels may occur with:

Marked elevations	Slight to moderate elevations
Hepatic necrosis	Cerebral infarction
Hepatitis, toxic and viral	Cirrhosis
Infectious mononucleosis	Crushing injuries

Hepatic carcinoma, metastatic	Pancreatitis, acute
Hepatitis, infectious	Toxemia of pregnancy
Jaundice, obstructive	Trauma, extensive
Myocardial infarction	

Decreased alanine aminotransferase levels may occur with pregnancy and renal dialysis.

Falsely elevated alanine aminotransferase levels may be caused by:

Acetaminophen

Alcohol

Opiates

(See Aspartate Aminotransferase—Variations for additional drugs that may interfere physiologically and chemically with transaminase test procedures.)

An **elevated AST/ALT ratio** (>1) may occur with:

Alcoholic liver disease	Muscular dystrophy, progressive
Carcinoma, metastatic	Myocardial infarction
Cirrhosis	Obstruction, extrahepatic

A **decreased AST/ALT ratio** (<1) may occur with:

Cholestasis, intrahepatic	Hepatitis, acute epidemic
Hepatic necrosis, acute	Infectious mononucleosis

Methodology

Alanine aminotransferase determinations require 5 mL of blood collected in a tube without anticoagulants (red-stoppered tube). Alanine aminotransferase remains stable in serum for 3 days at room temperature and for 1 week at refrigerator temperatures but is unstable when frozen because enzyme activity is altered during thawing.

Precautions

To ensure an accurate ALT analysis, do not collect blood if the patient has received any medications in the previous 24 hours. A number of hepatotoxic drugs and chemicals may produce falsely elevated ALT values as a result of slight liver damage or hepatic changes.

▶▶ Nursing Responsibilities and Implications

Stop all medications at least 12 hours before collecting the blood specimen because many hepatotoxic drugs and chemicals can produce falsely elevated test results; if medication cannot be withheld, list the medications on the laboratory slip.

Gamma-Glutamyl Transferase

Gamma-glutamyl transferase (GGT) is an enzyme found in highest concentrations in the liver, kidneys, and pancreas that also appears in the prostate, salivary glands, brain, and heart. Because GGT concentrations are highest in obstructive liver damage, laboratory determinations frequently are used in conjunction with other enzyme determinations to confirm and evaluate a diagnosis of liver disease. In addition, GGT values provide a useful screening tool for the detection of occult alcoholism because enzyme activity is the most sensitive indicator of chronic alcohol consumption. Gamma-glutamyl transferase determinations also have important medicolegal significance during the investigation of rape because seminal fluid contains high concentrations of this enzyme.

Clinical Significance

Significant GGT levels accompany most liver diseases, but the most striking elevations occur with obstructive liver disease, in which test values closely parallel alkaline phosphatase and 5'-nucleotidase elevations. Abnormal GGT values are a reliable indicator of the extent and severity of hepatic disorders because they persist for several weeks longer than elevations of other liver enzymes, including LDH, AST, ALT, and alkaline phosphatase. Gamma-glutamyl transferase activity also helps to differentiate biliary atresia from neonatal hepatitis because in biliary atresia, GGT values are three to four times higher (>300 U/L) than they are in neonatal hepatitis (<300 U/L).

Gamma-glutamyl transferase activity may increase following myocardial infarction, although concentrations remain normal for the first 3–4 days and peak about 10 days after the incident. Elevated test values persist for at least 1 month and reflect cellular healing rather than the death of muscle cells, which is indicated by CPK, AST, and LDH elevations.

Gamma-glutamyl transferase determinations recently have been used to evaluate and monitor chronic alcoholism because test values fall on withdrawal and rise with reexposure to alcohol. The GGT test currently is used by alcohol treatment centers to document the success of therapy and to identify patients who relapse following therapy. Thus, the test is helpful in preventive medicine because it provides early warning of alcohol-related liver damage and enables alcoholic patients with liver disease to seek help before the condition becomes acute.

Normal Values

The normal values for gamma-glutamyl transferase, depending on the test method used, are:

Children (<2 years)	<140 units
Premature infants	<250 units
Adults	1–70 U/L
	2–39 U/L
Men	7–40 units
	4–23 IU/L
	12–38 mU/mL
Women	4–25 units
	9–31 mU/mL
	3.5–13 IU/L

Variations

Elevated gamma-glutamyl transferase levels may occur with:

Marked elevations (>150 U/L)
    Cholestasis, intrahepatic (2000 U/L)
    Cirrhosis, biliary
    Hepatic carcinoma, metastatic
    Jaundice, obstructive
Slight to moderate elevations
(>45 U/L)
    Alcoholism, chronic

Cirrhosis, Laennec's
Congestive heart failure
Hepatitis, toxic and viral
Kidney diseases
Myocardial infarction
Pancreatic carcinoma
Pancreatitis

Falsely elevated gamma-glutamyl transferase levels may be caused by:

Barbiturates
Glutethimide

Methaqualone
Phenytoin

Methodology

Gamma-glutamyl transferase determinations require 5 mL of blood collected without anticoagulants (red-stoppered tube) and without excessive stasis or trauma. Gamma-glutamyl transferase remains stable for 5 days at room temperature, for about 1 week at refrigerator temperatures, and for up to 1 month when frozen.

Precautions

To ensure an accurate GGT analysis, the blood specimen, whenever possible, should not be collected if the patient has received any medications or used alcohol in the previous 24 hours. Certain drugs, particularly anticonvulsants, increase GGT activity and can produce as much as a fourfold rise above normal levels when taken for a long time.

▶▶ **Nursing Responsibilities and Implications**

1. Report all medications the patient has received during the previous 24 hours on the laboratory request slip.

2. Collect the blood specimen without incurring trauma or hemolysis, which can interfere with the test results.

5′-Nucleotidase

5′-Nucleotidase, an enzyme widely distributed throughout the body, appears in the blood almost exclusively during liver disease, with concentrations up to six times the normal levels frequently found in hepatobiliary obstruction. 5′-Nucleotidase determinations frequently are combined with alkaline phosphatase analysis to help distinguish liver disease from bone disease, in which high alkaline phosphatase levels accompany normal or marginally increased 5′-nucleotidase activity. Laboratory determinations of 5′-nucleotidase levels are most useful in differentiating hepatobiliary and skeletal abnormalities during the investigation of elevated alkaline phosphatase activity and provide a sensitive measure of obstructive biliary disease.

Normal Values
The normal values for 5'-nucleotidase, depending on the test method used, are:

0–17 U/L

2–15 mIU/mL

0–1.6 units

0.3–3.2 Bodansky units

Variations
Elevated 5'-nucleotidase may occur with:

Cholestasis, intrahepatic (resulting from chlorpromazine administration)

Cirrhosis, biliary

Jaundice, posthepatic

Metastatic liver disease

Obstruction, extrahepatic

Surgery

Methodology
5'-Nucleotidase determinations require 5 mL of blood collected without anticoagulants (red-stoppered tube) at 24- to 48-hour intervals to monitor changes that occur during the course of treatment. 5'-Nucleotidase remains stable in specimens for 5 days at room temperature, for about 1 week at refrigerator temperatures, and for up to 1 month when frozen.

LIPIDS

The term **lipid** refers to all fats and fatty acids present in the blood and body tissues that are derived from dietary fats or synthesized in the liver. Once formed, these lipids may be used immediately to meet energy demands, form steroid hormones, and build cell membranes, or they may be stored throughout the body for later use. A number of biologically important lipid compounds, such as cholesterol, cholesterol esters, triglycerides, phospholipids, and free fatty acids, may be found in the blood in varying concentrations.

These lipids are insoluble in serum and therefore circulate in the blood either combined with certain proteins, known as **lipoproteins**, or in an emulsified form known as **chylomicrons**. Thus, evaluation of lipid metabolism usually includes measurement of serum cholesterol, triglyceride, and total lipid levels together with a lipoprotein analysis to determine the relative amount of each lipoprotein type present. Additional tests for cholesterol esters, phospholipids, and free fatty acids also are requested occasionally to supplement the routine lipid profile.

Laboratory determinations of lipid concentrations are a valuable tool in the detection and diagnosis of patients with actual or suspected atherosclerosis and supplement other tests for liver and biliary tract diseases. Lipid concentration measurements also may be helpful in monitoring other conditions that affect lipid levels, including hypothyroidism, nephrotic syndrome, and diabetes mellitus. Lipoprotein electrophoresis, supplemented by cholesterol and triglyceride determinations, provides information necessary for the classification, management, and treatment of lipid diseases such as the hyperlipoproteinemias.

Cholesterol

Cholesterol, a fatlike substance formed in the liver or derived from the breakdown of dietary fats, is found throughout the body, especially in the blood, bile, and brain tissue. Most cholesterol is synthesized in the liver and flows with the bile into the small intestine, where it mixes with dietary cholesterol. This combined pool of free cholesterol is absorbed into the bloodstream and returned to the liver, where about 70% is combined with fatty acids to form cholesterol esters.

Both free and esterified cholesterol are used as building blocks to form many essential compounds, especially various steroid hormones. Free cholesterol and its esters are insoluble in plasma and therefore must be bound with various plasma proteins to be dispersed throughout the body. Thus, any liver disease that causes hepatocellular damage or obstructs the flow of bile from the liver affects the serum concentration of total cholesterol and alters the ratio of free cholesterol to esterified cholesterol.

The range of normal values for total cholesterol in adults appears to vary with many factors, including age, sex, race, geographic location, diet, seasonal changes, physical activity, and occupational stress. However, there is a general lack of agreement as to what constitutes an elevated value, how to determine when elevated values are physiologic or pathologic, and which values indicate a tendency toward atherosclerosis. Laboratory determinations of serum cholesterol are reliable indicators of a tendency toward atherosclerosis and are used mainly in the study of individuals who are prone to cardiovascular and coronary heart disease (CHD). Serum cholesterol and cholesterol ester studies are occasionally performed with other liver tests to aid in identifying the cause of jaundice.

Clinical Significance

Although cholesterol does not cause atherosclerosis, excess amounts of certain lipoproteins that contain cholesterol do contribute to the plaque deposits that occlude the coronary arteries. Normally, about two-thirds of the plasma cholesterol is transported as low-density lipoprotein (LDL), and a small but insignificant amount is bound to high-density lipoproteins (HDL) (see Lipoproteins). Because the concentration of HDL cholesterol appears to be inversely proportional to the tendency toward heart disease, higher levels may be associated with decreased coronary risk and increased longevity. The total cholesterol to HDL cholesterol ratio provides an index to the number of lipoproteins present and also can be used to evaluate the risk of future myocardial infarction. High ratios indicate a significant risk factor for CHD, whereas a low ratio is a favorable finding.

Total cholesterol levels, along with cholesterol ester determinations, provide a guide to the diagnosis and identification of various types of jaundice and liver disorders. For example, obstructive jaundice produces an elevated total cholesterol value with a normal ester ratio because adequate hepatic function is associated with the blockage of bile flow. On the other hand, liver diseases that damage liver cells and produce hepatic jaundice are accompanied by relatively normal or decreased total cholesterol levels and a decreased ester ratio. Cholesterol esters usually are decreased in patients with liver diseases such as infectious hepatitis and cirrhosis.

Normal Values
The normal and clinically significant values for total cholesterol, cholesterol esters, and HDL cholesterol are:

Total cholesterol (average)	120–270 mg/dL
Infants	50–100 mg/dL
1 year	70–175 mg/dL
Adolescence	135–240 mg/dL
20–29 years	144–275 mg/dL
30–39 years	165–295 mg/dL
40–49 years	170–315 mg/dL
50–69 years	175–340 mg/dL
>70 years	130–245 mg/dL
Free cholesterol	<50 mg/dL
Cholesterol esters	<210 mg/dL (68%–74% of total)
HDL cholesterol	29–77 mg/dL
Extreme risk of coronary heart disease	<25 mg/dL of HDL
High risk of coronary heart disease	26–35 mg/dL of HDL
Moderate risk of coronary heart disease	36–44 mg/dL of HDL
Average risk of coronary heart disease	45–59 mg/dL of HDL
Below-average risk of coronary heart disease	60–74 mg/dL of HDL
Probable protection	>75 mg/dL of HDL

Variations
Elevated total serum cholesterol levels (hypercholesterolemia) may occur with:

ACTH administration
Aplastic anemia
Atherosclerosis
Biliary obstruction
Cardiac disease
Celiac disease
Cirrhosis, biliary
Cushing's disease
Diabetes mellitus, uncontrolled or poorly managed

Eclampsia
Glomerulonephritis
Hepatitis
Hypercholesterolemia, familial or idiopathic
Hyperlipoproteinemia
Hypothyroidism
Jaundice, obstructive
Leukemia

Lipoidosis
Nephrosis
Nephrotic syndrome
Oral contraceptives
Pancreatitis, chronic
Pregnancy
Starvation, early
Stress

Decreased total serum cholesterol levels (hypocholesterolemia) may occur with:

Acanthocytosis	Gaucher's disease	Malnutrition
Cancer, terminal	Hepatic disease, extensive	Obstruction, intestinal
Cirrhosis, Laennec's or portal	Hepatitis, toxic or viral	Pernicious anemia
	Hyperthyroidism	Steatorrhea, idiopathic
Epilepsy	Infections, severe	Tuberculosis

Elevated cholesterol esters may occur with nephrotic syndrome and early starvation.

Decreased cholesterol esters may occur with:

Cirrhosis, portal	Hepatic necrosis	Malnutrition
Hepatic disease, chronic	Hepatitis, infectious	Steatorrhea, idiopathic

Decreased total cholesterol/HDL cholesterol ratio (<4.5:1) may occur with:

Alcoholism	Estrogens
Caloric restriction	Nicotinic acid
Drug therapy	Exercise, strenuous
β-adrenergic antagonists (e.g., terbutaline)	Ileal bypass, partial
	Obstructive lung disease, chronic
Clofibrate	

Elevated total cholesterol/HDL cholesterol ratio (>4.5:1) may occur with:

Androgens	Hyperlipoproteinemias (especially with increased very low-density lipoproteins and chylomicrons)
β-adrenergic blockers (e.g., propranolol)	
Carbohydrate feeding	Smoking
Diabetes mellitus	Uremia

Methodology

Total cholesterol and cholesterol ester determinations require 5 mL of unhemolyzed blood collected from a fasting patient in a tube without anticoagulants (red-stoppered tube). Measurement of HDL cholesterol requires 5 mL of blood collected in a tube containing EDTA (lavender-stoppered tube) or no anticoagulants (EDTA is preferred). Specimens for total cholesterol determinations remain stable for 1 week at room temperature and for 1 year or more when frozen. However, tests for cholesterol esters must be performed immediately because esters revert to free cholesterol when retained at room temperature for prolonged periods, producing inaccurate free cholesterol to ester ratios.

Precautions

To ensure an accurate cholesterol determination, the following precautions should be observed:

1. Do not collect blood specimens from patients who have received ACTH, bile salts, bromide, chlorpromazine, phenytoin, or vitamin A in the previous 24 hours because these substances produce elevated cholesterol test results.

2. Do not collect blood specimens from patients who have received heparin, thyroxine, or certain antibiotics such as tetracycline and neomycin in the previous 24 hours because these substances produce decreased cholesterol test results.

▶▶ *Nursing Responsibilities and Implications*

1. Instruct the patient to eat the evening meal no later than 6 PM on the day before testing. This meal should have a low to moderate fat content and should not include foods high in cholesterol such as eggs, organ meats, and shellfish.

2. Withhold medications whenever possible until the blood specimen is collected because many drugs may produce inaccurate test results or interfere with test interpretation.

3. Collect the blood specimen in the morning before the patient has eaten breakfast, following a 12- to 14-hour overnight fast.

4. Prevent hemolysis of the blood specimen during collection and transportation to the laboratory because the release of the cholesterol contained in the red blood cells can produce inaccurate test values.

Triglycerides

Triglycerides, or "true" fats, are composed of three fatty acids and one glycerol molecule, which are either absorbed from dietary fats or synthesized by the liver. Dietary fats enter the intestine, where they are partially broken down by bile. The components are then resynthesized into triglycerides, which are absorbed into the bloodstream as emulsified particles. These lipid particles, known as chylomicrons, are tiny fat droplets that give blood a turbid or milky appearance following a high-fat meal.

Triglycerides store energy and provide the main mechanism for transporting fats in the blood by linking themselves to various plasma protein fractions such as lipoproteins. Triglyceride levels vary considerably depending on the dietary consumption and the time interval since the last meal. Triglycerides usually are completely cleared from the bloodstream within 6 hours after a meal.

After a meal, when sources of energy such as carbohydrate and glucose are abundant, triglycerides are manufactured and stored in adipose tissue, where they can be called on later to provide energy for other tissues. Excess glucose and protein from the diet also are converted into triglycerides by the liver and transported to adipose tissue for storage and later use. Triglycerides currently are considered to be more important than cholesterol concentrations in the development of coronary artery diseases, and triglyceride determinations are used most frequently in the diagnosis of suspected atherosclerosis.

Clinical Significance

Measurement of serum triglyceride levels serves much the same purpose as cholesterol determinations in providing an index to the number of fatty lipoprotein particles associated with plaque deposits and atherosclerosis. Elevated triglyceride levels indicate the presence of any one of several lipid metabolism disorders, which are collectively referred to as hyperlipoproteinemias. Additional tests, such as serum cholesterol and lipoprotein electrophoresis, usually are performed along with triglyceride measurements to complete the lipid profile and make possible an exact diagnosis.

Elevated triglyceride levels also occur as a result of faulty glucose metabolism, in which the fatty acids are released from adipose tissues as an energy source when glucose is unavailable. Such an increase in triglyceride and fatty acid concentrations usually is associated with the ketosis frequently encountered in uncontrolled diabetes mellitus.

Normal Values
The normal values for serum triglycerides are:

0–29 years	20–140 mg/dL
30–39 years	20–150 mg/dL
40–49 years	20–160 mg/dL
>50 years	20–190 mg/dL

Variations
Elevated serum triglyceride levels may occur with:

Diabetes mellitus, uncontrolled	Hyperthyroidism
Glycogen storage disease	Nephrosis
Hemorrhage, chronic	Nephrotic syndrome
Hyperlipemias, idiopathic	Obstructive jaundice
Hyperlipoproteinemia	Starvation, early

Decreased serum triglyceride levels may occur with acanthocytosis, portal cirrhosis, and idiopathic steatorrhea.

Methodology
Triglyceride determinations require 5 mL of blood collected from a fasting patient in a tube without anticoagulants (red-stoppered tube) or containing EDTA (lavender-stoppered tube); serum concentrations are about 3% higher than plasma levels. Measurement of triglyceride levels is most accurate when specimens are collected in the morning following an overnight fast of 12–14 hours.

Precautions
To ensure accurate serum triglyceride determinations, the following precautions should be observed:

1. Do not collect blood specimens for serum triglyceride determinations if the patient has consumed any alcoholic beverage in the previous 24 hours.

2. Do not collect blood specimens if the patient has gained or lost any weight during the 2 weeks immediately preceding testing.

▶▶ Nursing Responsibilities and Implications

1. Instruct the patient to eat a normal diet during the 3 weeks before the test. No attempt to gain or lose weight should be made during this time.

2. Give the evening meal no later than 6 PM on the day before the test. This meal should

not contain excessive fat. The patient must continue to fast after this meal until the blood is collected the next morning, although water is permitted as desired.

3. Whenever possible, withhold all medications during the 24 hours preceding specimen collection because many drugs may affect serum triglyceride levels. It is best to discontinue all medications because it is not yet known exactly which drugs alter lipid levels.

Lipoproteins

Lipoproteins are a combination of various protein molecules and normally insoluble lipids such as cholesterol, triglycerides, phospholipids, and fatty acids, which are produced by the liver and transported in the bloodstream. As a general rule, lipoprotein density diminishes as lipid content increases and protein content decreases. Lipoproteins may be separated and identified according to their weight by ultracentrifugation. They also may be classified according to density based on the relative proportion of lipid to protein.

Lipids usually are separated in clinical practice by electrophoresis and have been divided into four classes on the basis of their density, flotation characteristics, and electrophoretic mobility patterns. Thus, lipoproteins may be categorized as high-density lipoproteins (HDL), low-density lipoproteins (LDL), very low-density lipoproteins (VLDL), and chylomicrons.

High-density lipoproteins, also known as α-lipoproteins, migrate electrophoretically as α_1-proteins. High-density lipoproteins are not associated with the development of atherosclerosis because they are high in protein, cholesterol, and phospholipids but low in triglycerides.

Low-density lipoproteins, also known as β-lipoproteins, migrate electrophoretically as β-proteins. An increase in the LDL level usually is related to the development of atherosclerosis. These lipoproteins are moderately high in protein and cholesterol but low in triglycerides.

Very low-density lipoproteins, also known as pre-β-lipoproteins, migrate electrophoretically as α_2-proteins. An increase in the VLDL level is thought to be consistent with the development of atherosclerosis because these lipoproteins are very high in triglycerides.

Chylomicrons do not migrate in an electrophoretic field but remain at the point of application and are composed almost entirely of triglycerides. Chylomicrons transport the triglycerides from foodstuffs and have no direct relationship to atherosclerosis.

Laboratory evaluation of lipoprotein distribution, in combination with serum cholesterol and triglyceride determinations, is extremely valuable in the identification of individuals who are likely to develop atherosclerosis or CHD. Lipoprotein electrophoresis also is employed to identify abnormal lipoproteins, classify hyperlipoproteinemias, and evaluate disorders of lipid metabolism that are secondary to other conditions such as diabetes, nephrotic syndrome, and hypothyroidism. A clear distinction between primary and secondary hyperlipoproteinemias is necessary and has important therapeutic and prognostic consequences because treatment of the secondary form usually is aimed at the underlying cause.

Clinical Significance
Electrophoretic analysis of lipoproteins has permitted the classification of five distinct patterns or abnormal types that can be correlated with clinical hyperlipemic states (Table

TABLE 4-6 Lipid Changes in Diseases with Hyperlipoproteinemia

Condition	Total Lipid	Cholesterol	Triglycerides	Chylomicrons	α-Lipoprotein	β-Lipoprotein	Pre-β-Lipoprotein
Primary hyperlipoproteinemia							
Type I	Marked increase	Normal to slight increase	Marked increase	Marked increase	Decreased to normal	Decreased to normal	Decreased to normal
Type II	Slight to moderate increase	Slight to marked increase	Normal to slight increase	Negligible	Decreased to normal	Slight to marked increase	Decreased to slight
Type III	Slight to moderate increase	Slight to marked increase	Slight to marked increase	Negligible	Decreased to normal	Slight to marked increase	Marked increase
Type IV	Slight to marked increase	Normal to slight increase	Slight to marked increase	Negligible	Decreased to normal	Decreased to normal	Slight to marked increase
Type V	Slight to marked increase	Normal to slight increase	Slight to marked increase	Slight to marked increase	Decreased to normal	Normal to slight increase	Slight to marked increase
Acquired hyperlipoproteinemia secondary to:							
Hypothyroidism	Slight increase	Moderate increase	Normal	Normal	Normal	Slight increase	Normal
Diabetes mellitus	Slight increase	Slight increase	Moderate increase	Normal	Normal	Normal	Slight increase
Nephrotic syndrome	Slight increase	Slight increase	Slight increase	Normal	Normal	Slight increase	Moderate increase
Alcoholism	Slight increase	Slight increase	Moderate increase	Normal	Normal	Normal	Slight increase
Obstructive liver disease	Slight increase	Moderate increase	Normal	Normal	Slight increase	Slight increase	Normal
Atherosclerosis	Slight increase	Moderate increase	Moderate increase	Normal	Normal	Slight increase	Normal

4-6). These disorders, known as primary hyperlipoproteinemias, refer specifically to electrophoretic patterns, although the addition of serum cholesterol and triglyceride measurements can help to classify the abnormality further. Accurate identification of lipoprotein disorders has important therapeutic significance because prognosis and management are different for each disorder. In addition, there are several secondary hyperlipoprotein disorders in which electrophoretic lipoprotein analysis provides both diagnostic and therapeutic assistance.

Type I primary hyperlipemia is a rare congenital disorder that is manifested in early childhood by bouts of abdominal pain. Individuals with this disorder are unable to adequately metabolize and transport dietary lipids because they lack sufficient concentrations of lipase. Drug therapy is ineffective, but the disorder responds dramatically to a low-fat diet, especially to a limited intake of triglycerides.

Type II primary hyperlipemia is a common inherited disorder that can appear at any age and produces a high risk of atherosclerosis or vascular complications early in life. Individuals with this disorder usually are treated with drugs such as clofibrate, cholestyramine, or probucol along with a low-fat, low-cholesterol, weight-reduction diet.

Type III primary hyperlipemia is a familial disorder that is manifested during adulthood by abnormal glucose tolerance curves and produces a high risk of atherosclerosis. This condition usually is controlled by weight reduction and a low-carbohydrate, low-cholesterol diet in which polyunsaturated fats are substituted for saturated fats, along with clofibrate, nicotinic acid, and dextrothyroxine.

Type IV primary hyperlipemia, the most common inherited hyperlipoproteinemia, is first manifested during adulthood and produces a risk of atherosclerosis or vascular disease. The condition is associated with an abnormal glucose tolerance curve, diabetes, and obesity and frequently is treated with a low-carbohydrate, low-lipid, weight-reduction diet, along with clofibrate or nicotinic acid.

Type V primary hyperlipemia is a rare familial disorder that is manifested during adulthood by abdominal pain. This condition usually is associated with diabetes and obesity and generally is accompanied by an abnormal glucose tolerance curve. Treatment for individuals with this disorder includes a low-carbohydrate, low-fat, weight-reduction diet, together with clofibrate or nicotinic acid therapy following weight loss.

Normal Values

The normal values for lipoprotein electrophoresis are:

High-density lipoproteins	80−310 mg/dL (12%−28%)
Low-density lipoproteins	160−400 mg/dL (50%−70%)
Very low-density lipoproteins	50−180 mg/dL (11%−29%)
Chylomicrons	0−50 mg/dL (0%−1%)

Variations

Type I secondary hyperlipoproteinemia may occur with:

Diabetes mellitus	Multiple myeloma
Dysglobulinemia	Pancreatitis
Macroglobulinemia	Systemic lupus erythematosus

Type II secondary hyperlipoproteinemia may occur with:

Biliary obstruction

Diet (excessive intake of carbohydrates, cholesterol, or fats)

Hypercalcemia, idiopathic

Hypoalbuminemia

Hypothyroidism

Liver disease, obstructive

Macroglobulinemia

Multiple myeloma

Nephrosis

Nephrotic syndrome

Porphyria, acute intermittent

Type III secondary hyperlipoproteinemia may occur with:

Diabetes mellitus (ketoacidosis)

Dysglobulinemia

Hepatic disease

Hypothyroidism

Myxedema

Systemic lupus erythematosus

Type IV secondary hyperlipoproteinemia may occur with:

Addison's disease

Alcoholism

Cushing's disease

Diabetes mellitus

Emotional stress

Gaucher's disease

Glycogen storage disease

Hepatic disease

Hyperestrogenemia

Nephrotic syndrome

Niemann-Pick disease

Obesity

Oral contraceptives

Pancreatitis

Pregnancy

Steroid therapy

Type V secondary hyperlipoproteinemia may occur with:

Addison's disease

Alcoholism

Cushing's disease

Diabetes mellitus, poorly controlled

Glycogen storage disease

Hepatic disease

Hypercalcemia

Hypothyroidism

Multiple myeloma

Nephrosis

Nephrotic syndrome

Pancreatitis

Methodology

Lipoprotein electrophoresis requires 5 mL of blood collected in a tube containing EDTA (lavender-stoppered tube) from a patient who has been fasting for 12–14 hours. Tests should be performed as soon as possible after specimen collection because lipoprotein values are inaccurate when plasma is left at room temperature for prolonged periods. Specimens also show irreversibly altered lipoprotein patterns and loss of the LDL and VLDL fractions when they are stored at refrigerator temperatures for more than 24 hours.

Precautions

To ensure an accurate lipoprotein analysis and lipid profile, the following precautions should be observed:

1. Do not collect specimens for lipoprotein evaluation if the patient has recently had any radiologic examination using x-ray contrast media.

2. Do not submit specimens for lipoprotein determination if the patient has had any alcoholic beverages in the previous 24–48 hours or has gained or lost a significant amount of weight during the preceding 2 weeks.

▶▶ *Nursing Responsibilities and Implications*

1. Give the patient the evening meal no later than 6 PM on the day before testing. The fat content of this meal should be moderate.

2. Collect the blood specimen, with a minimum of hemostasis, into a tube containing EDTA anticoagulant and deliver the specimen to the laboratory as soon as possible.

3. Schedule this test before any radiologic examination using x-ray contrast media.

Free Fatty Acids, Phospholipids, and Total Lipids

A complete laboratory profile of lipid metabolism occasionally may include determinations of less frequently analyzed substances such as phospholipids, free fatty acids, and total lipids.

Free fatty acids, the smallest lipid element, travel in the bloodstream joined to albumin. Although they are negligible in amount, they are the most important form in which lipids are mobilized from fatty tissues. Fat is released from adipose tissue in the form of free fatty acids under the influence of such hormones as ACTH, thyrotropin, growth hormone, and epinephrine. Since free fatty acids are the precursors of the ketones, high concentrations are accompanied by ketosis in the presence of hypoglycemia.

Phospholipids, the largest and most soluble of the lipid elements, play an important role in the metabolism of cellular membranes and are composed of lecithin, cephalin, and spingomyelin.

Total lipid determinations measure the concentration of all the lipid elements present in the circulating blood and may be used as a screening test to indicate abnormal levels of individual constituents.

Clinical Significance

Laboratory determinations of free fatty acids contribute relatively little diagnostic or prognostic information and are therefore not usually included in clinical lipid evaluations. Phospholipids are not related to atherosclerosis and are also therefore seldom included in routine clinical lipid evaluations.

Laboratory determinations of total lipids may routinely be included in a lipid profile, but measurement of individual elements such as lipoproteins, cholesterol, and triglycerides gives much more valuable diagnostic information.

Normal Values

The normal values for miscellaneous lipid studies are:

Free fatty acids	<25 mg/dL (0.3–1.0 mEq/L)
Phospholipids	125–380 mg/dL
Total lipids	
Adults	400–1000 mg/dL
Neonates	100–250 mg/dL
1 week	200–500 mg/dL
1 year	Adult levels

Variations
Elevated free fatty acid levels may occur with:

Diabetes mellitus, untreated	Hypoinsulinemia
Fasting, prolonged	Starvation
Glycogen storage disease	Stress
Hypoglycemia	

Elevated phospholipid levels may occur with:

Diabetes mellitus	Obstructive jaundice
Hypothyroidism	Starvation, early
Nephrotic syndrome	

Decreased phospholipid levels may occur with:

Cirrhosis, portal	Malnutrition
Malabsorption syndrome	Steatorrhea

Elevated total lipid levels may occur with:

Alcoholism	Hypothyroidism
Atherosclerosis	Nephrotic syndrome
Diabetes mellitus	Obstructive liver disease
Glycogen storage disease	Starvation, early
High-fat meal	

Decreased total lipid levels may occur with malabsorption syndrome and steatorrhea.

Methodology
Free fatty acid, phospholipid, and total lipid determinations require 5 mL of unhemolyzed blood collected without anticoagulants (red-stoppered tube) in the morning following a 12- to 14-hour fast. Test results are most significant when the blood specimen is drawn before the patient has received any medications.

Precautions
To ensure accurate free fatty acid, phospholipid, and total lipid determinations, the following precautions should be observed:

1. Do not collect specimens for lipoprotein evaluation if the patient has recently had any radiologic examination using x-ray contrast media.

2. Do not submit specimens for lipoprotein determination if the patient has had any alcoholic beverages in the previous 24–48 hours or has gained or lost a significant amount of weight during the preceding 2 weeks.

▶▶ *Nursing Responsibilities and Implications*

1. Give the patient the evening meal no later than 6 PM on the day before testing. The fat content of this meal should be moderate.

2. Collect the blood specimen, with a minimum of hemostasis, into a tube containing EDTA anticoagulant and deliver the specimen to the laboratory as soon as possible.

3. Schedule this test before any radiologic examination using x-ray contrast media.

LIVER FUNCTION TESTS

The liver is the largest organ in the body and performs many essential biochemical functions. It has a great reserve capacity because nearly four-fifths of the organ can be removed without seriously affecting its function. The following is a list of some of the liver's vital functions:

- Conjugation and excretion of bilirubin
- Detoxification of alcohol, drugs, and other toxic substances
- Metabolism of carbohydrates, fats, and protein
- Metabolism of iron
- Metabolism of steroid hormones
- Production of bilirubin
- Storage of glycogen
- Synthesis of coagulation factors

Damage to the liver or biliary tract may affect any or all of these functions, depending on the type and extent of the disease. Laboratory studies can help to determine the cause of hepatic disorders and assess their severity. Certain diseases affect different liver functions more than others, and the selection of an appropriate group of laboratory tests should be governed by the type of information desired to best identify the degree of liver dysfunction.

A complete clinical or diagnostic picture of liver disease requires a group of carefully selected tests because no single measurement yields all of the necessary information. The battery of liver tests most frequently ordered reflects the various functions of the liver and helps to establish the site, type, and extent of hepatic damage. Laboratory determination of liver function may be used for the differential diagnosis of jaundice, ascites, and hepatomegaly and also may be used to evaluate patients with known liver disease (Table 4-7). Liver function tests frequently help to monitor the convalescent period of conditions such as hepatitis and cirrhosis.

The following laboratory tests commonly are used to evaluate liver function. However, because these tests also frequently are used to investigate conditions other than liver disease, they are discussed elsewhere in this or other chapters.

α-Fetoprotein

Ammonia, blood

Bile pigments

    Bilirubin, serum (direct, indirect, and total) (Chapter 3)

    Bilirubin, urine (Chapter 1)

Urobilinogen, urine and fecal (Chapters 1, 3, and 8)

Cholesterol, serum (total and esters)

Enzymes, serum

    Alanine aminotransferase

    Alkaline phosphatase

TABLE 4-7 Summary of Frequently Used Liver Function Studies

Laboratory Test	Hemolytic Jaundice	Hepatic Jaundice	Obstructive Jaundice
Serum bilirubin (total)	Moderate increase	Marked increase	Marked increase
Serum bilirubin (direct)	Normal	Increased	Increased
Urine bilirubin	Negative	Positive	Positive
Urine urobilinogen	Increased	Increased	Decreased
Fecal urobilinogen	Increased	Normal	Decreased
Bromsulphthalein excretion	Normal	Increased retention	Increased retention
Flocculation and turbidity	Negative	Positive	Negative
Blood ammonia	Normal	Increased	Normal
Serum protein (albumin)	Normal	Decreased	Normal
Serum protein (globulin)	Normal	Increased	Normal
Serum cholesterol (total)	Normal	Decreased	Increased
Serum cholesterol (ester)	Normal	Decreased	Normal
Alkaline phosphatase	Normal	Slight increase	Marked increase
Transaminase enzymes	Normal	Marked increase	Slight increase
Lactic dehydrogenase	Increased	Increased	Normal
Pseudocholinesterase	Normal	Decreased	Decreased

Aspartate aminotransferase

Gamma-glutamyl transferase

Lactic dehydrogenase

5'-Nucleotidase

Pseudocholinesterase

Hepatitis-associated antigens and antibodies (Chapter 11)

Proteins, serum

Albumin

Albumin/globulin (A/G) ratio

Globulin

Fibrinogen (Chapter 10)

Serum protein electrophoresis

Prothrombin time (Chapter 10)

MISCELLANEOUS TESTS

Ascorbic Acid

Ascorbic acid (vitamin C), a natural substance present in many fruits and vegetables such as oranges, strawberries, tomatoes, potatoes, and leafy greens, plays an important role in the body's reaction to stress. Ascorbic acid is necessary for the maintenance of connective tissue and participates in a wide range of metabolic processes leading to the formation of collagen, norepinephrine, and homogentisic acid. Vitamin C also aids in the absorption of iron, activation of folic acid, and detoxification of poisonous substances.

The average intake of ascorbic acid ranges from 30 to 80 mg/day, with about half this amount normally excreted in the urine, depending on the dietary intake. Vitamin C levels in blood are lower in smokers than nonsmokers and may be depleted following prolonged stimulation of the adrenal glands and their hormones, such as occurs during stress. Severe vitamin C deficiency produces scurvy and is characterized by pathologic manifestations related to supportive tissue degeneration, including delayed wound healing, increased bone fracturability, edema, and hemorrhage.

Normal Values

The normal values for vitamin C are:

Plasma	0.2–2.0 mg/dL
Urine	1–7 mg/dL
	15–30 mg/24 hours

Variations

Elevated vitamin C levels may occur with massive ascorbic acid therapy and excessive dietary intake.

Decreased vitamin C levels may occur in the immediate postpartum period, during pregnancy, and with scurvy.

Elevated vitamin C excretion may occur with fever and infection.

Decreased vitamin C excretion may occur with ascorbic acid deficiency.

Methodology

Ascorbic acid determinations require 10 mL of blood collected with sodium oxalate (gray-stoppered tube) or without anticoagulants (red-stoppered tube). Urinary ascorbic acid determinations require a 50 mL random urine specimen, whereas evaluation of the ascorbic acid excretion rate requires a 50 mL aliquot of a 24-hour urine specimen. Plasma and urine specimens remain stable for ascorbic acid determinations for 6 days when frozen.

▶▶ Nursing Responsibilities and Implications

1. Inform the patient that there are no food or fluid restrictions required for ascorbic acid determinations.

2. Instruct the patient on the correct procedure for collecting a 24-hour urine specimen when evaluation of ascorbic acid excretion rate is requested.

Carotene and Vitamin A

Vitamin A, a naturally occurring substance, is required for normal cellular growth and development and may be metabolized from carotene or absorbed preformed from the diet. Vitamin A occurs principally in fish-liver oils, butter, cheese, liver, and tomatoes, as well as many other yellow and dark green vegetables. **Carotene** is a yellow pigment found in carrots, sweet potatoes, leafy vegetables, and egg yolks; following excessive dietary intake, the skin may turn yellow and resemble jaundice.

Vitamin A concentrations are influenced by the amount of carotene in the diet, whereas carotene levels reflect recent dietary intake but do not indicate the patient's overall vitamin A nutritional status. Laboratory determination of vitamin A is the most practical biochemical means of evaluating the patient's vitamin A nutritional status and aids in the differential diagnosis of hypercalcemia associated with bone resorption. Hypervitaminosis A should be considered as the cause of certain bone disorders because many food faddists may not admit to ingesting excessive amounts of vitamin A.

Clinical Significance

Vitamin A is essential for vision and also is required for bone growth, glycogen synthesis, maintenance of subcellular membranes, and spermatogenesis. Vitamin A intoxication (hypervitaminosis A) may produce varied clinical symptoms, including hair loss, bone pain, increased intracranial pressure, hepatic injury, and thyroid depression, and may lead to teratogenic effects in early pregnancy. Conversely, vitamin A deficiency (hypovitaminosis A) produces night blindness, hardening of the skin (resulting in lessened resistance to epithelial infections), and degeneration of mucous membranes with drying of the conjunctiva.

Normal Values
The normal values for carotene and vitamin A are:

Carotene	50–250 μg/dL (varies with diet)
	50–300 IU/L
Vitamin A	
Adults	20–80 μg/dL
	65–275 IU/dL
Infants	15–60 μg/dL

Variations

Elevated carotene levels may occur with:

Diabetes mellitus	Myxedema	Pregnancy
Hyperlipemia	Nephritis, chronic	

Decreased carotene levels may occur with:

Cystic fibrosis	Malabsorption syndrome	Steatorrhea
Low-fat diets	Pancreatic insufficiency	

Elevated vitamin A levels (hypervitaminosis A) may occur with chronic excessive dietary intake and oral contraceptive therapy.

Methodology

Carotene and vitamin A determinations each require 5 mL of blood collected without anticoagulants (red-stoppered tube) and protected from light. Specimens should be delivered to the laboratory as soon as possible and analyzed promptly because vitamin A is unstable when stored, although carotene remains stable for 4 days at room temperature.

▶▶ *Nursing Responsibilities and Implications*

1. Inform the patient that there are no fluid or food restrictions for vitamin A or carotene determinations.

2. Protect the blood specimen from a direct light source or direct sunlight which could cause deterioration of vitamin A.

Copper

Copper, an essential trace element contained in certain metalloenzymes and proteins, acts as an activator for many enzymes and is required for the formation of hemoglobin during hematopoiesis. Most copper is firmly bound to an α_2-globulin transport protein, known as **ceruloplasmin**, that helps to mobilize iron from storage sites. Abnormal copper metabolism produces Wilson's disease, which is characterized by degenerative changes of the liver and basal ganglia of the brain as a result of excessive copper deposition. Laboratory evaluation of serum copper levels aids in the diagnosis of Wilson's disease, allows the prompt institution of a low-copper diet, and helps to monitor therapy, which is aimed at promoting copper excretion.

Normal Values
The normal values for serum and urine copper are:

Serum copper	
Men	70–140 μg/dL
Women	80–155 μg/dL
Infants	15–65 μg/dL
Children	30–150 μg/dL
Urine copper	0–60 μg/24 hours

Variations
Elevated serum copper levels (hypercupremia) may occur with:

Cirrhosis	Myocardial infarction
Hodgkin's disease	Oral contraceptives (150–245 μg/dL)
Hyperestrogenemia	Pellagra
Infections, acute and chronic	Pregnancy
Lymphomas, various	Rheumatoid arthritis

Decreased serum copper levels (hypocupremia) may occur with:

Kwashiorkor	Nephrosis
Hypoproteinemia	Nutritional deficiencies, certain
Malabsorption syndrome, protein	Wilson's disease (40–60 μg/dL)
Menkes' kinky hair syndrome	

Elevated urine copper levels may occur with:

Aminoaciduria

Proteinuria

Hypoceruloplasminemia

Wilson's disease (500–1000 μg/dL)

Pellagra

Methodology

Serum copper measurements require 10 mL of blood collected in a plastic syringe and transferred to a tube without a rubber siliconized stopper (navy blue-stoppered tube). Determination of urinary copper excretion requires a 100 mL aliquot of a 24-hour urine specimen acidified to pH 2 with hydrochloric acid. Serum specimens for copper measurements remain stable for 4 days at room temperature; urine specimens remain stable for 11 days at room temperature.

Precautions

To ensure accurate serum and urine copper measurements, prevent the blood and urine specimens from coming in contact with the rubber stopper, which can interfere with test results.

▶▶ Nursing Responsibilities and Implications

1. Inform the patient that no food or fluid restrictions are required for copper determinations.

2. Instruct the patient on the procedure for collecting a 24-hour urine specimen.

3. Note on the laboratory request slip the total 24-hour urine volume.

Zinc

Zinc, a trace metal essential to cellular growth, is a constituent of many important enzymes and plays an important role in metabolism in neonates and children. Zinc-containing medications increase healing of extensive wounds, burns, and decubitus ulcers in patients with zinc depletion or inadequate dietary intake. Laboratory determination of zinc levels aids in the diagnosis of zinc intoxication and helps to monitor replacement therapy in zinc depletion.

Clinical Significance

Acute zinc intoxication may result from industrial exposure, consumption of acidic foods or beverages from galvanized containers, and children's toys and produces symptoms similar to lead toxicity. Toxic effects of accidental zinc exposure include cough and chest discomfort, tachycardia, hypertension, pulmonary edema, gastrointestinal irritation, fever, nausea, vomiting, diarrhea, abdominal pain, and a metallic taste in the mouth. Decreased zinc levels caused by dietary deficiency are accompanied by anorexia, impaired taste perception, mental lethargy, rough skin, failure to thrive (infants), growth retardation, and delayed sexual maturation.

> **Normal Values**
> The normal values for zinc are:
>
> Serum
> Men   75−160 μg/dL
> Women   50−110 μg/dL
> Urine   110−800 μg/24 hours

Variations
Decreased serum zinc levels may occur with:

Acrodermatitis enteropathica	Meat-deficient diets (children)
Alcoholic cirrhosis	Myocardial infarction, acute
Carcinoma of the lung	Oral contraceptives
Corticosteroid therapy	Pregnancy
Malabsorption syndrome	Sickle cell disease

Methodology
Zinc determinations require 10 mL of blood collected without hemolysis in a zinc-free plastic syringe or evacuated tube with no anticoagulants and a rubber siliconized stopper (navy blue-stoppered tube). Measurement of urinary zinc excretion requires a 50 mL aliquot of a 24-hour urine specimen; the 24-hour urine volume should be noted on the laboratory request slip.

Precautions
To ensure accurate serum and urine zinc measurements, the following precautions should be observed:

1. Prevent hemolysis during specimen collection because red blood cells contain approximately ten times as much zinc as plasma, and any appreciable hemolysis produces falsely elevated test results.

2. Collect a 24-hour urine specimen in a zinc-free container and prevent the specimen from coming in contact with rubber, which can produce falsely elevated test results.

▶▶ Nursing Responsibilities and Implications

1. Inform the patient that no food or fluid restrictions are required for zinc determinations.

2. Instruct the patient on the procedure for collecting a 24-hour urine specimen.

3. Note on the laboratory request slip the total 24-hour urine volume.

NONPROTEIN NITROGEN COMPOUNDS

Nonprotein nitrogen (NPN) compounds are a group of waste products in the blood that result from the metabolic breakdown of dietary or tissue protein. These nitrogen-containing compounds include urea (measured in blood as blood urea nitrogen, or BUN), creatinine, uric acid, amino acids, and ammonia. They are referred to collectively as the **nonprotein nitrogens** to distinguish them from the serum proteins, which also contain nitrogen. These waste products are removed from the body by the kidneys.

Simultaneous measurement of several of these substances helps to evaluate renal function because these compounds accumulate in the blood of patients with kidney disease due to a flaw in the filtering system. Nonprotein nitrogen concentrations reflect the degree and extent of renal involvement because uric acid is the first substance to become elevated in kidney disease and creatinine is usually the last. However, NPN determinations should not completely replace specific kidney function studies.

Blood Ammonia

Ammonia, a waste product of protein and amino acid metabolism, is derived mainly from bacterial action on the nitrogen contained in dietary protein within the gastrointestinal tract. Most ammonia in the blood normally is removed from the bloodstream by the liver, where it is converted to urea, which is excreted in the urine. Blood ammonia determinations are used to evaluate hepatic function because any damage to liver parenchymal cells may decrease urea synthesis by the liver and cause circulating levels of ammonia to rise. Laboratory determinations of blood ammonia levels therefore are useful in evaluating severe liver disease, recognizing impending or established hepatic coma, assessing the progress of therapy, and identifying gastrointestinal bleeding caused by esophageal varices.

Clinical Significance
Elevated blood ammonia levels (**hyperammonemia**) produce a variety of toxic effects on the central nervous system that may be characterized by lethargy, agitation, seizures, and coma; brain stem function is lost eventually. Acute hyperammonemia frequently produces hyperventilation, which leads to respiratory alkalosis, presumably because of stimulation of the central respiratory center. The major effect of chronic hyperammonemia, however, is impairment of intellectual function. A variety of neurologic symptoms, including coma, may result from the high blood ammonia levels that sometimes accompany liver diseases such as acute hepatitis, advanced cirrhosis, or Reye's syndrome.

Blood ammonia concentrations three to five times the upper limit of normal may be responsible for some toxic symptoms of hepatic coma that result from high ammonia levels in the cerebrospinal fluid. Hemorrhage from esophageal varices or any other gastrointestinal source in patients with cirrhosis generally is accompanied by elevated ammonia levels, whereas concentrations of ammonia in noncirrhotic individuals are usually normal. Blood ammonia levels in patients with impaired hepatic function may be lowered somewhat by controlling protein intake and by administering antibiotics to reduce the action of intestinal bacteria.

Normal Values
The normal blood ammonia levels, depending on the test method used, are:

Colorimetric method	70–200 μg/dL
Resin method	5–69 μg/dL

Variations

Elevated blood ammonia levels may occur with:

Azotemia

Cirrhosis, marked

Diabetic coma

Erythroblastosis fetalis

Esophageal varices, hemorrhagic

Heart failure, severe

Hepatic coma

Hepatitis, acute

Inborn errors of metabolism

Pneumonia, severe

Portacaval shunt

Premature infants (with severe neurologic symptoms)

Reye's syndrome

Shock

Falsely elevated blood ammonia levels may be produced by a number of drugs:

Acetazolamide

Ammonium salts

Chlorothiazide

Heparin (some brands)

Methicillin

Thiazide diuretics

Urea

Methodology

Blood ammonia determinations require 5 mL of blood collected in a tube containing potassium or sodium oxalate, EDTA, or heparin anticoagulant (gray-, lavender-, or green-stoppered tube, respectively) that is completely filled and mixed well to prevent clotting. (The ammonia salt of heparin should not be used because it will interfere with the accuracy of the test results.) Blood for ammonia determinations should be placed on ice and delivered immediately to the laboratory because specimens remain stable for no longer than 20–30 minutes when collected in heparin.

Precautions

To ensure accurate blood ammonia determinations, the following precautions should be observed:

1. Delay specimen collection, whenever possible, if the patient has received medications in the previous 24 hours because certain drugs may interfere with the test procedure.

2. Perform an accurate, swift venipuncture with minimal turbulence and minimal use of the tourniquet (use of a tourniquet for 10–15 seconds is acceptable).

3. Collect the blood directly into a cooled, heparinized, evacuated tube or transfer it immediately from a syringe into an open, cold, heparinized tube without using a needle.

4. Immerse the tube immediately in ice and rotate it to facilitate mixing and cooling. Deliver the blood specimen to the laboratory immediately because the amount of ammonia increases rapidly after the blood is drawn and can cause inaccurate test results.

▶▶ **Nursing Responsibilities and Implications**

1. Withhold the patient's breakfast after an overnight fast until the blood specimen is drawn because dietary intake of protein can cause ammonia concentrations to vary.

2. Caution the patient not to smoke during the morning before the blood specimen is collected.

3. Encourage the patient to relax before the test because extreme agitation or exercise can cause a marked elevation of the test values.

4. Notify the laboratory in advance that a blood ammonia determination has been requested so that the test can be performed without delay.

Blood Urea Nitrogen

Blood urea nitrogen (BUN) is the name traditionally applied to tests for urea concentrations in whole blood, although current methods measure serum or plasma levels because the difference is clinically insignificant. Urea, the chief waste product of protein and amino acid metabolism, is formed from the ammonia detoxified by the liver and is transported to the kidneys for excretion in the urine. Urea concentrations in the blood and urine therefore are directly influenced by the intake and breakdown of dietary protein, the rate of urea production in the liver, and the rate of urea removal by the kidneys.

The most common cause of increased urea concentrations is inadequate excretion, which is usually due to kidney disease or urinary obstruction, although other factors also may affect urea levels in the blood and urine. Elevated BUN concentrations may result from inadequate kidney function, which decreases the rate of urea removal, as well as excess protein ingestion or cellular protein catabolism. Laboratory determination of BUN generally is used as a screening test for renal disease, especially disorders of glomerular filtration, rather than as a measure of liver function or urea production.

Clinical Significance

The liver has the least influence on BUN values because at least 80%–85% of hepatic function must be lost before urea levels are affected. Elevated BUN values are a cause for grave concern because they indicate that other, more toxic substances are being retained in the blood in about the same proportion. Blood urea nitrogen concentrations are determined and reported in terms of urea nitrogen because urea is difficult to measure, although urea values can be obtained by multiplying BUN values by 2.14.

Normal Values

The normal and clinically significant values for blood and urine urea nitrogen are:

Blood

6–25 mg/dL	Normal
>26 mg/dL	Impaired renal function or gastro-intestinal bleeding
>50 mg/dL	Severe renal impairment

Urine

6–17 g/24 hours	Normal

Variations
Elevated blood urea nitrogen levels (azotemia) may be caused by:

Renal conditions

   Glomerulonephritis, acute and chronic

   Malignancy

   Nephritis, acute

   Nephrosclerosis, advanced

   Pyelonephritis

   Renal cortical necrosis

   Renal tuberculosis

   Suppuration

   Uremia

   Urinary obstruction (calculi, strictures, tumors, prostatic enlargement, scarring)

Extrarenal conditions

   Addison's disease

   Cachexia

   Cardiac failure

Dehydration (burns, water deprivation, profuse diarrhea, protracted vomiting, excessive perspiration, fever)

Diabetic ketoacidosis, severe

Gastrointestinal bleeding

Gout, chronic

Infection, sepsis, peritonitis

Intestinal obstruction

Metallic poisoning

Pancreatitis

Pneumonia

Postoperative state

Protein intake, excessive

Shock, hypovolemic or surgical

Starvation

Thyrotoxicosis

Tumor necrosis

Decreased blood urea nitrogen levels may be caused by:

Amyloidosis	Hemodialysis	Malnutrition
Cirrhosis	Liver destruction, acute	Nephrosis
Fluid intake, excessive	Low-protein diet	Pregnancy

Elevated urine urea nitrogen levels may be caused by febrile conditions, gastrointestinal bleeding, and starvation.

Decreased urine urea nitrogen levels may be caused by:

Acidosis

Cirrhosis

Dehydration

Glomerulonephritis, chronic

Liver destruction, acute

Nephritis, acute

Shock, hypovolemic or surgical

Urinary obstruction

Falsely elevated blood urea nitrogen levels may be caused by a number of drugs:

Anabolic steroids	Dextran	Mephenesin
Androgens	Furosemide	Methoxyflurane
Arginine	Gentamicin	Methsuximide
Calcium salts	Guanethidine	Methyldopa
Cephaloridine	Kanamycin	Metolazone
Chloral hydrate	Licorice	Neomycin
Clonidine	Marijuana	

Falsely decreased blood urea nitrogen levels may be caused by drugs that have a marked diuretic effect and by additional drugs:

Chloramphenicol	Paramethasone (during pregnancy)
Mercurial diuretics	Streptomycin

Methodology

Blood urea nitrogen determinations require 5 mL of blood collected without anticoagulants (red-stoppered tube). Although plasma specimens also may be used for urea nitrogen determinations, they should not be collected in double oxalate anticoagulant because it contains ammonium, which can cause inaccurate BUN results. Whole blood specimens for BUN may be refrigerated for up to 72 hours without changing the BUN concentration significantly. Serum and plasma specimens may be refrigerated for about 1 week after they are separated from their cells or frozen for 1 month without changing BUN values measurably.

Measurement of urine urea concentrations requires a 50–100 mL aliquot of a 24-hour urine specimen. Urine specimens are especially susceptible to urea loss due to bacterial decomposition, so specimens should be delivered to the laboratory immediately and the laboratory staff notified of its arrival so that BUN concentrations will be measured promptly.

Precautions

To ensure accurate BUN determinations, delay specimen collection, whenever possible, if the patient is receiving any medications that produce kidney toxicity.

▶▶ Nursing Responsibilities and Implications

1. Assess the patient for signs of over- or underhydration; dehydration may produce an elevated BUN level, whereas overhydration may produce a decreased BUN level.

2. Note on the laboratory slip any medications the patient is receiving that might interfere with the test results.

3. Institute the following steps if the BUN level is moderately severely elevated:
   a. Monitor urine hourly; notify the physician if hourly output is less than 50 mL.
   b. Provide safety measures because the patient's level of consciousness may be altered; institute seizure precautions.
   c. Observe for signs of anemia because elevated BUN destroys red blood cells.
   d. Observe the patient for signs of gastrointestinal bleeding, which might be associated with an elevated BUN level.

Creatinine

Creatinine is the chief waste product of the creatine produced when energy is released from phosphocreatine, an energy-storing compound, during skeletal muscle metabolism. The rate of creatinine formation is directly proportional to the total muscle mass and remains remarkably constant for each individual because it is not affected significantly by protein ingestion or muscular exercise. Creatinine is removed from the bloodstream by the kidneys and excreted in the urine at a rate that closely parallels its formation and is independent of water intake or the rate of urine production.

Serum and urine creatinine levels provide an index of renal function because individuals with uremia retain creatinine in their blood and develop grossly elevated serum concentrations as a result of incomplete renal clearance. Laboratory determinations of serum creatinine therefore are used almost exclusively in the diagnosis and follow-up of renal disease, whereas urine creatinine determinations usually are performed as part of the creatinine clearance test. (See Creatinine Clearance Test in Chapter 1.)

Clinical Significance

Serum creatinine levels indicate the balance between creatinine formation and excretion and reflect the efficiency of glomerular filtration and active tubular secretion. In kidney diseases in which 50% or more of the renal nephrons are destroyed, creatinine excretion is reduced and serum levels become increased in proportion to the decrease of renal function. However, although severe, long-standing renal impairment usually elevates serum creatinine values, normal test values may be obtained in some patients with mild chronic renal disease or even acute uremia.

Urine creatinine levels, on the other hand, reflect the amount of active muscle tissue in the body rather than body weight. Thus, individuals with an extra large muscle mass or increased tissue catabolism have higher urine creatinine values than those with less muscle mass. Urine creatinine concentrations are reported as milligrams per kilogram of body weight, but this figure may be distorted in excessively obese individuals because of the additional weight of adipose tissue.

Normal Values

The normal values for serum and urine creatinine are:

Serum	
Infants	<0.6 mg/dL
Men	0.6–1.5 mg/dL
Women	0.5–1.0 mg/dL
Urine	
Men	1.0–2.0 g/24 hours
	20–26 mg/kg of body weight/24 hours
Women	0.6–1.5 g/24 hours
	14–22 mg/kg of body weight/24 hours

Variations

Elevated serum creatinine levels may be caused by:

Acromegaly	Hypovolemic shock
Congestive heart failure	Nephritis
Glomerulonephritis, chronic	Obstruction, intestinal or urinary

Decreased serum creatinine levels may be caused by muscular dystrophy.
Elevated urine creatinine levels may be caused by fever and tissue catabolism.

Decreased urine creatinine levels may be caused by:

Glomerulonephritis, chronic	Muscular dystrophy or atrophy
Hyperthyroidism	Urinary obstruction
Hypovolemic shock	

Falsely elevated serum creatinine levels may occur immediately following tests using sodium bromsulphthalein (BSP) or phenolsulfonphthalein (PSP) dyes and in patients using the following drugs:

Amphotericin B	Cephalosporins	Doxycycline
Ascorbic acid (high levels)	Chlorthalidone	Dextran
	Clofibrate	Kanamycin
Barbiturates	Clonidine	L-dopa
Capreomycin	Colistin	Methyldopa
Carbutamide		

Falsely elevated urine creatinine levels may be reported in patients taking the following drugs:

Ascorbic acid	L-dopa	Nitrofuran
Corticosteroids	Methyldopa	Phenolsulfonphthalein

Falsely decreased urine creatinine levels may occur in patients taking anabolic steroids, androgens, and thiazide diuretics.

Methodology

Serum creatinine determinations require 7 mL of blood collected without anticoagulants (red-stoppered tube). Urine creatinine determinations require a 24-hour urine specimen, which must be kept refrigerated throughout the entire collection period because creatinine is unstable and readily decomposes at room temperature. Serum and urine specimens remain stable when refrigerated for about 1 week or at least 1 month when frozen.

Precautions

Delay specimen collection, whenever possible, if the patient has received any medications or has recently undergone tests utilizing certain dyes (BSP, PSP).

▶▶ Nursing Responsibilities and Implications

1. Inform the patient that there are no food or fluid restrictions before the test.

2. Note on the laboratory slip any medications the patient is receiving that might interfere with the test results.

3. Monitor the patient's urinary output to determine fluid balance; a decreased output may indicate renal insufficiency.

4. Provide safety measures because retained creatinine may cause an altered level of consciousness and confusion.

5. Teach the patient to limit the intake of beef, poultry, and fish if the serum creatinine level is severely elevated.

Blood Urea Nitrogen/Creatinine Ratio

Serum creatinine determinations are preferable to BUN values as a screening test for evaluating renal function because creatinine levels rise more slowly than BUN levels in the presence of renal disease. However, creatinine determinations are less useful than BUN values in assessing the effectiveness of hemodialysis because creatinine levels decrease slower than BUN values. The BUN/creatinine ratio adds sensitivity to the clinical interpretation of individual test results in assessing renal function and helps to evaluate the significance of an elevated BUN level.

Clinical Significance
The BUN/creatinine ratio may be decreased, increased, or disproportionate in certain conditions. For example, decreased BUN/creatinine ratios frequently develop in renal dialysis patients, because urea is dialyzed more readily than creatinine, and muscular individuals with renal failure because creatinine formation is greater. A decreased BUN/creatinine ratio also appears in individuals with diminished urea formation caused by a low-protein diet.

Conversely, an increased BUN/creatinine ratio develops during azotemia associated with inadequate blood flow to the kidneys caused by dehydration or shock and augmented tubular reabsorption of urea resulting from diminished glomerular filtration. An increased BUN/creatinine ratio also may develop because urea absorption is much greater than creatinine absorption, whether from the urinary tract in the case of acute obstructive uropathy or from tissues in the case of extravasation of urine.

Normal Values
The normal values for the BUN/creatinine ratio are:

<10:1	Diminished urea concentration
10:1–15:1	Normal
>15:1	Inadequate renal function

Variations
Elevated blood urea nitrogen/creatinine ratios may occur with:

Azotemia	Gastrointestinal bleeding	Protein intake, excessive
Burns	Glomerular disease	Shock
Cushing's disease	Heart failure	Tetracycline therapy
Dehydration	Hemorrhage	Thyrotoxicosis
Fever	Muscle, tissue destruction	Urinary tract obstruction

Decreased blood urea nitrogen/creatinine ratios may occur with:

Dialysis	Overhydration
Hyperammonemia syndromes, congenital	Phenacemide therapy
Liver disease, severe	Protein intake, decreased

Inappropriate blood urea nitrogen/creatinine ratios may occur with cephalosporin therapy and diabetic ketoacidosis.

Uric Acid

Uric acid is the nitrogen-containing end product of purine metabolism, which takes place in the bone marrow, muscles, and liver. Purines are synthesized in the body from the breakdown of cellular nucleic acids or are absorbed by the intestines from the complex nucleoproteins in foods. The uric acid derived daily from this purine-nucleoprotein metabolism passes into the bloodstream and is freely excreted in the urine.

Uric acid concentrations in serum and urine depend on renal function and the rate of purine formation and dietary intake of purine-rich foods such as legumes, mushrooms, spinach, coffee, tea, cocoa, and meats, particularly liver or sweetbreads. The quantities of uric acid excreted are governed by its rate of formation and the effectiveness of renal function, especially glomerular filtration and tubular secretion. Laboratory determinations of serum and urine uric acid levels are used to screen for renal disease and to detect nucleic acid metabolic disorders such as gout.

Clinical Significance

Abnormal purine metabolism and elevated serum or urine uric acid concentrations can cause serious consequences because uric acid is insoluble and crystallizes in the urinary tract. Severe kidney disease and impaired renal function, which depress uric acid excretion, are the most frequent causes of elevated serum concentrations (**hyperuricemia**). The secondary hyperuricemia associated with renal failure is a more common cause of elevated uric acid concentrations than the primary hyperuricemia that characterizes disorders involving purine metabolism such as gout.

However, elevated serum uric acid values are not sensitive or reliable enough to be used alone in evaluating therapy or the prognosis of gout. Normal uric acid levels, on the other hand, do not exclude the diagnosis of gout because serum levels often remain low during the early stages of this condition and become elevated only during acute episodes. Uric acid also appears in the synovial fluid of patients with gout and causes crystalline uric acid deposits (**tophi**) to form in cartilage and other tissues surrounding the joints.

Normal Values
The normal serum and urine uric acid values are:

Serum

Men	4.0–8.0 mg/dL
Women	2.5–7.5 mg/dL

Urine

Low-purine diet	250–500 mg/24 hours
Normal diet	400–800 mg/24 hours

Variations
Elevated serum uric acid levels may occur with:

Alcoholism, ethyl alcohol ingestion	Congestive heart failure
Arthritis	Diabetes, diabetic ketoacidosis

Drug therapy
  Acetazolamide
  Chlorthalidone
  Diazoxide
  Epinephrine
  Ethacrynic acid
  Furosemide
  Hydralazine
  6-Mercaptopurine
  Nitrogen mustard
  Phenothiazines
  Propylthiouracil
  Salicylates (prolonged low doses)
  Thiazide diuretics
Eclampsia
Exercise, strenuous
Glomerulonephritis, chronic
Gout
Hemolysis, prolonged
Hyperparathyroidism
Hypertension
Infections, acute
Infectious mononucleosis
Ketosis, nondiabetic
Lead poisoning
Leukemia
Lipoproteinemia, type III
Multiple myeloma
Nephritis
Obstruction, intestinal or urinary
Pernicious anemia
Pneumonia
Polycythemia vera
Pregnancy (during the onset of labor)
Psoriasis
Renal failure
Starvation
Toxemia of pregnancy
Uremia
von Gierke's syndrome

Decreased serum uric acid levels may occur with:

Acromegaly
Drug therapy
  Acetohexamide
  Allopurinol
  Azathioprine
  Chlorpromazine
  Chlorprothixene
  Cinchophen
Clofibrate
Corticosteroids
Corticotropin
Cortisone
Coumarin
Dicumarol
Phenylbutazone
Probenecid
Radiographic agents
Salicylates (prolonged large doses)
Fanconi's syndrome
Wilson's disease
Yellow atrophy of liver
Xanthinuria

Elevated urine uric acid levels may occur with:

Fanconi's syndrome
Drug therapy
  Cytotoxic drugs
Salicylates (prolonged high doses)
Gout
Leukemia
X-ray contrast media

Decreased urine uric acid levels may occur with:

Drug therapy (see elevated serum uric acid)
Eclampsia
Glomerulonephritis, chronic
Nephritis
Renal failure
Toxemia of pregnancy
Uremia
Urinary obstruction

Methodology

Serum uric acid determinations require 5 mL of blood collected without anticoagulants (red-stoppered tube). Determination of urine uric acid values requires a 50 mL aliquot of a 24-hour urine specimen that has been kept refrigerated during the entire collection period. When uric acid determinations cannot be performed immediately, serum and urine specimens remain stable for at least 1 week when refrigerated or 1 month when frozen.

Precautions

To ensure accurate uric acid test results, delay specimen collection, whenever possible, in patients who have received certain medications within the past 24 hours. Falsely elevated uric acid values may occur with certain test methods in the presence of excess reducing substances, such as nonglucose sugars, and a variety of drugs, including ascorbic acid, L-dopa, and methyldopa.

▶▶ **Nursing Responsibilities and Implications**

1. Inform the patient that although there are no food or fluid restrictions prior to the test, it is advisable to limit the intake of foods high in purine such as organ meats, scallops, sardines, anchovies, asparagus, mushrooms, and spinach.

2. Keep 24-hour urine specimens refrigerated during the entire collection period.

3. If uric acid levels are elevated, teach the patient to avoid foods high in purine.

SERUM PROTEINS

Serum proteins are composed of at least 100 individual substances synthesized in the liver and reticuloendothelial system and divided into several different fractions classified as albumin and globulins. As a group, these proteins perform many vital and varied physiologic functions that are entirely different from those of tissue proteins, including:

- Production of antibodies against disease-causing organisms in the body's immunologic defense system.
- Provision of coagulation factors necessary for hemostasis.
- Provision of many vital enzymes and hormones.
- Maintenance of osmotic pressure and water balance between blood and tissue.
- Maintenance of a reserve of protein for tissue growth and repair.
- Service as precursors for the synthesis of tissue protein and source of rapid replacement during tissue depletion.
- Service as pH buffers for acid-base balance.
- Transportation of other blood constituents, including bilirubin, calcium, certain enzymes, steroid and thyroid hormones, lipids, metals, oxygen, and vitamins.
- Contribution to the body's nitrogen needs.

Albumin, the smallest protein molecule, plays an important role in regulating the osmotic pressure of plasma, stabilizing blood volume, and controlling the distribution of water between blood and tissues. In addition, albumin aids in the transportation of vital physiologic substances that are not soluble in water such as bilirubin, fatty acids, cortisol, and thyroxine. Albumin also contributes to the solubility of many drugs and antibiotics, including sulfonamides and barbiturates, by aiding their diffusion into tissues as loosely bound albumin complexes.

Globulins, a family of unrelated proteins, represent the total of all protein fractions classified by serum protein electrophoresis as α_1-, α_2-, β-, and γ-globulins. Although their function is not fully understood, serum globulins are vital to the immune defense system, the conservation of free hemoglobin and iron, and the transportation of specific hormones and lipids. Globulin molecules also help to maintain the osmotic pressure of blood, even though they are larger than albumin molecules and less efficient for this purpose. The γ-globulin fraction may be separated further by radial diffusion studies into several immunoglobulins, each with a specific immunologic function.

Laboratory tests for serum proteins may include measurement of total protein (albumin plus globulins) and albumin, calculation of total globulin fractions, and expression of the albumin/globulin (A/G) ratio. Although these determinations may still be requested, their significance has largely been replaced by serum protein electrophoresis and immunoelectrophoresis, which reveal the distribution of protein fractions more clearly than quantitative methods. Protein studies usually are performed on serum specimens to avoid measuring the fibrinogen fraction, which is utilized during the clotting process and can interfere with test interpretation.

Total Protein, Albumin, and Globulins

Total protein concentrations represent the sum of the albumin and globulin fractions present in the blood; this test has limited significance as a sensitive or specific indicator of disease when performed alone. Total protein concentrations are most meaningful when accompanied by albumin determinations because in many pathologic conditions protein levels are more significantly affected by changes in albumin than changes in other protein fractions. Accurate interpretation of total protein values, as well as information concerning protein synthesis and depletion, requires the measurement of albumin and globulin fractions.

The **A/G ratio** expresses the distribution of the two main protein fractions and, until the development of accurate protein electrophoresis, was considered a useful measurement. However, the A/G ratio is of little help in specific diagnosis because normal ratios can be obtained with abnormal quantities of albumin or globulin or both. Moreover, the calculation is now considered imprecise at best because total protein, albumin, globulin, and the A/G ratio may change independently of one another in many disease states.

Laboratory determinations of total protein are used to screen for diseases that alter protein balance and are required to calculate absolute values for each fraction from the relative percentages detected. Albumin and globulin measurements indicate the state of body hydration and abnormalities in the rate of protein synthesis and aid in the assessment of systemic diseases, including hepatic and renal disorders. Abnormal test results frequently indicate the need for more specific electrophoretic or immunoelectrophoretic studies to identify abnormalities of individual fractions.

Clinical Significance

Total protein values represent true plasma concentrations when body fluids and electrolytes are in balance, whereas water intoxication produces low total protein levels because of simple dilution. Conversely, dehydration produces total protein values that are higher than normal because of the loss of plasma water and a relative increase in the concentration of all proteins. Abnormal total protein concentrations may result from changes in one, several, or all protein fractions, although changes may occur in these fractions without producing a corresponding change in total protein values.

Changes in albumin concentrations closely parallel changes in total protein concentrations in many pathologic conditions because albumin composes such a large portion of total protein values. Thus, decreased total protein values resulting from actual protein loss often are accompanied by lower than normal albumin levels. Markedly low albumin levels often indicate significant liver disorders, which reduce albumin synthesis, abnormal albumin loss through the kidneys or gastrointestinal tract, or a variety of protein-altering colloid diseases. Any sizable loss of albumin from the vascular circulation reduces the density of the blood and allows water to flow toward the tissues, resulting in edema.

Total globulin values are so generalized that slight abnormalities in any of the fractions may be overlooked, or a decrease in one fraction may be offset by an elevation in another fraction and pass unnoticed. An increase in globulin concentration usually occurs in the γ-globulin fraction (**hypergammaglobulinemia**) and generally is accompanied by a corresponding increase in the total protein concentration.

Normal Values

The normal values for total protein, albumin, globulin, and the A/G ratio are:

Total protein	
Infants	4.7–7.4 g/dL
Adults	6.0–8.3 g/dL
Albumin	3.5–5.5 g/dL
Globulin	1.5–3.7 g/dL
A/G ratio	1.5:1–2.5:1
Average	2:1

Variations

Diagnostically significant protein disturbances are summarized in Table 4-8.

Elevated total serum protein levels (hyperproteinemia) may occur with:

Addison's disease	Multiple myeloma
Dehydration	Protozoal diseases (kala-azar)
Diarrhea	Sarcoidosis
Hemoconcentration	Vomiting
Macroglobulinemia	

Decreased total serum protein levels (hypoproteinemia) may occur with:

Burns, severe	Colitis, ulcerative	Hepatitis, infectious
Cirrhosis	Hemorrhage, severe	Hodgkin's disease

TABLE 4-8 Diagnostically Significant Protein Disturbances

Total Protein	Albumin	Globulin	A/G Ratio	Usual Disorders
High	Normal to low	High	1:1–1:2	Multiple myeloma Macroglobulinemia Sarcoidosis
High	High	High	2:1	Dehydration
Normal	Low	High	1:2	Acute and chronic infections Hepatitis Lupus erythematosus
Low	Low	Normal	1:1	Renal disease Ulcerative colitis
Low	Low	Low	2:1	Severe burns Water intoxication Scleroderma

Inadequate diet	Malnutrition, prolonged	Renal disease
Kwashiorkor	Nephrosis	Sprue
Liver disease	Nephrotic syndrome	Starvation
Malabsorption	Protein-losing enteropathies	Water intoxication

Elevated serum albumin levels (hyperalbuminemia) may occur with:

Dehydration	Hemoconcentration
Diarrhea, severe	Vomiting, prolonged

Decreased serum albumin levels (hypoalbuminemia) may occur with:

Beriberi	Lymphoma	Protein-losing enteropathies
Brucellosis	Macroglobulinemia	Rheumatic fever
Burns, severe	Malabsorption syndrome	Rheumatoid arthritis
Cirrhosis	Malnutrition	Sarcoidosis
Colitis, ulcerative	Multiple myeloma	Scleroderma
Diabetes mellitus	Myasthenia	Starvation
Glomerulonephritis	Myocardial infarction	Sprue
Heart failure, congestive	Myxedema	Steatorrhea
Hepatitis, viral	Nephrosis	Trauma, accidental and surgical
Hodgkin's disease	Nephrotic syndrome	Tuberculosis
Infections, acute and chronic	Oral contraceptives (estrogen-progestin combinations)	Uremia
Leukemia	Pregnancy, early	Water intoxication
Lupus erythematosus		

Elevated serum globulin levels (hyperglobulinemia) may occur with:

Connective tissue disease

Dehydration

Hemoconcentration

Hepatic carcinoma

Hepatitis, toxic or viral

Hodgkin's disease

Hypergammaglobulinemia

Infections and inflammations, chronic

Leukemia

Multiple myeloma

Obstructive jaundice, prolonged

Rheumatoid arthritis

Sarcoidosis

Decreased serum globulin levels (hypoglobulinemia) may occur with agammaglobulinemia, severe burns, and water intoxication.

Methodology

Total protein and albumin determinations generally are performed simultaneously on the same serum specimen and require 5 mL of blood collected without anticoagulants (red-stoppered tube). Serum globulin values are calculated by subtracting the albumin concentration from the total protein test value (total protein − albumin = globulin). A more specific evaluation of individual protein fractions is obtained by serum electrophoresis and immunoelectrophoresis. Serum specimens for protein determinations remain stable for at least 1 week at refrigerator temperatures.

Precautions

To ensure an adequate serum specimen for reliable protein determinations, do not submit blood specimens for protein determination if the patient's blood contains substances that can interfere with laboratory test procedures and give inaccurate test results. Serum protein values are falsely elevated by the presence of the bromsulphthalein (BSP) dye used in liver function studies, free hemoglobin, bilirubin, or other pigments, as well as turbidity from lipemic sera.

▶▶ Nursing Responsibilities and Implications

1. Wait at least 48 hours to collect the blood specimen if the patient has had a BSP test.
2. Collect the blood specimen before giving the patient a high-fat meal.
3. Prevent hemolysis of the blood specimen while it is being collected and transported to the laboratory.
4. If total protein, albumin, and globulin levels are decreased, observe the patient for signs of dependent edema because fluid shifts from the intravascular compartment to interstitial spaces when serum proteins are reduced.
5. If total protein, albumin, and globulin levels are decreased, encourage the patient to increase the intake of dietary protein.
6. Monitor the patient's fluid intake and urinary output.

Immunoglobulins

Immunoglobulins (Ig), produced by B-lymphocytes and plasma cells, are a group of functionally and chemically related γ-globulins that act as antibodies in the body's immune defense system. These antibodies migrate together during serum electrophoresis as a single wide globulin band that can be separated further by radial immunodiffusion or immunoelectrophoresis into several classes identified as IgG, IgA, IgM, IgD, and IgE.

IgG. IgG contains antibodies against most bacteria, viruses, and toxins. These antibodies pass through the placental barrier and thus provide much of the early immunity to newborns.

IgA. IgA includes antitoxins, antibacterial agglutinins, cold agglutinins, antinuclear antibodies, and allergic reagins. This immunoglobulin is an important factor in respiratory, genitourinary, and gastrointestinal secretions.

IgM. IgM contributes the ABO blood group isoantibodies, Rh antibodies, rheumatoid factor, and heterophil antibodies. Complement is needed for these immunoglobulins to combine with and destroy antigenic substances or cells.

IgD and IgE. IgD and IgE comprise such a small portion of the total γ-globulin fraction that their exact roles have not yet been specifically defined.

Individuals with very low or totally absent γ-globulin levels (**hypogammaglobulinemia** or **agammaglobulinemia**) are highly susceptible to any infection because they lack the ability to produce antibodies. Increased immunoglobulin levels, on the other hand, indicate infectious diseases or other processes that cause antibody formation; increased IgM levels at birth usually indicate intrauterine infections such as toxoplasmosis, herpes, cytomegalovirus, or rubella. Laboratory studies of immunoglobulins are especially useful in identifying abnormal globulins, such as cryoglobulins and macroglobulins, and in investigating the characteristic changes in the various fractions that accompany a variety of disorders.

Clinical Significance

The electrophoretic migration patterns of immunoglobulin fractions vary in many complex ways during disease states, depending on the disorder, because each immunoglobulin group has its own specific immunologic functions. Therefore, it is not always possible to draw specific diagnostic conclusions from these altered immunoelectrophoretic patterns. However, the two most common variations that indicate immunoglobulin overproduction (**dysgammaglobulins**) or abnormalities are the monoclonal and polyclonal patterns.

The **monoclonal pattern**, a single, well-defined globulin peak migrating at a uniform rate, usually is associated with increases in any one of the immunoglobulins and a decrease in the others. Monoclonal gammopathies result from antibody-producing cells and neoplasms, including malignant conditions such as multiple myeloma, plasma cell leukemia, lymphoma, Waldenström's macroglobulinemia, heavy-chain disease, amyloidosis, and cold agglutinins.

The **polyclonal pattern** shows a broad, irregularly contoured band of globulin material, with various rates of migration reflecting the stimulation of several or all of the immunoglobulin classes from many different cells. These multispecific electrophoretic patterns are produced by several immunoglobulins with different characteristics, resulting in multiple antibodies against even a single bacterial antigen. A recognizable polyclonal pattern is produced by chronic infections with specific antigens such as parasitic infestations, tuberculosis, leprosy, lymphogranuloma venereum, intrauterine syphilis, or viral hepatitis. Polyclonal gammopathies also include chronic liver diseases such as hepatitis and cirrhosis, collagen diseases such as lupus erythematosus and rheumatoid arthritis, infectious mononucleosis, sarcoidosis, autoimmune diseases, and far-advanced carcinoma.

Normal Values
The normal values for the immunoglobulins are:

IgG

Birth	620–1300 mg/dL
3–6 months	225–750 mg/dL
1 year	340–1180 mg/dL
3 years	440–1300 mg/dL
6 years	600–1450 mg/dL
12 years	700–1580 mg/dL
Adults	650–1600 mg/dL (80%)

IgA

Birth	0–6 mg/dL
3–6 months	5–80 mg/dL
1 year	2–100 mg/dL
3 years	40–120 mg/dL
6 years	50–200 mg/dL
12 years	100–280 mg/dL
Adults	50–400 mg/dL (15%)

IgM

Birth	5–18 mg/dL
3–6 months	20–95 mg/dL
1 year	20–100 mg/dL
3 years	20–165 mg/dL
6 years	40–175 mg/dL
12 years	50–180 mg/dL
Adults	18–280 mg/dL

IgD	0.5–3.0 mg/dL (0.2%)
IgE	0.01–0.04 mg/dL (0.0002%)

Radioimmunoassay

1–3 years	<10 U/mL
4–6 years	<24 U/mL
7–8 years	<46 U/mL
9–12 years	<116 U/mL
13–14 years	<63 U/mL
Adults	<41 U/mL

Variations

Abnormal immunoglobulin levels may occur with:

Agammaglobulinemia	Psittacosis
Cirrhosis, biliary or Laennec's	Pyelitis
Cholecystitis	Rheumatoid arthritis
Cystitis	Rubella
Cytomegalovirus	Subacute bacterial endocarditis
Dysgammaglobulinemia	Syphilis
Hepatitis, viral	Systemic lupus erythematosus
Hodgkin's disease	Telangiectasia
Infectious mononucleosis	Thyroiditis, autoimmune
Leukemia, acute and chronic	Toxoplasmosis
Lymphogranuloma venereum	Trichinosis
Lymphoid aplasia	Trypanosomiasis
Macroglobulinemia	Tuberculosis
Nephrotic syndrome	Typhus
Pneumonia	

Methodology

Identification and measurement of specific immunoglobulins by immunoelectrophoresis or radial immunodiffusion require 5 mL of blood collected without anticoagulants (red-stoppered tube).

Precautions

To ensure accurate immunoglobulin patterns, delay testing, whenever possible, if the patient recently has received active immunization, passive antisera, or blood transfusion therapy, which may produce confusing or variable test results.

▶▶ Nursing Responsibilities and Implications

1. Record any vaccination or immunization, including toxoids, that the patient has received in the previous 6 months. These should be noted on the patient's chart and reported to the laboratory on the request slip.

2. Record on the patient's chart any blood transfusions, blood component therapy, or passive antisera, such as γ-globulin or tetanus antitoxin, that the patient has received in the previous 6 weeks. These globulin-containing treatments also should be reported to the laboratory on the request slip.

Serum Protein Electrophoresis and Immunoelectrophoresis

Electrophoresis, currently the most common form of protein testing, is a sensitive method for separating serum protein into its various component fractions and determining their identity. Individual proteins migrate as charged particles in an electric field, each moving at a different rate according to characteristic molecular size, shape, and electrical charge. This movement causes individual protein fractions to separate into a recognizable pattern of distinct layers that may be identified as albumin and α_1-, α_2-, β-, and γ-globulins.

Albumin. Albumin comprises the single largest component of total serum proteins. Albumin accounts for 75% of the osmotic pressure control between blood and tissues and acts as a vital transport media for several pigments, dyes, and drugs.

Globulin. Globulin is a family of several proteins that are unlike in chemical structure but similar in electrophoretic mobility. The α- and β-globulins serve as transport media for specific hormones and lipids. As a group they also reflect liver function, although their concentrations change in relatively few diseases. The γ-globulins represent the body's antibody system and are subject to considerable variations in many disease states.

α_1-Globulin consists of transcortin, which binds and transports the hormone cortisol; thyroid-binding globulin; antitrypsin; acid glycoprotein; and α-lipoprotein, which transports some lipids in plasma.

α_2-Globulin includes ceruloplasmin, which transports copper; haptoglobin, which binds free hemoglobin; macroglobulin; many glycoproteins; and the enzymes lactic dehydrogenase, cholinesterase, and alkaline phosphatase.

β-Globulin includes hemopexin, which binds heme but not hemoglobin; complement; plasminogen, which is the precursor to plasmin in fibrin clot lysis; transferrin, which binds and transports iron; and β-lipoprotein, which transports additional lipids.

γ-Globulin consists of the family of immunoglobulins indicated by the notation Ig, which contribute to immunity and antibody activity. γ-Globulin may be separated further into its immunoglobulin components by the specialized process of immunoelectrophoresis.

Immunoelectrophoresis combines the migration of protein molecules with immune reactions using a group of known antibodies against specific protein antigens to separate the major fractions into more detailed and specific patterns. This process identifies the constituent protein subcategories by the characteristic pattern of precipitin arcs and helps to determine their relative concentrations. The absolute value of individual protein fractions can be calculated by comparing the relative percentage of each protein band with total protein concentrations.

Laboratory procedures for serum protein electrophoresis provide a valuable initial screening tool for identifying diseases in which the distribution and amount of one or more of the primary protein fractions are altered. Identification and measurement of specific protein subcategories by immunoelectrophoresis help to document suspected protein deficiencies and investigate abnormal globulin concentrations but should be supplemented, whenever indicated, by quantitative immunoglobulin determinations.

Clinical Significance

Electrophoresis provides an initial screening test for a number of disorders because the technique readily demonstrates the existence of abnormal proteins or normal proteins in characteristically abnormal proportions. Immunoelectrophoresis, on the other hand, is a highly specific and sensitive method that often is used as a confirmatory test to help identify the nature and specificity of protein disorders. Immunoelectrophoresis is used to screen for a variety of immunoglobulin abnormalities, including antibody deficiency syndromes, monoclonal gammopathies such as myeloma and macroglobulinemia, or polyclonal gammopathies such as chronic infections, liver diseases, and collagen diseases. The combination of electrophoresis and immunoelectrophoresis has uncovered and clarified many previously puzzling or overlooked immunologic disorders and is now preferred for determining the quantity of specific immunoglobulin fractions.

Normal Values

The normal values for serum protein fractions, as determined by electrophoresis and immunoelectrophoresis, are:

Albumin	3.5−5.5 g/dL (53%−74%)
Globulin, total	1.5−3.0 g/dL (27%−55%)
α_1	0.1−0.4 g/dL (1%−5%)
α_1-Glycoprotein	30−130 mg/dL
α_1-Antitrypsin	80−260 mg/dL
α_2	0.4−1.0 g/dL (4.6%−14%)
Ceruloplasmin	15−50 mg/dL
α_2-Macroglobulin	105−575 mg/dL
Haptoglobin	25−215 mg/dL
β	0.5−1.5 g/dL (7.3%−15%)
Complement (C3)	65−20 mg/dL
Complement (C4)	10−40 mg/dL
Transferrin	200−435 mg/dL
γ	0.5−1.7 g/dL (8%−21%)
IgA	70−440 mg/dL
IgG	700−1800 mg/dL
IgM	60−290 mg/dL

Variations

The changes in protein fractions that occur during various diseases are summarized in Table 4-9. (See Total Protein, Albumin, and Globulins—Variations.)

Elevated α-globulin levels may occur with:

Carcinomatosis	Hodgkin's disease	Myxedema
Diabetes mellitus	Hypoalbuminemia	Nephrosis
Dysproteinemia, familial idiopathic	Infection, acute	Nephrotic syndrome
	Lupus erythematosus	Sarcoidosis
Glomerulonephritis	Myocardial infarction	Ulcerative colitis

Decreased α-globulin levels may occur with:

Hepatitis, viral	Malabsorption syndrome	Starvation
Liver disease	Scleroderma	Steatorrhea

Elevated β-globulin levels may occur with:

Acute phase reactants	Hepatitis, viral	Nephrotic syndrome
Diabetes mellitus, uncontrolled	Hypercholesterolemia	Obstructive jaundice
	Hyperlipemia, idiopathic	Sarcoidosis
Dysproteinemia, familial idiopathic	Macroglobulinemia	

TABLE 4-9   Summary of Electrophoretic Protein Fraction Changes in Various Diseases

Condition	Total Protein	Albumin	α_1-Globulin	α_2-Globulin	β-Globulin	γ-Globulin
Acute infection	—	Decreased	—	Increased	—	—
Asthma, allergies with poor response to therapy	—	Decreased	—	Increased	—	Decreased
Carcinomatosis	—	Decreased	Increased	Increased	—	—
Chronic infection	—	Decreased	—	—	—	Increased
Cryoglobulinemia	—	—	—	—	—	Increased
Dehydration	Increased	Increased	Increased	Increased	Increased	Increased
Diabetes mellitus	—	Decreased	Increased	Increased	Increased	—
Glomerulonephritis	Decreased	Decreased	Increased	—	—	—
Hepatic cirrhosis	Decreased	Decreased	—	—	—	Increased
Hepatitis, viral	—	Decreased	Decreased	Decreased	Increased	Increased
Hodgkin's disease	Decreased	Decreased	—	Increased	—	Increased
Hypogammaglobulinemia	Decreased	—	—	—	—	Decreased
Leukemia (myelogenous)	—	Decreased	—	—	—	Increased
Lupus erythematosus	—	Decreased	—	Increased	—	Increased
Lymphoma and lymphatic leukemia	Decreased	Decreased	—	—	—	Decreased
Macroglobulinemia	Increased	Decreased	—	—	Increased	Increased
Malabsorption, starvation	Decreased	Decreased	Decreased	Decreased	Decreased	Decreased
Myeloma	Increased	Decreased	—	—	—	Increased
Myasthenia	—	Decreased	—	—	—	Increased
Myxedema	—	Decreased	—	Increased	—	Increased
Nephrosis	Decreased	Decreased	Decreased	Increased	—	Decreased
Rheumatic fever	—	Decreased	—	Increased	—	—
Rheumatoid arthritis	—	Decreased	—	Increased	—	Increased
Sarcoidosis	Increased	Decreased	—	Increased	Increased	Increased
Scleroderma	Decreased	Decreased	Decreased	Decreased	Decreased	Decreased
Ulcerative colitis, exudative enteropathies	Decreased	Decreased	Increased	Increased	Decreased	Decreased

Decreased β-globulin levels may occur with:

Autoimmune disorders	Starvation	Systemic lupus erythematosus
Malabsorption syndrome	Steatorrhea	
Scleroderma		Ulcerative colitis

Elevated γ-globulin levels may occur with:

Amyloidosis	Hypergamma-globulinemia	Liver disease
Carcinoma, advanced		Lupus erythematosus
Cirrhosis	Infections (chronic bacterial, fungal, or protozoal)	Macroglobulinemia
Cryoglobulinemia		Multiple myeloma
Hashimoto's disease	Leukemia, myelocytic and monocytic	Rheumatoid arthritis
Hepatitis, viral		Sarcoidosis
Hodgkin's disease		

Decreased γ-globulin levels may occur with:

Hypogamma-globulinemia	Nephrosis	Starvation
	Nephrotic syndrome	Steatorrhea
Leukemia, lymphocytic	Malabsorption	Ulcerative colitis
Lymphoma	Scleroderma	

Methodology

Separation and measurement of serum protein fractions by electrophoresis and immunoelectrophoresis require 7 mL of blood collected without anticoagulants (red-stoppered tube).

▶▶ Nursing Responsibilities and Implications

1. Prevent hemolysis of the blood specimen while it is being collected and transported to the laboratory.

2. Record any vaccination or immunization, including toxoids, that the patient has received in the previous 6 months. These should be noted on the patient's chart and reported to the laboratory on the request slip.

3. Record on the patient's chart any blood transfusions, blood component therapy, or passive antisera, such as γ-globulin or tetanus antitoxin, that the patient has received in the previous 6 weeks. These globulin-containing treatments also should be reported to the laboratory on the request slip.

TUMOR MARKERS

Characteristic biochemical substances secreted into the bloodstream recently have been identified in patients with certain neoplastic diseases and may be used as markers to help detect the presence of specific tumors. Most commonly included in this group are such substances as α-fetoprotein, β-chain human chorionic gonadotropin, carcinoembryonic antigen, and prostatic acid phosphatase. Unfortunately, the production of these compounds is not sufficiently reliable for tumor marker tests to be used independently to establish a diagnosis of cancer; they must be combined with other clinical data. The most significant application of tumor marker tests therefore is in assessing the status of patients with cancer, evaluating their response to therapy, and monitoring for the early detection of recurrent disease.

α-Fetoprotein

α-Fetoprotein (AFP) is a globulin normally secreted into the bloodstream in huge quantities by the fetal liver until approximately the thirty-second week of gestation. Appreciable amounts of AFP normally appear in the blood of neonates and pregnant females but decrease to very low levels soon after birth and delivery. However, because AFP synthesis resumes when hepatic cells multiply rapidly, as in neoplasms, prolonged elevation of AFP levels in the serum of children and nonpregnant adults strongly indicates primary liver carcinoma.

Laboratory determination of AFP levels provides a useful clue to the presence of hepatocellular carcinoma and aids in the differential diagnosis of hepatomegaly, jaundice, and hepatocellular dysfunction. α-Fetoprotein determinations also provide a useful index for monitoring the efficacy of therapy because the disappearance of AFP indicates the elimination of malignant cells, whereas rising AFP levels reflect the recurrence of hepatic carcinoma. The greatest significance of AFP determinations, however, may be in helping to detect fetuses with neural tube defects such as spina bifida and anencephaly. (See Amniotic Fluid Analysis in Chapter 8.)

Normal Values

The normal values for α-fetoprotein in serum are:

Men	<10 ng/mL
Women	
Nonpregnant	<10 ng/mL
Pregnant	
8 weeks' gestation	<75 ng/mL
12 weeks' gestation	<130 ng/mL
16 weeks' gestation	<210 ng/mL
20 weeks' gestation	<300 ng/mL
24 weeks' gestation	<400 ng/mL
28 weeks' gestation	<450 ng/mL
32 weeks' gestation	<450 ng/mL
36 weeks' gestation	<400 ng/mL
40 weeks' gestation	<375 ng/mL
Children (>1 year)	<30 ng/mL

Variations
Elevated α-fetoprotein levels may occur with:

Alcoholic cirrhosis (40−500 ng/mL)

Ataxia telangiectasia

Cirrhosis (40−500 ng/mL)

Germ cell tumors (>400 ng/mL)

Gonadal teratoblastoma in children (>3000 ng/mL)

Hepatocellular carcinoma (>1000 ng/mL)

Hepatitis, acute and chronic (40−500 ng/mL)

Hepatitis, neonatal

Pancreatic carcinoma

Testicular carcinoma (>400 ng/mL)

Tyrosinemia, hereditary

Ulcerative colitis

Methodology
Measurement of AFP requires 5 mL of blood collected without anticoagulants (red-stoppered tube) or 2 mL of amniotic fluid. (See Amniotic Fluid Analysis in Chapter 8.)

Carcinoembryonic Antigen

Carcinoembryonic antigen (CEA), a glycoprotein produced by the fetus and secreted into the adult gastrointestinal tract, normally appears in trace amounts in the blood of healthy adults. Secretion of CEA increases during the rapid multiplication of epithelial cells, especially those in the digestive tract, producing elevated concentrations in the bloodstream of patients with colorectal adenocarcinoma. However, although elevated CEA levels are noted in patients with extensive disease, determinations are not recommended to establish a diagnosis of cancer or as an absolute test for malignancy.

Laboratory determinations of CEA levels provide a valuable guide to the management of cancer and help to evaluate the success of surgery and other forms of therapy in known cancer patients. Elevated CEA values usually decrease to normal following successful treatment, so any subsequent rise suggests tumor recurrence, metastases, or resistance to treatment. Tests are most valuable for the early detection of recurrent colorectal cancer because values may rise 3 months before clinical symptoms of recurrent disease appear.

Clinical Significance
In patients with elevated CEA levels, circulating CEA values usually decrease following surgical removal of malignant colorectal tumors. Therefore, a baseline determination should be established for each patient prior to surgery to aid in the interpretation of subsequent postsurgical values and identify any significant subsequent changes. Measurements are not reliable, however, if they are collected during the first 2−4 weeks after surgery because the normal postsurgical rise in CEA can prevent the accurate interpretation of test results.

Follow-up CEA tests to monitor patients after surgery should be performed 4−6 weeks after surgery and at regular intervals thereafter as part of overall clinical management. A period of 2−6 months generally is required before CEA values return to normal after the complete removal of gastrointestinal tumors. However, postoperative CEA values that continue to rise during subsequent follow-up studies suggest incomplete resection, tumor recurrence, or metastatic disease. A rising postsurgical CEA titer correlates with metastasis up to 19 months before clinical evidence of disease.

The interpretation of CEA values and other tumor markers for assessing the effects of therapy is more involved than their interpretation for monitoring disease recurrence. Because CEA values may vary significantly in some patients during therapy, clinical interpretation of single determinations is meaningless, and serial determinations are needed for an accurate assessment. Therefore, when an elevated value is found during subsequent follow-up, CEA tests should be repeated until a definite trend is established, usually three elevated values. Conversely, test results within the normal range do not guarantee the absence of malignancy because CEA values may decrease when patients are responding to therapy but are not yet in complete remission.

Normal Values
The normal and clinically significant values for carcinoembryonic antigen are:

Normal

Nonsmokers	<2.5 ng/mL
Smokers	<3.0 ng/mL
Inflammatory disorders	10–15 ng/mL (falls after acute phase)
Neoplastic disease	>15 ng/mL (continues to rise)

Variations
Elevated carcinoembryonic antigen levels may occur with:

Breast carcinoma	Pancreatic carcinoma
Gastrointestinal carcinoma	Prostatic carcinoma
Hypothyroidism	Pulmonary carcinoma
Inflammatory bowel disease	Smoking
Neuroblastoma	

Methodology
Carcinoembryonic antigen determinations require 7 mL of blood collected without hemolysis in a tube without anticoagulant or with EDTA (red- or lavender-stoppered tube). Specimens should be delivered to the laboratory as soon as possible so that serum or plasma can be separated from the cells within 6 hours. Serum and plasma remain stable for CEA determinations for 3 days at room temperature and for 1 week when refrigerated.

Precautions
To ensure accurate CEA determinations, the following precautions should be observed:

1. Collect blood without trauma because hemolysis can interfere with the test results.

2. Heparin interferes with test results; therefore, do not collect the blood in a tube containing that anticoagulant.

REFERENCES

Annino, J. S. 1976. *Clinical laboratory principles and procedures.* 4th ed. Boston: Little, Brown, & Co.

Batsakis, J. G. 1982. Serum alkaline phosphatase: refining an old test for the future. *Diagn. Med.* 5(3): 25.

Bauer, J. D. 1982. *Clinical laboratory methods.* 9th ed. St. Louis: The C. V. Mosby Co.

Becton-Dickinson and Co. 1976. *A guide to the Vacutainer blood collection system.* Rutherford, N.J.: Becton-Dickinson, and Co.

Bio-Science Laboratories. 1984. *Directory of services.* Van Nuys, Calif: Bio-Science Laboratories.

————. 1982. *The Bio-Science handbook.* 13th ed. Van Nuys, Calif: Bio-Science Laboratories.

Bologna, C. V. 1971. *Understanding laboratory medicine.* St. Louis: The C. V. Mosby Co.

Castelli, W. P. 1982. *Hypercholesterolemia.* Teterboro, N.J.: MetPath.

Collins, R. D. 1975. *Illustrated manual of laboratory diagnosis.* 2nd ed. Philadelphia: J. B. Lippincott Co.

Doucet, L. D. 1981. *Medical technology review.* Philadelphia: J. B. Lippincott Co.

Duncan, T. G. 1982. *The diabetes fact book.* New York: Charles Scribner's Sons.

Eilers, R. J. 1980. *Laboratory aids in diabetes mellitus.* Van Nuys, Calif.: Bio-Science Laboratories.

Freeman, J. A., and Beehler, M. F. 1983. *Laboratory medicine—clinical microscopy.* 2nd ed. Philadelphia: Lea & Febiger.

French, R. M. 1980. *Guide to diagnostic procedures.* 5th ed. New York: McGraw-Hill Book Co.

Fritsche, H. A. 1982. Tumor marker tests in patient monitoring. *Lab. Med.* 13(9): 528.

Galen, R. S. 1978. Isoenzymes and myocardial infarction. *Diagn. Med.* 1(1): 40.

Garb, S. 1976. *Laboratory tests in common use.* 6th ed. New York: Springer Publishing Co.

Garg, A. K., and Nanji, A. A. 1982. The anion gap. *Diagn. Med.* 5(3): 33.

————. 1982. Ratios and calculated values in laboratory medicine. *Diagn. Med.* 5(8): 28.

Glasgow, A. M. 1981. Clinical applications of blood ammonia determinations. *Lab. Med.* 12(3): 151.

Hammons, G. T. 1981. Glycosylated hemoglobin and diabetes mellitus. *Lab. Med.* 12(4): 213.

Helena Laboratories. 1972. *Protein electrophoresis test report sheet.* Beaumont, Texas: Helena Laboratories.

————. 1973. *LDH isoenzyme electrophoresis test report sheet.* Beaumont, Texas: Helena Laboratories.

————. 1973. *Lipoprotein electrophoresis test report sheet.* Beaumont, Texas: Helena Laboratories.

————. 1974. *CPK isoenzyme electrophoresis test report sheet.* Beaumont, Texas: Helena Laboratories.

————. 1980. *Glycosylated hemoglobin test method.* Beaumont, Texas: Helena Laboratories.

Henry, J. B. 1984. *Clinical diagnosis and management by laboratory methods.* 17th ed. Philadelphia: W. B. Saunders Co.

Isolab, Inc. 1978. *Glycohemoglobin determination.* Akron, Ohio: Isolab, Inc.

Killingsworth, L. M., Cooney, S. K., and Tyllia, M. M. 1980. Protein analysis: the closer you look, the more you see. *Diagn. Med.* 3(1): 47.

Lamb, L. E. 1973. Cholesterol, triglycerides, blood fats, atherosclerosis. *Health Lett.* 1(2): 1.

Larson, F. C. 1983. *Clinical significance of tests available on the DuPont Automatic Clinical Analyzer.* Wilmington, Del.: DuPont Industries.

MetPath. 1983. *Reference manual.* Teterboro, N.J.: MetPath.

Naito, H. K. 1983. Lipoprotein abnormalities because of gout. *Diagn. Med.* 6(7):9.

Peterson, C. K. 1980. What we are learning from glycosylated hemoglobin. *Diagn. Med.* 3(4):73.

Princeton Biomedix. 1979. *GlucoHemoglobin product information.* Princeton, N.J.: Becton-Dickinson and Co.

Raphael, S. S., et al. 1983. *Medical laboratory technology.* 4th ed. Philadelphia, W. B. Saunders Co.

Reynoso, G. 1981. CEA: basic concepts, clinical applications. *Diagn. Med.* 4(4):41.

Shaw, L. M. 1982. Keeping pace with a popular enzyme: GGT. *Diagn. Med.* 5(3):62.

Slockbower, J. M. 1979. Venipuncture procedures. *Lab. Med.* 10(12):747.

Slockbower, J. M., and Blumenfeld, T. A. 1983. *Collection and handling of laboratory specimens.* Philadelphia: J. B. Lippincott Co.

Statland, B. E. 1980. Turning lab values into action. *Diagn. Med.* 3(5):56.

———. 1981. Tumor markers. *Diagn. Med.* 4(4):21.

Stehling, L., and Brown, D. 1983. Malignant hyperthermia: more than a rising temperature. *Diagn. Med.* 6(3):59.

Stirton, M. S., and Batjer, J. D. 1982. Acid phosphatase and other biochemical markers for prostatic carcinoma: current status. *Lab. Med.* 13(8):506.

Strand, M. M., and Elmer, L. A. 1983. *Clinical laboratory tests.* 3rd ed. St. Louis: The C. V. Mosby Co.

Tilkian, S. M., Conover, M. B., and Tilkian, A. G. 1983. *Clinical implications of laboratory tests.* 3rd ed. St. Louis: The C. V. Mosby Co.

VanLente, F., and Shamberger, R. J. 1982. Diagnosing acute pancreatitis the enzymatic way. *Diagn. Med.* 5(5):50.

White, W. L., Erickson, M. M., and Stevens, S. C. 1976. *Chemistry for the clinical laboratory.* 4th ed. St. Louis: The C. V. Mosby Co.

Widmann, F. K. 1983. *Clinical interpretation of laboratory tests.* 9th ed. Philadelphia: F. A. Davis Co.

Wolf, P., et al. 1974. Identification of CPK isoenzymes MB in myocardial infarction. *Lab. Med.* 5(7):48.

5

Chemistry: Serum Electrolytes and Blood Gas Studies

FLUID AND ELECTROLYTE BALANCE   248
Total Body Fluid   ·   Electrolyte Studies   ·   Sodium   ·   Potassium   ·   Carbon Dioxide   ·   Chloride   ·   Calcium   ·   Phosphorus   ·   Magnesium   ·   Anion Gap   ·   Osmolality
ACID-BASE BALANCE AND BLOOD GASES   278
Bicarbonate-Carbonic Acid Buffers   ·   Blood Gas Studies   ·   Blood Gas Specimen Collection and Handling   ·   pH   ·   Partial Pressure of Carbon Dioxide   ·   Base Excess   ·   Partial Pressure of Oxygen   ·   Oxygen Saturation   ·   Acid-Base Imbalance

FLUID AND ELECTROLYTE BALANCE

Concentrations of fluid and electrolytes in the body must remain within narrow ranges to preserve the delicate balance required for good health. Because the roles of water and electrolytes are widely diverse and yet totally intertwined, electrolyte imbalance generally is associated with conditions that significantly change fluid levels. Thus, the vital balance is threatened by almost every illness or disease process if fluid and electrolyte intake is not adequate.

For example, excessive fluid accumulation and overhydration of the fluid compartments may occur in patients with cardiac failure, cirrhosis, and nephrotic syndrome. On the other hand, excessive fluid loss occurs during vomiting, diarrhea, surgical drainage, renal disease, severe burns, fevers, diabetes insipidus, and adrenocortical insufficiency (Addison's disease). In addition, fluid and electrolyte imbalances may occur with normal daily situations or environmental changes and many therapeutic regimens, including diuretic therapy or the administration of large volumes of intravenous fluids.

Total Body Fluid

Body fluids result from the oxidation of cellular metabolism as well as from the ingestion of solids and liquids and normally comprise 60%–70% of the total adult body weight. These fluids usually remain at a relatively constant volume distributed between two major compartments: intracellular and extracellular. The **intracellular fluid reservoir** contributes two-thirds to three-quarters of the total fluid volume and is composed of the fluid found within all body cells. The **extracellular fluid reservoir** is found outside the cell walls and is subdivided further into **interstitial fluid**, which surrounds and bathes all cells, and **intravascular fluid**, which also is called blood plasma. Health usually is maintained if the relative volume and chemical composition of all fluid compartments remain constant within narrow, safe limits.

The nutrient composition of intracellular and extracellular fluids is similar, although the electrolyte composition of these fluids varies from one compartment to another. (The electrolyte composition of the three fluid compartments is shown in Figure 5-1.) The composition in one compartment is maintained in proportion to the amount of electrolytes and the quantities of fluid contained in the other compartments. Because there are no laboratory tests that directly measure fluid volume, imbalance can be detected only through its effects on other tests, including the hematocrit, total protein, blood urea nitrogen (BUN), and osmolality. For example, a fluid deficiency concentrates blood constituents and produces elevated test results, whereas a fluid excess causes dilution and lowers many test results.

Electrolyte Studies

Electrolytes are inorganic substances in the body that conduct an electrical current and can dissociate into positively and negatively charged particles or ions called **cations** and **anions**. These ions are distributed throughout the body to help maintain osmotic pressure, control fluid volumes in various compartments, regulate pH, and participate as cofactors in many enzymatic reactions. The body contains the following cations and anions in varying concentrations in all tissues and fluids:

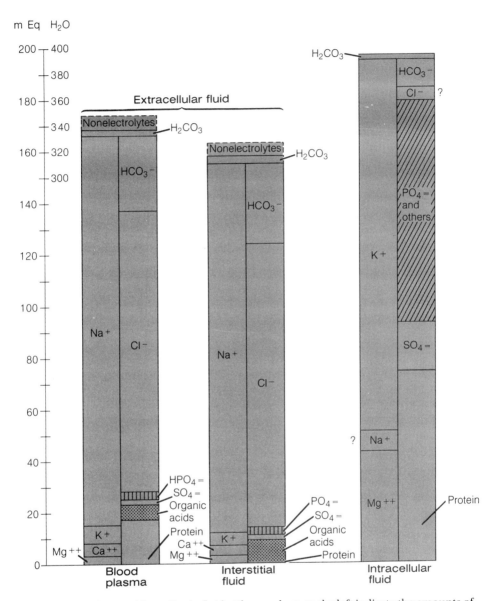

Figure 5-1 Composition of body fluids. The numbers on the left indicate the amounts of cations or anions. The numbers on the right indicate the sum of cations and anions. (From Spence, A. P., and Mason, E. B. 1979. HUMAN ANATOMY AND PHYSIOLOGY. Menlo Park, Calif.: Benjamin/Cummings Publishing Co., Inc., p. 737.)

Positive Ions (Cations)	*Negative Ions (Anions)*
Sodium	Chloride
Potassium	Bicarbonate
Calcium	Phosphate
Magnesium	Sulfate
	Protein
	Organic acids

Although the specific numbers may vary, the total of all cations must equal the sum of all anions in each fluid compartment to maintain electrical neutrality. Unfortunately, if electrolyte measurements are reported in terms of milligrams per deciliter, the number of electrical charges may falsely appear to be unequal. Thus, electrolyte concentrations must be expressed as milliequivalents per liter (mEq/L) to compare values more accurately and evalute the overall balance. However, electrolyte ion balance and body fluid levels are so closely interrelated that electrolyte values alone can be misleading unless the overall state of hydration also is known. For example, serum electrolyte concentrations may appear low in individuals with edema or congestive heart failure because of the increased extracellular fluid volume, which dilutes the concentration of electrolytes.

The electrolyte concentrations usually measured are sodium, potassium, carbon dioxide (bicarbonate), and chloride because they are the most variable and frequently fluctuate, along with water, in many diseases. These ions routinely are measured in blood serum and urine to determine the acid-base and electrolyte status of body fluids. However, serum and urine electrolyte levels may vary from moment to moment and at best offer only a rough indication of the body's total ion concentration. Therefore, all of the electrolytes should be studied together to determine an individual's electrolyte status accurately.

Normally, 80%–90% of the ingested sodium, potassium, and chloride is excreted by the kidneys in the urine. The kidneys also excrete bicarbonate and water in varying amounts according to the body's needs. Variable amounts of electrolytes and fluid also are lost through the sweat glands and intestinal tract, although these organs are unable to adjust their rate of secretion to meet immediate body requirements.

The kidneys and lungs, along with the endocrine system, primarily are responsible for regulating the distribution of body fluids and the proper balance among electrolytes. Renal filtration and reabsorption of necessary ions, along with adequate excretion of excess electrolytes and water in the urine, are essential to maintain electrical neutrality and the optimum state of overall hydration. Extrarenal stimuli, such as the antidiuretic and adrenocortical hormones (ADH and ACTH, respectively), also govern electrolyte and water balance by influencing urine volume and concentration. The urine volume and concentration control the osmotic equilibrium between body fluids and tissues.

Sodium

Sodium (Na^+) is the main cation of extracellular fluid and plays a major role in controlling acid-base equilibrium and the balance of water between blood and body tissue cells. Sodium is absorbed into the bloodstream from the small intestine and excreted in the urine in amounts that vary depending on dietary sodium chloride intake. Laboratory determinations of serum sodium concentration are used to detect changes in water and sodium balance in patients with certain endocrine disorders and body fluid imbalances or those receiving electrolyte infusion therapy. However, urine sodium determinations are a much more sensitive guide to fluctuations in sodium balance because serum values are of little help in detecting early or subtle electrolyte changes. (Data regarding fluid and electrolytes are summarized in Table 5-1.)

Signs and Symptoms

The nurse should be aware of the signs and symptoms associated with decreased serum sodium levels (**hyponatremia**) or increased serum sodium levels (**hypernatremia**). Individuals with mild to moderate hyponatremia may demonstrate fatigue, weakness, confusion, stupor, anorexia, and apprehension, and they may complain of headache, nausea, vomiting, diarrhea, and abdominal cramps. Severe sodium depletion may cause hypovolemic shock and convulsions, which can result in death.

Individuals with mild to moderate hypernatremia may have dry, sticky mucous membranes, fever, sweating, firm, rubbery tissue turgor, intense thirst, oliguria, flushed skin, agitation, restlessness, and decreased reflexes. Severe sodium excess may cause the individual to become hypermanic and convulse.

Clinical Significance

The body's tendency to maintain a consistent osmotic pressure with constant cation levels in fluids and tissues causes serum sodium concentrations to remain close to normal in most pathologic conditions. For example, when sodium is lost from the body, there is a corresponding loss of extracellular fluid; when sodium is retained by the body, there is a corresponding increase in extracellular fluid. In addition, the kidneys excrete the concentrations of sodium needed to maintain serum sodium levels within the narrow limits required for osmotic equilibrium and electrolyte balance. Thus, when serum sodium levels fall below the renal threshold of 110 mEq/L, all the sodium filtered by the kidneys is reabsorbed and urine excretion decreases. Therefore, to obtain a complete picture of whole body sodium concentrations, both serum and urine sodium determinations are necessary because the value of either alone can be misleading.

Normal Values
The normal values for sodium are:

Serum sodium	135–145 mEq/L
Urine sodium (intake of 100–250 mEq/day of sodium)	75–200 mEq/24 hours

---

Variations

Serum electrolyte responses in selected conditions are summarized in Table 5-2.

Elevated serum sodium levels (hypernatremia) may be found in:

Corticosteroid administration	Bicarbonate
Cushing's disease (aldosteronism)	Clonidine
Drug therapy	Estrogens
Anabolic steroids	Guanethidine

TABLE 5-1 Overview of Data Regarding Fluid and Electrolytes

Clinical Factor	Body Normal	Predisposing Conditions	Deficit Symptoms	Excess Symptoms	Food Source
Extracellular fluid	Infant: 29% of body weight Adult: 15% of body weight	*Deficit* Insufficient fluid intake, vomiting, diarrhea *Excess* Excessive administration or intake of fluid with sodium chloride	Weight loss, dry skin and mucous membranes, thirst, oliguria, low blood pressure, plasma pH above 7.45, urine pH above 7.0	Weight gain, edema, puffy eyelids, high blood pressure	Meats, fruits, vegetables, liquids
Base bicarbonate (HCO_3)	Plasma bicarbonates, 25–29 mEq/L, urine pH 5.0–7.0, plasma pH 7.35–7.45	*Deficit* Uncontrolled diabetes mellitus, starvation, severe infectious diseases, renal insufficiency *Excess* Loss of chloride or potassium through vomiting, gastric suction, hyperadrenalism, prolonged insertion of alkali	Metabolic acidosis, disorientation, weakness, shortness of breath, sweet, fruity odor to breath, plasma pH below 7.35, bicarbonate concentration below 25 mEq/L	Metabolic alkalosis, slow, shallow respirations, tetany, hypertonic muscles, plasma pH above 7.45, bicarbonate concentration above 30 mEq/L	
Carbonic acid (H_2CO_3)		*Deficit* Oxygen lack, fever, encephalitis, hyperventilation *Excess* Pneumonia, emphysema, barbiturate poisoning	Respiratory alkalosis, deep rapid breathing, tetany, convulsions, plasma pH above 7.45, low P_{CO_2}	Respiratory acidosis, disorientation, respiratory embarrassment, cyanosis, weakness, plasma pH below 7.35, high P_{CO_2}	

Nutrient	Normal value	Causes	Deficit symptoms	Excess symptoms	Food sources
Protein	14–18 g/dL in plasma (women), 12–16 g/dL in plasma (men)	*Deficit* Hemorrhage, burns, inadequate protein intake, draining wounds	Mental depression, fatigue, pallor, weight loss, loss of muscle tone, edema	No adverse effects	Dairy products, meat, fish, grains, poultry
Sodium (Na⁺)	135–145 mEq/L (plasma)	*Deficit* Excessive perspiration, gastrointestinal suction, diarrhea *Excess* Inadequate water intake	Apprehension, abdominal cramps, rapid weak pulse, oliguria, plasma sodium below 135 mEq/L	Dry, sticky mucous membranes, fever, thirst, firm, rubbery tissue turgor, plasma sodium above 145 mEq/L	Table salt, cheese, butter and margarine, processed meat (ham, bacon, pork), canned vegetables, vegetable juice
Potassium (K⁺)	3.5–5 mEq/L (plasma)	*Deficit* Diarrhea, vomiting, some kidney diseases, diuretic therapy, increased stress *Excess* Renal failure, burns, excessive administration	Muscle weakness, abnormal heart rhythm, anorexia, abdominal distention	Oliguria, intestinal colic, irritability, irregular pulse, diarrhea	Nuts, fruits, vegetables, poultry, fish

TABLE 5-1 Overview of Data Regarding Fluid and Electrolytes *(continued)*

Clinical Factor	Body Normal	Predisposing Conditions	Deficit Symptoms	Excess Symptoms	Food Source
Calcium (Ca^{++})	5 mEq/L (plasma)	*Deficit* Removal of parathyroid glands, excessive loss of intestinal fluids, massive infections *Excess* Overactive parathyroid gland, excessive ingestion of milk	Muscle cramps, tingling in the fingers, tetany, convulsions	Relaxed muscles, flank pain, kidney stones, deep bone pain	Dairy products, meat, fish, poultry, whole grain cereals
Magnesium (Mg^{++})	3 mEq/L (plasma)	*Deficit* Diarrhea, vomiting, chronic alcoholism, gastric suction, renal disease *Excess* Chronic renal disease	Hallucinations, tremor, disorientation, hyperreflexia, rapid pulse, hypertension	Central nervous system depression, cardiac irregularities	Nuts, wheat bran, chocolate

From Kozier, B., and Erb, G. L. 1979. FUNDAMENTALS OF NURSING: CONCEPTS AND PROCEDURES. Menlo Park, Calif.: Addison-Wesley Publishing Co.

TABLE 5-2 Serum Electrolyte Responses in Selected Conditions

Condition	Sodium	Potassium	Bicarbonate	Chloride
Vomiting, gastric suction	Increased	Decreased	Increased	Decreased
Diarrhea	Decreased	Decreased	Decreased	Variable
Diabetic ketoacidosis	Decreased	Increased	Decreased	Decreased
Uremia	Increased	Increased	Decreased	Increased
Cushing's disease, Aldosteronism	Increased	Decreased	Normal	Increased
Addison's disease	Decreased	Increased	Normal	Decreased
Hyperventilation, coma	Increased	Decreased	Decreased	Increased
Hypoventilation, emphysema	Decreased	Increased	Increased	Decreased
Diuresis	Decreased	Decreased	Increased	Decreased

Methoxyflurane

Oral contraceptives

Phenylbutazone

Prolactin

Tetracycline

Excess sodium intake with insufficient fluid intake

Hypercorticoadrenalism

Hypernatremic dehydration (fluid loss exceeds sodium loss)

   Coma

   Diabetes insipidus

Diaphoresis

Diarrhea, prolonged severe

Diuresis

Draining intestinal wounds

Fever

Head trauma

Hyperventilation

Salicylate intoxication

Vomiting, severe

Impaired renal function

Decreased serum sodium levels (hyponatremia) may be found in:

Addison's disease

Alkali deficit

Diabetic acidosis

Dilution hyponatremia

   Cirrhosis with ascites

   Congestive heart failure

   Hypoalbuminemia

   Pregnancy

   Renal insufficiency (oliguria)

   Uremia

   Water intoxication

Diuretic therapy

Drug therapy

   Ammonium chloride

Cathartics, excessive

Chlorpropamide

Ethacrynic acid

Furosemide

Mannitol

Metolazone

Spironolactone

Triamterene

Emphysema

Fasting

Glomerulonephritis

Hyponatremia dehydration (sodium loss exceeds fluid loss)

Burns

Diaphoresis, severe

Diarrhea, prolonged severe

Nasogastric suction

Vomiting

Malabsorption syndrome

Metabolic acidosis

Nephritis, severe

Paracentesis

Polyuria, severe

Pulmonary infection

Pyelonephritis

Pyloric obstruction

Sprue

Starvation

Thoracocentesis

Elevated urine sodium levels may be found in:

Adrenocortical insufficiency

Dehydration

Diabetic acidosis

Diuretic therapy

Fever

Head trauma

Salicylate intoxication

Starvation

Decreased urine sodium levels may be found in:

Acute renal failure

Diarrhea

Emphysema

Fluid retention

Hypernatremic dehydration (fluid loss exceeds sodium loss)

  Diaphoresis

  Diuresis

Hyperventilation

Vomiting, severe

Increased aldosterone production

  Cirrhosis

  Congestive heart failure

  Shock

Malabsorption syndrome, sprue

Pyloric obstruction

Methodology

Serum sodium determinations require 3 mL of blood collected without anticoagulant (red-stoppered tube) and delivered promptly to the laboratory for swift processing. Urine sodium determinations require a 24-hour urine specimen collected without preservatives and sent to the laboratory in its entirety so that the total volume can be measured.

▶▶ Nursing Responsibilities and Implications

1. Collect a venous blood specimen in a clean container free of sodium chloride or sodium-containing solutions.

2. Collect the blood from a vein as far away as possible from the site of intravenous saline or electrolyte infusion.

3. Note on the laboratory slip any diuretic that the patient is taking.

4. Observe the patient for signs of hyponatremia or hypernatremia.

5. Encourage the intake of foods high in sodium if the patient is hyponatremic; encourage the avoidance of foods high in sodium if the patient is hypernatremic. (High-sodium foods include bacon, ham, cheese, celery, cold cuts, pickles, olives, catsup, and tomato juice.)

Potassium

Potassium (K^+), the predominant intracellular cation, is present in large concentrations in all tissue cells and in much smaller amounts in blood plasma and serum. It is absorbed into the bloodstream from the small intestine following the ingestion of many foods, including those high in potassium such as bananas, meat broths, prunes, milk, boiled meats, oranges, and tomatoes. To preserve electrolyte balance, the kidneys excrete potassium in the urine in concentrations that vary according to dietary potassium intake.

Potassium plays a major role in influencing the body's water balance, controlling acid-base equilibrium, and regulating the electrical potential in all muscle cells. Serum and whole body potassium levels must remain within narrow limits to maintain osmotic pressure and proper electrical conduction in cardiac and skeletal muscles. Laboratory determinations of serum potassium concentrations are performed to assess changes in water and electrolyte balance in patients with certain endocrine disorders or those receiving intravenous potassium infusions. Urine potassium determinations are performed to help evaluate potassium levels, detecting variations that can cause cardiac toxicity and death (see Table 5-1).

Signs and Symptoms

The nurse should be aware of the signs and symptoms associated with decreased serum potassium levels (**hypokalemia**) or increased serum potassium levels (**hyperkalemia**). Individuals with mild hypokalemia may complain of malaise, thirst, anorexia, and polyuria. Moderate hypokalemia is characterized by muscle weakness, decreased reflexes, cardiac arrhythmias, weak pulse, falling blood pressure, nausea, vomiting, and decreased respiratory functioning. Severe untreated hypokalemia can result in death from respiratory or cardiac arrest.

Individuals with mild hyperkalemia may complain of irritability, nausea, diarrhea, and abdominal cramps. Moderate hyperkalemia is characterized by weakness, flaccid paralysis, difficulty in speaking and breathing, and oliguria, which can progress to anuria. Severe hyperkalemia slows the transmission of stimuli through the heart and can result in heart muscle weakness, ventricular fibrillation, and death if untreated.

Clinical Significance

Serum potassium levels are especially important to cardiac muscle because elevated concentrations cause a toxic state that disrupts the muscle contraction sequence and can result in death. Patients with impaired renal function or those receiving dialysis are at greater risk of an increased potassium concentration and should avoid high-potassium foods. On the other hand, decreased serum potassium concentrations also cause cardiac abnormalities, which are particularly dangerous in patients receiving digitalis glycosides because these drugs can contribute to cardiac dysrhythmias when levels are elevated. Because the kidneys cannot conserve potassium, hypokalemia can occur rapidly in patients receiving diuretics or on a low-potassium diet if their potassium intake is not at least 30–45 mEq/day.

The body's tendency to preserve electrolyte neutrality and maintain a constant level of cations in body fluids causes plasma potassium levels to remain within nearly normal limits even in many pathologic conditions. For example, when massive amounts of extracellular potassium ions are lost from the body through long-term diuretic use, large amounts of potassium ions leave the cells to support plasma concentrations and maintain a normal osmotic pressure. Thus, the patient's serum concentrations may be normal while the whole body potassium levels may actually be deficient and produce profound metabolic consequences. The range of normal values may vary slightly according to the specific method used to perform the test; therefore, the nurse should be familiar with the normal potassium values identified by the laboratory.

Normal Values

The normal values for potassium are:

Serum potassium	3.6–5.0 mEq/L
Urine potassium (intake of 60 mEq/day of potassium)	25–100 mEq/24 hours
Urine sodium to urine potassium ratio	2:1

Interpretation

The urine sodium to urine potassium ratio may be useful in evaluating certain endocrine abnormalities. With decreased aldosterone production, the relationship between sodium and potassium excretion can be increased to a ratio of 10:1. With increased aldosterone production, the excretion ratio may be reversed to 1:2.

Variations

Potassium concentrations in selected conditions are presented in Table 5-2.

Elevated serum potassium levels (hyperkalemia) may be found in:

Addison's disease	Hypoventilation
Adrenocortical insufficiency	Infections, acute
Asthma, acute bronchial	Intestinal obstruction, acute
Burns	Pneumonia
Drug therapy	Potassium therapy, excessive
Ephedrine	Renal failure, acute
Heparin	Sepsis
Histamine, intravenous	Tissue damage and destruction, severe
Methicillin	Trauma, severe accidental or surgical
Spironolactone	Uremia
Tetracycline	Wasting diseases

Decreased serum potassium levels (hypokalemia) may be found in:

ACTH or cortisol therapy	Diaphoresis, severe
Alkalosis	Diarrhea, chronic
Anorexia	Dieting, crash
Congestive heart failure, chronic	Diuretic therapy
Cushing's disease	Drug therapy
Dehydration	Bicarbonates

Ethacrynic acid

Furosemide

Gentamicin

Fever, chronic

Glucose administration

Hyperaldosteronism

Hypercorticoadrenalism

Hypertensive disease

Insulin administration

Liver disease with ascites

Low-sodium diet

Malabsorption syndrome

Malignant tumors

Malnutrition

Metabolic acidosis, ketoacidosis

Nephritis, chronic

Pyloric obstruction

Renal tubular acidosis

Salicylate intoxication

Sprue

Starvation

Stress, chronic

Surgery

Vomiting, severe

Elevated urine potassium levels may be found in:

Cushing's disease, primary and secondary aldosteronism

Dehydration, fever

Head trauma

Mercurial and chlorothiazide therapy

Salicylate intoxication

Starvation

Decreased urine potassium levels may be found in:

Acute renal failure

Addison's disease, adrenocortical insufficiency

Diarrhea

Malabsorption syndrome

Methodology

Serum or plasma potassium measurements require 3 mL of blood collected without anticoagulants (red-stoppered tube) or with heparin (green-stoppered tube). Specimens must be free of hemolysis. Even in the absence of visible hemolysis, potassium may shift from red blood cells into the serum or plasma and falsely elevate test values; therefore, the cells should be removed from the specimen within 1 hour after collection.

Urine potassium determinations require a 24-hour urine specimen collected without preservatives and sent to the laboratory in its entirety so that the total volume can be measured. Serum, plasma, and urine specimens for potassium determinations are stable for at least 7 days at room temperature.

Precautions

To ensure adequate serum specimens for potassium determinations, the following precautions should be observed:

1. Collect the blood specimen from an arm or hand opposite to the site of an intravenous electrolyte infusion.

2. Do not allow the patient to pump the hand with a tourniquet in place; if possible, do not use a tourniquet, or if a tourniquet is used, it should be released after the needle enters the vein, and 2 minutes should elapse before the sample is withdrawn because forearm exercises and restricted blood flow can increase potassium levels in the specimen by 10%–20%.

3. Deliver the blood specimen to the laboratory shortly after it is collected so that serum can be separated from the cells as soon as possible.

▶▶ *Nursing Responsibilities and Implications*

1. Inform the patient that there are no food or fluid restrictions.

2. Note on the laboratory slip the time the specimen is obtained because potassium values may vary by 0.2–0.4 mEq/L depending on the time of day, with the highest concentrations obtained in the afternoon and early evening.

3. Observe the patient for signs of hypokalemia or hyperkalemia.

4. Encourage the intake of foods high in potassium if the patient is hypokalemic; encourage the avoidance of foods high in potassium if the patient is hyperkalemic. (High-potassium foods include orange juice, bananas, prunes, apricots, meats, tomatoes, and potatoes.)

5. Monitor T waves if the patient is on a cardiac monitor; peaked T waves occur in individuals with hyperkalemia, and depressed T waves occur in patients with hypokalemia.

Carbon Dioxide

The **carbon dioxide** (CO_2) concentrations measured during electrolyte and blood gas studies reflect the total amount of carbon dioxide formed in the body as the end product of food metabolism and cellular activity. Carbon dioxide dissolves in and combines with body water, forming carbonic acid, which partially dissociates into bicarbonate ions. Thus, the carbon dioxide content of plasma is a combination of the gas dissolved in the body fluid plus the vital carbonic acid-bicarbonate buffer pair. (The role of the bicarbonate-carbonic acid buffer system in preserving the pH of extracellular fluid is discussed under Bicarbonate-Carbonic Acid Buffers later in this chapter.)

In the past, carbon dioxide content was determined as carbon dioxide-combining power. This test measures the amount of carbon dioxide gas that can be absorbed by a plasma specimen. However, carbon dioxide-combining power is not an accurate measurement because the plasma specimen is saturated with carbon dioxide gas at a constant pressure of 40 mm Hg rather than the varying pressures that actually exist in the patient. Carbon dioxide-combining power gradually is being replaced by other tests of electrolyte balance and pH status.

Carbon dioxide content currently is determined from the bicarbonate ion concentration because bicarbonate is an important anion as well as being the major transport form of carbon dioxide in the body. Test results offer a valuable guide to the efficiency of the body's buffering capacity and permit a more accurate assessment of clinical problems involving gas exchange. Laboratory determinations of carbon dioxide content routinely are included in the measurement of overall electrolyte balance and reflect the body's ability to control pH and abnormalities in acid-base equilibrium. Test values for carbon dioxide content are most significant when evaluated with the entire electrolyte panel and carbon dioxide partial pressure (P_{CO_2}), pH, and oxygen partial pressure (P_{O_2}) values (see Table 5-1).

Signs and Symptoms

The nurse should be aware that abnormal carbon dioxide concentrations accompany acid-base imbalances and are characterized by the symptoms of acidosis and alkalosis. (See Acid-Base Balance later in this chapter.)

Clinical Significance

The carbon dioxide content of plasma frequently is evaluated in patients with respiratory insufficiency because higher than normal concentrations may reflect inadequate gas exchange. For example, emphysema reduces carbon dioxide excretion and disturbs the plasma equilibrium by increasing the carbonic acid concentration and stimulating the kidneys to conserve bicarbonate to preserve a normal pH. The result is an elevated total carbon dioxide concentration due to increases in both carbonic acid and bicarbonate levels and a corresponding change in other electrolyte values to preserve electrical neutrality.

Measurement of total carbon dioxide levels also is necessary for the overall evaluation of acid-base imbalance because it provides a guide to the nature of pH disturbances. For example, a lower than normal concentration of carbon dioxide may be caused by a respiratory carbonic acid decrease accompanied by a secondary bicarbonate loss, as in hyperventilation, which produces alkalosis. Because both increased and decreased carbon dioxide levels may be associated with either acidosis or alkalosis, total carbon dioxide values must be interpreted along with pH values for maximum clinical significance.

Normal Values

The normal values for carbon dioxide are:

Arterial blood	21–30 mEq/L
Venous blood	22–34 mEq/L

Variations

Carbon dioxide (bicarbonate) concentrations in selected conditions are presented in Table 5-2.

Elevated carbon dioxide levels may be found in:

ACTH or cortisone therapy	Drug therapy	Pneumonia
	Ethacrynic acid	Pulmonary dysfunction
Adrenal cortex hormone imbalance	Metolazone	Pyloric obstruction
	Tromethamine	Renal disorders
Airway obstruction	Viomycin	Respiratory acidosis
Aldosteronism, primary	Emphysema	Sodium bicarbonate ingestion, prolonged
Alkali ingestion, excessive	Hypoventilation	
Cardiac disorders	Metabolic alkalosis	Stomach drainage
Diarrhea, severe	Peptic ulcer therapy	Vomiting, severe
Diuretic therapy		

Decreased carbon dioxide levels may be found in:

Acetazolamide administration	Drug therapy	Lactic acidosis
Alcoholic ketosis	Phenformin	Malabsorption syndrome
Ammonium chloride administration	Tetracycline	Metabolic acidosis
	Triamterene	Renal disorders
Dehydration	Fever, high	Renal failure
Diabetic acidosis	Head trauma	Renal tubular acidosis
Diarrhea, severe	Hepatic disorders	Respiratory alkalosis
Drainage of intestinal fluids	High altitude	Salicylate intoxication
	Hyperventilation	Starvation
	Hysteria	Uremia

Methodology

Carbon dioxide content determinations require 5 mL of blood collected in a heparinized tube or syringe (green stopper). The specimen should be placed on wet ice at once and delivered to the laboratory immediately. The specimen should be maintained anaerobically by capping the syringe tip or leaving the vacuum tube stopper in place because a significant amount of carbon dioxide escapes from the blood sample if it is freely exposed to the atmosphere. When the specimen must be stored and refrigerated before testing, the plasma should be removed from the cells shortly after collection with as little exposure to the atmosphere as possible. (Because carbon dioxide pressure in the atmosphere is far lower than it is in the alveoli, carbon dioxide leaves the blood freely. Thus, significant amounts of carbon dioxide are allowed to escape when the blood specimen is exposed to the air, and the longer the blood is exposed to outside air, the less accurate the test results will be.) Plasma specimens remain stable for up to 24 hours when refrigerated in a tightly sealed tube or container.

Precautions

To ensure an adequate specimen for carbon dioxide content determinations, the following precautions should be observed:

1. Instruct the patient not to pump the fist immediately before or during specimen collection because exercise of the hand and forearm may falsely elevate the test results.

2. Collect the blood without a tourniquet whenever possible to prevent stasis or with the tourniquet in place for as little time as possible. When the tourniquet must be used, instruct the patient to maintain a fist without straining.

▶▶ Nursing Responsibilities and Implications

1. Note if the patient is receiving nitrofurantoin, which may falsely decrease test values, or dimercaprol, lipomul, or methicillin, which will cause test values to be unreliable.

2. Place the specimen on ice and deliver the unopened tube to the laboratory immediately.

Chloride

Chloride (Cl^-), the most abundant anion of extracellular fluid, is absorbed into the bloodstream from dietary sodium chloride intake and is a vital factor in preserving electrical neutrality. Its main function is to counterbalance sodium, the major extracellular cation, and act as a buffer during oxygen and carbon dioxide exchange in red blood cells. The kidneys excrete chloride in the urine in amounts regulated by the concentrations of other electrolyte ions to preserve the body's overall electrolyte balance. Laboratory determinations of serum chloride are performed to assess the acid-base and water equilibrium of the body and evaluate the influence of chloride on osmotic pressure. (Spinal fluid chloride levels are discussed in Chapter 9.)

Signs and Symptoms
Although increased serum chloride levels (**hyperchloremia**) and decreased serum chloride levels (**hypochloremia**) do develop, they occur along with hypernatremia and hyponatremia, respectively. The symptoms associated with the sodium excess or deficiency overshadow those associated with chloride excess or deficiency.

Clinical Significance
Changes in serum chloride concentration are usually a secondary response to fluctuations in one or more of the other electrolytes. Thus, chloride levels ordinarily are measured along with sodium, potassium, and carbon dioxide concentrations to correctly interpret the important anion-cation interrelationship of these ions. For example, chloride helps to maintain the overall anionic charge of extracellular fluid by moving into red blood cells to replace bicarbonate as it responds to changing concentrations of carbon dioxide.

As bicarbonate ions accumulate in the plasma, chloride ions are displaced into cells in substantial numbers to preserve the anion total, decreasing serum chloride values. Urine chloride excretion falls to low levels whenever the serum chloride value is much below 100 mEq/L. Any increase in sodium ions increases chloride concentrations proportionately and also decreases urine chloride levels as the kidneys reabsorb larger quantities of chloride and water to preserve osmotic equilibrium.

Normal Values
The normal chloride values are:

Serum chloride	95–108 mEq/L
Urine chloride (intake of 70–210 mEq/day of chloride)	110–254 mEq/24 hours

---

Variations
Chloride concentrations in selected conditions are presented in Table 5.2.
Elevated serum chloride levels (hyperchloremia) may be found in:

Acute renal failure

Anemia

Cardiac conditions

Cushing's disease (primary hyperaldosteronism)

Diabetes insipidus

Drug therapy
  Chlorothiazide
  Guanethidine
  Phenylbutazone
Eclampsia
Fever
Head trauma
Hypercorticoadrenalism
Hyperparathyroidism
Hyperventilation

Hypoproteinemia
Injudicious ammonium chloride or acetazolamide administration
Nephritis
Prostatic obstruction
Salicylate intoxication
Serum sickness
Severe dehydration
Uremia
Urinary obstruction

Decreased serum chloride levels (hypochloremia) may be found in:

Acute infections
Addison's disease (adrenocortical insufficiency)
Alkalosis
Burns
Central nervous system disorders
Chronic renal failure
Congestive heart failure
Diabetic ketoacidosis, lactic acidosis
Diaphoresis, profuse
Diarrhea, prolonged
Diuretic therapy
Drug therapy
  Aldosterone
  Bicarbonates
  Corticotropin
  Prednisolone

Edema
Extracellular fluid excess
Fasting
Fever
Heat exhaustion, heat cramps
Hypoventilation, pneumonia, emphysema, ether anesthesia
Intestinal fistula
Metallic poisoning
Pyloric obstruction, gastrointestinal obstruction
Tubular acidosis
Typhus fever
Ulcerative colitis
Uremia
Vomiting, severe

Methodology

Serum chloride determinations require 3 mL of blood collected without anticoagulants (red-stoppered tube). Urine chloride measurements require a 24-hour urine specimen collected without preservatives and sent to the laboratory in its entirety so that the total volume can be measured.

Precautions

To ensure adequate specimens for accurate chloride determinations, the following precautions should be observed:

1. Collect blood and urine specimens in clean, dry containers that are free of saline or chloride-containing solutions.

2. Collect the blood specimen from the arm or hand opposite to the site of saline or electrolyte infusion.

3. Note if the patient is receiving any medications containing bromide because large quantities of these drugs may cause falsely elevated test results.

▶▶ *Nursing Responsibilities and Implications*

1. Inform the patient that there are no food or fluid restrictions.

2. Observe the patient for signs and symptoms of hypochloremia or hyperchloremia.

Calcium

Calcium (Ca^{++}), the most abundant cation in the body, is absorbed into the bloodstream from the small intestine following dietary intake of milk, cheese, butter, and certain meats and vegetables. Calcium is utilized in bone and tooth formation and is essential to the transmission of nerve impulses, skeletal and cardiac muscle contractility, and efficient blood clotting. Approximately 50% of the circulating calcium exists as the physiologically active free calcium ion; the remainder is bound to protein, mainly albumin, or to certain organic compounds, mainly citrate.

Calcium concentrations in the serum are controlled by the parathyroid hormone, which releases calcium salts from bone when blood levels fall, and by the kidneys, which excrete excess calcium in the urine. Laboratory determinations of serum calcium levels are helpful in the diagnosis of bone diseases and parathyroid disorders, and serum calcium concentrations frequently are monitored following thyroid or parathyroid surgery to detect deficiencies (see Table 5-1). (Urine calcium levels are discussed in Chapter 1.)

Signs and Symptoms
The nurse should be aware of the signs and symptoms associated with decreased serum calcium levels (**hypocalcemia**) or increased serum calcium levels (**hypercalcemia**). The individual with mild to moderate hypocalcemia may complain of a tingling sensation in the fingertips and around the mouth, abdominal and skeletal muscle cramping, carpopedal spasms (Trousseau's sign), and facial muscle spasms (Chvostek's sign). Severe calcium depletion produces tetany, which may lead to convulsions.

The individual with mild to moderate hypercalcemia may have deep bone pain, pathologic fractures, relaxed muscles, and flank pain caused by renal stones. Severe calcium excess causes a hypercalcemic crisis, which is heralded by intractable nausea and vomiting, dehydration, stupor, and coma and leads to cardiac arrest if untreated.

Clinical Significance
Calcium concentrations must remain within a narrow range because substantially reduced values result in a state of neuromuscular excitability, and higher than normal values result in muscular weakness. Calcium ion levels are influenced directly by protein concentration and blood pH as the body preserves ionic neutrality. For example, the percentage of available ionized calcium is higher than normal with alkalosis or increased protein levels, although these conditions are not always indicated by total calcium values alone.

Total calcium concentration is regulated by the parathyroid hormone, which releases calcium and phosphorus from bone and increases calcium absorption from the intestine. Because calcium levels usually vary inversely with phosphorus values, the parathyroid hormone also acts on the renal tubules to conserve calcium and excrete phosphorus ions. However, there are exceptions to this relationship. Calcium and phosphorus values may be increased in children during periods of active bone formation or with healing bone fractures, whereas they may be decreased in individuals with rickets. As a rule of thumb, the product of calcium and phosphorus concentrations should remain at approximately 40 mg/dL, although this value may be as high as 50 mg/dL in children and may fall below 30 mg/dL in individuals with rickets.

Normal Values

The normal values for calcium are:

Serum calcium—total	
Adults	4.3–5.3 mEq/L
	8.5–10.5 mg/dL
Children	6.0 mEq/L
	12.0 mg/dL
Serum calcium—ionized	48%–56% of total
	4.7–5.5 mg/dL
Urine calcium (intake of 200–500 mg/day of calcium)	25–200 mEq/24 hours
	50–250 mg/24 hours

Variations

Serum calcium and phosphorus concentrations in selected conditions are presented in Table 5-3.

Elevated serum calcium levels (hypercalcemia) may be found in:

Alkalosis

Drug therapy

    Anabolic steroids

    Antacids

    Calcium gluconate

    Estrogens

    Secretin

Hyperparathyroidism

Hyperproteinemia

Hypervitaminosis, vitamin D intoxication

Immobilization, prolonged

Leukemia

Lymphoma

Metastatic bone cancer

Multiple myeloma

Paget's disease

Peptic ulcer diet

Polycythemia vera

Respiratory disease

Sarcoidosis

Thiazide diuretics

TABLE 5-3   Serum Calcium and Phosphorus Concentrations in Selected Conditions

Condition	Calcium	Phosphorus
Hyperparathyroidism	Increased	Decreased
Hypoparathyroidism	Decreased	Increased
Renal insufficiency	Decreased	Increased
Osteomalacia, rickets	Decreased	Decreased
Multiple myeloma	Increased	Normal
Milk-alkali syndrome	Increased	Increased
Vitamin D intoxication	Increased	Increased
Metastatic carcinoma	Increased	Normal
Sarcoidosis	Increased	Increased

Decreased serum calcium levels (hypocalcemia) may be found in:

Acute pancreatitis

Drug therapy

  Corticosteroids

  Diuretics, mercurial

  Gastrin

  Insulin

  Mestranol

  Phenytoin sodium

Excessive laxative use

Fanconi syndrome

Hypoparathyroidism, parathyroidectomy

Hypoproteinemia

Increased magnesium or phosphorus intake

Liver disease

Malnutrition, malabsorption syndrome, sprue, celiac disease

Massive transfusions without calcium replacement

Newborns

Osteomalacia

Pregnancy

Renal failure, nephritis, nephrosis, renal tubular acidosis

Rickets

Vitamin D deficiency

Methodology

Serum calcium measurements require 3 mL of blood collected without anticoagulants (red-stoppered tube). Serum specimens for calcium determinations remain stable for 24 hours when refrigerated and for 1 year when frozen.

Urine calcium measurements require a 24-hour urine specimen collected in a bottle containing 10 mL of concentrated hydrochloric acid or glacial acetic acid. Specimens must be sent to the laboratory in their entirety so that total volume can be measured. Urine specimens remain stable for 7 days at room temperature.

▶▶ Nursing Responsibilities and Implications

1.   Withhold the patient's breakfast before collecting the blood specimen because dietary calcium may elevate the test results slightly.

2. Collect the blood specimen before administering such medications as heparin, insulin, and magnesium salts, which interfere with the test results.

3. Collect the blood specimen carefully to avoid any hemolysis, which can invalidate the test results.

4. Delay collecting the blood specimen if the patient has had a BSP (bromsulphthalein) retention test within the previous 48 hours. The presence of this dye in the bloodstream can cause calcium test results to appear falsely decreased.

5. Deliver blood to the laboratory immediately so that the serum can be removed from the clot within 1 hour after the blood is drawn.

6. Observe the patient for signs and symptoms of hypocalcemia and hypercalcemia.

7. Encourage the intake of foods high in calcium if the patient is hypocalcemic; encourage the avoidance of foods high in calcium if the patient is hypercalcemic. (High-calcium foods include milk and milk products, eggs, and fish.)

8. Note on the laboratory slip if the patient has been consuming a diet high in calcium.

9. Encourage the patient who is hypercalcemic to increase the daily fluid intake to 3000 mL to prevent renal calculi formation.

Phosphorus

Phosphorus (P), an inorganic element that is found mainly in bones and teeth, appears in body cells as both organic and inorganic compounds and esters. It is absorbed from the small intestine into the bloodstream, where the largest portion exists as the physiologically active free phosphate anion (HPO_4-) and the remainder is bound to protein. Phosphorus compounds are essential to the formation of bone, storage and liberation of energy, metabolism of carbohydrates and lipids, and regulation of serum pH. The kidneys excrete excess phosphorus in the urine to maintain plasma concentrations within optimum levels or to help elevate the plasma calcium level when it falls below normal.

Phosphorus metabolism is associated directly with calcium metabolism under the control of the parathyroid hormone. However, laboratory determinations of serum phosphorus levels alone are of limited usefulness to clinical diagnosis because there are only a few rare conditions that affect phosphorus metabolism directly. Thus, tests for calcium and phosphorus usually are ordered simultaneously because each value is important to the proper evaluation and interpretation of the other.

Signs and Symptoms
There are no clinical symptoms directly associated with decreased serum phosphorus levels (**hypophosphatemia**) or increased serum phosphorus levels (**hyperphosphatemia**).

Clinical Significance
The product of phosphorus and calcium concentrations (Ca × P) usually remains relatively constant because a decrease in the level of one of these two elements generally is accompanied by an increase in the level of the other. Urine phosphate excretion, which helps to regulate the phosphorus-calcium equilibrium, is affected by such factors as dietary phosphorus intake, acid-base balance, and endocrine production. Abnormal phos-

phate metabolism and excretion usually are accompanied by endocrine system disorders, bone diseases, or renal dysfunction and commonly are accompanied by corresponding changes in serum calcium concentrations.

Normal Values

The normal values for phosphorus are:

Serum phosphorus

Adults	1.8−2.6 mEq/L
	2.5−4.8 mg/dL
Children	25%−50% higher than adults
	4.1 mEq/L
	4.0−7.0 mg/dL
Urine phosphorus	0.2−0.6 mEq/24 hours
	0.9−1.3 g/24 hours

Variations

Serum calcium and phosphorus concentrations in selected conditions are presented in Table 5-3.

Elevated serum phosphorus levels (hyperphosphatemia) may be found in:

Acromegaly

Acute osteoporosis

Administration of enemas or purgatives containing large amounts of sodium phosphate

Administration of heparin, phenytoin, pituitary extract (Pituitrin)

Diabetic acidosis, hyperinsulinism

Healing bone fractures

Hyperthyroidism

Hypervitaminosis D

Hypoparathyroidism

Multiple blood transfusions

Nephritis, severe

Peptic ulcer diet, milk-alkali syndrome

Pyloric obstruction, starvation

Renal failure, renal disease

Sarcoidosis

Uremia

Decreased serum phosphorus levels (hypophosphatemia) may be found in:

Administration of insulin and adrenalin

Excessive use of antacids

Hyperalimentation

Hyperparathyroidism

Hypopituitarism

Hypovitaminosis D

Lobar pneumonia

Malnutrition, malabsorption syndrome, steatorrhea, sprue

Myxedema

Renal tubular acidosis, Fanconi's syndrome

Rickets, osteomalacia

Treatment of diabetic acidosis (coma)

Methodology

Serum phosphorus determinations require 3 mL of blood collected without anticoagulants (red-stoppered tube) and delivered immediately to the laboratory so that serum and cells can be separated within 30 minutes of specimen collection. Red blood cells contain high levels of phosphates, which can cause falsely elevated test results if allowed to remain in contact with the serum. Serum specimens remain stable for approximately 3 days at room temperature or when refrigerated and for 1 year when frozen.

Urine phosphorus determinations require a 24-hour urine specimen collected without preservatives and sent to the laboratory in its entirety so that the total volume can be measured.

Precautions

The use of purgatives or enemas containing large amounts of sodium phosphate can increase serum phosphorus levels by 5 mg/dL within 1–2 hours after the dose. Although this increase rarely lasts more than 4–6 hours, this effect should be considered when abnormal results are obtained that cannot otherwise be explained.

▶▶ **Nursing Responsibilities and Implications**

1. Collect the blood specimen in the morning after the patient has fasted overnight because increased carbohydrate metabolism lowers serum phosphorus levels due to movement of phosphate into body cells along with glucose.

2. Wait at least 4 hours to collect the blood specimen if the patient has received an intravenous glucose infusion.

3. Deliver the blood specimen to the laboratory immediately.

4. Prevent hemolysis of the blood specimen because ruptured red blood cells release high levels of phosphates and produce markedly increased test results.

5. Encourage the intake of foods high in phosphorus if the patient's serum phosphorus level is low; encourage the avoidance of foods high in phosphorus if the patient's serum phosphorus level is high. (High-phosphorus foods include milk, cheese, poultry, whole grain cereals, and fish.)

Magnesium

Magnesium (Mg^{++}), an abundant intracellular cation, is absorbed into the bloodstream from the small intestine following the ingestion of practically all foods. It is a vital coenzyme in the metabolism of carbohydrates, lipids, and proteins and is essential to the maintenance of the macromolecular structure of DNA and RNA. About 50% of serum magnesium exists as the physiologically active magnesium ion, and the remainder is bound to protein. Laboratory determinations of magnesium levels are used to detect early magnesium deficiency, assess its severity, and monitor patients following prolonged intravenous therapy with magnesium-free solutions (see Table 5-1).

Signs and Symptoms

The nurse should be aware of the signs and symptoms associated with decreased serum magnesium levels (**hypomagnesemia**) or increased serum magnesium levels (**hypermagnesemia**). Individuals with mild to moderate hypomagnesemia may experience tremors, painful paresthesia, weakness, nerve and muscle irritability, and tetany. Severe magnesium depletion causes increased blood pressure and heart rate, disorientation, and convulsions.

Individuals with mild to moderate hypermagnesemia may demonstrate reduced nerve and muscle activity, which impairs respiration and produces lethargy. Severe magnesium excess produces coma and may result in cardiac arrest if uncorrected.

Clinical Significance

Plasma magnesium levels are regulated by the endocrine and urinary systems, which help to maintain the concentrations necessary to preserve neuromuscular irritability and the function of many enzymes. Little is known about the significance of urine magnesium levels, although its measurement may be useful in assessing magnesium deficiency. Magnesium deficiencies are rare in well-nourished individuals, with plasma levels usually remaining above 1 mEq/L until at least 25% of cellular magnesium has been lost.

Normal Values

The normal values for magnesium are:

Serum magnesium	
Adults	1.5–2.5 mEq/L
	1.8–3.0 mg/dL
Neonates	0.2 mEq/L lower than adults
Urine magnesium (intake of 360 mg/day of magnesium)	6.0–9.0 mEq/24 hours

---

Variations

Elevated serum magnesium levels (hypermagnesemia) may be found in:

Acidosis

Addison's disease

Adrenalectomy

Antacid therapy, large doses

Dehydration

Diabetic coma, severe untreated

Milk of magnesia therapy accompanied by renal insufficiency

Renal failure

Thyroxine administration, excessive

Uremia

Decreased serum magnesium levels (hypomagnesemia) may be found in:

Acidosis

Acute pancreatitis

Chronic alcoholism, alcoholic cirrhosis, alcohol intoxication

Cirrhosis

Continuous bowel or gastric aspiration

Dialysis therapy

Diarrhea

Digitalis intoxication

Ethacrynic acid administration

Hyperaldosteronism, primary

Hypercalcemia

Hyperparathyroidism

Intravenous feeding, prolonged

Malabsorption syndrome, severe malnutrition	Thiazide diuretics
	Ulcerative colitis
Pathologic diuresis	Vomiting

Methodology

Serum magnesium measurements require 3 mL of blood collected without anticoagulants (red-stoppered tube) and delivered to the laboratory immediately so that serum and cells can be separated promptly. Urine magnesium determinations require a 24-hour urine specimen collected without preservatives and delivered to the laboratory in its entirety so that the total volume can be measured. Serum and urine specimens remain stable for 7 days at room temperature and for even longer when refrigerated or frozen.

▶▶ Nursing Responsibilities and Implications

1. Collect the blood specimen with as little trauma and hemolysis as possible. Hemolysis releases high levels of intracellular magnesium and falsely elevates the test results.

2. Notify the laboratory if the patient is receiving gluconic acid therapy, usually in the form of calcium gluconate, which interferes with the color reaction in some laboratory methods and falsely decreases the test results.

3. Note on the laboratory slip if the patient is taking medications that cause hypermagnesemia (laxatives and antacids containing magnesium) or hypomagnesemia (diuretics, calcium gluconate, and insulin).

4. Observe the patient for signs and symptoms of hypomagnesemia or hypermagnesemia.

5. Encourage the intake of foods high in magnesium if the patient has hypomagnesemia; encourage the avoidance of foods high in magnesium if the patient has hypermagnesemia. (High-magnesium foods include fish, meats, seafood, green vegetables, nuts, and whole grains.)

6. Observe the patient for signs of hypokalemia, hyponatremia, and hypocalcemia if the patient has hypomagnesemia.

Anion Gap

For optimum health, the body must preserve a state of electrical neutrality or electrolyte equilibrium between anion and cation groups in extracellular fluids. Therefore, information about the interrelationship of electrolyte values is extremely important in the diagnosis of acute illness. However, because simultaneous measurement of all electrolytes is seldom requested, a calculation of the difference between the unmeasured serum anions and cations (**anion gap**) can demonstrate this interrelationship.

A simple formula using the electrolyte values most frequently performed (sodium, potassium, bicarbonate [carbon dioxide], and chloride) can measure the anion gap and help analyze the anion-cation balance. The most commonly used formula is as follows:

Anion gap = (sodium + potassium) − (chloride + bicarbonate)

The anion gap value obtained from this calculation is approximately the difference between unmeasured calcium and magnesium ions minus the sum of unmeasured protein, phosphate, organic acid, and sulfate ions. (Table 5-4 presents the approximate nor-

TABLE 5-4 Approximate Normal Concentrations of Serum Electrolytes

Cations	mEq/L	Anions	mEq/L
Sodium	143.0	Chloride	104
Potassium	4.5	Bicarbonate	29
Calcium	5.0	Proteinate	16
Magnesium	2.5	Organic acids	3
		Phosphate	2
		Sulfate	1
Total cations	155	Total anions	155

mal concentrations of serum electrolytes.) Laboratory calculation of the anion gap is helpful in the differential diagnosis of metabolic acidosis and alkalosis, monitoring therapy for excess anion accumulation, and screening for paraproteinemias.

Clinical Significance
The calculation of the anion-cation balance allows an overall evaluation of patient status and alerts the physician to seek out the cause of any imbalance or abnormality. A normal anion-cation balance does not necessarily exclude the possibility of one or more abnormal values for individual ions. Electrolyte equilibrium only indicates that for each abnormal value, several compensations may have occurred to preserve neutrality. Thus, a decreased cation value may be accompanied by a corresponding decrease in one or more unmeasured anions, an increase in some unmeasured cation, or a combination of these two effects. The kidneys regulate this equilibrium by selectively excreting and retaining varying amounts of sodium, potassium, hydrogen, and bicarbonate ions.

Normal Values

The normal values for the anion gap, obtained from a balanced electrolyte panel, are:

$(Na^+ + K^+) - (Cl^- + HCO_3^-) = 11–17$ mEq/L

Interpretation
The difference between the sum of the two largest cation values (sodium and potassium) and the sum of the two largest anion values (chloride and bicarbonate) should equal approximately 14 mEq/L, plus or minus 2–3 mEq/L. A difference of less than 10 mEq/L or more than 17 mEq/L between these values indicates a serious illness or pathologic condition.

The following is an example of a balanced electrolyte panel:

$$
\begin{array}{lll}
\text{Sodium} & = & 143 \text{ mEq/L} \\
\text{Potassium} & = & \underline{4 \text{ mEq/L}} \\
& & 147 \text{ mEq/L} \\
\\
\text{Minus} \\
\text{Chloride} & = & 104 \text{ mEq/L} \\
\text{Bicarbonate} & = & \underline{29 \text{ mEq/L}} \\
& & 133 \text{ mEq/L} = 14 \text{ mEq/L}
\end{array}
$$

The electrolyte panel for a patient with hypokalemic, hypochloremic alkalosis may have the following values:

Sodium	=	131 mEq/L
Potassium	=	2 mEq/L
		133 mEq/L

Minus		
Chloride	=	88 mEq/L
Bicarbonate	=	35 mEq/L
		123 mEq/L = 10 mEq/L

Although this patient has a near-normal anion-cation equilibrium, indicating adequate compensation, the precariously low potassium value is an indication for replacement therapy.

On the other hand, the electrolyte panel for a diabetic with uncontrolled disease might read as follows:

Sodium	=	135 mEq/L
Potassium	=	4 mEq/L
		139 mEq/L

Minus		
Chloride	=	95 mEq/L
Bicarbonate	=	10 mEq/L
		105 mEq/L = 34 mEq/L

Although this patient has several normal electrolyte values, the imbalanced anion-cation calculation indicates a deficit in some unmeasured anion.

Variations

An **increased anion gap** (greater than 17 mEq/L) may occur with:

Antibiotic therapy, high-dose (penicillin, carbenicillin)

Dehydration, volume depletion (increased plasma protein)

Hypocalcemia

Hypomagnesemia

Metabolic acidosis (endogenous acid accumulation)

    Ethylene glycol poisoning

    Ketoacidosis (starvation, uncontrolled diabetes)

Lactic acidosis (shock)

Methyl alcohol intoxication

Paraldehyde poisoning

Salicylate intoxication

Renal failure (phosphate, sulfate, proteinate retention)

Therapy with acetate, citrate, or lactate

A **normal anion gap** can help classify hyperchloremic metabolic acidosis resulting from:

Anion-exchange resins

Diarrhea

Dilutional acidosis

Gastrointestinal loss of bicarbonate

Hyperalimentation acidosis	Obstructed ileal loop conduit
Renal loss of bicarbonate	Pancreatic drainage
Carbonic anhydrase inhibitors	Small-bowel fistula
Renal tubular acidosis	Ureterosigmoidostomy

A **decreased anion gap** (less than 10 mEq/L) may occur with:

Bromism	Hyperviscosity	Lithium intoxication
Dilution	Hypoalbuminemia (renal disease)	Multiple myeloma
Hypercalcemia		Polyclonal gammopathy
Hypermagnesemia	Hypophosphatemia	Polymyxin B therapy
Hypernatremia		

Osmolality

Osmolality is a sensitive and reliable indicator of the concentration or number of particles dissolved in serum and urine. These particles include electrolyte ions, glucose, urea, creatinine, and protein molecules. Osmolality determinations help diagnose fluid and electrolyte imbalances by measuring changes in urine or serum freezing points, which vary according to the number of particles in solution. For example, during intravenous fluid therapy, increased osmolality values may indicate that the patient is receiving too many electrolytes for the amount of fluid. Conversely, decreased osmolality values may indicate that the patient is receiving too much water for the amount of electrolytes.

Serum osmolality values reflect the balance of osmotic pressure between tissue cells and body fluids and are used to measure the extent of dehydration. Urine osmolality values vary widely with diet and fluid intake and provide a more sensitive index of renal function than specific gravity readings. Laboratory tests of serum and urine osmolality frequently are ordered to evaluate the effect of dialysis therapy and intravenous fluid administration, monitor the course of uremia, and interpret disturbances in sodium levels.

Clinical Significance

Plasma osmolality levels are the main regulator of antidiuretic hormone (ADH) release, which in turn controls the rate of water reabsorption by the kidneys and thus urine osmolality. For example, increased plasma osmolality levels stimulate ADH secretion, which causes more water to be reabsorbed from the renal tubules, thus producing a more concentrated urine and increasing urine osmolality. Simultaneous urine and serum determinations are often valuable in assessing renal response to circulating ADH.

Solute concentrations are reported as milliosmoles of solute per kilogram of fluid, which is usually water in a biologic system (mOsm/kg), and are roughly equivalent to the significance of specific gravity readings. Each 40 mOsm/kg is approximately equal to one specific gravity unit; thus, urine specific gravity values of 1.010 and 1.020 equal 400 and 800 mOsm/kg, respectively. Test values reported as milliosmoles per liter (mosM/L) are measuring osmolarity rather than osmolality. However, when the solvent is water, the osmolality and osmolarity are the same because 1 L of water weighs 1 kg.

Normal Values
The normal values for osmolality are:

Serum osmolality	275–300 mOsm/kg
Urine osmolality	
Healthy males	390–1090 mOsm/kg
	770–1630 mOsm/24 hours
Healthy females	300–1090 mOsm/kg
	430–1150 mOsm/24 hours
Infants	213 mOsm/kg
Hospital patients on bedrest	280–900 mOsm/kg
	300–900 mOsm/24 hours
Ratio	
$\dfrac{\text{Urine osmolality}}{\text{Serum osmolality}}$	1.0–3.0
$\dfrac{\text{Serum sodium}}{\text{Serum osmolality}}$	0.43–0.50

Interpretation
The relationship between urine and serum osmolality values is important in interpreting the significance of abnormal urine or serum osmolality values. The ratio of urine osmolality to serum osmolality should exceed 1.0, with values greater than 3.0 normally occurring after an overnight fast (concentrated urine). A ratio close to 1.0 (dilute urine) usually indicates advanced renal disease and a loss of concentrating ability by the kidneys. A ratio below 1.0 commonly occurs following excessive water intake or disproportionate water loss in diabetes insipidus, in which the urine is extremely dilute.

Because at least 90% of the serum osmolality level is due to sodium ions and their accompanying chloride, the relationship between sodium concentrations and serum osmolality is also useful in clinical assessments. The ratio of serum sodium in milliequivalents per liter to serum osmolality in milliosmoles per kilogram usually falls in the range of 0.43–0.50, with values below 0.43 generally carrying an unfavorable prognosis. Patients with hypernatremia may have an elevated ratio without a change in the level of any other serum metabolite. Patients with true hyponatremia have a decreased ratio, which helps to differentiate them from patients with dilution hyponatremia, in whom the ratio is normal.

Variations
Elevated serum osmolality may be found in:

Acidosis	Dehydration, hemoconcentration from any cause
Advanced liver disease	
Alcohol ingestion	High-protein diet
Aldosteronism, primary	Hyperbilirubinemia
Chronic wasting disease	Hypercalcemia

Hyperglycemia, severe diabetes mellitus, diabetes insipidus	Shock
Hypokalemia	Sodium overload
Methanol poisoning	Trauma
	Uremia

Decreased serum osmolality may be found in:

Acute illness	Hyponatremia
Addison's disease	Increased ADH secretion
Chronic wasting disease	Post surgery
Congestive heart failure	Water overload, compulsive water drinking
Hepatic cirrhosis, hepatic failure with ascites	

Elevated urine osmolality may be found in:

Addison's disease	Increased ADH secretion
Congestive heart failure	Post surgery
Dehydration	Sodium overload
Hepatic cirrhosis	Uremia
Hyperglycemia	

Decreased urine osmolality may be found in:

Aldosteronism, primary	Hypokalemia
Diabetes insipidus	Renal failure, chronic progressive
High-protein diet	Water overload, compulsive water drinking
Hypercalcemia	

Methodology

Serum osmolality determinations require 3 mL of blood collected without anticoagulants (red-stoppered tube). A 10 mL random urine specimen is needed for urine osmolality measurements. Serum specimens are stable for up to 10 hours when refrigerated; urine specimens are not stable and must be collected without preservatives and delivered to the laboratory promptly for immediate testing.

▶▶ Nursing Responsibilities and Implications

1. Collect the blood specimen with a clean, dry syringe or vacuum tube.

2. Collect blood with a tourniquet in place as briefly as possible to prevent hemostasis.

3. Deliver the blood to the laboratory promptly or, if the determination cannot be performed immediately, separate the serum from the clot as soon as possible. Refrigerate the serum in a small tube, which should be filled to the top and tightly sealed.

4. If serum osmolality is decreased, observe the patient for signs of overhydration such as cough, dyspnea, weight gain, vein engorgement, and rales.

5. If serum osmolality is increased, observe the patient for signs of dehydration such as thirst, dry mucous membranes, and poor skin turgor.

ACID-BASE BALANCE AND BLOOD GASES

The normal life-preserving equilibrium between the acidity and alkalinity of all body fluids requires the interrelated function of three physiologic mechanisms. The body regulates the acid-base balance of its fluid through (1) a combination of electrolytes and chemical buffers; (2) the respiratory function of the lungs; and (3) the excretory function of the kidneys. Blood gas studies are helpful in evaluating the ability of the lungs and kidneys to preserve the acid-base balance of body fluid and in monitoring alveolar efficiency in gas exchange. These procedures usually are ordered during or immediately following conditions that subject the body to unusual stress such as renal malfunction, cardiac failure, shock, major surgery, drug overdose, and uncontrolled diabetes mellitus.

Bicarbonate-Carbonic Acid Buffers

The bicarbonate-carbonic acid buffer pair normally constitutes approximately 60% of the total buffering capacity of the body and is largely responsible for regulating the pH of body fluid. Together with the electrolytes, this buffer system helps to prevent the accumulation of metabolic acid and facilitates its elimination from the body. The bicarbonate-carbonic acid buffer system may be represented by the following equation:

$$CO_2 \quad + \quad H_2O \leftrightarrow H_2CO_3 \leftrightarrow H^+ \quad + \quad HCO_3^-$$

| Carbon dioxide from metabolism (controlled by lungs) | Water | Carbonic acid | Hydrogen cation | Bicarbonate anion (controlled by kidneys) |

The bicarbonate and carbonic acid of this buffer system normally exist in a 20 : 1 ratio, and any disturbance of this ratio results in a blood pH that is too acid or alkaline. These buffers effectively regulate pH by neutralizing and eliminating excess acids while attempting to maintain a normal balance between the individual components of the system. Bicarbonate concentrations, known as the metabolic factor, are regulated by the kidneys, whereas carbonic acid levels, known as the respiratory factor, are controlled by the lungs.

The lungs are able to rapidly alter the rate and depth of carbon dioxide excretion to compensate for malfunctioning kidneys. Because this mechanism regulates the carbonic acid levels to maintain the bicarbonate-carbonic acid ratio, alteration of respiratory activity significantly changes the pH of body fluids. For example, hyperventilation increases the amount of carbon dioxide that is exhaled, causing a greater than normal loss of carbonic acid and increasing the pH to a more alkaline level. Conversely, hypoventilation retains carbon dioxide, which is then available to form excess amounts of carbonic acid and reduces the pH to a more acid level.

The kidneys' role in maintaining the acid-base balance is more complex. The kidneys respond more slowly, over several hours or days, compensating for malfunctioning lungs by adjusting the rate of bicarbonate excretion, reabsorption, and regeneration. The kidneys normally maintain acid-base equilibrium by excreting specific amounts of bicarbonate and hydrogen ions according to the current pH level. However, as carbonic acid accumulates and the plasma pH becomes more acidic, the kidneys excrete more hydrogen ions and retain the bicarbonate ions as a buffer. Conversely, when the plasma pH becomes too alkaline, the kidneys retain hydrogen ions and excrete bicarbonate ions to produce more acidity.

An abnormal pH level becomes evident after disturbances of body chemistry deplete the buffering ability of either bicarbonate or carbonic acid. However, a normal pH can exist during disorders that affect the acid-base balance if the disturbance of one buffer component is exactly neutralized or compensated for by the same degree of imbalance in the other component. Investigation and evaluation of acid-base imbalance require a battery of studies and calculations that are known collectively as **blood gas studies**.

Blood Gas Studies

Investigation of acid-base balance and whole-blood buffering capacity routinely includes measurement of pH, P_{CO_2} (carbonic acid concentration), total carbon dioxide (bicarbonate plus carbonic acid), P_{O_2}, and oxygen saturation. This battery of tests reflects the efficiency of alveolar ventilation, alveolar-capillary diffusion, and pulmonary circulation, and helps evaluate the effectiveness of gas exchange in the lungs. The concentration of oxygen and carbon dioxide in the blood also is influenced by other factors, including hemoglobin content, percent saturation, and the hemoglobin dissociation curve.

Although pH and P_{CO_2} values reveal most about acid-base balance, P_{O_2} values provide additional information about the status of the buffering mechanism. When any two of these values are known, the third may be calculated from a special nomograph (Figure 5-2). However, it is risky to report a prediction as if it were an actual measurement when gas exchange does not always react normally or predictably and can be altered by many factors.

Analysis of blood gas values helps to recognize any disturbance of acid-base regulation, identify its probable cause, determine the extent of the disturbance, and monitor the effects of treatment. Blood gas determinations also are required to regulate therapy in patients receiving mechanical respiratory assistance and evaluate respiratory difficulties that are sufficiently prolonged and severe to alter acid-base equilibrium. For a complete investigation of acid-base disturbances, base excess also may need to be calculated to assess the buffering capacity of whole blood caused by buffers other than bicarbonate-carbonic acid.

Blood Gas Specimen Collection and Handling

Arterial blood provides the most accurate results for blood gas studies involving pulmonary dysfunction, arterial oxygen saturation, and alveolar oxygen tension. It also is preferred when evaluating patients in cardiovascular collapse in whom venous blood may be stagnant or oxygenation compromised and when monitoring the effectiveness of mechanical respiratory therapy. However, at times it is either undesirable or impractical to obtain arterial blood from patients such as obese individuals or neonates. Under these circumstances, venous blood and arterialized capillary blood are suitable substitutes for pH, P_{CO_2}, and base excess determinations and should be used to diagnose and monitor most acid-base disturbances.

Because venous blood varies greatly from arterial blood in oxygen content, it is not adequate for the measurement of P_{O_2} and oxygen saturation but may be used for other blood gas studies. Test results on venous blood depend on the gas content of arterial blood

SIGGAARD-ANDERSEN ALIGNMENT NOMOGRAM

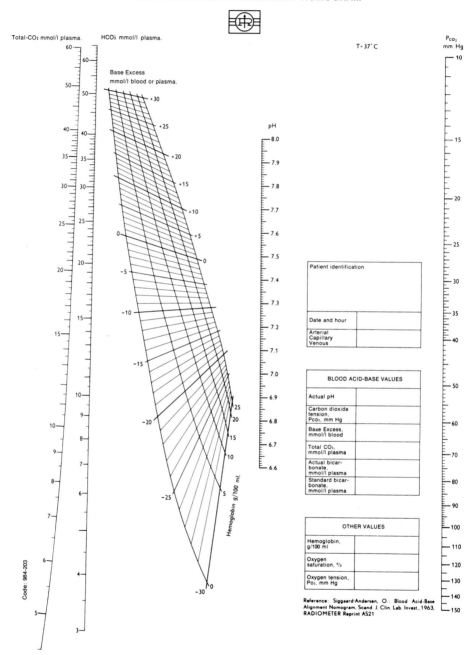

Figure 5-2   Siggaard-Andersen nomograph. (Copyright by Radiometer A/S.)

entering the capillary bed and are determined by the metabolic rate and relative blood flow in surrounding tissues.

Capillary blood is acceptable for evaluating acid-base status if blood flow at the puncture site is not impaired by shock, low cardiac output, vasoconstriction, or systolic pressure below 95 mm Hg. Specimens are most suitable if the blood is arterialized immediately before collection by warming the area to promote vasodilation, increase the blood flow, and narrow the arterial-venous differences. Infants with respiratory distress syndrome may be monitored using serial specimens of arterialized capillary blood to evaluate arterial oxygen tension only if blood from an indwelling umbilical catheter is not available. The earlobe commonly is used to obtain arterialized capillary blood specimens because it is a vascular area with low metabolic requirements that can be arterialized easily. When collecting capillary blood from the earlobe is impractical, as in neonates and infants, specimens may be obtained from the distal edge of the heel.

Precautions
To ensure accurate test results, the following precautions should be observed:

1. Do not use plastic syringes for collecting arterial blood because they require aspiration, which causes air leaks through even the smallest space between the needle hub and syringe fitting. Vacuum tubes also are unsuitable for collecting arterial specimens for blood gas studies because they expose the blood to subatmospheric pressure, which alters the test results.

2. Immerse the syringe containing the specimen in wet ice immediately to slow cellular metabolism, which continues to consume oxygen and liberate carbon dioxide at a temperature-dependent rate. Specimens left at room temperature lose 0.01 pH units every 15 minutes.

▶▶ Nursing Responsibilities and Implications
Before specimens for blood gas studies are collected, several important factors should be noted on the laboratory slip to aid in the interpretation of the test data:

Patient temperature—each centigrade degree above or below normal temperature causes a potential 7% error in Po_2 values, 3% error in Pco_2 values, and 0.014 units of error in pH levels.
Patient age—normal oxygen tensions gradually decrease with increasing age.
Ventilator settings—failure to report these settings limits the usefulness of test values because arterial blood gas levels are helpful in determining the proper respirator settings for volume, pressure, and frequency.
Inspired oxygen concentration—assessment of the patient's condition in relation to the test values is difficult without knowing the oxygen flow rate.

To help the physician obtain an arterial blood specimen that is suitable for blood gas studies, the nurse should proceed as follows:

1. Check the patient's chart to see if the physician has requested that mechanical respiratory devices or oxygen therapy be discontinued before the specimen is drawn.

2. Allow 10–30 minutes (depending on the patient's respiratory abnormalities) after suctioning or changing either respirator settings or inspired oxygen concentrations for the patient to reach steady-state ventilation before testing.

3. Prepare a syringe with a small amount of local anesthetic (0.5–1.0 mL of 1% Xylocaine without epinephrine), using a 25-gauge needle, for the physician to use in infiltrating the test site.

4. Reassure the patient that arterial blood collection is relatively painless to help prevent acute hyperventilation or hypoventilation from anxiety. Every attempt must be made to minimize changes in the patient's ventilatory pattern because blood gas test results immediately reflect the status of gas exchange in the lungs.

5. Assemble a 5 mL glass syringe with a short-beveled 20-gauge or 21-gauge needle. The use of a glass syringe prevents aspiration and avoids subatmospheric pressure within the barrel because arterial pressure usually is high enough to freely push up the plunger.

6. Rinse the barrel with an anticoagulant by drawing 0.5 mL of sodium or lithium heparin (1000 U/mL) into the syringe. Invert the syringe and pull the plunger back to wet the inside of the barrel with the liquid.

7. Eliminate all of the heparin left in the syringe by pushing the plunger to its end stop. The quantity of heparin remaining in the needle and the dead space of the syringe is sufficient to anticoagulate 5 mL of blood.

8. Assist the physician as necessary to obtain an arterial blood specimen.

9. Remove the needle and cap the syringe immediately to prevent the specimen from being exposed to the atmosphere.

10. Immerse the syringe in wet ice immediately.

11. Deliver the unopened specimen to the laboratory at once because the blood must be analyzed within 10–15 minutes to prevent oxygen consumption by continuing metabolism. When very high oxygen tensions are anticipated, such as occurs during cardiopulmonary bypass or shunt measurements, the specimen should be tested within 3–5 minutes of collection.

To obtain a capillary blood specimen suitable for blood gas determinations, the nurse should proceed as follows:

1. Arterialize the capillary blood by increasing the blood flow at the test site. The earlobe can be arterialized by applying heat or by flicking it with the index finger until a definite flushing is observed. Arterialized capillary blood can be obtained from neonates and pediatric patients by immersing the heel in warm water for 5–10 minutes.

2. Prepare the puncture site and perform a deep skin prick to obtain a free flow of blood. (See Specimen Collection and Handling in Chapter 2.)

3. Fill two 100 μL heparinized capillary tubes to capacity without bubbles. Exposure of the specimen to outside air is minimized by placing the capillary tube into the center of a large drop of blood.

4. Insert a rustproof metal stirrer into the capillary tube.

5. Seal both ends of the capillary tube tightly with clay to prevent exposure to the atmosphere.

6. Stir the blood in the tubes by using a magnet to mix the specimen with the heparin.

7. Immerse the specimen tubes immediately in wet ice and deliver them to the laboratory at once for analysis within 10−15 minutes.

pH

The **pH** is a measurement of the body's concentration of hydrogen ions, the active component of all acids, and provides a guide to the acidity and alkalinity of the blood. Values for pH represent the ratio between the bicarbonate and carbonic acid components of the acid-base buffer system and reflect the interaction of many elements and electrolytes within the body. Any disturbance of the buffering process caused by the abnormal accumulation or loss of either bicarbonate or carbonic acid results in a variation from the optimum pH range.

Adequate functioning of the body's buffering ability is vital to maintain the acid-base balance, protect a stable pH, and guard against drastic changes in pH, which can result in death (Figure 5-3). Laboratory determination of the pH level provides important dynamic information about the continuing process of compensation and is helpful in the diagnosis, monitoring, and treatment of numerous disorders. Blood pH may be measured directly or calculated from a special chart or nomogram based on the relationship between pH, bicarbonate (frequently calculated from the total carbon dioxide content), and carbonic acid (measured as P_{CO_2}). (Urine pH levels are discussed in Chapter 1.)

Clinical Significance

Measurement of pH can reveal acidosis or alkalosis, but it cannot give diagnostic information concerning the exact cause of the pH disturbance. Analysis of additional information concerning the individual buffers, such as provided by P_{CO_2} and total carbon dioxide values, is necessary to distinguish the nature of the imbalance. For example, any pH rise is termed alkalosis but may result either from a loss of respiratory carbon dioxide (carbonic acid) or from a metabolically induced accumulation of bicarbonate. On the other hand, a low pH is termed acidosis but may have either a respiratory origin, such as carbon dioxide retention, or a metabolic origin such as a loss of bicarbonate.

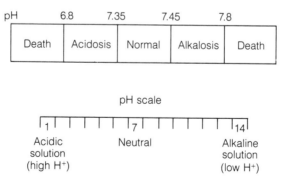

Figure 5-3 The pH of body fluids is maintained at a slightly alkaline state between the precise values of 7.35 and 7.45. (From Kozier, B., and Erb, G. L. 1983. FUNDAMENTALS OF NURSING: CONCEPTS AND PROCEDURES. Menlo Park, Calif.: Addison-Wesley Publishing Co., p. 804.)

Normal Values
The normal values for pH in the blood are:

Arterial blood	7.35−7.45
Venous blood	7.36−7.41

Variations
Elevated pH levels may occur with:

Alkali, overmedication	Hyperventilation	Renal disorders
Cushing's disease	Hysteria	Respiratory alkalosis
Diarrhea, severe	Metabolic alkalosis	Salicylate intoxication
Fever	Peptic ulcer therapy, excessive	Vomiting, excessive
High altitude		

Decreased pH levels may occur with:

Addison's disease	Emphysema	Pneumonia
Asthma	Hepatic dysfunction	Pulmonary dysfunction
Cardiac disorders	Hypoventilation	Renal disorders
Diabetic acidosis	Metabolic acidosis	Respiratory acidosis
Diarrhea, severe		

Methodology
Measurement of pH requires 5 mL of arterial or venous blood collected anaerobically and with a minimum of stasis into an airtight syringe containing heparin or a green-stoppered tube. Samples should be packed in wet ice to slow the rate of cellular metabolism and delivered to the laboratory immediately.

▶▶ Nursing Responsibilities and Implications

1. Collect the blood specimen without a tourniquet, if possible, to prevent stasis. If a tourniquet is necessary, it should remain in place as the blood is withdrawn.

2. Instruct the patient not to pump the fist, either before or during specimen collection, because this causes metabolic acids to accumulate, which can affect the pH level.

3. Collect venous or arterial blood into a vacuum tube with a green stopper or a syringe that has been rinsed with heparin. Heparin should always be the anticoagulant used for pH measurement because any other anticoagulant may have a significant effect on the pH level. Venous blood has a pH value approximately 0.03 units lower than arterial blood because of the accumulation of metabolic acids, but in most cases venous blood is suitable.

4. Maintain the blood anaerobically by inserting the needle into a cork or rubber stopper or by removing the needle and immediately capping the tip of the syringe. The contents of a vacuum tube remain anaerobic when the tube is removed from the adapter before the needle is withdrawn from the vein and the stopper is left in place.

5. Deliver the specimen to the laboratory immediately so that analysis can begin at once. As time passes, glycolytic activity, which is accelerated at room temperature, produces metabolic acids that can lower the pH. However, when the test cannot be performed immediately, the pH will remain virtually unchanged for as long as 2 hours if the sample is refrigerated or immersed in ice.

Partial Pressure of Carbon Dioxide

The **partial pressure of carbon dioxide** (Pco_2), which is a measure of the pressure or tension exerted by dissolved carbon dioxide gas in the blood, is directly related to the carbon dioxide produced by the tissues. Pco_2 levels are regulated by the lungs and indicate the amount of carbonic acid available to the body's acid-base buffer system. Laboratory determinations of Pco_2 are used to evaluate whether the cause of acidosis or alkalosis is metabolic or respiratory. A thorough interpretation of abnormal values requires a careful correlation of clinical findings, serum electrolyte levels, and blood pH levels.

Clinical Significance

The body strives to maintain an optimum pH level and to compensate for acid-base imbalances by stimulating or depressing respiration to regulate Pco_2 and carbonic acid concentrations. Thus, because Pco_2 values are indirectly proportional to respiration, the more rapidly or deeply an individual breathes, the greater the amount of carbon dioxide exhaled and the lower the Pco_2 level. The reverse is also true because the Pco_2 level is increased when the individual's breathing is more shallow or slower than normal. A constant level depends on the lungs removing the same amount of carbon dioxide from the blood as was added to it by the tissues.

Normal Values

The normal values for Pco_2 in the blood are:

Arterial blood	35–45 mm Hg
Venous blood	35–50 mm Hg

Variations

Elevated Pco_2 levels may occur with:

Asthma	Hypoventilation	Renal disorders
Congenital cardiovascular defects	Metabolic alkalosis	Respiratory acidosis
	Pneumonia	Vomiting, severe
Emphysema	Pulmonary disorders	

Decreased Pco_2 levels may occur with:

Diabetic acidosis	Hyperventilation, hysteria	Respiratory alkalosis
Fever	Metabolic acidosis	Salicylate intoxication
High altitude		

Methodology

Measurement of P_{CO_2} requires 5 mL of blood collected anaerobically with heparin anti-coagulant (green-stoppered tube), packed in wet ice, and maintained anaerobically for immediate delivery to the laboratory. (See Blood Gas Specimen Collection and Handling.)

▶▶ Nursing Responsibilities and Implications

1. Instruct the patient to rest quietly for at least 15 minutes before the blood specimen is drawn.

2. Assist in collecting a sample of arterial blood in a heparinized vacuum tube (green stopper) or a heparinized syringe. Maintain the specimen anaerobically by completely filling the container with blood and placing the needle into a rubber stopper or capping the syringe with a metal cap. Contents of vacuum tubes remain anaerobic if they are removed from the adapter while the needle is still in the vein and the rubber stopper is left in place.

3. Pack the specimen in ice and deliver it to the laboratory immediately. Test results are most accurate when the determinations are performed within 10 minutes after the blood is drawn.

Base Excess

Base excess, a calculated value also known as **buffer base capacity** and **delta base**, reflects the degree of acid-base imbalance by indicating the status of the body's total buffering capacity. It represents the amount of acid (or base) that can accumulate in the body before depleting the buffering ability of the blood and significantly changing the pH level. The total buffering capacity of whole blood, the buffer base capacity, is composed of the bicarbonate-carbonic acid buffer pair plus hemoglobin, plasma proteins, and phosphate compounds, and normally equals 46–52 mEq/L (average of 49.0 mEq/L). Laboratory calculation of base excess reflects the difference between this average normal buffer capacity and the actual buffer base of the patient at the time of testing.

Clinical Significance

Although base excess might be understood more easily if it were expressed as milliequivalents of buffering capacity per liter of blood, it commonly is expressed in abstract terms of positive or negative deviation from normal values. For example, a blood specimen with a total buffering capacity of 40.5 mEq/L is indicated by a base excess of −8.5 (40.5 mEq/L − 49.0 mEq/L = −8.5). Another sample with a buffering capacity of 53.0 mEq/L is indicated by a base excess of +4.0 (53.0 mEq/L − 49.0 mEq/L = +4.0). A sample with a buffering capacity of 49.0 mEq/L is indicated by a base excess value of 0.

Normal Values

The normal values for base excess are:

Arterial blood	−3.0 to +3.0
Venous blood	−2.5 to +2.5

Variations

Because base excess indicates the degree of deviation from acid-base balance, abnormal values may occur with conditions characterized by an electrolyte imbalance, acidosis, or alkalosis such as renal disease, diabetic acidosis, pneumonia, severe dehydration, congestive heart failure, and others.

Methodology

Because actual buffer base values are never measured directly in the clinical laboratory, base excess must be derived from the effects of the total buffering capacity on other test results. Base excess is calculated from a special nomogram (see Figure 5-2), using test results for pH and total carbon dioxide content to measure the amount of deviation from the average buffering capacity.

Partial Pressure of Oxygen

The **partial pressure of oxygen** (Po_2) is a measure of the tension or pressure exerted by the small amount of oxygen in its free form that is dissolved in the plasma. Most of the oxygen in the blood is carried by hemoglobin, and this amount, together with that represented by the Po_2 value, provides a measure of the total oxygen content. Laboratory determinations of Po_2 are useful in the evaluation of cardiopulmonary disorders in which respiratory exchange is affected. A complete interpretation of abnormal Po_2 values must depend on correlation with clinical findings, pH, and Pco_2 values.

Clinical Significance

The Po_2 of venous and arterial blood regulates the movement of oxygen out of the lungs and into the body tissues. Because gas diffuses from a place in which its partial pressure is high to one in which it is low, venous blood flowing through the lungs receives oxygen from the alveolar air, which has a greater Po_2. The diffusion of alveolar air into the blood oxygenates it. The blood is then transported to body tissues, where the Po_2 is lower. The difference in oxygen tension between tissues and arterial blood diffuses the oxygen from the blood into the tissues. A steady Po_2 level depends on the ability of the lungs to supply as much oxygen to the alveolar air as the tissues remove from the blood.

Normal Values

The normal values for Po_2 in the blood are:

Arterial blood	80–100 mm Hg
Venous blood	20–49 mm Hg

Variations

Decreased Po_2 (hypoxia) may occur with:

Arteriovenous shunt	Emphysema	Pneumonia
Asthma	Hypoventilation	Pulmonary dysfunction
Congenital heart defects		

Methodology

Measurements of Po_2 require 5 mL of blood collected anaerobically with heparin anticoagulant, packed in wet ice, and delivered to the laboratory immediately. (See Blood Gas Specimen Collection and Handling.)

Precautions

Test values for Po_2 may be affected by many variables, including sex, age, physical activity, and smoking habits.

▶▶ **Nursing Responsibilities and Implications**

1. Instruct the patient to lie quietly for at least 15 minutes before the specimen is collected.

2. Assist in collecting an arterial blood specimen in a syringe that has been rinsed in heparin, making sure that the tube is filled to capacity.

3. Maintain the specimen anaerobically, place it in ice at once, and deliver it to the laboratory immediately. Test results are most significant when the test is begun within 5–10 minutes after the specimen is drawn.

Oxygen Saturation

Oxygen saturation is the ratio of the amount of oxygen present in the blood compared with the total or maximum amount of oxygen the blood is capable of holding. This ratio is related to the ability of hemoglobin in the red blood cells to form oxyhemoglobin when exposed to oxygen in alveolar air or when completely saturated with oxygen under test conditions. Laboratory determinations of oxygen saturation are of great value in monitoring the patient's ventilation during and immediately following open-heart surgery. Oxygen saturation also aids in establishing a diagnosis during special examinations, such as cardiac catheterization or respiratory function tests, and may contribute to the planning of appropriate therapy.

Normal Values

The normal values for oxygen saturation are:

Arterial blood	95%–98%
Venous blood	60%–85%

Variations

Decreased oxygen saturation may occur with:

Arteriovenous shunt	Emphysema	Pneumonia
Asthma	Hypoventilation	Pulmonary dysfunction
Congenital heart defects		

Methodology

Oxygen saturation may be calculated from the ratio of laboratory measurements for oxygen content and oxygen-carrying capacity, but it recently has been calculated automatically from the values for pH and Po_2 by the laboratory apparatus used to determine blood gases.

Acid-Base Imbalance

The body strives to preserve an optimal pH level and maintain the normal $20:1$ ratio of bicarbonate to carbonic acid buffers through corrective responses by the kidneys and lungs. Some of these corrective changes occur rapidly, whereas others may take several days. If the body reserves of either buffer component are completely consumed, the buffering capacity of both is lost and the condition becomes uncompensated, resulting in abnormal pH values.

Four main acid-base disturbances have been recognized and classified as (1) acid or alkaline according to pH and (2) metabolic or respiratory according to cause. Conditions that cause a metabolically induced bicarbonate increase or a respiratory carbonic acid loss result in a pH rise and are termed **alkalosis**. Conditions that produce a respiratory carbonic acid increase or a metabolically diminished bicarbonate concentration lower the pH and are known as **acidosis**. (The laboratory indications of acid-base imbalance are presented in Table 5-5.)

Analysis of acid-base disorders also should include a review of total electrolyte balance because various ions are affected by abnormal buffer concentrations. Laboratory values are more informative than the clinical signs and symptoms of acid-base imbalance, which are subtle but increase in severity as compensation decreases. The nurse should recall that major clinical symptoms include respiratory changes such as hypoventilation or hyperventilation and changes in mental alertness such as disorientation leading to stupor and coma.

Respiratory Acidosis

Respiratory acidosis is produced by the carbonic acid excess that results when pulmonary disorders affect respiratory function and impede carbon dioxide excretion. Carbon dioxide accumulates in the blood, raising Pco_2 levels and causing the pH to become more acid (lower than normal). Impaired ventilation also increases the total carbon dioxide content as the kidneys retain bicarbonate ions to compensate for a persistently elevated carbonic acid concentration.

Signs and Symptoms

The nurse should be particularly alert for signs of respiratory acidosis, which include impaired and shallow respirations, poor exhalation, generalized weakness, loss of mental alertness, and disorientation leading to stupor and coma.

Respiratory acidosis may be caused by:

Anesthesia

Asthma

Bronchiectasis

Carbon dioxide overbreathing, prolonged

Head trauma

Morphine intoxication

Obesity

Oversedation

Pneumonia

TABLE 5-5   Laboratory Indications of Acid-Base Imbalance

Clinical Conditions	Plasma pH	Urine pH	P$_{CO_2}$	Carbon Dioxide Content	Base Excess	Common Cause
Respiratory acidosis (carbonic acid excess)						
Early	<7.35	<6.0	Moderate increase	Slight increase	Positive	Hypoventilation
Compensated	≦Normal	<6.0	Moderate increase	Marked increase	Positive	
Metabolic acidosis (bicarbonate deficit)						
Early	<7.35	<6.0	Slight decrease	Slight decrease	Negative	Loss of gastrointestinal alkali
Compensated	≦Normal	<6.0	Marked decrease	Slight decrease	Negative	Increased organic acids
Respiratory alkalosis (carbonic acid deficit)						
Early	>7.45	>7.0	Moderate decrease	Slight decrease	Negative	Hyperventilation
Compensated	≧Normal	>7.0	Moderate decrease	Marked decrease	Negative	
Metabolic alkalosis (bicarbonate excess)						
Early	>7.45	>7.0	Slight increase	Moderate increase	Positive	Alkali ingestion
Compensated	≧Normal	>7.0	Slight increase	Moderate increase	Positive	Loss of gastrointestinal acids

Cardiac disorders

Central nervous system respiratory depression

Emphysema

Pulmonary edema

Respiratory paralysis (Guillain-Barré syndrome, poliomyelitis)

Sleep apnea

Respiratory Alkalosis

Respiratory alkalosis is produced by the carbonic acid deficiency that results when respiratory stimulation increases the rate of carbon dioxide excretion. Prolonged pulmonary loss of carbon dioxide lowers Pco_2 levels, causing the pH to become more alkaline (higher than normal). Increased ventilation also depletes both buffer components and decreases the total carbon dioxide content as the kidneys increase bicarbonate ion excretion to compensate for excessive carbonic acid loss.

Signs and Symptoms

The nurse should be particularly alert for signs of respiratory alkalosis, which include deep and rapid breathing, lightheadedness, carpopedal spasms, and tetany leading to convulsions and unconsciousness.

Respiratory alkalosis may be caused by:

Anemia

Anxiety

Drug reactions

    Antihistamine

    Phenol

    Quinine

    Sulfanilamide

Encephalitis

Hepatic coma

High altitude

High environmental temperature

High fever

Hyperventilation

Hysteria

Infections

Medullary tumors of the respiratory center

Pulmonary fibrosis

Salicylate intoxication (early)

Metabolic Acidosis

Metabolic acidosis is produced by the bicarbonate ion deficiency that results when organic acids accumulate in the blood faster than they can be buffered or excreted by the kidneys. The body buffers organic acid by converting bicarbonate ions to carbonic acid, which can be eliminated through the increased respiratory excretion of carbon dioxide. Decreased bicarbonate concentration, produced by actual bicarbonate ion loss or excessive bicarbonate consumption, causes the pH to become more acid (lower than normal). Pulmonary compensation for excess nonvolatile acids decreases Pco_2 levels, depletes both bicarbonate and carbonic acid buffering capacity, and causes a tremendous loss of total carbon dioxide content.

Signs and Symptoms

The nurse should be particularly alert for signs of metabolic acidosis, which include weakness, Kussmaul respirations (deep, rapid breathing), shortness of breath (may be absent in infants), and disorientation leading to coma.

Metabolic acidosis may be caused by:

Addison's disease (terminal)	Lactic acidosis caused by shock or phenformin therapy
Circulatory failure, advanced	
Diabetic ketoacidosis, uncontrolled diabetes mellitus	Low-carbohydrate diet
	Malnutrition
Diarrhea, severe	Methanol intoxication
Duodenal fistulas	Renal failure, acute
Fat metabolism, excessive	Renal tubular acidosis
Hepatic dysfunction	Salicylate intoxication (late)
Hypothyroidism	Starvation
Intestinal intubation	Vomiting, severe

Metabolic Alkalosis

Metabolic alkalosis is produced by the bicarbonate ion excess that results when more base is retained in the blood than can be neutralized or excreted. Increased bicarbonate concentration, caused by the uncompensated loss of gastric acids or the improper intake of antacids, causes the pH to become more alkaline (higher than normal). Pulmonary compensation for acid deficiency reduces respiration to increase Pco_2 and conserve carbonic acid in an attempt to buffer the bicarbonate accumulation. However, this mechanism can only succeed to a certain point because increasing Pco_2 levels stimulate the respiratory center and promote respiration, although the net result is still an elevated total carbon dioxide content.

Signs and Symptoms

The nurse should be particularly alert for signs of metabolic alkalosis, which include mental dullness, depressed respirations, and muscular hypertonicity leading to tetany.

Metabolic acidosis may be caused by:

Adrenocorticosteroid imbalance	Peptic ulcer therapy
Alkalizing agents, overmedication	Potassium deficiency
Antacid therapy	Renal disorders
Cushing's disease	Sodium bicarbonate overmedication
Diuretic therapy, prolonged	Steroid therapy
Gastric fistulas	Vomiting, prolonged
Gastric suction or gavage, prolonged	

REFERENCES

Bauer, J. D. 1982. *Clinical laboratory medicine*. 9th ed. St. Louis: The C. V. Mosby Co.

Browning, R. J. 1982. Pulmonary disease: putting blood gas tests to work. *Diagn. Med.* 5(2):55.

Collins, R. D. 1975. *Illustrated manual of laboratory diagnosis*. 2nd ed. Philadelphia: J. B. Lippincott Co.

Doucet, L. D. 1981. *Medical technology review.* Philadelphia: J. B. Lippincott Co.

French, R. M. 1980. *Guide to diagnostic procedures.* 5th ed. New York: McGraw-Hill Book Co.

Garb, S. 1976. *Laboratory tests in common use.* 6th ed. New York: Springer Publishing Co.

Garg, A. K., and Nanji, A. A. 1982. The anion gap. *Diagn. Med.* 5(5):33.

Henry J. B. 1984. *Clinical diagnosis and management by laboratory methods.* 17th ed. Philadelphia: W. B. Saunders Co.

Kozier, B., and Erb, G. L. 1979. *Fundamentals of nursing: concepts and procedures.* Menlo Park, Calif.: Addison-Wesley Publishing Co.

Larson, F. C. 1982. *Clinical significance of tests available on DuPont Automatic Clinical Analyzer.* Wilmington, Del.: DuPont Industries.

Lee, C. A., Stroot, V. R., and Schaper, C. A. 1975. What to do when acid-base problems hang in the balance. *Nursing '75* 5:32.

Raphael, S. S., et al. 1983. *Medical laboratory technology.* 4th ed. Philadelphia: W. B. Saunders Co.

Slockbower, J. M., and Blumenfeld, T. A. 1983. *Collection and handling of laboratory specimens.* Philadelphia: J. B. Lippincott Co.

Soloway, H. B. 1978. Things your mother never told you about acid-base. *Diagn. Med.* 1(4).

———. 1981. Interpretation of tests: the anion gap. *Diagn. Med.* 4(6):15.

Strand, M. M., and Elmer, L. A. 1983. *Clinical laboratory tests.* 3rd ed. St. Louis: The C. V. Mosby Co.

Tilkian, S. M., Conover, M. H., and Tilkian, A. G. 1983. *Clinical implications of laboratory tests.* 3rd ed. St. Louis: The C. V. Mosby Co.

VanKessel, A. L. 1979. The blood gas laboratory. An update: 1979. *Lab. Med.* 10(7):419.

Weisberg, H. F. 1981. Osmolality. *Lab. Med.* 12(2):81.

Widmann, F. K. 1983. *Clinical interpretation of laboratory tests.* 9th ed. Philadelphia: F. A. Davis Co.

6

Chemistry: Tests of Endocrine Function

ADRENAL HORMONE STUDIES 295
Aldosterone · Catecholamines · Cortisol
· 17-Hydroxycorticosteroids · 17-Ketogenic Steroids
· 17-Ketosteroids · Vanillylmandelic Acid

MISCELLANEOUS HORMONE STUDIES 312
Calcitonin · 5-Hydroxyindoleacetic Acid · Parathyroid
Hormone · Renin · Vitamin D

PITUITARY HORMONE STUDIES 319
Adrenocorticotropic Hormone · Follicle-Stimulating
Hormone · Growth Hormone · Luteinizing
Hormone · Prolactin · Thyroid-Stimulating Hormone

REPRODUCTIVE HORMONE STUDIES 330
Estrogens · Human Chorionic Gonadotropin · Human Placental
Lactogen · Pregnanediol · Progesterone · Testosterone

THYROID HORMONE STUDIES 344
Triiodothyronine · Thyroxine · T_3 Uptake and T_3 Uptake
Ratio · Free Thyroxine Index

Hormones, vital substances secreted by a number of endocrine glands, act as a chemical communications system and exert a specific metabolic influence on target organs or body processes. Hormones are highly active substances, and exceedingly small amounts are sufficient to stimulate or inhibit cellular metabolism and control body functions. The endocrine glands and their hormones do not function as discrete units but comprise an integrated system that helps to maintain homeostasis and control general body metabolism. Endocrine glands, or tissues with endocrine function, include the adrenals, islet cells of the pancreas, ovaries, parathyroids, pineal body, pituitary, placenta, testes, thymus, thyroid, and gastrointestinal mucosa (Figure 6-1).

The various hormones produced by these endocrine glands play an essential role in triggering the cellular responses required for growth, reproduction, structural and biochemical differentiation, and adaptation to environmental or nutritional stress. Thus, any endocrine system disorder produces a hormone deficiency or excess that in turn may alter body function and the activity of other glands. Although glands that compose the endocrine system secrete many vital hormones, only a few are analyzed routinely.

Because the majority of hormones are carried to their sites of action by the bloodstream, the concentration of each hormone in the circulation reflects the activity of the endocrine gland that secreted it. Most hormones are present in the blood in such small amounts that it is difficult to analyze endocrine function. In addition, blood specimens only measure the hormone levels present at the time of collection and do not reflect diurnal changes or variations occurring in the patient.

However, many hormones and their metabolites are present in greater quantities in the urine, and measuring urinary levels is helpful in estimating the amount of hormones present in the blood. Thus a 24-hour urine specimen is more accurate than a single random urine specimen for the analysis of hormone and metabolite levels, because it allows for the normal fluctuation of hormone secretion during the day. Laboratory analysis of hormones and their metabolites in blood and urine aids in the diagnosis of diseases associated with abnormal hormone secretion and helps to identify increased or decreased levels associated with a number of pathologic conditions.

ADRENAL HORMONE STUDIES

The **adrenal glands**, reddish-brown organs located on top of the kidneys, are composed of two structurally different portions: an outer cortex surrounding an inner medulla, each with separate, completely independent functions. The adrenal cortex secretes nearly 50 steroid hormones that are essential to life; the medulla produces hormones that are not vital to life but are important to the management of stress situations. The most important adrenocortical hormones include **cortisol**, a glucocorticoid that influences carbohydrate metabolism; **aldosterone**, a mineralocorticoid that controls water and electrolyte balance; and **androgens** (sex hormones that also are produced by the ovaries and testes), which affect the development of primary and secondary sexual characteristics.

Routine measurement of adrenocortical hormones or their metabolites in urine provides an estimate of related groups of compounds rather than an analysis of individual steroids. The usual screening procedures for evaluating adrenocortical function determine the levels of plasma cortisol and its urinary metabolites, measured as 17-hydroxycorticosteroids (17-OHCS) and 17-ketogenic steroids (17-KGS). However, measurement of 17-OHCS and 17-KGS may be ordered infrequently as determination of urinary free cortisol levels is currently the most sensitive and specific evaluation of cortisol excretion. The urinary metabolites of the androgens are also measured as 17-ketosteroids (17-KS). It is

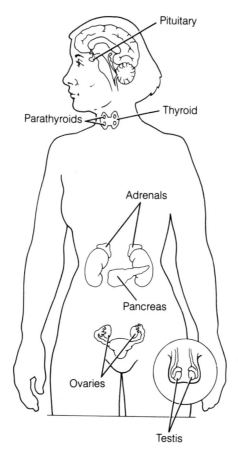

Figure 6-1 The major endocrine glands. (From Spence, A. P., and Mason, E. B. 1979. HUMAN ANATOMY AND PHYSIOLOGY. Menlo Park, Calif.: Benjamin/Cummings Publishing Co., Inc., p. 433.)

unfortunate that these terms are so similar because the substances are quite different and each provides unique clinical information.

The adrenal medulla secretes epinephrine, norepinephrine, and dopamine, hormones collectively known as the **catecholamines** that control the fight or flight response to various nervous and physiologic stimuli. Epinephrine is particularly important to the sympathetic nervous system response to stress situations by participating in liver and muscle glycogenesis and the release of lipids from adipose tissue. Norepinephrine and dopamine regulate the response of the vascular system to stress through peripheral sympathetic nerve activity.

Although small amounts of catecholamines are secreted continuously into the bloodstream, they are metabolized so rapidly that only minimal amounts normally remain in the plasma. Thus, the majority of the catecholamines are excreted in the urine as vanillylmandelic acid (VMA), a metabolite, and metanephrine, an end product of catecholamine degradation. The usual tests for evaluating adrenal medullary function therefore include blood and urinary catecholamine levels and VMA determinations, which are vital to the diagnosis of certain tumors.

Aldosterone

Aldosterone, a potent mineralocorticoid produced by the adrenal cortex, regulates the transport of electrolyte ions across renal tubular membranes, controlling blood volume and maintaining blood pressure through the retention of extracellular fluid. Although the actual mechanism that controls aldosterone production is not fully understood, the amount of hormone produced varies according to the state of electrolyte balance and the total body sodium concentration. Aldosterone secretion is stimulated by the renin-angiotensin system to adjust the extracellular fluid volume through the retention of sodium and chloride and the excretion of potassium.

Adrenal secretion of aldosterone is stimulated by angiotensin. Angiotensin is formed when diminished blood volume causes specialized kidney cells to release renin, which initiates a complex series of reactions that trigger angiotensin production. Elevated aldosterone levels increase sodium concentration and cause water to be retained, expanding blood volume; restoration of extracellular fluid and blood volume reverses this sequence and aldosterone production is decreased. Excessive aldosterone secretion may result from primary adrenal hyperfunction, as in adrenal cortex tumors (primary aldosteronism), or pathologic changes, as in the regulation of blood volume and electrolyte balance (secondary aldosteronism). Laboratory analysis of aldosterone levels helps to determine the cause and significance of hypertension, polyuria, tetany, alkalosis, hypernatremia, and hypokalemia and aids in the differential diagnosis of primary and secondary aldosteronism.

Clinical Significance

Aldosterone levels are influenced by posture as well as the state of salt balance, which often may cause normal and abnormal values to overlap. For example, patients who remain upright for 4 hours have aldosterone levels that are approximately 50% of those collected from patients who are supine. In addition, a low salt intake (10 mEq/day) and potassium administration generally double aldosterone secretion, whereas sodium administration and potassium deficiency reduce aldosterone secretion. Thus, it is important for the patient to have a normal sodium diet immediately prior to and during the test.

Normal Values

The normal and clinically significant values for aldosterone are:

Blood

  Upright

Men	6–22 ng/dL
Women, nongravid	4–31 ng/dL
Women, pregnant	18–100 ng/dL
Supine	<16 ng/dL

Urine

Normal salt diet	2–26 μg/24 hours
Low-salt diet	17–44 μg/24 hours
High-salt diet	0–6 μg/24 hours
Adrenal tumor	20–100 μg/24 hours

Variations

Decreased aldosterone secretion may occur with Addison's disease, systemic infections, and severe stress.

Elevated aldosterone secretion (aldosteronism) may occur with:

ACTH (adrenocorticotropic hormone) administration, large doses

Adrenal tumors

Cardiac failure

Cirrhosis

Hemorrhage

Hypovolemia

Potassium loading

Pregnancy

Nephrosis, lower nephron

Salt depletion

Methodology

Serum or plasma aldosterone determinations require 5 mL of blood collected without anticoagulants (red-stoppered tube) or with heparin or EDTA anticoagulant (green- or lavender-stoppered tube). Specimens should be delivered to the laboratory immediately after collection, promptly separated from the cells, and frozen. The laboratory request slip should specify if the specimen was obtained from the peripheral circulation or from adrenal vein catheterization.

Urinary aldosterone determinations require a 100 mL aliquot of a 24-hour urine specimen collected in a bottle containing 10 g of boric acid and refrigerated during the collection period. Urine specimens for aldosterone analysis remain stable for 7 days at room temperature. The total 24-hour urine volume should be recorded on both the laboratory request slip and the urine collection container.

Catecholamines

The **catecholamines**, mainly epinephrine (adrenaline), norepinephrine (noradrenaline), and dopamine, are a group of hormones secreted by the adrenal medulla that act on peripheral arteries and affect cardiac output. Collectively, the catecholamines exert a profound effect on the nervous system, increasing blood pressure and initiating adaptive responses to such physiologic stress conditions as hypoxia, hemorrhage, hypotension, or strenuous muscle activity. These hormones remain unaltered in the bloodstream for a brief period of time, are rapidly metabolized to vanillylmandelic acid (VMA) and metanephrine, and are excreted in the urine in very small amounts.

Catecholamines normally are secreted in episodic bursts and the concentrations vary greatly throughout the day, with the highest levels occurring during the day and the lowest levels occurring during sleep. Catecholamine secretion increases significantly in the presence of pheochromocytoma, a rare tumor of the adrenal medulla that often is accompanied by an elevated blood pressure. Thus, single plasma catecholamine values reflect the physiologic state only at the time of testing and are subject to misinterpretation because of intermittent epinephrine and norepinephrine secretion by tumors.

Epinephrine and norepinephrine values are most significant when measured in a 24-hour urine specimen that reflects total daily excretion. However, analysis of random or timed urine specimens also may be requested following an episode of hypertension because catecholamine levels of this nature can pass undetected when diluted in a 24-hour urine specimen. Laboratory determinations of plasma and urinary catecholamine levels are helpful in the clinical evaluation of adrenal function and are used almost exclusively to diagnose pheochromocytoma in patients with otherwise unexplained hypertension.

Clinical Significance

Measurement of the catecholamines and their metabolites provides a reliable index to the presence of pheochromocytoma and neuroblastoma when the presence of these adrenal tumors is suspected in hypertensive patients. (See Vanillylmandelic Acid later in this chapter.) Because catecholamine secretion accompanying pheochromocytoma is usually 3–100 times greater than normal, urinary catecholamine analysis is a more reliable aid in diagnosing this condition than blood levels, which exhibit appreciable diurnal variation. Slightly increased urinary catecholamine levels also may occur in some patients with psychiatric disorders, although these levels are not high enough to interfere with the diagnosis of pheochromocytoma if this condition is present.

Normal Values

The normal and clinically significant values for the catecholamines are:

Plasma	140–650 pg/mL
Dopamine	0–90 pg/mL
Epinephrine	0–55 pg/mL
Norepinephrine	65–320 pg/mL
Urine	
Total	0–18 μg/dL (random)
	1.4–7.3 μg/hour (during daylight hours)
	0–135 μg/24 hours
Epinephrine	0–20 μg/24 hours
Norepinephrine	10–80 μg/24 hours
Borderline	100–200 μg/24 hours
Pheochromocytoma	>200 μg/24 hours

Variations

Decreased plasma catecholamine levels may occur with anorexia nervosa and orthostatic hypotension.

Falsely decreased plasma catecholamine levels may occur with the administration of anticonvulsants, antiarrhythmics, and barbiturates.

Decreased urinary catecholamine levels may occur with familial dysautonomia, malnutrition, and transection of the cervical spinal cord.

Elevated plasma and urinary catecholamine levels may occur with:

Anger, severe	Ganglioneuroma
Anxiety, severe	Medications (see falsely elevated plasma and urinary catecholamine levels)
Burns, extensive	
Exercise, strenuous	

Muscular dystrophy, progressive	Neuroblastoma
Myasthenia gravis	Pheochromocytoma

Falsely elevated plasma catecholamine levels may occur with:

Amphetamines	Dopamine	Levarterenol
Bronchodilators	Isoproterenol	Vasodilators

Falsely elevated urinary catecholamine levels may occur with:

Adrenaline	Ethanol	Methyldopa
Aminophylline	Exercise, strenuous	Nicotinic acid
Amphetamines	Guanethidine	Quinidine
Antihypertensive agents	Histamine	Quinine
Bananas	Hydralazine	Reserpine
Caffeine	Hypoglycemia	Riboflavin
Chlorpromazine	Isoproterenol	Salicylates
Cocaine	L-dopa	Stress, emotional
Ephedrine	Metanephrine	Tetracycline
Epinephrine inhalation, excessive	Methenamine	Tyramine
Erythromycin	Methenamine mandelate	Vitamin B complex, large doses

Methodology

Plasma catecholamine determinations require 5 mL of blood collected with heparin (green-stoppered tube), placed in an ice bath, and delivered to the laboratory immediately. When prompt delivery to the laboratory is not possible, the plasma should be separated from the cells and frozen immediately. Because plasma catecholamine levels may be spuriously elevated by anxiety, specimens should be collected after the patient has remained in a seated or supine position for 30 minutes in a tranquil surrounding. Test results are most significant when specimens are collected between 8 AM and noon to minimize the effects of circadian rhythm.

Urinary catecholamine measurements require a 100 mL aliquot of a 24-hour urine sample collected in a dark bottle containing 10–15 mL of concentrated (6N) hydrochloric acid and kept under refrigeration. Random urine specimens also may be used for the investigation of suspected pheochromocytoma when they are collected during or immediately following an episode of hypertension and acidified with a small amount of concentrated hydrochloric acid. Urine specimens acidified to a final pH below 3.0 remain stable for catecholamine determinations for several days at room temperature and for several months when refrigerated.

Precautions

To ensure significant results, the following precautions should be observed when obtaining specimens for catecholamine determinations:

1. Withhold for at least 1 week before testing, if possible, any substances that might interfere with accurate catecholamine determinations or interpretation, including bananas, coffee, and the drugs listed under Variations, which may falsely elevate catecholamine levels.

2. Caution the patient to avoid strenuous activity during the test period because vigorous exercise prior to blood or urine collection can increase the output of catecholamines as much as sevenfold.

▶▶ *Nursing Responsibilities and Implications*

1. Provide a quiet environment and caution the patient to avoid any activity for at least 30 minutes before the test period begins.

2. Collect the blood sample in a calm, reassuring manner, pack the specimen in ice, and deliver it to the laboratory immediately.

3. Place 10 mL of 6N hydrochloric acid in a dark urine collection bottle at the start of the test, collect the urine in that container, and refrigerate the container during the entire 24-hour collection period. It is essential that the urine be kept acid during the entire urine collection period.

4. Add additional hydrochloric acid as needed after urine collection is completed to achieve a urine pH of less than 3.0.

5. Record the total urine volume on the laboratory request slip and send a 100 mL aliquot for analysis.

Cortisol

Cortisol, also known as hydrocortisone or compound F, is the principal and most abundant steroid hormone secreted by the adrenal cortex. This potent glucocorticoid exerts several physiologic effects, helping to maintain constant blood pressure, depress inflammatory responses to injury, increase renal blood flow, and synthesize carbohydrates from protein. Cortisol synthesis is controlled by ACTH from the pituitary gland, which stimulates cortisol production in response to a normal circadian rhythm and supresses production through a negative feedback inhibition. The rate of cortisol secretion also is affected by physical and psychologic stress as well as low blood glucose levels.

The physiologic activity of cortisol is produced by the 10% that is not bound to protein which leaves the bloodstream to affect target cells and is excreted in the urine. The amount of free (unbound) cortisol in urine therefore is derived from and reflects the amount of free cortisol in the blood. Laboratory measurement of plasma cortisol is used to evaluate adrenocortical function and aids in the diagnosis of abnormal states such as Addison's disease or Cushing's disease. A combination of morning and evening plasma cortisol determinations, supplemented by stimulation (ACTH) or suppression (dexamethasone, metyrapone) tests, can offer strong evidence for the diagnosis of specific diseases related to adrenal dysfunction. Measurement of urinary free cortisol is one of the best screening tests for confirming the diagnosis of Cushing's disease because there is very little overlap between normal and abnormal values.

Clinical Significance

Plasma cortisol secretion normally exhibits diurnal variation, with maximum levels generally occurring between 5 and 10 AM and decreasing as the day progresses. Lowest plasma cortisol values occur between 4 PM and midnight, falling to approximately one-third to one-half of the morning level. A midday surge of cortisol levels normally occurs in women that is coincident with food intake but is markedly attenuated by food deprivation. Extreme elevations of plasma cortisol levels accompanied by a disruption of this diurnal variation appear in patients with Cushing's disease and also may suggest lesions in the adrenal glands.

Normal Values
The normal values for cortisol are:

Plasma cortisol

8 AM	5–25 μg/dL
8 PM	2–18 μg/dL
Urine free cortisol	20–100 μg/24 hours
ACTH stimulation	Two to three times the morning levels
Suppression tests	<5 μg/dL

Variations
Decreased plasma cortisol levels may occur with:

Addison's disease	Dexamethasone administration
Adrenal insufficiency	Hypopituitarism
Adrenogenital syndrome	Hypothyroidism

Elevated plasma cortisol levels may occur with:

ACTH administration	Hyperthyroidism	Shock
Burns	Infectious disease	Stress, extreme
Cushing's disease	Obesity	Surgery
Eclampsia	Oral contraceptives	Vasopressin administration
Estrogen administration	Pancreatitis, acute	Virilism
Hyperpituitarism	Pregnancy	
Hypertension, severe		

Falsely elevated plasma cortisol levels may occur with:

Alcohol, large doses	Oral contraceptives
Amphetamines, oral	Smoking, heavy
Estrogen administration	Spironolactone administration
Methamphetamines, parenteral	

Methodology
Plasma cortisol measurements require 5 mL of blood collected with heparin or EDTA anti-coagulants (green- or lavender-stoppered tube), although serum specimens (red-stoppered tube) also may be used. Plasma and serum specimens for cortisol determinations remain stable for 7 days at room temperature and for longer when frozen.

Urinary free cortisol measurements require a 25 mL aliquot of a 24-hour urine specimen collected in a bottle containing 10 g of boric acid for each liter of urine. Urine specimens for free cortisol determinations should be frozen as soon as the collection period has ended to prevent the hormone from deteriorating. The total volume of urine collected should be noted on both the specimen container and the laboratory request slip.

Precautions
To ensure significant test results, the following precautions should be observed when collecting specimens for plasma cortisol determinations.

1. Collect blood specimens at the same time each day, usually in the early morning and late afternoon, to allow a valid comparison of plasma cortisol levels for the diagnosis of adrenal dysfunction.

2. Encourage bedrest for at least 2 hours before specimen collection because physical activity affects cortisol levels.

3. Collect blood specimens from patients who have fasted for 3 or more hours because there is less interference from lipids in these specimens.

4. Deliver the blood specimens to the laboratory as soon as possible so that plasma can be separated from the cells promptly to prevent spuriously decreased test results.

5. Withhold the administration of estrogen or oral contraceptives for at least 6 weeks before plasma cortisol analysis to prevent falsely elevated test results.

▶▶ Nursing Responsibilities and Implications

1. Collect morning specimens for plasma cortisol determinations from a fasting patient between 7 and 9 AM; obtain afternoon specimens between 4:30 and 5 PM, before the evening meal.

2. Note the time of blood specimen collection on the laboratory request slip as a guide to the normal diurnal variation of cortisol secretion.

17-Hydroxycorticosteroids

The **17-hydroxycorticosteroids** (17-OHCS), also known as the Porter-Silber chromogens, are a group of compounds that are metabolized from the adrenocortical steroid hormones, mainly cortisol, and excreted in the urine. Because the rate of excretion of corticosteroid metabolites fluctuates, complete 24-hour urine specimens are needed for accurate 17-OHCS determinations. Analysis of urinary 17-OHCS levels, next to the determination of plasma cortisol values, provides the best assessment of adrenocortical function. Laboratory measurement of urinary 17-OHCS aids in the diagnosis of clinical conditions related to hypofunction and hyperfunction of the adrenal cortex. However, measurement of 17-OHCS may be ordered infrequently as determination of urinary free cortisol levels currently provides a more sensitive and specific index to the rate of cortisol secretion.

Clinical Significance
The excretion of abnormally large amounts of 17-OHCS generally indicates a state of hyperadrenalism because urinary concentrations of 17-OHCS accurately reflect adrenocortical activity. Unfortunately, the diminished 17-OHCS excretion that is expected to accompany hypoadrenalism is not always apparent, and diagnosis requires additional tests that measure functional cortisol reserves. Urinary 17-OHCS measurements are used in

dynamic testing procedures involving suppression (dexamethasone) in the evaluation of adrenocorticol status and alterations in the pituitary-adrenal axis. Urinary excretion levels of 17-OHCS vary according to muscle mass and body weight, causing higher values to appear in men than in women. Concentrations of 17-OHCS tend to increase following muscular activity.

Normal Values

The normal values for 17-hydroxycorticosteroids are:

Men

<70 years	5–23 mg/24 hours
>70 years	3–12 mg/4 hours

Women

<70 years	2–15 mg/24 hours
>70 years	3–12 mg/24 hours

Children

<1 year	<1 mg/24 hours
1–5 years	1–2 mg/24 hours
5–10 years	<5 mg/24 hours

Variations

Decreased urinary 17-hydroxycorticosteroid levels may occur with:

Addison's disease	Hypoadrenalism	Hypothyroidism
Adrenogenital syndrome	Hypopituitarism	Oral contraceptives

Falsely decreased 17-hydroxycorticosteroid levels may occur with:

Dexamethasone	Promethazine
Glycosuria	Reserpine
Phenytoin	

Elevated 17-hydroxycorticosteroid levels may occur with:

Acromegaly	Obesity
Adrenal cancer	Pancreatitis (marked increase)
Burns (moderate increase)	Pregnancy, first trimester (slight increase)
Cushing's disease (marked increase)	
Eclampsia (marked increase)	Pregnancy, third trimester (moderate increase)
Hyperadrenalism	
Hyperpituitarism	Stress, extreme (marked increase)
Hypertension, severe (slight increase)	Surgery (moderate increase)
Hyperthyroidism	Virilism (slight increase)
Infectious diseases (moderate increase)	

Falsely elevated 17-hydroxycorticosteroid levels may occur with:

Chloral hydrate	Etryptamine	Methenamine
Chlordiazepoxide	Fructose	Oleandomycin
Chlorthiazide	Hydroxyzine	Paraldehyde
Chlorpromazine	Iodides	Piperidines
Colchicine	Monoamine oxidase	Prochlorperazine
Cortisone	(MAO) inhibitors	Spironolactone
Erythromycin	Meprobamate	Quinidine

Methodology

Measurement of 17-OHCS requires a 100 mL aliquot of a 24-hour urine specimen collected in a bottle containing 10 g of boric acid and kept refrigerated during the collection period. Laboratories occasionally require that alternate preservatives such as 15 mL of toluene or 10 mL of 6N hydrochloric acid be added to prevent bacterial decomposition of the steroids. Acidified urine specimens for 17-OHCS assays remain stable for 14 days at room temperature. The total 24-hour urine volume should be recorded on both the laboratory request slip and the specimen container.

Precautions

To ensure accurate results, the following precautions should be observed when collecting specimens for 17-OHCS determinations:

1. Whenever possible, withhold all medications for at least 3 days before testing because many drugs and substances interfere with the measurement of urinary 17-OHCS and have a significant effect on the test results (see Variations). Additional substances that interfere with 17-OHCS results include:

Acetazolamide	Estrogens	Phenothiazines
Bilirubin	Nitrofurantoin	Propoxyphene
Coffee	Penicillin	Quinine
Digitoxin, digoxin	Phenazopyridine	Sulfonamide

2. Do not schedule any kidney or liver function studies during the urine collection period as these tests may interfere with the formation or excretion of 17-OHCS.

17-Ketogenic Steroids

The **17-ketogenic steroids** (17-KGS) are those 17-hydroxycorticosteroids (17-OHCS) and adrenal cortex hormones that can be converted to 17-ketosteroids (17-KS) and measured in the urine. Urinary 17-KGS levels therefore indicate the total 17-OHCS concentration, including cortisol and its many metabolites, along with those glucocorticoids that normally are not measured as 17-OHCS by the Porter-Silber procedure. Thus, because more compounds are being estimated, the 17-KGS technique yields higher values than other tests of adrenocortical function that measure only 17-OHCS. To accurately interpret 17-KGS levels, however, any 17-KS present in the urine before testing must be inactivated or measured separately. Laboratory determinations of urinary 17-KGS provide a sensitive index of adrenocortical secretion and glucocorticoid metabolism and aid in the diagnosis of Cushing's disease when 17-OHCS levels are within the normal range. As indicated earlier, urinary free cortisol has replaced tests for 17-KGS in many laboratories.

Clinical Significance

The maximum rate of 17-KGS excretion occurs between 20 and 50 years of age and decreases steadily thereafter. Measurement of urinary 17-KGS aids in the diagnosis of some pathologic conditions in which evaluation of the total steroid level is significant because 17-OHCS contributes only 40% of the 17-KGS values. Because of abnormal adrenal hormone metabolites that are not measured by the Porter-Silber technique, elevated 17-KGS levels occur in some cases of adrenal carcinoma or hyperplasia even when 17-OHCS levels are within the normal range. A 17-KGS value that is more than 5 mg/24 hours over the test level for 17-OHCS signifies some hormone abnormality and warrants further investigation.

Normal Values

The normal values for 17-ketogenic steroids are:

Men	5–23 mg/24 hours
Women	3–15 mg/24 hours
Children	
<1 year	<1 mg/24 hours
<5 years	<2 mg/24 hours
5–10 years	3–6 mg/24 hours

Variations

Decreased urinary 17-ketogenic steroid levels may occur with:

Addison's disease	Morphine administration
Corticosteroid therapy	Oral contraceptives
Cretinism	Simmonds' disease
Hypoadrenalism	Wasting disorders, generalized
Hypopituitarism	

Falsely decreased urinary 17-ketogenic steroid levels may occur with:

Chlorothiazide	Paraldehyde	Reserpine
Cortisone derivatives	Quinine	Thiazine
Metyrapone		

Elevated urinary 17-ketogenic steroid levels may occur with:

ACTH therapy	Cushing's disease	Stress, severe
Adrenal carcinoma	Hyperadrenalism	Surgery
Adrenogenital syndrome	Infectious diseases	Virilism
Burns	Obesity	

Falsely elevated urinary 17-ketogenic steroid levels may occur with:

Acetazolamide	Glucuronide	Phenothiazines
Acetophenone	Hydralazine	Phenaglycodol
Chlorpromazine	Meprobamate	Spironolactone
Cortisone	Oleandomycin	Triacetyloleandomycin
Ethinamate	Penicillin	

Methodology

Measurement of urinary 17-KGS excretion requires a 100 mL aliquot of a 24-hour urine specimen collected in a bottle containing 10 g of boric acid and stored on ice or refrigerated during the entire collection period. Laboratories occasionally require that alternate preservatives such as 10 mL of 6N hydrochloric acid be added to prevent the production of extraneous compounds from bacterial decomposition of the steroids. Acidified urine specimens for 17-KGS determinations remain stable for 14 days at room temperature. The total 24-hour urine volume should be recorded on both the laboratory request slip and the specimen container.

Precautions

To ensure accurate urinary 17-KGS measurements, withhold all medications, whenever possible, for at least 48 hours before the specimen collection period because many medications interfere with the 17-KGS test results and make accurate interpretation impossible. Drugs that might interfere with 17-KGS test results include many of those listed in Variations plus:

Betamethasone	Methyprylon	Pyrazinamide
Chlordiazepoxide	Phenazopyridine	Quinidine
Dexamethasone	Piperidine	Secobarbital
Estrogens	Probenecid	

17-Ketosteroids

The **17-ketosteroids** (17-KS) are a group of organic compounds that are metabolized from androgenic hormones and excreted in the urine. Androgens are biologically active compounds of adrenal and testicular origin that stimulate the development of male secondary sexual characteristics. Approximately two-thirds of the urinary 17-KS in men is derived from the adrenal cortex, with the remainder derived from the testicular steroids. Virtually all of the urinary 17-KS in women and children directly reflects adrenal androgen production, with just a trace (if any) produced by the gonads.

Assays of 17-KS provide a rough guide to androgenic hormone secretion but are not a true index of androgenic activity because the most powerful androgen, testosterone, is not a 17-KS. Thus, although the 17-KS determination in males reflects testicular and adrenocortical activity, 17-KS measurements are more valuable for diagnosing adrenal dysfunction than testicular disorders. Laboratory determinations of 17-KS may be used to screen for marked changes in adrenocortical activity and to indicate pituitary and gonadal dysfunction.

Clinical Significance

Urinary 17-KS excretion varies from day to day and is influenced in adults by age and sex; normal levels in men are significantly higher than those in women. The levels of 17-KS are generally low in both sexes before puberty, and the usual difference because of gender is absent. Excretion of 17-KS begins to decrease after 50 years of age, and by 65 years of age levels have fallen below the normal adult range for both men and women. Levels of 17-KS usually correlate closely with 17-OHCS values, except in certain pathologic conditions involving benign tumors in which 17-OHCS levels are elevated but 17-KS levels are within normal limits.

Normal Values

The normal values for 17-ketosteroids are:

Men

<65 years	7−25 mg/24 hours
>65 years	4−8 mg/24 hours

Women

<65 years	4−15 mg/24 hours
>65 years	4−8 mg/24 hours

Children

<1 year	<1 mg/24 hours
1−4 years	<2 mg/24 hours
5−8 years	<3 mg/24 hours
9−12 years	3 mg/24 hours
12−16 years	4−9 mg/24 hours

Variations

Decreased urinary 17-ketosteroid levels may occur with:

Addison's disease	Hypothyroidism
Adrenocortical insufficiency	Klinefelter's syndrome
Anorexia nervosa	Liver disease, advanced
Debilitating illness, chronic	Myxedema
Diabetes mellitus	Nephrosis
Estrogen therapy	Nephrotic syndrome
Gout	Salicylate therapy, prolonged
Hypogonadism	Simmonds' disease
Hypopituitarism	Thyrotoxicosis

Falsely decreased urinary 17-ketosteroid levels may occur with:

Chlorothiazide	Paraldehyde	Reserpine
Cortisone derivatives	Probenecid	Thiazides
Metyrapone	Quinine	

Elevated urinary 17-ketosteroid levels may occur with:

ACTH therapy	Hyperpituitarism
Adrenocortical carcinoma, adenoma	Infectious diseases
Adrenocortical hyperplasia	Ovarian tumors, certain
Adrenogenital syndrome	Precocious puberty
Burns	Stress, severe
Cushing's disease	Surgery
Hirsutism	Testicular tumors, certain

Falsely elevated urinary 17-ketosteroid levels may occur with:

Acetazolamide	Ethinamate	Penicillin
Acetophenone	Hydralazine	Phenaglycodol
Chloramphenicol	Glucuronide	Phenazopyridine
Chlorpromazine	Meprobamate	Phenothiazines
Cloxacillin	Nalidixic acid	Spironolactone
Cortisone	Oleandomycin	Triacetyloleandomycin
Erythromycin		

Methodology

Measurement of 17-KS requires a 100 mL aliquot of a 24-hour urine specimen collected in a bottle containing 10 g of boric acid and stored on ice or refrigerated during the entire collection period. Laboratories occasionally require that alternate preservatives such as 3 mL of acetic acid, 15 mL of toluene, or 10 mL of 6N hydrochloric acid be added to prevent bacterial decomposition of the steroids. Urine specimens for 17-KS determinations remain stable for 14 days at room temperature and for longer when frozen. The total 24-hour urine volume should be noted on both the laboratory request slip and the specimen container.

Precautions

To ensure significant results, the following precautions should be observed when collecting specimens for 17-KS determinations:

1. Whenever possible, withhold all medications for at least 48 hours before the urine specimen collection period is begun. Numerous medications may interfere with 17-KS test results and make accurate interpretation difficult, including:

Betamethasone	Methyprylon	Probenecid
Chlordiazepoxide	Oral contraceptives	Pyrazinamide
Dexamethasone	Phenazopyridine	Quinidine
Estrogens	Piperidine	Secobarbital

2. Do not schedule liver or kidney function tests during the urine specimen collection period as these tests may interfere with formation or excretion of 17-KS.

Vanillylmandelic Acid

Vanillylmandelic acid (VMA), the chief metabolite of catecholamines secreted by the adrenal medulla, is excreted in the urine and provides a reliable index of epinephrine and norepinephrine production. Vanillylmandelic acid is excreted, along with its metabolic precursor metanephrine, in concentrations that are 10–100 times greater than total catecholamines, 95% of which are metabolized before they appear in the urine. Urinary VMA and metanephrine excretion increase significantly in the presence of pheochromocytoma and neuroblastoma, the rare adrenal tumors that frequently are accompanied by an elevated blood pressure.

Laboratory determinations of urinary VMA have the same physiologic significance as total catecholamine measurements in the diagnosis of pheochromocytoma and neuroblastoma and provide a useful indication of hormone secretion in individuals with unexplained hypertension and normal catecholamine levels. Vanillylmandelic acid determinations also may be used to confirm elevated catecholamine secretion or as an alternate method when interfering substances yield falsely elevated catecholamine results. Measurement of total metanephrine concentrations provides a reliable indicator of total catecholamine synthesis, which is particularly helpful in suspected cases of pheochromocytoma when VMA and total catecholamine levels are normal.

Clinical Significance

Vanillylmandelic acid and epinephrine levels accurately and reliably elevate hormone secretion because urine concentrations of these hormones are considerably higher than total catecholamines, and test results are influenced by fewer interfering substances. To obtain diagnostic VMA values, a complete 24-hour urine specimen is needed to avoid misinterpretation caused by the diurnal variation of catecholamine secretion. Test results must be closely correlated with the patient's physical status because persistent and transient hypertension may occur in conditions other than pheochromocytoma. In patients exhibiting paroxysmal hypertension, the urine collection period should be started during a paroxysm of hypertension regardless of the time of day.

Normal Values

The normal values for vanillylmandelic acid and metanephrine are:

Vanillylmandelic acid	0.5–14 mg/24 hours
Metanephrine	0.3–1.3 mg/24 hours

Variations

Elevated metanephrine levels may occur with:

Chlorpromazine	Monoamine oxidase inhibitors
Dopamine	Stress, severe

Decreased vanillylmandelic acid levels may occur with:

α-Methyldopa	Imipramine
Clofibrate	Methyldopa
Guanethidine analogs	Monoamine oxidase inhibitors

Elevated vanillylmandelic acid levels may occur with:

Burns	Pheochromocytoma
Carcinoid tumors	(150 mg/24 hours)
Carotid body tumors	Retinoblastoma
Childbirth	Stress, severe
Ganglioneuroma	Surgery
Neuroblastoma	Trauma

Falsely elevated vanillylmandelic acid levels may occur with:

Anileridine hydrochloride	Methocarbamol
Antihypertensive agents	Methyldopa
Aspirin	Oxytetracycline
Bananas	Phenazopyridine
Bromsulphthalein (BSP) dye	Phenolsulfonphthalein (PSP) dye
Chocolate	Reserpine
Citrus fruits	Stibophen
Coffee	Tea
Glyceryl guaiacolate	Vanilla flavoring
Mephenesin	

Methodology

Analysis of urinary VMA and metanephrine excretion requires a 100 mL aliquot of a complete 24-hour urine specimen collected in a brown plastic bottle containing 25 mL of concentrated (6N) hydrochloric acid and kept refrigerated. Urine specimens acidified to a final pH of 3.0 remain stable for VMA and metanephrine determinations for 4−8 weeks at room temperature and for 6 months when refrigerated. The total volume of urine collected should be recorded on the laboratory request slip.

Precautions

To ensure reliable results, the following precautions should be observed when collecting specimens to measure VMA and metanephrine excretion:

1. Whenever possible, withhold for at least 3 days before and during the test period any foods and drugs that are known to interfere with VMA analysis (these substances may raise test results by 10%–15%; see Variations). Additional medications that might interfere with VMA test results include:

Clofibrate	Penicillin
Nalidixic acid	Sulfa drugs
Para-aminosalicylic acid	

2. Discontinue the use of monoamine oxidase (MAO) inhibitors for 3 days before metanephrine analysis because these drugs may interfere with the conversion of metanephrine to VMA and produce falsely elevated test results.

MISCELLANEOUS HORMONE STUDIES

Calcitonin

Calcitonin, also known as thyrocalcitonin, is a potent hormone secreted by parafollicular or C cells of the thyroid gland that helps to maintain normal serum calcium and phosphorus levels. Although its physiologic role is poorly understood, calcitonin is secreted in response to high serum calcium levels (hypercalcemia) to diminish calcium mobilization from bone and soft tissue and inhibit its resorption. Calcitonin functions as a physiologic antagonist to parathyroid hormone (PTH) and vitamin D to regulate the activity of osteoclasts in bone and increase the clearance of calcium by the kidneys. (See also Parathyroid Hormone and Vitamin D in this chapter; calcium also is discussed in Chapters 1 and 5.)

Because increased calcitonin secretion also decreases the synthesis of vitamin D to diminish the transport of intestinal calcium and phosphorus, thyroid gland impairment or hyperactivity alters the ratio of calcium to phosphate. Thus, excess calcitonin secretion occurs in medullary carcinoma of the thyroid, a neoplasm of parafollicular or C cells, although the fasting calcitonin level is normal in a significant number of patients with medullary carcinoma. Laboratory determinations of calcitonin concentration are valuable in the diagnosis of medullary thyroid tumors and the investigation of ectopic calcitonin production in patients with carcinoma of the lung or breast.

Normal Values
The normal value for calcitonin is:

Normal   <100 pg/mL

Variations
Elevated calcitonin levels may occur with:

Breast cancer	Pernicious anemia
Cushing's disease, Type II	Pheochromocytoma
Hypercalcemia	Renal failure, chronic
Lung cancer	Uremia
Medullary carcinoma of the thyroid	Zollinger-Ellison syndrome
Parathyroid hyperplasia or adenoma	

Methodology
Calcitonin determinations require 10 mL of blood collected with heparin or EDTA (green- or lavender-stoppered tube) or without anticoagulants (red-stoppered tube) from a fasting patient. Serum and plasma specimens should be sent to the laboratory promptly for immediate analysis or frozen to prevent deterioration.

5-Hydroxyindoleacetic Acid

5-Hydroxyindoleacetic acid (5-HIAA), the urinary metabolite of serotonin, is produced by certain cells of the gastrointestinal tract and acts as a local vasoconstrictor. Normally, 90%–95% of serotonin is located within the intestinal mucosa, while the remainder is converted to 5-HIAA and excreted in very low concentrations in the urine. Abnormally large amounts of serotonin are produced by rare carcinoid tumors arising mainly from the argentaffin cells in the appendix and result in a marked increase of 5-HIAA excretion. Laboratory determination of urinary 5-HIAA provides an indication of excessive serotonin production and is the most useful tool for diagnosing carcinoid tumors.

Clinical Significance

Qualitative measurements of urinary 5-HIAA excretion usually are performed as a screening procedure because of the low incidence of carcinoid tumors, and quantitative evaluations are used to investigate positive results. Prompt diagnosis and removal of carcinoid tumors generally result in a favorable prognosis; complete cures are frequent because many intestinal tumors have a low degree of malignancy. However, although serotonin overproduction is characteristic of carcinoid tumors, some patients with carcinoid syndrome may not exhibit elevated urinary 5-HIAA levels. Occasionally, patients without the carcinoid syndrome or those with noncarcinoid tumors also may have increased concentrations of urinary 5-HIAA.

A number of foods and drugs may inhibit 5-HIAA excretion or interfere chemically with the test procedure, resulting in falsely increased or decreased test values. It is not clear, however, whether the inhibition produced by these foods and drugs is sufficient to interfere with the diagnosis of carcinoid tumors.

Normal Values

The normal and clinically significant values for urinary 5-HIAA are:

Normal	1–10 mg/24 hours
Doubtful	10–100 mg/24 hours
Suggestive of metastatic tumor	>100 mg/24 hours

Variations

Elevated urinary 5-hydroxyindoleacetic acid levels may occur with argentaffin tumors, carcinoid tumors, and nontropical sprue.

Falsely elevated urinary 5-hydroxyindoleacetic acid levels may occur with:

Acetanilid	Glyceryl guaiacolate	Pineapples
Avocados	Mephenesin	Plums
Bananas	Methocarbamol	Reserpine
Eggplants	Phenacetin	Walnuts

Falsely decreased urinary 5-hydroxyindoleacetic acid levels may occur with:

Chlorpromazine, large doses	Methenamine
Imipramine	Methyldopa

Phenothiazines, large doses

Promazine, large doses

Phenylalanine

Promethazine

Prochlorperazine

Methodology

Urinary 5-HIAA determinations require 100 mL of a 24-hour urine specimen collected in a bottle containing 12 g of boric acid or 25 mL of 6N hydrochloric acid and refrigerated during the test period. Acidification of the urine specimen is necessary to prevent decomposition of the hormone metabolite. The acidified specimen remains stable for 5-HIAA analysis for 1 week at room temperature and for longer when refrigerated.

Precautions

To ensure significant test results when measuring 5-HIAA, withhold any foods and drugs that might interfere with 5-HIAA levels, whenever possible, for at least 3 days before as well as during the test period (see Variations).

Parathyroid Hormone

Parathyroid hormone (PTH), also called parathormone or parathyrin, is an essential hormone secreted by the parathyroid gland that helps to maintain normal plasma concentrations of calcium and phosphate. Secretion of PTH is stimulated by low plasma calcium levels (hypocalcemia) to raise calcium and lower phosphate concentrations by releasing calcium from bone, increasing tubular resorption of calcium ions, and reducing phosphate resorption. Parathyroid hormone also enhances the synthesis of active vitamin D metabolites in the kidneys, which then raises plasma calcium levels by increasing absorption from the small intestine and mobilizing reserves from bone and soft tissue. Conversely, high plasma calcium levels suppress parathyroid activity, inhibit PTH secretion, and stimulate the release of calcitonin to decrease calcium concentrations and increase phosphate levels. (See Calcitonin and Vitamin D in this chapter; calcium also is discussed in Chapters 1 and 5.)

Thus, hyperactivity of the parathyroid gland is manifested by increased PTH secretion, whereas impaired parathyroid function decreases PTH secretion. Laboratory determination of PTH concentrations is useful in the differential diagnosis of hypercalcemia associated with hyperparathyroidism resulting from adenoma or hyperplasia and also may be used to detect hypoparathyroidism. Parathyroid hormone levels do not change in individuals with pseudohypoparathyroidism.

Clinical Significance

Two clinically significant forms of PTH, a biologically inert C-terminal fragment and a biologically active N-terminal fragment, have proven to be useful in the differential diagnosis of parathyroid disorders. Measurement of either fragment may be used to detect chronic hypersecretion of the parathyroid glands, although C-terminal assays generally have higher values and provide a better indication of hyperparathyroidism. Conversely, acute changes in the secretion of PTH by the parathyroid glands are reflected more clearly by assays of N-terminal fragments.

The concomitant measurement of serum calcium concentrations and PTH levels usually provides adequate diagnostic information in the differential diagnosis of hypercalcemia in clearly pathologic parathyroid states. However, both assays as well as other diagnostic aids often are needed to clearly establish the diagnosis in patients with early or borderline disorders. For example, many patients with elevated serum calcium concentrations caused by malignancy may have increased C-terminal assays and normal or suppressed N-terminal assays (except in hyperparathyroidism). Measurement of N-terminal PTH therefore is probably superior to C-terminal assays in determining whether the hypercalcemia associated with a malignancy is caused by the neoplasm or by an underlying parathyroid disorder.

Normal Values
The normal and clinically significant values for parathyroid hormone are:

C-terminal parathyroid hormone

Normal	400−885 pg/mL
Hypercalcemia, nonparathyroid	<600 pg/mL
Hyperparathyroidism, primary	>900 pg/mL
Hyperparathyroidism, secondary	>2000 pg/mL
Hypoparathyroidism	<800 pg/mL
N-terminal parathyroid hormone	230−630 pg/mL

Variations
Decreased C-terminal parathyroid hormone levels may occur with nonparathyroid hypercalcemia and hypoparathyroid hypocalcemia.

Decreased N-terminal parathyroid hormone levels may occur with:

Hypercalcemia

Neoplasm

Pseudohyperparathyroidism

Hypocalcemia, hypoparathyroidism

Elevated C-terminal parathyroid hormone levels may occur with:

Hypercalcemia

Neoplasm

Primary hyperparathyroidism

Pseudohyperparathyroidism

Hypocalcemia

Pseudohypoparathyroidism

Secondary hyperparathyroidism

Elevated N-terminal parathyroid hormone levels may occur with:

Hypercalcemia, primary hyperparathyroidism

Hypocalcemia

Pseudohypoparathyroidism

Secondary hyperparathyroidism

Methodology
Parathyroid hormone measurements require 10 mL of blood collected without anticoagulants (red-stoppered tube) and delivered to the laboratory for immediate analysis.

Although serum specimens remain stable for C-terminal PTH determinations for 7 days at room temperature, specimens for N-terminal PTH determinations are extremely unstable and must be frozen if immediate analysis is not possible.

Renin

Renin is an enzyme secreted by specialized kidney cells in response to decreased intravascular fluid volume caused by sodium depletion or a postural change from supine to upright. Renin secretion initiates sequential steps that stimulate the production of angiotensin II, which acts as a powerful vasopressor and directly stimulates the synthesis of aldosterone by the adrenal cortex. Aldosterone in turn promotes the increased retention of sodium and water in an effort to expand blood volume and return arterial pressure to normal (see Aldosterone earlier in this chapter).

Renin levels vary widely in normal individuals and are specifically affected by a number of factors, including salt intake, time of day, posture, and medications. For example, renin levels are increased in patients on a low-salt diet, highest early in the day, and higher in the upright position than in the recumbent position. Thus, correct interpretation of renin values requires detailed knowledge of the patient's electrolyte status, diet over the preceding several days, exposure to diuretic agents, and posture for the 4 hours preceding the test. Laboratory determinations of renin often are included as a valuable screening test for patients with hypertension of renal origin and also may be used to distinguish primary from secondary hyperaldosteronism.

Clinical Significance

The renin-angiotensin-aldosterone system controls reabsorption of sodium and potassium by the kidneys, which helps to regulate intravascular fluid volume and blood pressure. Low plasma volume and sodium levels stimulate renin secretion, resulting in marked stimulation of aldosterone; conversely, increased blood volume or acutely elevated blood pressure suppresses renin and aldosterone secretion, resulting in subsequent sodium loss. Thus, the presence of increased plasma renin activity and elevated aldosterone levels in a hypertensive patient suggests overactivity of the renin-angiotensin system associated with secondary aldosteronism or a renin-secreting tumor.

Normal Values

The normal values for renin are:

Normal salt intake

Recumbent (6 hours)	0.5–1.6 ng/mL
Upright (4 hours)	1.9–3.6 ng/mL

Low salt intake

Recumbent (6 hours)	2.2–4.4 ng/mL
Upright (4 hours)	4.0–8.1 ng/mL
Upright with diuretics	6.8–15.0 ng/mL

Variations

Decreased renin levels may occur with:

Aldosteronism, primary

Antidiuretic hormone (ADH) therapy

Diabetes mellitus

Excess sodium intake

Salt-retaining steroid therapy

Elevated renin levels may occur with:

Addison's disease, untreated

Cushing's disease

Diuretics

Estrogens

Glucocorticoids

Hemorrhage

Low-sodium diet

Malignant hypertension

Oral contraceptives

Pregnancy

Renal failure, chronic

Renin-secreting tumors

Renovascular hypertension

Salt-losing nephropathy, primary

Vasodilating agents

Methodology

Renin measurements require 10 mL of blood collected in a plastic or glass syringe and transferred immediately to a prechilled tube containing EDTA anticoagulant (lavender-stoppered tube). Specimens must be mixed, cooled promptly in an icewater bath, and delivered to the laboratory immediately because renin is very unstable at room temperature.

▶▶ Nursing Responsibilities and Implications

1. Provide the patient with a regular diet containing 180 mEq of sodium and 100 mEq of potassium for 3 days before the specimen is collected; instruct the patient to avoid eating licorice.

2. Withhold medications that interfere with the test results for at least 4 days prior to the test, if possible; note on the laboratory slip any medications the patient is receiving.

3. Note on the laboratory slip and chart the exact time of day the specimen is drawn and the patient's position for the 4 hours prior to the test.

4. Deliver the specimen to the laboratory immediately.

5. Monitor the patient's blood pressure, especially if antihypertensive medications have been withheld.

Vitamin D

Vitamin D, a general term for a group of fat-soluble sterols, is obtained from the diet as well as through the action of sunlight on certain compounds present in the skin. Because vitamin D_3, the principal form (also called cholecalciferol), is produced by ultraviolet irradiation of a precursor in the skin, appreciable seasonal fluctuations of vitamin D levels may result from variable exposure to sunlight. Vitamin D_3 becomes physiologically active only after successive hydroxylation, first to 25-hydroxycholecalciferol in the liver and finally to the most biologically important metabolite, 1,25-dihydroxycholecalciferol in the kidneys.

Vitamin D_3 is required to maintain serum calcium and phosphorus levels and, together with PTH and calcitonin, acts as a hormone to help regulate calcium and phosphate homeostasis through intestinal absorption. Because vitamin D is also essential to the mobilization of skeletal calcium and maintenance of normal skeletal mineralization, children with vitamin D deficiency develop rickets and adults develop osteomalacia. Laboratory determinations of 25-hydroxycholecalciferol provide a useful indication of vitamin D_3 status in the differential diagnosis of hypercalcemia and aid in the evaluation of vitamin D deficiency as a cause of bone disease. The most direct indication of calcium metabolic disorders, however, is the 1,25-dihydroxycholecalciferol level, which also may be used to ensure an adequate intake of 25-hydroxycholecalciferol in individuals with vitamin D deficiency and to guard against possible overdosage.

Clinical Significance
1,25-Dihydroxycholecalciferol is considered the only active form of vitamin D with respect to calcium and phosphorus control and plays an essential role in maintaining concentrations in the bloodstream within normal limits. Thus, when plasma values fall below acceptable levels, 1,25-dihydroxycholecalciferol enhances the effects of PTH in mobilizing skeletal calcium and phosphorus to bring about a return to normal concentrations. Its precursor, 25-hydroxycholecalciferol, on the other hand, has no calcium-controlling function and probably serves as a storage pool for active 1,25-dihydroxycholecalciferol. However, because the kidney converts inactive 25-hydroxycholecalciferol to biologically active 1,25-dihydroxycholecalciferol in the presence of PTH, this normal conversion is compromised and calcium control affected by renal dysfunction.

Normal Values
The normal and clinically significant values for vitamin D are:

25-Hydroxycholecalciferol	
Normal	10–55 ng/mL
Toxic	>100 ng/mL
1,25-Dihydroxycholecalciferol	20–76 pg/mL

Variations
Decreased 25-hydroxycholecalciferol levels may occur in:

Diminished intestinal absorption	Hepatobiliary disease
Drug therapy, long-term	Intestinal malabsorption disease
Ethosuximide	Nephrotic syndrome
Phenytoin	Osteomalacia
Primidone	Pregnancy
Steroids, high-dose	Rickets
Elderly individuals during winter	Thyrotoxicosis
Gastrectomy	Vitamin D deficiency, dietary

Decreased 1,25-dihydroxycholecalciferol levels may occur in:

Hyperthyroidism

Hypoparathyroidism

Lead poisoning in children

Parenteral nutrition, total (prolonged, 3 months)

Pseudohypoparathyroidism

Renal failure, chronic

Renal osteodystrophy

Rickets

Rickets, vitamin D-dependent

Vitamin D deficiency, severe

Elevated 25-hydroxycholecalciferol levels may occur in vitamin D intoxication.
Elevated 1,25-dihydroxycholecalciferol levels may occur in:

Acromegaly

Hypercalcemia

Hyperparathyroidism

Hypothyroidism

Pregnancy

Rickets, vitamin D-dependent

Sarcoidosis

Methodology

Measurements of 25-hydroxycholecalciferol and 1,25-dihydroxycholecalciferol require 10 mL of blood collected without anticoagulants (red-stoppered tube) and delivered to the laboratory immediately for prompt analysis. Serum specimens for 25-hydroxycholecalciferol analysis remain stable for 7 days at room temperature; specimens for 1,25-dihydroxycholecalciferol measurements are unstable and must be frozen if testing cannot be performed immediately.

PITUITARY HORMONE STUDIES

The pituitary gland, often called the master control gland, is a spherical nubbin of tissue at the base of the brain that is divided into two lobes and produces numerous hormones. The anterior lobe, or **adenohypophysis**, produces two groups of hormones, somatotropins and gonadotropins, that stimulate endocrine secretion in several target organs and tissues to regulate various physiologic processes. The somatotropins include growth hormone (GH), which affects skeletal and muscle growth, plus adrenocorticotropic hormone (ACTH) and thyroid-stimulating hormone (TSH), which stimulate adrenal and thyroid hormone secretion, respectively. The gonadotropins include follicle-stimulating hormone (FSH) and luteinizing hormone (LH), which stimulate maturation and the release of germinal cells in the ovaries and testes, together with prolactin (PRL), which acts on the mammary gland to initiate the flow of milk. The posterior lobe, or **neurohypophysis**, secretes oxytocin, which triggers the release of milk from the lactating breast, and antidiuretic hormone (ADH), or vasopressin, which regulates the rate of water excretion.

The pituitary gland, however, is not an autonomous master gland; its function is governed by a delicate negative feedback mechanism that is controlled by the effects of various hormones produced in the target organs. For example, when thyroxine (T_4) and triiodothyronine (T_3) are being produced by the thyroid at an optimal level, the pituitary production of TSH ceases. This same process also occurs in the other endocrine glands. Likewise, pituitary function increases when body needs require additional quantities of a specific hormone or when circulating levels are lower than normal.

Clinical hypopituitarism refers to any decrease of anterior pituitary function; the condition is characterized by entities ranging from an isolated lack of one tropic hormone to the complete absence of all hormones. The clinical symptoms of hypopituitarism depend largely on the patient's age as well as on the nature of the deficiency. For example, GH deficiency in children produces easily recognized clinical manifestations, whereas the same deficiency in adults may not produce a distinctive clinical picture.

Adrenocorticotropic Hormone

Adrenocorticotropic hormone (ACTH), also known as corticotropin, is an anterior pituitary hormone that regulates the production and secretion of glucocorticosteroids by the adrenal cortex. Adrenocorticotropic hormone secretion is controlled by the corticotropin-releasing hormone of the hypothalamus and depends on the amount of adrenal hormones, predominantly cortisol, in the bloodstream. The amount of cortisol produced by the adrenal cortex is in turn controlled by ACTH secretion, which exerts a negative feedback effect when cortisol concentrations reach optimal levels.

These integrated regulatory factors are stimulated by stress and cycles of sleeping and waking to produce a diurnal rhythm of ACTH secretion. Thus, the pattern of ACTH secretion is episodic, with the highest levels appearing in the morning, between 8 AM and 10 AM, and the lowest levels occurring at night. Laboratory determinations of ACTH levels are helpful in the differential diagnosis of primary and secondary adrenocortical insufficiency and in monitoring response to therapy.

Clinical Significance
Adrenocorticotropic hormone levels are useful in the diagnosis of certain adrenocortical disorders. Low to normal levels accompany secondary insufficiency caused by pituitary dysfunction or indicate autonomous adrenal activity. Increased ACTH values, on the other hand, occur in individuals with primary adrenocortical insufficiency, whereas persistently high values combined with high cortisol levels indicate pituitary hyperactivity or ectopic ACTH production. Adrenocorticotropic hormone assays also are helpful in determining the cause of Cushing's disease, which results from the overproduction of cortisol due to adrenocortical tumors with low ACTH levels or hypothalamic-pituitary lesions and elevated ACTH levels.

Normal Values
The normal and clinically significant values for adrenocorticotropic hormone are:

8 AM–10 AM	15–100 pg/mL
Primary adrenal insufficiency	>200 ng/mL
Secondary adrenal insufficiency	<75 ng/mL

Variations
Decreased adrenocorticotropic hormone levels may occur in congenital adrenal hyperplasia, secondary adrenal insufficiency, and hypopituitarism.

Elevated adrenocorticotropic hormone levels may occur in:

Addison's disease (pri-
mary adrenal atrophy)

Menstrual cycle

Pregnancy

Electroshock therapy

Pituitary tumors follow-
ing adrenalectomy

Pyrogens

Hypoglycemia

Surgery

Methodology

Measurement of ACTH requires 5 mL of blood collected between 8 and 10 AM in a plastic syringe and transferred to a plastic tube containing EDTA or heparin anticoagulant (lavender- or green-stoppered tube). Specimen containers should be immersed in ice as soon as the blood is drawn and transported to the laboratory immediately so that plasma can be separated from the cells promptly. If ACTH determinations cannot be performed within 15 minutes after specimen collection, plasma should be frozen at −20 C or lower. For accurate evaluation of ACTH secretion, sequential determinations are often needed because values change significantly with episodes of secretion or inactivity, and a single measurement may be misleading.

Follicle-Stimulating Hormone

Follicle-stimulating hormone (FSH), also known as follitropin, is an anterior pituitary hormone that stimulates the development and function of the gonads in both men and women. In females FSH promotes the proliferation and growth of ovarian follicle cells, ripening of the graafian follicle, and maturation of the ovum in preparation for ovulation. In males FSH promotes the development of seminiferous tubules, production and matura- tion of spermatozoa, and synthesis of testosterone by the Leydig cells of the testes.

Follicle-stimulating hormone is released from the pituitary, in conjunction with the luteinizing hormone (LH), by the gonadotropin-releasing hormone of the hypothalamus, which is under the feedback-inhibitory control of the sex steroid hormones. Thus, estro- gens, particularly estradiol, which are secreted by the developing ovarian follicle and by the corpus luteum after ovulation, control the circulating level of FSH by negative feed- back on the hypothalamus. Likewise, testosterone, along with estradiol produced by the testes, helps to maintain circulating FSH levels by controlling pituitary response to gonadotropin-releasing hormones from the hypothalamus. Laboratory determinations of FSH therefore are helpful in evaluating pituitary-hypothalamic-gonadal function, distin- guishing primary from secondary gonadal failure, and determining the causes of infertility.

Clinical Significance

Follicle-stimulating hormone appears in the bloodstream at all ages; the concentration is approximately the same in men and women except for the midcycle ovulatory peak in women. Children have low levels of FSH, which increase to about twice their previous levels at puberty. Although little change in the level of FSH occurs as males age, a marked elevation occurs in postmenopausal women, usually beginning in the fifth decade of life.

Increased FSH production occurs during primary failure of the gonads, whereas de- creased values accompany gonadal failure secondary to diminished pituitary function. However, rapid fluctuations in FSH concentrations have been noted in normal individuals due to episodic release of the hormone from the pituitary gland. Thus, single FSH deter- minations may not be diagnostic, and several specimens may be required to establish a baseline value.

Normal Values

The normal values for follicle-stimulating hormone are:

Serum

Children, prepubertal	5–13 mIU/mL
Men	
Uncastrated	4–25 mIU/mL
Castrated	30–200 mIU/mL
Women	
Follicular phase	2–25 mIU/mL
Midcycle peak	12–30 mIU/mL
Luteal phase	2–25 mIU/mL
After menopause	40–250 mIU/mL

Urine

Men	2–15 IU/24 hours
Women	
Follicular phase	2–15 IU/24 hours
Midcycle peak	8–60 IU/24 hours
Luteal phase	2–10 IU/24 hours
After menopause	35–100 IU/24 hours

Variations

Decreased follicle-stimulating hormone levels may occur in:

Adrenal hyperplasia and neoplasms

Amenorrhea, secondary (caused by pituitary failure)

Anorexia nervosa

Anovulatory menstrual cycle

Delayed puberty

Estrogen administration

Hypogonadotropinism

Hypophysectomy

Hypopituitarism

Hypothalamic dysfunction

Oral contraceptives

Ovarian neoplasms

Prepubertal children

Testicular neoplasms

Testosterone administration

Elevated follicle-stimulating hormone levels may occur in:

Amenorrhea, primary (caused by ovarian failure)

Anorchism

Castration

Hypothalamic tumor

Hysterectomy

Klinefelter's syndrome

Male climacteric

Menopause

Orchiectomy

Ovarian failure

Pituitary tumors, certain

Precocious puberty

Premature menopause

Seminiferous tubule failure

Testicular agenesis

Methodology

Measurement of circulating FSH requires 5 mL of blood collected without anticoagulants (red-stoppered tube) or with EDTA (lavender-stoppered tube). Specimens must be collected without trauma because grossly hemolyzed or lipemic samples may cause inaccurate test results.

Measurement of urinary FSH requires a 50 mL aliquot of a 24-hour urine specimen collected in a container to which 10 g of boric acid has been added prior to the test period. The entire 24-hour urine volume should be noted on both the laboratory request slip and the specimen container.

Precautions

To ensure accurate results, the following precautions should be observed when collecting specimens for FSH determinations:

1. Note on the laboratory request slip if the patient has received any diagnostic or therapeutic procedures requiring the administration of radioisotopes because these agents will interfere with the test procedures and may cause falsely decreased FSH levels.

2. Handle the blood specimen gently to prevent hemolysis.

▶▶ **Nursing Responsibilities and Implications**

1. Note on the laboratory slip if the patient is postmenopausal. If the patient is premenopausal, note the phase of the menstrual cycle.

2. Note on the laboratory slip if the patient is receiving hormones, including oral contraceptives.

Growth Hormone

Growth hormone (GH), an anterior pituitary hormone that plays an important role in adult metabolism, is essential to the regulation of bone and muscle growth in children. Growth hormone secretion stimulates the production of RNA, increasing the rate of anabolism. In the absence of GH, growth in children proceeds at one-third to one-half the normal rate. Normal GH function in adults has not been fully clarified, although its activity is intimately connected with that of insulin, and it is an important mobilizer of fatty acids from stored lipids.

Growth hormone secretion occurs intermittently and at varying rates; increases are associated with several events, including hypoglycemia, amino acid infusion or protein ingestion, major surgery, periods of deep sleep, and exercise. Growth hormone is secreted into the bloodstream in substantial amounts during the first 2 hours of sleep, and bursts of secretion also may occur with exercise, especially in fasting individuals. Laboratory determination of GH may be used to confirm the diagnosis of acromegaly and helps to diagnose hypopituitarism in adults earlier than is possible with other conventionally measured pituitary hormones.

Clinical Significance

Hyposecretion of GH by the pituitary gland during the growth phase in children results in less than normal growth or dwarfism; hypersecretion of GH during this phase causes pituitary gigantism. Hypersecretion of GH following the growth phase, when the epiphyses of the long bones have closed, results in acromegaly, or abnormal bone growth, which is characterized by gradual deformation of the face, hands, and feet.

Growth hormone concentrations in the bloodstream are subject to wide, rapid fluctuations during the day, and test results may be greatly altered by normal physiologic events. Therefore, test results obtained from a single random blood specimen often are difficult to interpret, and challenge testing may be required to establish a diagnosis. A deficiency of GH can be detected by a subnormal test response to appropriate stimulation such as TRH (thyrotropin releasing hormone), arginine or glucagon infusion, or L-dopa administration.

Normal Values
The normal values for growth hormone are:

Baseline values

Adults

Men	0–10 ng/mL
Women	0–15 ng/mL
Children	0–20 ng/mL

Challenge testing

Borderline	>5 ng/mL
Normal	>7 ng/mL

Variations
Decreased growth hormone levels may occur in dwarfism and hyperglycemia in adults.

Elevated growth hormone levels may occur in:

Acromegaly	Pituitary gigantism
Infants, premature and newborn	Surgery, major

Methodology
Measurement of GH requires 5 mL of blood collected without anticoagulants (red-stoppered tube) from a patient who is in the postabsorptive state following an 8- to 10-hour fast. To obtain a true basal GH level, the patient should be unstressed and at complete rest in a quiet environment for at least 30 minutes prior to specimen collection. Specimens should be delivered to the laboratory immediately because GH is not stable in serum at room temperature. When immediate analysis is not possible, serum specimens should be frozen.

Luteinizing Hormone

Luteinizing hormone (LH), also known as lutropin, is an anterior pituitary hormone that stimulates the development and function of the gonads in both men and women. In women LH exerts a variety of effects on the ovary and, together with FSH, is responsible for a number of changes that occur during the menstrual cycle. A temporary fourfold increase in LH secretion occurs about 24 hours before ovulation to stimulate maturation of the graafian follicle, which is followed by follicular rupture and release of the mature ovum. This normal, sharp, midcycle upsurge of LH also is necessary for the development of a functioning corpus luteum as well as the production of progesterone and estrogens.

In men LH, which is properly referred to as interstitial cell-stimulating hormone (ICSH), is required along with FSH for the complete development and maturation of spermatozoa in the seminiferous tubules. Luteinizing hormone also promotes testosterone production through its role in the maintenance and stimulation of testicular interstitial cells or Leydig cells.

The circulating level of LH is controlled by the gonadotropin-releasing hormone from the hypothalamus, which is under the negative-feedback influence of estradiol in females and testosterone in males. Thus, LH is released when estradiol or testosterone concentrations in the peripheral circulation fall below a certain level. Conversely, increased estradiol and testosterone levels inhibit the secretion of LH-releasing hormone, which in turn prevents the pituitary release of LH and delays the maturation of another ovarian follicle and ovum. Laboratory determinations of LH levels are valuable in evaluating pituitary-hypothalamic-gonadal function and determining the causes of infertility.

Clinical Significance

The LH assay is helpful in evaluating infertility in both men and women; high values are associated with primary gonadal dysfunction and low values occur with pituitary or hypothalamic failure. Thus, the absence of a midcycle LH peak helps to identify women with anovulatory fertility problems, whereas elevated LH levels occur in women with amenorrhea caused by ovarian failure. The normal midcycle LH peak completely disappears in women using oral contraceptives but reappears during the first full cycle after the oral contraceptives are discontinued.

Normal Values

The normal values for luteinizing hormone are:

Serum

Children	4−20 mIU/mL

Men

Uncastrated	6−30 mIU/mL
Castrated	30−200 mIU/mL

Women

Follicular phase	2−30 mIU/mL
Midcycle peak	40−200 mIU/mL
Luteal phase	0−25 mIU/mL
After menopause	20−200 mIU/mL

Urine

Men	5−18 IU/24 hours

Women

Follicular phase	2−25 IU/24 hours
Midcycle peak	30−95 IU/24 hours
Luteal phase	2−20 IU/24 hours
After menopause	40−110 IU/24 hours

Variations
Decreased luteinizing hormone levels may occur with:

Adrenal hyperplasia and neoplasms

Amenorrhea, secondary (caused by pituitary failure)

Delayed puberty

Estrogen administration (in postmenopausal women)

Hyperprolactinemia

Hypogonadotropinism

Hypophysectomy

Hypopituitarism

Hypothalamic dysfunction

Oral contraceptives

Testicular failure, secondary (caused by pituitary failure)

Testosterone administration (in postmenopausal women)

Elevated luteinizing hormone levels may occur with:

Adrenogenital syndrome

Advancing age

Amenorrhea, primary (caused by ovarian failure)

Anorchism

Central nervous system dysfunction

Hypothalamic tumors

Hysterectomy

Klinefelter's syndrome

Menopause, premature

Ovarian agenesis

Pituitary tumors

Precocious puberty

Stein-Leventhal syndrome

Testicular failure, primary

Testicular tumors

Methodology
Measurement of circulating LH levels requires 5 mL of blood collected without trauma and without anticoagulants (red-stoppered tube) or with EDTA (lavender-stoppered tube). However, a single determination may not be diagnostic because rapid or episodic fluctuations have been noted in both sexes, caused by characteristic bursts of LH released from the pituitary gland. Thus, evaluating several specimens obtained on the same day can increase the reliability of test results and more fully indicate the true LH status of the patient. A series of daily specimens is required to establish the presence or absence of a midcycle LH peak in the assessment of infertility.

Measurement of urinary LH requires a 50 mL aliquot of a 24-hour urine specimen. The entire 24-hour urine volume should be noted on the laboratory request slip.

Precautions
To ensure reliable results, the following precautions should be observed when collecting specimens for LH determinations:

1. Do not submit lipemic or grossly hemolyzed blood samples to the laboratory because they may yield inaccurate test results.

2. Handle the specimen carefully to prevent hemolysis.

Prolactin

Prolactin (PRL), an anterior pituitary hormone, acts directly on the mammary gland to stimulate its growth and development and is essential for the initiation and maintenance of lactation. Prolactin levels rise progressively during pregnancy to induce milk production in a breast already stimulated by high estrogen levels, peak when lactation begins, and surge each time the infant nurses. In nonpregnant adults a normal fluctuation in prolactin secretion begins 60–90 minutes after the onset of sleep and reaches a sleep-induced peak 4–5 hours later. Physiologic prolactin increases also occur in nonpregnant adults during exercise, surgical trauma, pain, insulin-induced hypoglycemia, and other stresses.

Prolactin secretion is uniform in both sexes until puberty, when increased estrogen production causes higher prolactin levels in females, and again after menopause, when concentrations in females decrease. Laboratory determination of prolactin is useful in differentiating functional galactorrhea from pituitary or hypothalamic tumors, evaluating the effectiveness of surgical removal of pituitary tumors, and monitoring the course of therapy. The role of prolactin in sexual dysfunction is becoming increasingly apparent; prolactin values also aid in the diagnosis and management of pathologic hyperprolactinemias that result in nonpuerperal galactorrhea and ovulatory suppressant-induced lactation.

Clinical Significance

The unstimulated pituitary secretes prolactin at a high, continuous rate unless circulating levels are controlled by dopamine, a hypothalamic inhibitor; any agent that antagonizes or depletes dopamine causes prolactin levels to rise. Excessive levels of circulating prolactin (**hyperprolactinemia**) disturb gonadal function in both men and women, causing men to become impotent, even in the presence of adequate testosterone levels, and women to experience amenorrhea and anovulation. Prolonged prolactin elevations in nonpregnant women often stimulate inappropriate milk production and secretion (**galactorrhea**).

Hyperprolactinemia combined with clinical symptoms of secondary amenorrhea or galactorrhea suggests a pituitary tumor, whereas prolactin deficiency (**hypoprolactinemia**) usually is seen following pituitary necrosis or infarction. The significance of hypoprolactinemia is poorly defined; the condition is rare, and the only demonstrable clinical correlation is the absence of postpartum lactation in females with an isolated prolactin deficiency. Prolactin also has been detected in amniotic fluid, where levels approximately two to ten times higher than corresponding serum levels appear to be crucial for fetal development.

Normal Values

The normal and clinically significant values for prolactin are:

Men	0–28 ng/mL
Women	
Follicular phase	0–28 ng/mL
Luteal phase	5–40 ng/mL
After menopause	0–12 ng/mL
Pituitary tumor	>100 ng/mL

Variations
Decreased prolactin levels may occur with:

Apomorphine	Dopamine	L-dopa
Bromocriptine	Ergot alkaloids	Lergotrile

Elevated prolactin levels may occur with:

Acromegaly	Thioridazine
Amenorrhea	Tricyclic antidepressants
Breast-feeding	Ectopic tumors
Breast stimulation	Endometriosis
Bronchogenic carcinoma	Exercise
Chiari-Frommel syndrome	Forbes-Albright syndrome
Coitus	Galactorrhea
Del Castillo syndrome	Hyperestrogen states
Drug therapy	Hypothalamic disorders
Aldomet	Hypothyroidism, primary
Benzamides	Hysterectomy
Estrogens	Nelson's syndrome
Haloperidol	Oral contraceptives
Meprobamate	Pituitary tumors
Methyldopa	Pregnancy
Metoclopramide	Renal failure, chronic
Phenothiazines	Sleep
Procainamide derivatives	Stress
Reserpine	Thyroid-stimulating hormone

Methodology
Prolactin determinations require 5 mL of blood collected without trauma and without anticoagulants (red-stoppered tube) or with EDTA (lavender-stoppered tube). Serum and plasma specimens for prolactin analysis remain stable for 4 days at room temperature but must be frozen if analysis is delayed beyond that period.

Precautions
To ensure reliable results, the following precautions should be observed when collecting specimens for prolactin determinations:

1. Do not submit lipemic or grossly hemolyzed blood specimens to the laboratory because they may yield inaccurate test results.

2. Note on the laboratory request slip if the patient has had any diagnostic or therapeutic procedures requiring the administration of radioisotopes because these substances may cause a falsely decreased level of prolactin.

Thyroid-Stimulating Hormone

Thyroid-stimulating hormone (TSH), also known as thyrotropin, is an anterior pituitary hormone that stimulates and accelerates nearly all aspects of thyroid activity, including the production and secretion of thyroid hormones. The thyroid gland, like the gonads and adrenal cortex, is controlled by a negative feedback mechanism between the hypothalamus and anterior pituitary that monitors the secretion of thyroxine (T_4) and triiodothyronine (T_3). Thus, the thyrotropin-releasing hormone (TRH) secreted by the hypothalamus stimulates the pituitary to release TSH, which in turn activates the thyroid gland.

For example, when the circulating levels of T_3 and T_4 fall below optimal values, the pituitary feedback mechanism increases the secretion of TSH and accelerates thyroid activity. Conversely, a decrease in the levels of circulating T_3 and T_4 suppresses TSH secretion and reduces the synthesis of these thyroid hormones. Laboratory determination of TSH aids in the differentiation of primary thyroid failure and secondary hypothyroidism (caused by pituitary disorders) and is useful during therapy to help prevent the undertreatment of primary hypothyroidism or overtreatment of hyperthyroidism.

Clinical Significance
A marked elevation in TSH secretion frequently is observed in patients with primary hypothyroidism before any other measurable disturbance of thyroid function caused by decreased thyroid hormone feedback. Conversely, TSH concentrations are normal or undetectable in patients with hypothyroidism secondary to pituitary or hypothalamic disorders and are inconclusive in patients with hyperthyroidism when interpreted alone.

Hypothyroidism secondary to pituitary disorders may be differentiated from the hypothyroidism associated with hypothalamic deficiency by evaluating TSH response to exogenous thyrotropin-releasing hormone (TRH) administered intravenously. In individuals with a normal hormone response, TSH levels rise promptly, peaking 20–40 minutes after an intravenously administered TRH test dose. However, if previously undetectable or normal TSH levels increase following TRH stimulation, the defect is at the hypothalamic level; if TSH does not respond, the defect is at the pituitary level.

The TRH stimulation test also provides an excellent supplement to TSH determinations in the diagnosis of hyperthyroidism because the TSH response to TRH is inhibited by an excess of thyroid hormones. Thus, TRH stimulation separates euthyroid and hyperthyroid patients, particularly those who are symptomatic and have borderline routine laboratory tests, and serves as an excellent confirmatory test for thyrotoxicosis. Stimulation tests also eliminate the possibility of administering T_3 to patients whose thyroid hormone levels already may be elevated, to elderly individuals, or to those with coexisting cardiac disease who are suspected of having thyrotoxicosis.

Normal Values
The normal values for thyroid-stimulating hormone are:

Adults	1.9–6.7 μU/mL
Neonates	
<1 week	<25 μU/mL
>2 weeks	<4.6 μU/mL

Variations

Decreased thyroid-stimulating hormone levels may occur with:

Hyperthyroidism	Thyrotoxicosis
Hypothyroidism, secondary	Triiodothyronine (T₃) therapy

Elevated thyroid-stimulating hormone levels may occur in:

Antithyroid therapy for hyperthyroidism	Lymphocytic thyroiditis
Hypothyroidism, primary	Newborn infants, umbilical cord blood
Iodine deficiency, severe	

Methodology

Measurement of TSH in adults and children requires 5 mL of blood collected without anticoagulants (red-stoppered tube) or with heparin (green-stoppered tube). Measurement of neonatal TSH levels requires several drops of blood collected from the infant's heel on a special filter paper form. All circles on the filter paper must be completely filled with blood, and the blood must soak through the paper completely.

Precautions

To ensure accurate results, the following precautions should be observed when collecting specimens for TSH determinations:

1. Note on the laboratory slip if the patient has had any diagnostic or therapeutic procedures requiring the administration of radioisotopes because these substances will affect the choice of a testing method.

2. Note on the laboratory slip if the patient has recently ingested foods high in iodine (shellfish, iodized salt) because this will decrease TSH concentrations.

REPRODUCTIVE HORMONE STUDIES

The organs of the reproductive system are responsible for the growth and release of mature germ cells and for the production of various hormones that govern the development of primary and secondary sexual characteristics. Thus, the testes (in men) and the ovary and placenta (in women) secrete numerous steroid hormones, classified as androgens, progesterone, and estrogens, that control certain physiologic and emotional changes. For example, the continuous production of the androgens, primarily testosterone, in men is essential for spermatogenesis and is responsible for the appearance and maintenance of characteristic masculine physical and behavioral patterns. Likewise, the production of varying concentrations of estrogens and progesterone during the menstrual cycle in women is responsible for cyclic changes in the ovary and uterine mucosa that play a vital role in fertility and pregnancy. The reproductive hormones usually measured include testosterone to help diagnose infertility in men, human chorionic gonadotropin (HCG) to detect pregnancy, human placental lactogen (HPL) and estriol (see the following section on Estrogens) to evaluate fetal status during pregnancy, and progesterone or its urinary metabolite pregnanediol to pinpoint ovulation.

Estrogens

The **estrogens** are a group of hormones secreted by the ovaries and placenta in women and by the adrenal cortex and testes in men that control the development of female secondary sexual characteristics. Estrogen is produced primarily by the ovary during the normal menstrual cycle in nonpregnant females, reaching peak concentrations just before midcycle and again during the luteal phase. These hormones act on the female genitals during the menstrual cycle to produce an environment suitable for the fertilization, implantation, and nutrition of the early embryo. Estrogen also is produced by the fetoplacental unit during pregnancy, increasing progressively from the eighth week of gestation until birth.

Three clinically significant estrogen fractions—estradiol, estrone, and estriol—may be measured, along with total estrogen, to evaluate ovarian function as well as other gynecologic conditions. **Estradiol**, the most physiologically active estrogen, is helpful in diagnosing gonadal dysfunction such as prepubertal feminization, primary amenorrhea, induction of ovulation, and estrogen-producing tumors in men. **Estrone**, the immediate metabolite of estradiol, serves as the principal precursor for the formation of the other significant estrogens and is seldom analyzed alone. **Estriol**, the metabolic end product of estradiol and estrone, reflects the functional integrity of the fetoplacental unit because it is derived partly from the placenta and partly from the fetal adrenal gland.

Laboratory measurement of total estrogen and estrogen fractions may be used in nonpregnant women to indicate ovarian function, evaluate infertility, and establish the time for ovulation to optimize the chance of conception. Total estrogen and estriol determinations also provide a valuable guide in the assessment of fetal status during pregnancy, diagnosis of fetal distress, and management of high-risk pregnancies. In addition, estrogen concentrations recently have been used to help determine the presence of estrogen receptors in cancerous breast tumors. During estrogen receptor studies, significant binding of estrogen on tumor tissue indicates a 60%–80% probability that follow-up hormone therapy will be effective.

Clinical Significance

Measurement of estriol values helps to evaluate the competency of the developing fetoplacental unit and indicates the state of fetal well-being because estriol excretion increases progressively during normal fetal growth. Estriol values are most significant for evaluating fetoplacental function in problem pregnancies when serial measurements are made on at least two different days to determine the trend in excretion. Any sharp decrease in maternal estriol levels or a failure of these levels to rise as rapidly as expected is a warning of impending fetal jeopardy or serious placental dysfunction. This can be defined as a decrease of 35%–50% in plasma or urinary estriol values on two consecutive days or a drop of at least 35% in the average of the three preceding values.

Serial estriol measurements also are helpful in monitoring high-risk pregnancies when toxemia, diabetes mellitus, preeclampsia, placental insufficiency, or hypertension are threatened. Determinations under these conditions should be performed two or three times each week after the thirty-third week of gestation because urinary values below 4 mg/24 hours or plasma values below 3 ng/mL indicate increased fetal risk. Persistently low or failing values after the thirty-second week of gestation strongly suggest that premature delivery is needed to ensure fetal survival. However, diabetic patients who exhibit lower than normal estriol concentrations with a constant tendency to increase generally may be allowed to continue the pregnancy to term.

Normal Values

The normal values for total estrogen and estrogen fractions are:

Blood

Total Estrogen	Men	35−225 pg/mL
	Women (nonpregnant)	
	Follicular phase	60−350 pg/mL
	Midcycle	120−650 pg/mL
	Luteal phase	75−560 pg/mL
Estrone (E1)	Men	100−175 pg/mL
	Women (nonpregnant)	
	Follicular phase	80−250 pg/mL
	Midcycle	130−375 pg/mL
	Luteal phase	100−400 pg/mL
Estradiol (E2)	Men	10−50 pg/mL
	Women (nonpregnant)	
	Follicular phase	10−170 pg/mL
	Midcycle	50−770 pg/mL
	Luteal phase	40−340 pg/mL
	After menopause	10−50 pg/mL
	Oral contraceptives	12−50 pg/mL
	Children	3−10 pg/mL
Estriol (E3) (Pregnancy)	25−28 weeks gestation	25−140 ng/mL
	29−32 weeks gestation	31−180 ng/mL
	33−34 weeks gestation	40−270 ng/mL
	35−36 weeks gestation	50−340 ng/mL
	37−38 weeks gestation	75−410 ng/mL
	39−40 weeks gestation	98−450 ng/mL

Urine

Total Estrogen	Men	4−25 μg/24 hours
	Women (nonpregnant)	4−60 μg/24 hours
	Onset of menstruation	4−25 μg/24 hours
	Ovulation peak	28−99 μg/24 hours
	Luteal peak	12−105 μg/24 hours
	Menopause	1.4−19.6 μg/24 hours

(continued)

Normal Values (Continued)

	Women (pregnant)	
	10 weeks gestation	0.4–1.0 mg/24 hours
	15 weeks gestation	1.6–3.5 mg/24 hours
	20 weeks gestation	3–7 mg/24 hours
	24 weeks gestation	4–10 mg/24 hours
	28 weeks gestation	5–15 mg/24 hours
	32 weeks gestation	8–20 mg/24 hours
	36 weeks gestation	10–30 mg/24 hours
	40 weeks gestation	15–42 mg/24 hours
	Children	<1 μg/24 hours
Estrone (E1)	Men	3.4–8.2 μg/24 hours
	Women	
	Follicular phase	4–7 μg/24 hours
	Luteal phase	11–32 μg/24 hours
	Menopause	0.8–7.1 μg/24 hours
	Children	0.2–1.0 μg/24 hours
Estradiol (E2)	Men	0–0.4 μg/24 hours
	Women	
	Follicular phase	0–3 μg/24 hours
	Luteal phase	4–14 μg/24 hours
	Menopause	0–2.3 μg/24 hours
	Children	0–0.2 μg/24 hours
Estriol (E3)	Men	0.3–2.4 μg/24 hours
	Women (nonpregnant)	
	Follicular phase	0–15 μg/24 hours
	Luteal phase	13–54 μg/24 hours
	Menopause	0.6–6.8 μg/24 hours
	Women (pregnant)	
	<16 weeks gestation	1–4 mg/24 hours
	16–24 weeks gestation	2–6 mg/24 hours
	25–32 weeks gestation	6–32 mg/24 hours
	33–36 weeks gestation	10–45 mg/24 hours
	37–38 weeks gestation	15–53 mg/24 hours
	39–40 weeks gestation	18–62 mg/24 hours
	Children	0.3–2.4 μg/24 hours

Variations

Decreased plasma estradiol levels may occur with:

Anorexia nervosa

Gonadal dysfunction or failure, primary

Hyperprolactinemia

Hypopituitarism

Hypothalamic disorders

Masculinizing tumors

Menopause

Pituitary disorders

Polycystic ovarian disease

Decreased plasma estriol levels may occur with:

Down's syndrome

Fetal adrenal hypoplasia or insufficiency

Fetal death, intrauterine

Fetal liver deficiency

Malnutrition, maternal

Retarded intrauterine growth

Steroid therapy, maternal

Ulcerative colitis

Decreased urinary estriol levels may occur with:

Anencephaly

Choriocarcinoma

Congenital anomalies

Diabetes

Fetal growth retardation

Hydatidiform mole

Preeclampsia

Rh immunization

Decreased total urinary estrogen levels may occur with:

Arrhenoblastoma

Fetal distress

Infantilism

Liver impairment, maternal

Lutein cell tumors

Renal impairment, maternal

Ovarian agenesis

Ovarian dysfunction

Simmonds' disease

Elevated plasma estradiol levels may occur with:

Adrenal tumors

Dysfunctional bleeding with anovulation

Ovarian tumors

Precocious puberty

Elevated total urinary estrogen levels may occur with:

Adrenocortical hyperplasia

Adrenocortical tumors

Ovarian tumors, certain

Pregnancy

Testicular tumors, certain

Methodology

Measurement of total estrogen or estrogen fractions in the bloodstream requires 10 mL of blood collected without anticoagulants (red-stoppered tube) or with EDTA or heparin (lavender- or green-stoppered tube). Serum and plasma specimens obtained to monitor the estradiol surge prior to ovulation should be collected in the morning because estrogen secretion exhibits diurnal variation. Specimens must be delivered to the laboratory promptly so that plasma and serum can be separated from cells immediately because serum and plasma for total estrogen or estrogen fraction determinations are not stable at room temperature.

Measurement of urinary estrogens requires a 100 mL aliquot of a 24-hour urine specimen collected in a bottle containing 10 g of boric acid. Laboratories occasionally require that alternate preservatives such as 15 mL of 6N concentrated hydrochloric acid or glacial acetic acid be added to produce a urine pH of 3-5 to prevent bacterial decomposition. Urine specimens for estrogen excretion analyses remain stable for 7 days at room temperature and for longer periods when refrigerated or frozen. The entire 24-hour urine volume should be recorded on both the laboratory request slip and the specimen container.

Precautions

To ensure accurate results, the following precautions should be observed when collecting specimens for estrogen determinations:

1. Withhold any drugs that might interfere with the measurement of urinary estrogens, whenever possible, for several days before as well as during the specimen collection period. Drugs that significantly affect the measurement of urinary estrogens include:

Ampicillin	Hydrochlorothiazide	Phenolphthalein
Cascara	Meprobamates	Prochlorperazine
Cortisone (large doses)	Methenamine mandelate	Senna
Diethylstilbestrol	Phenazopyridine	Tetracyclines
Hexamine		

2. Ensure that the 100 mL urine specimen is obtained from a well-mixed 24-hour urine collection.

▶▶ Nursing Responsibilities and Implications

1. Record the age of the patient on the laboratory request slip as well as the phase of the menstrual cycle (in nonpregnant women) to aid in the interpretation of total estrogen test results.

2. Record the trimester of pregnancy or the number of weeks of gestation on the laboratory request slip to aid in the interpretation of estrogen and estriol test results in pregnant women.

Human Chorionic Gonadotropin

Human chorionic gonadotropin (HCG), a hormone produced by the placenta following the implantation of the fertilized ovum into the uterine wall, is the first substance associated with pregnancy and is detectable prior to the onset of clinical symptoms of pregnancy. The primary function of HCG is to maintain the corpus luteum during the first trimester of pregnancy to ensure the adequate production of estrogen and progesterone until the placenta can provide these hormones. Increased concentrations of HCG may be detected in serum and urine 6–8 days after conception, increase dramatically throughout the first trimester of pregnancy, and reach peak concentrations at 8–12 weeks of gestation.

Levels of HCG in maternal serum gradually decrease during the second and third trimesters and usually return to normal levels 2–4 days after completion of a full-term pregnancy. The rate of decrease is slower following a first-trimester abortion. Levels of HCG remain elevated in ectopic pregnancy until death of the placenta. Although HCG is not present in the serum or urine of healthy men and nonpregnant women, it may be detected in both men and women with certain malignant tumors.

Clinical Significance

Laboratory determinations of HCG generally are used to detect pregnancy within 10–14 days of conception but also may be used to diagnose and monitor a number of other conditions. Knowledge of the characteristic patterns of HCG secretion during normal pregnancy makes it possible to diagnose ectopic pregnancy, evaluate threatened or incomplete abortion, and verify the early interruption of pregnancy. Measurement of HCG levels also may identify the need for precautionary measures in women who are prone to miscarriage and help to monitor the effectiveness of therapy to induce ovulation and conception. Likewise, elevated HCG levels may aid in the diagnosis and management of malignant neoplasms because HCG often appears in patients with hydatidiform moles and certain testicular and ovarian germ-cell tumors. In addition, tests for HCG occasionally are used to assess the effectiveness of therapy following surgical removal of these tumors and to monitor the response of certain carcinomas to chemotherapy.

Normal Values
The normal values for HCG are:

Blood

Men	<0.01 IU/mL
Women (nonpregnant)	<0.01 IU/mL

Women (pregnant)

1 week	0.010–0.04 IU/mL
2 weeks	0.03–0.1 IU/mL
3 weeks	0.1–1.0 IU/mL
4 weeks	1–10 IU/mL
5–12 weeks	10–100 IU/mL
13–24 weeks	10–30 IU/mL
25 weeks to term	5–15 IU/mL

Urine

Men	Undetectable
Women (nonpregnant)	Undetectable

Women (pregnant)

1–12 weeks	6000–500,000 IU/24 hours
13–24 weeks	5000–350,000 IU/24 hours
25 weeks to term	2500–150,000 IU/24 hours

Variations
Elevated human chorionic gonadotropin levels may occur with:

Abortion, threatened	Hydatidiform moles
Breast cancer	Malignant melanoma
Bronchogenic carcinomas	Multiple myeloma
Choriocarcinoma	Pancreatic cancer
Ectopic pregnancy	Pregnancy
Embryonal carcinomas	Seminomas
Gastrointestinal carcinoma, certain	Teratomas
Hepatocarcinoma	Trophoblastic tumors

Methodology
Serum HCG determinations require 5 mL of blood collected without trauma in a tube without anticoagulants (red-stoppered tube) and delivered promptly to the laboratory so that serum can be separated promptly from the cells. Serum specimens for HCG determinations remain stable for 2 days when refrigerated and for 3 months when frozen. However, repeated freezing and thawing of serum specimens may cause deterioration of the hormone and erroneous test results.

Measurement of urinary HCG may be performed on any morning urine specimen with a specific gravity greater than 1.010 or a 50 mL aliquot of a 24-hour urine specimen. Urine specimens should be delivered to the laboratory as soon as possible for prompt analysis to prevent interference from bacterial overgrowth.

Precautions
To ensure accurate results, the following precautions should be observed when collecting specimens for HCG determinations:

1. Do not submit hemolyzed, lipemic, or icteric serum specimens to the laboratory because these variables interfere with the test procedures.

2. Do not submit urine specimens with hematuria or heavy proteinuria (3+ or 4+) because these conditions may interfere with the test procedures and produce false-positive test results.

3. Whenever possible, withhold any medications for several days before testing because many drugs are cleared by the kidneys and appear in the urine. Drugs that might interfere with urine HCG tests include:

Anticonvulsants	Phenothiazine derivatives
Antiparkinsonism drugs	Psychotropic drugs
Chlorpromazine derivatives	Thioridazine
Hypnotic drugs	

4. Do not eliminate the possibility of a pregnancy when a screening test for HCG produces negative or borderline results shortly after the last menstrual period. Significant test results may be obtained by quantitatively retesting the same sample or testing a fresh sample at least 48 hours after the initial analysis.

▶▶ *Nursing Responsibilities and Implications*

1. Collect serum and urine specimens for pregnancy testing at least 2 weeks after the last menstrual period.

2. Note the patient's age, sex, and time of gestation on the laboratory request slip as an aid to interpreting the test results.

Human Placental Lactogen

Human placental lactogen (HPL), a hormone normally produced by the placenta, is detectable in maternal blood after 5 weeks of gestation and gradually increases, reaching peak concentrations at 35−36 weeks' gestation. This hormone is rapidly metabolized by the maternal liver and kidneys and has a half-life of only 20 minutes, which causes it to disappear rapidly from the bloodstream. Any changes in placental integrity therefore are rapidly reflected by circulating levels of HPL because serum concentrations precisely indicate its rate of synthesis and release at the time of testing. Although the role of HPL in pregnancy is not fully understood, it is involved in fetal carbohydrate metabolism and therefore is an indicator of fetal health.

Concentrations of HPL fluctuate widely from day to day in most pregnancies but follow a steadily increasing pattern until near term, when a precipitous drop normally occurs. A dramatic decrease in HPL concentrations occurring earlier in gestation that clearly reverses the upward trend is an ominous indication and warrants tests for other signs of fetal distress. Laboratory measurement of HPL is the most sensitive and accurate test for assessing placental function and is used to monitor high-risk pregnancies. When combined with urinary estriol excretion determinations, HPL measurements provide a valuable guide to the management of difficult pregnancies.

Clinical Significance

Assessment of maternal concentrations of HPL is helpful in detecting impending abortion during the first half of pregnancy because low values often precede spontaneous abortion by 5−10 days. Human placental lactogen measurements during the final trimester of pregnancy detect values within the fetal danger zone and indicate the degree of risk for the fetus. For example, HPL values of 4 μg/mL or less after 30 weeks of gestation frequently are associated with the risk of stillbirths, fetal distress in labor, or neonatal asphyxia, especially in pregnancies complicated by severe maternal hypertension related to pregnancy.

All HPL assays should be interpreted in conjunction with appropriate physical examination and total clinical evaluation of the pregnant woman and unborn fetus. Serum HPL values usually are higher in multiple-birth pregnancies than in single-offspring pregnancies because of the correlation between HPL levels and placental mass. Human placental lactogen measurements combined with serum estriol determinations provide information about the fetoplacental unit that neither test alone can provide (see Estrogens earlier in this chapter).

Normal Values
The normal values for human placental lactogen are:

Men	<0.5 μg/mL
Women (nonpregnant)	<0.5 μg/mL
Women (pregnant)	
<5 weeks gestation	<0.5 μg/mL
5–27 weeks gestation	<4.6 μg/mL
28–31 weeks gestation	2.4–6.1 μg/mL
32–35 weeks gestation	3.7–7.7 μg/mL
36 weeks to term	5.0–11 μg/mL

Variations
Decreased human placental lactogen levels may occur with or indicate:

Fetal distress in labor

Hypertensive toxemia

Neonatal asphyxia

Spontaneous abortion, threatened

Stillbirth, imminent

Methodology
Measurement of HPL requires 5 mL of blood collected without anticoagulants (red-stoppered tube) or with heparin (green-stoppered tube). Serial assays of specimens obtained over several days are more valuable than single readings for predicting the course of a pregnancy. Serum and plasma specimens for HPL determinations remain stable for 3 days at room temperature, 7 days at refrigerator temperatures, and up to 6 months when frozen.

Pregnanediol

Pregnanediol, the chief urinary metabolite of progesterone, is derived from progesterone secreted by the corpus luteum of the ovary and by the placenta after the second month of pregnancy (see the following section on Progesterone). Pregnanediol excretion increases rapidly within 24 hours after ovulation and increases for 3–10 days with the development of the corpus luteum; excretion decreases precipitously with degeneration of the corpus luteum and the onset of menstruation. Urinary excretion of pregnanediol provides an index of progesterone secretion; progesterone is the hormone responsible for changes in the uterus following ovulation, for maintaining the pregnancy after fertilization, and for placental development.

Clinical Significance
Urinary pregnanediol values normally increase steadily during pregnancy, reaching peak levels in the third trimester. Human placental lactogen levels reflect the condition of the placenta, but they provide little information about the condition of the fetus. Thus, life-

threatening fetal disorders may exist in the presence of normal pregnanediol levels. A decrease in pregnanediol levels during pregnancy, however, indicates placental dysfunction and may signal the threat of spontaneous abortion. A decrease in pregnanediol excretion together with a rapid drop in urinary estriol values generally accompany fetal death (see Estrogens earlier in this chapter).

Laboratory determinations of urinary pregnanediol levels reflect the status of placental function and can be used in instances of threatened abortion to determine if progesterone therapy will ensure a full-term pregnancy. Urinary pregnanediol analyses also provide an index of progesterone production, help to evaluate menstrual disturbances, and may be used to verify the time of ovulation in patients who are attempting to become pregnant.

Pregnanediol determinations are most accurate when performed on 24-hour urine specimens because progesterone secretion normally fluctuates from day to day and with different activities, although bedrest does help to minimize these fluctuations. Serum pregnanediol values, on the other hand, seldom are measured because they reflect the HPL secretion only at the moment of testing and fail to establish a trend in production levels.

Normal Values
The normal values for urinary pregnanediol are:

Men	0.1–1.8 mg/24 hours
Women (nonpregnant)	0.2–7.0 mg/24 hours
Follicular phase	0.1–2.3 mg/24 hours
Luteal phase	1.2–9.5 mg/24 hours
After menopause	0.1–1.5 mg/24 hours
Women (pregnant)	
10–12 weeks gestation	5–15 mg/24 hours
12–18 weeks gestation	5–25 mg/24 hours
18–24 weeks gestation	13–33 mg/24 hours
24–28 weeks gestation	20–42 mg/24 hours
28–32 weeks gestation	27–47 mg/24 hours
Children	0.4–1.0 mg/24 hours

Variations
Decreased urinary pregnanediol levels may occur with:

Amenorrhea	Placental failure
Anovular menstruation	Preeclampsia
Fetal death	Threatened abortion
Luteal deficiency	Toxemia of pregnancy
Menstrual abnormalities	

Elevated urinary pregnanediol levels may occur with:

Adrenocortical hyperplasia

Corpus luteum cysts

Ovarian neoplasms, certain

Placental tissue, retained following parturition

Methodology

Measurement of urinary pregnanediol requires a 100 mL aliquot of a 24-hour urine specimen collected without preservatives in a glass or polyethylene bottle and kept refrigerated during the collection period. Urine specimens for pregnanediol analysis remain stable for 7 days at room temperature and for longer periods when refrigerated or frozen. The entire 24-hour urine volume should be noted on the laboratory request slip.

▶▶ *Nursing Responsibilities and Implications*

1. Note the date of the patient's last menstrual period on the laboratory request slip as an aid to the interpretation of the test results.

2. State the number of weeks of gestation on the laboratory request slip if the patient is pregnant because normal pregnanediol excretion values vary with the length of gestation.

Progesterone

Progesterone is a steroid hormone produced primarily by the corpus luteum of the ovary in women and, to a lesser extent, by the adrenal cortex in men, postmenopausal women, and children. Secretion of this hormone helps to control the normal cyclic alterations of cervical and vaginal cellular morphology as well as the uterine changes required for attachment and growth of the embryo. Low levels of progesterone appear in the plasma during the preovulatory (follicular) phase of the normal menstrual cycle, increase after the midcycle peak in LH activity, and return to baseline values after the onset of menstruation. However, only minute amounts of progesterone may be detected in the blood because it is metabolized rapidly into its major urinary metabolite, pregnanediol, and little remains in the bloodstream (see the previous section on Pregnanediol).

Laboratory measurements of progesterone are used to confirm corpus luteum formation and to evaluate its functional status in infertile patients. Progesterone analysis also may be used to indicate the day of ovulation, to determine, retrospectively, if ovulation has occurred, and to assess placental function during pregnancy.

Clinical Significance

The diagnostic significance of progesterone evaluations is increased by comparing several determinations performed on serial specimens collected at specific times during the normal menstrual cycle or pregnancy. For example, progesterone assays performed at the midpoint of the follicular phase (days 5–10) or luteal phase (days 19–23) help to assess the formation and functional state of the corpus luteum. In addition, serial assays performed on alternate days (days 10, 12, 14, and 16) of the normal cycle help pinpoint the day of ovulation. Likewise, the time of specimen collection for progesterone assays during pregnancy depends on the diagnostic purpose of the test as well as the patient's status.

Normal Values

The normal values for progesterone are:

Men	0–1.0 ng/mL
Women (nonpregnant)	
Follicular phase	0.1–1.5 ng/mL
Luteal phase	1.2–28.1 ng/mL
Midluteal phase	5.7–28.1 ng/mL
After menopause	0–0.2 ng/mL
Oral contraceptives	0.1–0.3 ng/mL
Women (pregnant)	
1–12 weeks	9–47 ng/mL
13–24 weeks	16.8–146 ng/mL
25 weeks to term	55–255 ng/mL

Variations

Decreased progesterone levels may occur with:

Amenorrhea	Luteal deficiency	Preeclampsia
Anovular menstruation	Menstrual abnormalities	Threatened abortion
Fetal death	Placental failure	Toxemia of pregnancy

Elevated progesterone levels may occur with:

ACTH administration

Adrenal hyperplasia, congenital (in males)

Corpus luteum cysts

Ovarian neoplasms, certain

Placental tissue, retained following parturition

Methodology

Progesterone determinations require 10 mL of blood collected without anticoagulants (red-stoppered tube) or with heparin (green-stoppered tube). Serum and plasma specimens for progesterone determinations remain stable for 7 days at room temperature and for longer periods when refrigerated or frozen. The phase of the patient's menstrual cycle or the number of weeks of gestation should be noted on the laboratory request slip to aid in the interpretation of the test results.

Testosterone

Testosterone, the most active androgen and the primary male sex hormone, is produced by the testes and adrenal cortex in men and by ovarian and adrenal tissue in women. Testosterone exerts a widespread effect on the development and maintenance of male secondary sexual characteristics, including a generalized increase in total body mass, geni-

growth, altered patterns of body hair growth, and vocal changes. The amount of physiologically active testosterone, which crosses the blood-brain barrier to act on target tissues, is best represented by the concentration of free or weakly bound testosterone.

Approximately two-thirds of the testosterone in males is produced in the testes and appears to be more potent than the testosterone produced by the adrenal cortex (see the sections on Luteinizing Hormone and 17-Ketosteroids earlier in this chapter). Laboratory measurement of testosterone levels is helpful in evaluating decreased or absent testicular function, diagnosing testicular tumors, and assessing the adequacy of hormone function in impotent males. Analysis of free testosterone levels correlates better with the clinical signs of androgenicity in females than the measurement of total testosterone levels and is useful in determining the cause of female hirsutism.

Clinical Significance

Distinctly subnormal testosterone values in adult males generally reflect testicular hypofunction and suggest that deficient hormone secretion is an important factor in the development of impotence. Conversely, overproduction of testosterone in women may result from hyperplasia or tumors of the adrenals or ovaries and causes readily observable changes such as excessive hair growth and masculinization. Excessive secretion of testosterone in males, however, is difficult to recognize clinically unless it occurs before puberty.

Normal Values

The normal values for testosterone are:

Blood

Men		
	Free	75−390 ng/dL (15%−55% of total testosterone)
	Total	300−1200 ng/dL
Women		
	Free	1−11 ng/dL (6%−21% of total testosterone)
	Total	10−100 ng/dL
Children		12−16 ng/dL
Urine		
Men		500−800 ng/24 hours
Women		20−80 ng/24 hours

Variations

Decreased testosterone levels in men may occur with:

Antineoplastic agents	Hypogonadism, primary and secondary	Orchiectomy
Estrogen therapy		Renal disease, chronic
Ethanol ingestion	Hypopituitarism	Testicular feminization
Hepatic cirrhosis	Klinefelter's syndrome	Testicular infection
	Obesity, extreme	Testicular trauma

Decreased testosterone levels in women may occur with oral contraceptive therapy.

Elevated testosterone levels in men may occur with adrenal hyperplasia, adrenal tumors, and central nervous system lesions.

Elevated testosterone levels in women may occur with:

Adrenal hyperplasia	Arrhenoblastoma	Ovarian tumors
Adrenal tumors	Female hirsutism	Polycystic ovarian disease

Methodology

Measurement of circulating testosterone requires 5 mL of blood collected without anti-coagulants (red-stoppered tube) or with heparin (green-stoppered tube). Serum and plasma specimens for testosterone determinations remain stable for 4 days at room temperature and for 6 months when frozen.

Measurement of urinary testosterone requires a 50 mL aliquot of a 24-hour urine specimen, which should be kept refrigerated during the collection period. The 24-hour urine volume should be noted on both the laboratory request slip and the specimen container.

▶▶ Nursing Responsibilities and Implications

1. Record the patient's age, sex, and information about prior hormone therapy on the laboratory request slip as an aid to accurate interpretation of the test results.

2. Handle the specimen gently to prevent hemolysis, which can affect the test results.

THYROID HORMONE STUDIES

The thyroid gland secretes two hormones, triiodothyronine (T_3) and thyroxine (T_4), that influence the general metabolic rate and control normal growth, development, and tissue differentiation. These hormones are required to regulate carbohydrate, protein, and fat metabolism as well as electrolyte mobilization and play an important role in reproduction. Because thyroid hormones are also essential for the development of the central nervous system, thyroid-deficient infants suffer irreversible mental damage, whereas hypothyroid adults may exhibit slowed deep-tendon reflexes and diffuse psychomotor retardation.

Control of T_3 and T_4 concentrations depends not only on the thyroid gland but also on the interaction of these hormones with the hypothalamus and anterior pituitary through negative feedback. Thyroid hormones are synthesized and released in response to a hypo-thalamic signal that reacts to variations in the circulating hormone level by altering the release of thyrotropin-releasing hormone (TRH). Thyrotropin-releasing hormone in turn stimulates the pituitary to release thyroid-stimulating hormone (TSH), which also is controlled by a feedback mechanism that is sensitive to circulating levels of thyroid hormones. Once in the bloodstream, T_3 and T_4 are bound to several proteins, mainly thyroxine-binding globulin (TBG), except for a small fraction of each that remains free and physiologically active.

Because any malfunction of the hypothalamic-pituitary-thyroid system influences circulating hormone levels, measurement of T_3 and T_4 is a useful method for assessing thyroid activity and diagnosing hypothalamic-pituitary disorders. A series of laboratory determinations have been developed to assess thyroid function and help differentiate euthyroid patients from those with hyperthyroid or hypothyroid disorders. The most useful tests for hyperthyroidism are total T_3, total T_4, free T_4 (measured as T_3 uptake), and the free thyroxine index. The most clinically useful tests to confirm or exclude a diagnosis of hypothyroidism include total T_4, free T_4 (measured as T_3 uptake), the free thyroxine index, and TSH (see the section on Thyroid-Stimulating Hormone earlier in this chapter).

The values obtained for thyroid function measurements, however, may be influenced by factors other than thyroid disease, including age, intercurrent illness, drug therapy, and the binding capacity of serum proteins. Therefore, the final diagnosis and treatment of patients with thyroid disorders must be based on a clinical evaluation of the patient as well as the careful consideration of laboratory values (Table 6-1).

TABLE 6-1 Summary of Thyroid Values in Selected Conditions

Clinical Condition	Triiodothyronine	Thyroxine	T_3 Uptake Ratio	Thyroid-Stimulating Hormone
Thyroid disease				
Hyperthyroidism	High	High	High	Low
Triiodothyronine toxicosis	High	Normal	Normal	Normal to low
Graves' disease	High	High	High	Normal
Antithyroid drug therapy	Normal	High	Low	Normal to high
Hypothyroidism	Low	Low	Low	High
Pituitary	Low	Low	Low	Normal to low
Thyroxine therapy	Normal	High	Normal	Normal
Triiodothyronine therapy	High	Low	Normal	Normal
Pregnancy	High	High	Low	Normal
Hormone therapy				
Estrogens	High	High	Low	Normal
Oral contraceptives	High	High	Low	Normal
Androgens	Low	Low	High	Normal
Anabolic steroids	Low	Low	High	Normal
Nephrosis, cirrhosis	Low	Low	High	Normal
Idiopathic thyroxine-binding globulin states				
Thyroxine-binding globulin deficiency, genetic	Low	Low	High	Normal
Thyroxine-binding globulin excess, genetic	High	High	Low	Normal

Triiodothyronine

Triiodothyronine (T$_3$), the principal thyroid hormone, is more biologically active than thyroxine (T$_4$) and plays an important role in the maintenance of optimum health and the development of pathologic thyroid conditions. Although T$_3$ circulates in extremely small quantities, it is bound to thyroid-binding proteins much less firmly than T$_4$, and a relatively greater proportion (approximately 0.4%) exists in the free state. Therefore, changes in the binding capacity of TBG are reflected by concomitant changes in the total serum concentration of T$_3$.

Laboratory determination of T$_3$ levels is the preferred test in the evaluation of patients suspected of having T$_3$ thyrotoxicosis. Triiodothyronine determinations also may be extremely useful in confirming the diagnosis of hyperthyroidism in patients with minimal T$_4$ elevations or ambiguous clinical manifestations. However, T$_3$ values are not useful in the diagnosis of hypothyroidism because levels may be low in a variety of nonthyroid diseases, and T$_3$ concentrations are within normal limits in many patients with clinical hypothyroidism.

Clinical Significance

Triiodothyronine values provide the most sensitive indication of classic hyperthyroidism because T$_3$ values appear to rise before T$_4$ levels and reach greater concentrations. Measurement of T$_3$ concentrations also may aid in the diagnosis of a hyperthyroid variant, termed T$_3$ thyrotoxicosis, in which thyrotoxic individuals exhibit elevated T$_3$ values and normal T$_4$ levels. In this form of hyperthyroidism, other routine screening tests for thyroid dysfunction may give normal results.

Patients treated with thyroid preparations will have uninterpretable T$_3$ results unless the time of hormone administration is known. Patients treated with T$_3$ alone, synthetic T$_3$ and T$_4$ combinations, or thyroid preparations such as desiccated thyroid exhibit elevated T$_3$ concentrations and peak values within 2−4 hours.

Normal Values
The normal values for total and free T$_3$ are:

Total T$_3$

Adults	70−200 ng/dL
Neonates (<1 week)	180−240 ng/dL
Free T$_3$	250−390 pg/mL

Variations
Decreased triiodothyronine levels may occur with:

Advanced age	Illness, acute
Anabolic steroid therapy	Phenytoin, large doses
Androgen therapy	Salicylates, large doses
Decreased TBG levels, idiopathic	Starvation
Hypothyroidism	

Elevated triiodothyronine levels may occur with:

Elevated TBG levels, idiopathic

Estrogen therapy

Graves' disease

Hyperthyroidism

Oral contraceptives

Pregnancy

Thyroiditis, acute

Thyroxine therapy

Triiodothyronine therapy

Triiodothyronine thyrotoxicosis

Methodology

Triiodothyronine determinations require 5 mL of blood collected without anticoagulants (red-stoppered tube). Specimens for T_3 analysis remain stable for 4 days at room temperature and for 1 month when frozen.

▶▶ Nursing Responsibilities and Implications

1. Inform the laboratory if the patient has recently had any diagnostic or therapeutic procedures using radioactive substances because significant quantities of radioactivity in the serum can produce serious test errors.

2. If the patient is receiving thyroid medications, note the dose and time administered on the laboratory slip.

3. Handle the specimen gently to prevent hemolysis.

Thyroxine

Thyroxine (T_4) is a thyroid hormone present in the bloodstream in protein-bound and free (unbound) forms, which together are used to evaluate thyroid function. Thyroxine concentrations, however, are affected by abnormal levels of the thyroid-binding globulin (TBG) and rise or fall in direct proportion to TBG levels even in individuals with normal thyroid function. Thus, T_4 values generally are elevated by situations in which drugs or other factors increase protein binding, whereas decreased total T_4 levels accompany decreased protein-binding capacity. Thus, because a number of conditions alter TBG concentrations, measurement of T_4 levels alone can give misleading information about the patient's thyrometabolic status and an erroneous impression of thyroid function.

On the other hand, a small fraction of the circulating T_4 (about 0.05%) is not bound to serum proteins and is unaffected by TBG concentrations. This physiologically active free T_4 (FT_4) fraction correlates more closely with a patient's thyroid status than T_4 because it penetrates tissues to exert its metabolic effect. Laboratory determination of T_4 levels may be used to screen for thyroid disorders, evaluate therapy in patients with hyperthyroidism, and establish a maintenance dose level in the treatment of hypothyroidism. Measurement of T_4 levels, together with FT_4 (estimated by T_3 uptake), provides a more useful index of thyrometabolic status than T_4 alone and is essential to the evaluation of thyroid function (see the following section on T_3 Uptake and T_3 Uptake Ratio).

Clinical Significance

Normal growth and development of the brain, both before and after birth, cannot take place in the absence of adequate thyroid hormone. Thus, thyroid gland failure or extreme

T_4 deficiency in newborn infants is characterized by low circulating levels of T_4 and results in neurologic impairment, growth deficit, and mental retardation (cretinism). The severity of these disorders depends on the stage of development during which the defect arises as well as the age at which the diagnosis is established and treatment begun. For example, permanent disorders result from early stage T_4 defects, whereas transient abnormalities, especially in premature infants, accompany later-phase development of primary hypothyroidism.

Diagnosis and initiation of appropriate therapy within the first 3 months of life appear to be necessary to prevent neurologic deficits and can improve both the intellectual and physical prognosis of neonates with hypothyroid conditions. Infants whose hypothyroid condition is not recognized at birth and who are not treated will be both physically and mentally retarded. Thus, neonatal T_4 screening for primary hypothyroidism is essential to early diagnosis and neonatal management because the clinical or radiologic criteria of congenital defects are not clearly evident at birth.

The use of T_4 values as a guide to establishing a maintenance dose of thyroid hormone is unreliable when L-triiodothyronine therapy is administered to correct hypothyroidism. Because it is more potent than T_4, very small amounts of L-triiodothyronine suppress normal T_4 secretion, causing T_3 to become the major circulating thyroid hormone. The net result is a decreased circulating T_4 level, even though clinically normal thyroid function has been achieved.

Normal Values

The normal and clinically significant values for total and free T_4 are:

Total T_4

Adults	4.5–13.5 μg/dL
Infants	
<1 month	7.8–23 μg/dL
>1 month	9–18 μg/dL
>1 year	Adult levels
Hyperthyroidism	15–35 μg/dL
Hypothyroidism	
Adults	0–4 μg/dL
Infants	<7.0 μg/dL
Alert limits	
1–5 days	<4.9 μg/dL
6–8 days	<4.0 μg/dL
9–11 days	<3.5 μg/dL
12–120 days	<3.0 μg/dL
Free T_4	0.8–2.3 ng/dL
Hyperthyroidism	>2.3 ng/dL
Hypothyroidism	<0.8 ng/dL

Variations
Decreased total thyroxine levels may occur with:

Acute illness	Propranolol	Hypothyroidism
Cretinism	Salicylates (large doses)	Myxedema
Decreased TBG, idiopathic	Sulfonamides	Nephrosis
Drug therapy	Triiodothyronine	Nephrotic syndrome
Androgens	Goiter (not all forms)	Pancreatic malabsorption
Cortisone (long-term)	Hashimoto's disease	Simmonds' disease
Phenytoin	Hepatic disease, chronic	Surgical stress
Prednisone	Hypoproteinemia	Thyroiditis, chronic

Elevated total thyroxine levels may occur with:

Drug therapy	Intermittent porphyria, acute	Pregnancy
Estrogen	Neonates	TBG elevations, idiopathic
Prednisone	Oral contraceptives	Thyroiditis, acute
Hepatic disease, early		Thyrotoxicosis
Hyperthyroidism		

Decreased free thyroxine levels may occur with untreated hypothyroidism, hypothyroidism treated with T_3, and phenytoin therapy.
Elevated free thyroxine levels may occur with:

Fever	Hypothyroidism treated with L-thyroxine
Heparin therapy	Malignancy
Hyperthyroidism	Terminal illness

Methodology
Total T_4 determinations require 5 mL of blood collected without trauma and without anticoagulants (red-stoppered tube). Measurement of free T_4 requires 5 mL of blood collected in a tube without anticoagulants (red-stoppered tube) or with EDTA (lavender-stoppered tube). Specimens for both T_4 determinations remain stable for 6 days at room temperature and for 30 days when frozen.

Measurement of neonatal T_4 requires several drops of blood obtained from a heel puncture during the first week of life and collected on a special filter paper form. It is important that the blood soak completely through the paper and that all the test circles on the filter paper be completely filled with blood. Specimens for neonatal T_4 determinations remain stable for 6 days at room temperature.

Precautions
To ensure accurate results, the following precautions should be observed when collecting specimens for T_4 determinations:

1. Discontinue thyroid treatment for 1 month prior to testing, whenever possible, to obtain a true picture of the base T_4 level without therapy.

2.   Do not submit hemolyzed or grossly lipemic serum for T_4 determinations because this may produce spuriously elevated test results.

▶▶ *Nursing Responsibilities and Implications*

1.   Collect specimens for T_4 determinations before the patient receives any diagnostic or therapeutic procedures requiring the administration of radisotopes because the presence of these substances in the blood may produce misleading test results. When this is not possible, at least 48 hours should elapse following the administration of radioactive material before the test specimen is collected.

2.   Inform the laboratory of the possibility of interfering radioactivity so that they can determine the suitability of the specimen.

3.   Note on the laboratory slip if the patient is pregnant; thyroxine levels increase during the second or third month of pregnancy.

4.   Indicate on the laboratory slip any medications the patient is receiving that might interfere with the test results.

T_3 Uptake and T_3 Uptake Ratio

The **T_3 uptake test** is an indirect measurement of free T_4 that reflects the quantity of TBG in the bloodstream and the amount of thyroid hormone attached to it. Ordinarily, TBG is not fully saturated with thyroid hormone, and about two-thirds of its binding sites remain free to combine with any additional hormone available. The greater the amount of hormone present in the plasma, the smaller the number of sites available for binding by a radioactively labeled thyroid hormone test reagent. In this context the term T_3 refers to the radioactive triiodothyronine (T_3) reagent used in the uptake test and has nothing to do with measuring the actual T_3 serum level.

Thus, determination of the relative number of unoccupied TBG binding sites is an inverse measure of the amount of thyroid hormone already present in the patient's bloodstream. For example, the increased hormone production that accompanies hyperthyroidism increases the saturation of TBG, decreases its binding capacity, and results in a lower than normal binding of the labeled T_3 reagent. Conversely, the decreased hormone secretion and saturation of TBG that accompany hypothyroidism increase TBG binding capacity and the higher than normal binding of radiolabeled T_3 reagent.

However, T_3 uptake results are inversely proportional to the unsaturated thyroid-binding capacity of the patient's TBG and usually are reported as the percentage of radioactivity remaining after complete saturation of TBG. Thus, clinical conditions accompanied by a decrease in the number of available TBG binding sites (hyperthyroidism) produce an increased amount of residual T_3 reagent and elevated test results. On the other hand, conditions that produce a large excess of unsaturated TBG binding sites (hypothyroidism) yield a decreased amount of residual radioactivity and low test results.

Test results also may be expressed as the **T_3 uptake ratio**, which compares the patient's T_3 uptake to that of normal control serum. The T_3 uptake ratio is required to calculate the free T_4 index. Laboratory determinations of T_3 uptake and the T_3 uptake ratio provide an indication of thyroid function and may be used in conjunction with T_4 results to calculate the free T_4 index (see the following section on Free Thyroxine Index).

Clinical Significance

The T_3 uptake test and T_3 uptake ratio are more useful in the evaluation of the free thyroid hormone levels than more specific methods and have become essential components of a detailed thyroid investigation. Free hormone levels customarily are calculated from the measured values for total hormone and the information about TBG binding capacity derived from T_3 uptake, using the T_3 uptake ratio instead of raw figures for T_3 uptake. Evaluation of the free thyroid hormone level or free T_4 index, using the T_3 uptake ratio, correlates most significantly with thyroid status in patients with slightly, but not markedly, abnormal TBG concentrations.

T_3 uptake determinations are less subject than many thyroid studies to interference by various iodine compounds in medications or diagnostic agents such as x-ray contrast media, foods, and other substances. However, test values can be affected significantly by previous diagnostic or therapeutic procedures involving radioactive substances that interfere with the radioactively labeled reagent and produce misleading test results.

Normal Values

The normal and clinically significant values for T_3 uptake and the T_3 uptake ratio are:

T_3 uptake	25%–40%
Hyperthyroidism	>40%
Hypothyroidism	<25%
T_3 uptake ratio	0.8–1.35
Hyperthyroidism	>0.8
Hypothyroidism	<1.35

Variations

Decreased T_3 uptake and T_3 uptake ratio may occur with:

Cretinism	Myxedema
Elevated TBG concentrations	Oral contraceptives
Estrogen therapy	Pregnancy
Hyperestrogenic states	Propylthiouracil therapy
Hypothyroidism	Triiodothyronine therapy

Elevated T_3 uptake and T_3 uptake ratio may occur with:

ACTH therapy	Metastatic malignancy, severe
Anticoagulant therapy (dicumarol, heparin)	Nephrosis
	Phenylbutazone
Corticosteroids	Phenytoin
Decreased TBG concentrations	Pulmonary insufficiency
Hyperandrogenic states	Salicylates (large doses)
Hyperthyroidism	Thyroxine therapy
Liver disease, severe	

Methodology

Measurements of T_3 uptake and the T_3 uptake ratio require 5 mL of blood collected without trauma and without anticoagulants (red-stoppered tube).

Precautions

To ensure accurate results for T_3 uptake and the T_3 uptake ratio, grossly lipemic serum should not be submitted to the laboratory because it may produce low test results.

▶▶ Nursing Responsibilities and Implications

1. Notify the laboratory if the patient recently has received any diagnostic or therapeutic procedures requiring the administration of radioactive substances because significant quantities of radioactivity in the serum may produce unreliable test results.

2. Collect and handle the specimen gently to prevent hemolysis.

3. Note on the laboratory slip any medications the patient is receiving that might interfere with the test results.

Free Thyroxine Index

The **free thyroxine index** (FTI) is a simple calculation that accurately reflects the concentration of circulating thyroid hormone by correcting the total T_4 values for abnormal amounts of TBG present. Free thyroxine index values correlate closely with concentrations of the physiologically active portion of T_4 in healthy individuals as well as those with thyroid disorders and provide the same diagnostic significance as specific measurements of free (unbound) T_4. However, determinations of free T_4 are seldom performed in hospital laboratories because the methods are expensive and technically exacting.

The FTI, also known as the adjusted T_4, can be calculated by multiplying the test results for total T_4, usually determined by radioimmunoassay, and the T_3 uptake ratio. Free thyroxine index determinations provide a better measure of thyroid function than T_4 levels or the T_3 uptake ratio, either singly or together, because the FTI is influenced less by pregnancy or the administration of estrogen or oral contraceptives. Laboratory calculations of the FTI are more valuable in evaluating true thyroid function than individual thyroid studies. They can therefore detect a thyroid abnormality that previously was missed because the values for either test alone were within the normal range.

Clinical Significance

The FTI is used to assess the degree of nonthyroid influence on laboratory values for thyroid hormones and to place apparently abnormal values into proper perspective. The FTI also is useful in the diagnosis of hyperthyroidism and hypothyroidism, especially in patients with known or suspected abnormalities in TBG levels. In such cases laboratory findings and clinical evaluations may seem to be contradictory unless both T_4 and TBG are considered as interrelated parameters of thyrometabolic status.

For example, low T_4 levels may occur in euthyroid patients with correspondingly low TBG levels (high T_3 uptake ratio) and produce a normal FTI. Conversely, high T_4 levels accompanied by low TBG levels produce FTI values above the normal range and indicate clinical hyperthyroidism. On the other hand, the same high level of circulating T_4 induced by any condition that produces increased TBG levels (identified by a low T_3 uptake ratio) yields a normal FTI and indicates normal thyroid function.

Normal Values

The normal and clinically significant values (in arbitrary units) for the free thyroxine index are:

Normal	5.8–10.6
Hyperthyroidism	>11.0
Hypothyroidism	<5.0

Variations

A **decreased free thyroxine index** may occur with:

Cretinism	Low free T_4 levels
Hypothyroidism	Myxedema

An **elevated free thyroxine index** may occur with high free T_4 levels, hyperthyroidism, and thyrotoxicosis.

Methodology

Calculation of the FTI (expressed in arbitrary units) requires accurate results for total T_4 values and the T_3 uptake ratio. Free thyroxine index levels cannot be expressed in objective units because values represent the product of total T_4 values (which are expressed in micrograms per deciliter) and the T_3 uptake ratio (which is expressed as a decimal). Values falling outside this range indicate an abnormality of the active thyroid hormone level.

REFERENCES

Annino, J. S. 1976. *Clinical chemistry.* 4th ed. Boston: Little, Brown, and Co.

Bauer, J. D. 1982. *Clinical laboratory methods.* 9th ed. St. Louis: The C. V. Mosby Co.

Becton-Dickinson. 1982. *B-HCG radioimmunoassay.* Orangeburg, N.J.: Becton-Dickinson, Inc.

Bio-Science Laboratories. 1981. Vitamin D metabolites. *Bio-Science reports.* Van Nuys, Calif.: Bio-Science Laboratories.

———. 1982. *The Bio-Science handbook.* 13th ed. Van Nuys, Calif.: Bio-Science Laboratories.

Bologna, C. V. 1971. *Understanding laboratory medicine.* St. Louis: The C. V. Mosby Co.

Braunstein, G. 1981. Hormones: new potential for tumor markers. *Diagn. Med.* 4(4):59.

Clinical Assays, Inc. 1981. *B-HCG RIA kit for the detection of human chorionic gonadotropin.* Cambridge, Mass.: Clinical Assays, Inc.

———. 1981. *Cortisol RIA kit.* Cambridge, Mass.: Clinical Assays, Inc.

———. 1981. *T₃ uptake kit for the assessment of unsaturated thyroid-binding globulin.* Cambridge, Mass.: Clinical Assays, Inc.

———. 1981. *T₄ RIA test kit for determination of total and/or free thyroxine.* Cambridge, Mass.: Clinical Assays, Inc.

Consolidated Biomedical Laboratories. 1981. *Reference manual.* Richmond, Va.: Consolidated Biomedical Laboratories.

Finley, P. R. (ed.). 1980. Interpretation of tests: thyroid function tests. *Diagn. Med.* 3(2):21.

Finley, P. R., and Soloway, H. B. (eds.). 1982. Interpretation of tests: testosterone. *Diagn. Med.* 5(2):19.

French, R. M. 1980. *Guide to diagnostic procedures.* 5th ed. New York: McGraw-Hill Book Co.

Garb, S. 1976. *Laboratory tests in common use.* 6th ed. New York: Springer Publishing Co.

Henry, J. B. 1984. *Clinical diagnosis and management by laboratory methods.* 17th ed. Philadelphia: W. B. Saunders Co.

Hybritech, Inc. 1982. *HCG test for the detection of human chorionic gonadotropin.* San Diego, Calif.: Hybritech, Inc.

Hycel, Inc. 1974. *Cuvette cortiset.* Houston, TX: Hycel, Inc.

———. 1974. *Mandelic acid test.* Houston, TX: Hycel, Inc.

———. 1974. *Serotonin test.* Houston, TX: Hycel, Inc.

———. 1974. *17-Hydroxy set.* Houston, TX: Hycel, Inc.

Immuno Nuclear Corporation. 1981. *Calcitonin: human calcitonin by RIA.* Stillwater, Minn.: Immuno Nuclear Corp.

Kallestad Laboratories, Inc. 1980. *T₃ RIA kit protocol.* Austin, TX: Kallestead Laboratories, Inc.

Kumar, R. 1982. Vitamin D activation and receptor sites. *Diagn. Med.* 5(6):77.

LaGanga, T. S. 1981. *Laboratory aids in thyroid problems.* Van Nuys, Calif.: Bio-Science Laboratories.

MetPath Laboratory. 1983. *Reference manual.* Teterboro, N.J.: MetPath Laboratory.

Olds, S. B., et al. 1980. *Obstetric nursing.* Menlo Park, Calif.: Addison-Wesley Publishing Co.

Serono Laboratories, Inc. 1980. *FSH—RIA kit for the quantitation of human follicle-stimulating hormone.* Braintree, Mass.: Serono Laboratories, Inc.

———. 1980. *LH—RIA kit for the quantitation of human luteinizing hormone.* Braintree, Mass.: Serono Laboratories, Inc.

———. 1980. *PRL kit for the quantitation of prolactin.* Braintree, Mass.: Serono Laboratories, Inc.

Stanbio Laboratory, Inc. 1977. *Total pregnancy estrogen test set.* San Antonio, Tex.: Stanbio Laboratory, Inc.

Statland, B. E., and Freer, D. E. 1979. Assessing fetal health and maturity. *Diagn. Med.* 2(6):73.

Strand, M. M., and Elmer, L. A. 1983. *Clinical laboratory tests.* 3rd ed. St. Louis: The C. V. Mosby Co.

Tilkian, S. M., Conover, M. B., and Tilkian, A. G. 1983. *Clinical implications of laboratory tests.* 3rd ed. St. Louis: The C. V. Mosby Co.

Warkentin, D. 1983. Infertility: how RIAs can point to the cause. *Diagn. Med.* 6(5):57.

White, W. L., Erickson, M. M., and Stevens, S. C. 1976. *Chemistry for the clinical laboratory.* 4th ed. St. Louis: The C. V. Mosby Co.

Widmann, F. K. 1983. *Clinical interpretation of laboratory tests.* 9th ed. Philadelphia: F. A. Davis Co.

7

Clinical Toxicology and Therapeutic Drug Monitoring

CLINICAL TOXICOLOGY   356
Specimen Collection and Handling   ·   Medicolegal Specimen Collection and Handling

THERAPEUTIC DRUG MONITORING   358
Factors Affecting Drug Response   ·   Test Interpretation   ·   Specimen Collection and Handling

ALCOHOL   360
Ethanol   ·   Isopropanol   ·   Methanol

AMINOGLYCOSIDES   366

AMPHETAMINES   367

ANALGESICS   369
Acetaminophen   ·   Acetylsalicylic acid

ANTICONVULSANTS   372
Carbamazepine   ·   Ethosuximide   ·   Phenobarbital   ·   Phenytoin   ·   Primidone   ·   Valproic Acid

BARBITURATES   379

CARDIAC DRUGS   382
Digitoxin and Digoxin   ·   Lidocaine   ·   Disopyramide   ·   Procainamide   ·   Propranolol   ·   Quinidine

HEMOGLOBIN DERIVATIVES   391
Carbon Monoxide   ·   Methemoglobin   ·   Sulfhemoglobin

HEAVY METALS   397
Arsenic   ·   Iron   ·   Lead   ·   Mercury

MISCELLANEOUS SUBSTANCES   404
Bromide   ·   Methotrexate   ·   Theophylline

PSYCHOTHERAPEUTIC DRUGS   409
Lithium   ·   Phenothiazines   ·   Tricyclic Antidepressants

MINOR TRANQUILIZING AGENTS   415
Benzodiazepines   ·   Other Sedative/Tranquilizing Agents

DRUG ABUSE   418

DRUG SCREENING   420

CLINICAL TOXICOLOGY

Clinical toxicology includes the investigation of acute intoxication from accidental exposure to or intentional abuse of medications, illicit drugs, poisons, household products, and industrial compounds. Identification and measurement of toxic substances in body fluids are often vital for accurate diagnosis and help to determine when certain treatment regimens, such as dialysis, should be employed. Because acute and chronic poisonings with many toxic agents often mimic many serious diseases, laboratory analysis can help to establish the cause of undetermined clinical conditions, including coma. Laboratory testing in forensic toxicology may be required for the medicolegal investigation of drug or alcohol abuse, intentional poisoning, and suicide. A variety of drugs and substances may be responsible for toxic poisonings, but the majority of cases are caused by alcohol, barbiturates, chlordiazepoxide, diazepam, glutethimide, imipramine, narcotics, phenothiazines, and salicylates.

When the toxic agent cannot be identified immediately on the basis of clinical symptoms, patient history or tests for individual substances, broad-spectrum screening tests that detect entire drug groups can be helpful. Screening tests can identify the presence of prescribed and abused drugs, including amphetamines, barbiturates, benzodiazepines, hallucinogens, meperidine, methadone, narcotics, phenothiazines, propoxyphene, and tranquilizers. Laboratory screening for abused drugs is used frequently in public health settings or treatment facilities to diagnose addiction, assess drug use patterns, and select patients for admission to treatment programs.

Specimen Collection and Handling

Laboratory tests to identify and measure toxic drugs or chemical agents implicated in emergency intoxication require samples of blood, urine, or gastric aspirate collected in clean containers without preservatives. Specimens must be properly labeled and delivered to the laboratory immediately. When this is not possible, the specimens should be refrigerated promptly to prevent chemical deterioration.

Laboratory screening tests for drug abuse generally are performed on urine or gastric specimens. However, the nurse also should collect one or two blood samples at the same time and refrigerate them, with complete identification and labeling, for possible later quantitative analysis.

▶▶ *Nursing Responsibilities and Implications*

To ensure the most rapid and significant emergency toxicology and drug screening test results, the nurse should record the following pertinent information on the laboratory request slip:

1. Patient's name and hospital identification number.

2. Patient's medical history, including cardiac, renal, gastrointestinal, or hepatic conditions that could affect drug metabolism and excretion.

3. Suspected drug or toxic agent involved.

4. Estimate of amount ingested.

5. Time of drug ingestion.

6. When the symptoms began and their progression.

7. Clinical observations.

8. Patient's level of consciousness.

9. Current medications the patient is taking.

10. Nature of the patient's work or hobbies.

11. Test requested.

12. Type of specimen.

13. Time of specimen collection.

Medicolegal Specimen Collection and Handling

When blood and urine specimens are collected for medicolegal investigations of toxicity, the chain of possession must remain unbroken from the time the specimen is collected until court testimony is completed. Anyone having access to or custody of a medicolegal specimen at the scene of the incident, in the examination or autopsy room, in the laboratory, and in the courtroom must maintain this continuity of possession. Each step in the collection, processing, and transportation of a medicolegal specimen should be performed in the presence of a witness.

▶▶ *Nursing Responsibilities and Implications*
To help ensure the legal credibility of laboratory test results, the nurse must observe the following additional precautions during the collection and transportation of medicolegal specimens:

1. Obtain a signed consent form before collecting the specimen.

2. Collect the specimen in the presence of a witness, using appropriate collection containers and equipment.

3. Have the witness sign the laboratory request slip, noting the time the specimen was collected.

4. Seal the collection container with tape to prevent tampering.

5. Label the container with the date, contents, and subject's name. Be sure to sign the label.

6. Complete the laboratory request slip, including the type, source, and weight or volume of the specimen, date obtained, and test requested. Sign the laboratory request slip.

7. Maintain a continuous record of the chain of possession for the specimen. Each person who receives the specimen must sign the laboratory request slip, recording the exact time and date the exchange took place. Keep the number of people who handle each specimen to a minimum.

8. Seal the specimen and laboratory request slip in a package and label it "Medicolegal Case" on all sides.

9. Deliver the specimen to the laboratory immediately. If transportation is delayed, lock the specimen in a container and refrigerate the entire container and its contents.

THERAPEUTIC DRUG MONITORING

Laboratory toxicologic investigation also includes therapeutic drug monitoring to help maintain dosages within their beneficial range and prevent toxic side effects. In general, as serum drug levels rise above the therapeutic range, the frequency and severity of toxic side effects increase. When serum drug levels fall below the lower limits of this range, the substance loses its effectiveness, resulting in therapeutic failure. Drug monitoring is especially useful when the margin of safety between effective and toxic levels is narrow. Drugs commonly monitored for therapeutic effectiveness include analgesics, antiarrhythmics, antibiotics, anticonvulsants, bronchodilators, and tricyclic antidepressants.

The drug dosage necessary to produce the maximum therapeutic effect differs widely among patients; therefore, dosage requirements must be interpreted according to test results and observations of the patient's response. Depending on the individual patient, the standard drug dosage may have a therapeutic effect, produce toxicity, or be ineffective. Serum drug levels below the therapeutic range are usually inadequate but may exert beneficial effects in some patients, whereas other patients require levels above the therapeutic range for a fully satisfactory response.

Factors Affecting Drug Response

Individual response to drug therapy is affected by the interaction of many factors that must be considered when interpreting serum drug levels.

Patient Noncompliance.   Failure to maintain a consistent regimen through poor motivation or forgetfulness is the most common cause of inappropriately low serum drug levels. Such noncompliance frequently occurs with chronically administered drugs or those that cause unpleasant side effects. Noncompliance also may be the cause of unexpectedly high serum drug levels because some patients mistakenly believe that they cannot take too much of a good thing.

Disease.   Any change in a patient's normal physiologic status from disease or some other cause can affect the absorption, distribution, metabolism, and excretion of drugs. Thus, drug levels may be elevated or depressed depending on the severity of the disease or changes in the body system involved. For example, gastrointestinal disorders, such as severe diarrhea, can impair drug absorption and result in decreased serum drug levels. On the other hand, certain cardiac, hepatic, and renal diseases interfere with drug clearance rates and can cause toxic drug accumulation.

Age.   Drugs that are cleared by metabolic breakdown are especially sensitive to the age of the patient. In general, young children metabolize drugs twice as quickly as adults; newborn infants and adolescents clear drugs more slowly, at rates comparable to those of adults. Thus, frequent monitoring and appropriate dosage adjustments are required for children on prolonged drug regimens to compensate for age variations. On the other hand, geriatric patients metabolize drugs more slowly than younger adults; in older patients clearance patterns change gradually, becoming significantly altered after 70 years of age. Because of their increased susceptibility to multiple drug interactions, geriatric patients commonly experience clinical intoxication, even when serum concentrations of each drug are within the optimum therapeutic range.

Physiologic Status. Individual response to a therapeutic drug regimen may be altered by physiologic factors such as sex, stress, weight, state of hydration, menstrual cycle, and thyroid function.

Metabolic Rate. A patient's genetic makeup can influence the rate of drug metabolism, producing atypically fast or slow drug responses and causing serum drug levels to be consistently higher or lower than expected. Genetically induced fast drug metabolism appears to be more common than slow drug metabolism.

Drug Interactions. Drug interactions may occur any time different classes of drugs are administered together. However, the greatest risk of drug interaction occurs whenever medications, including over-the-counter drugs, are added to or removed from a patient's existing therapeutic drug regimen. Such changes affect a patient's clinical status by accelerating or retarding the action of certain drugs on the metabolism and excretion of other drugs. Unfortunately, the presence of therapeutic levels of all drugs in a patient's serum does not rule out potential drug interaction or intoxication because the side effects of similar agents can be cumulative.

Dosage. Variations in serum drug levels may result from individual dosage requirements, the route of drug administration, and changes in the metabolism rates among different formulations of the same drug. Therefore, it can be difficult to determine the drug dosage and dosing regimen needed to achieve therapeutic levels in each patient. The drug dose per unit of body weight that leads to toxicity in one patient may be therapeutically inadequate in the next patient. The risk of adverse drug-related side effects may be minimized by calculating a dosage regimen according to the patient's body weight and the desired total daily drug dose (mg/kg/day).

Test Interpretation

Laboratory tests to monitor serum drug levels do not reliably indicate a patient's drug status until a balance is reached between daily drug intake and excretion. Most therapeutic drugs are administered in a given dose at regular intervals over an extended period to allow the drug to accumulate gradually to effective levels. Thus, the maximum therapeutic effect of any new or adjusted drug regimen is not observed until after that balance, or steady-state level, has been reached.

The time required to reach this steady-state level varies according to the drug administered, dosage regimen employed, and individual differences in each drug. Most therapeutic drugs are administered at **half-life** intervals (the time required to eliminate half the plasma concentration of the drug) to minimize fluctuations in serum drug levels between doses. A pharmacologic steady state usually is reached after five oral doses administered at half-life intervals.

The nurse can calculate the steady-state level of any new or adjusted therapeutic drug regimen by multiplying the half-life of the drug by five. For example, during the administration of quinidine, which has a half-life of 4–7 hours, the steady-state level will be reached approximately 20–35 hours after the first dose (4–7 hours × 5 doses = 20–35 hours).

Even with steady-state conditions, intermittent drug administration causes serum concentrations to fluctuate between maximum (peak) and minimum (trough) levels during the dose cycle. Drugs administered by constant infusion or at comparatively short dosage intervals in relation to their elimination half-life produce relatively constant blood levels.

Specimen Collection and Handling

Laboratory tests to monitor therapeutic drug regimens are influenced by the timing of specimen collection with regard to dosage administration. Therefore, the time interval between dosage administration and specimen collection must be consistent when comparing serial samples from the same patient.

Peak Drug Levels. Blood specimens for peak drug levels, which are used to screen for drug intoxication, must be collected when the highest serum concentration of each drug is expected. Toxic drug levels and clinical intoxication also may be evaluated by collecting a blood specimen when toxic symptoms first appear.

Trough Drug Levels. Specimens for trough drug levels must be collected at the lowest serum concentration of the dose cycle, generally immediately before the next scheduled dose or after an overnight fast. Monitoring of trough levels ensures that serum drug concentrations remain within the therapeutic range at all times.

▶▶ *Nursing Responsibilities and Implications*

To ensure the most accurate interpretation of therapeutic drug levels, the nurse should record the following information on the laboratory request slip:

1. Patient's name and hospital identification number.

2. Patient's condition.

3. Test requested.

4. Other current medications the patient is taking.

5. Exact time the last drug dose was administered.

6. Exact time of specimen collection.

7. Specific drug and dosage given.

ALCOHOL

Ethanol

Measurement of ethyl alcohol (ethanol) concentrations in the blood is probably one of the most frequently requested tests in the clinical or forensic laboratory. The amount of ethanol in 1 oz of whiskey is about the same as that contained in 10 oz of beer or 4 oz of wine. On an empty stomach, at least 50% of the ingested alcohol load is absorbed within 15 minutes, and peak blood ethanol levels are reached in 40–70 minutes. Severe, fatal alcohol intoxication may occur not only from the ingestion of large amounts of ethanol but also from breathing concentrated ethanol fumes, which can occur in a distillery.

Ethanol determinations may be requested for medical or legal purposes and generally are included with other screening tests when an unconscious patient arrives at the hospital. Alcohol must be investigated as the possible cause of coma of unknown etiology because alcohol intoxication mimics certain pathologic conditions such as diabetic coma, cerebral trauma, and drug overdose. Laboratory determinations of blood ethanol levels are used to diagnose alcohol intoxication, establish its degree, and help determine appropriate therapy.

Signs and Symptoms

Ethanol is a central nervous system depressant and anesthetic that initially causes mild intoxication, evidenced by sleepiness, poor coordination and reflexes, loss of inhibition and judgment, and slurred speech. As blood concentrations increase, moderate intoxication develops, causing nausea, vomiting, disorientation, personality changes, impaired memory, stupor, diuresis, weak, rapid pulse, and dyspnea. Further alcohol ingestion results in severe intoxication, which is characterized by cyanosis, acidosis, respiratory depression, coma, and finally circulatory collapse and death.

Clinical Significance

Blood ethanol determinations generally are performed in the investigation of traffic accidents in which alcohol is suspected to have been a contributing factor. However, an alcoholic odor on the breath, which can result from the ingestion of a small amount of alcohol, may lead to a misdiagnosis of alcohol intoxication if it is accompanied by symptoms of another physiologic condition. Thus, to reliably and legally diagnose alcohol intoxication, laboratory analysis by accurate chemical methods is needed to substantiate subjective impressions of drunkenness.

The amount of alcohol required to produce a given degree of intoxication varies among individuals according to body weight, time interval since ingestion, individual tolerance, previous experience with alcohol, and the presence of food in the stomach (which affects the speed of absorption). In general, 1 oz of whiskey (10 oz of beer or 4 oz of wine) raises the blood ethanol level to approximately 25–35 mg/dL, and it takes the average 70 kg person approximately 1 hour to metabolize this amount of ethanol. Chronic alcoholics metabolize ethanol almost twice as quickly as nonalcoholic persons and develop a degree of tolerance to ethanol that enables them to survive potentially lethal levels.

The presence of other drugs in the body interferes with the hepatic degradation of ethanol and causes a variation in the blood levels necessary to produce observable symptoms. Drugs such as barbiturates, chlordiazepoxide, diazepam, glutethimide, guanethidine, isoniazid, meprobamate, and phenytoin have increased half-lives and prolonged effectiveness in the presence of ethanol. The interaction of combined ethanol and barbiturate ingestion enhances the depressant effects of both substances and frequently causes dangerously high levels that can result in coma and death. Thus, the combination of ethanol and drugs such as antihistamines, anticonvulsants, barbiturates, morphine derivatives, and tranquilizers should be considered in cases of accidental or intentional poisoning.

The relationship between blood and urine alcohol levels is usually constant and can provide a reliable index to blood ethanol concentrations. The average ratio of urine alcohol to blood alcohol is 1.35. Because the kidneys cannot concentrate ethanol, this ratio means that serum ethanol levels must have been at least 1.35 times the urine level. The urine to blood ethanol ratio is valid, however, only if the peak blood alcohol content has already been passed and the bladder was emptied in the 30 minutes prior to specimen collection.

Normal Values

Normally, no ethanol is present in the blood or urine; the blood concentrations that produce varying degrees of intoxication are:

Ounces of Whiskey	Concentration	Effects
1–2	10–50 mg/dL (0.01%–0.05%)	Subclinical, with no intoxication; mild euphoria; sedation; tranquility
3–4	50–100 mg/dL (0.05%–0.1%)	Sociability; talkativeness; mild influence on stereoscopic vision and dark adaptation; lack of coordination; slurred speech
	100 mg/dL (0.1%)	Decreased attention; diminished control; slow mental response; legal intoxication
5	100–150 mg/dL (0.1%–0.15%)	Emotional instability; euphoria; disappearance of inhibition; loss of critical judgment; prolonged reaction time; driving ability significantly reduced; some incoordination
6–7	150–200 mg/dL (0.15%–0.2%)	Decreased sensory response; obvious intoxication; slightly disturbed equilibrium and coordination; poor color perception; loss of inhibition; reaction time greatly prolonged; moderately severe poisoning
8–9	200–250 mg/dL (0.2%–0.25%)	Disorientation; decreased sense of pain; disturbances of equilibrium and coordination; exaggerated emotional states; retardation of thought processes; clouding of consciousness
10–14	250–350 mg/dL (0.25%–0.35%)	Apathy; inability to stand; unconsciousness; tremors; sweating; incontinence; vomiting; beginning stupor; confusion; marked intoxication; severe degree of poisoning
15–20	350–500 mg/dL (0.35%–0.5%)	Anesthesia; unconsciousness; decreased reflexes; deep, possibly irreversible or fatal coma; incontinence; circulatory and respiratory collapse
20–30	500–800 mg/dL (0.5%–0.8%)	Fatal concentration

Methodology

Ethanol determinations require 5 mL of serum, plasma, urine, or gastric fluid. It is not always known when a blood ethanol measurement is requested whether the results eventually will be used in litigation. Therefore, the strict regulations imposed by the laboratory regarding specimen collection for blood alcohol concentrations must be followed precisely. It is essential that alcohol not be used to prepare the patient's arm for venipuncture and that the exact time of specimen collection and delivery to the laboratory be noted.

When urine alcohol levels also are requested, the most reliable results are obtained by collecting two urine specimens exactly 30 minutes apart. The alcohol concentration of the second urine specimen usually correlates closely with the blood alcohol level. Both blood and urine alcohol specimens remain stable for 2 days at refrigerator temperatures and for much longer periods when frozen.

▶▶ ### Nursing Responsibilities and Implications

1. Cleanse the patient's arm for the venipuncture with an aqueous germicidal solution rather than the usual alcohol swab or antiseptic. For example, a solution of benzalkonium chloride may be used to cleanse the skin, but a tincture should not be used because it contains alcohol and may contaminate the test specimen. Note the substance used on the laboratory slip.

2. Collect 5 mL of venous blood in a tube containing EDTA or oxalate anticoagulant (vacuum tube with a lavender or black stopper); a serum specimen tube (red-stoppered tube) also may be used.

3. Label the tube carefully, recording the exact time the specimen was drawn and the time it was sent to the laboratory. Each step of specimen collection eventually may become part of the legal evidence (see the section on Medicolegal Specimen Collection and Handling earlier in this chapter).

Isopropanol

Isopropyl alcohol (isopropanol) is an antiseptic substance that is widely used as an external disinfectant (known as rubbing alcohol). Although isopropanol has no noticeable harmful effects on human skin, it can cause toxicity when ingested or inhaled. Isopropanol is a common ingredient of antifreeze and industrial solvents for gums, metal degreasers, shellac, stains, and polish. It also is used in drugs and cosmetic substances, including liniments, friction rubs, aftershave lotions, and perfumes. Workers in occupations involving the manufacture of or extensive exposure to any of these substances should be suspected of isopropanol intoxication when toxic symptoms occur. Laboratory determination of isopropanol levels helps to identify and confirm the degree of isopropanol intoxication and serves as a guide for treatment.

Signs and Symptoms

Ingestion of isopropanol results in symptoms similar to those of ethanol intoxication, including gastritis with pain, cramps, nausea, and vomiting. Continued or acute isopropanol ingestion results in central nervous system depression, with symptoms ranging from dizziness to confusion, coma, respiratory paralysis, and death. Prolonged inhalation of concentrated isopropanol vapors can produce rhinitis and bronchitis.

Clinical Significance

Isopropanol is twice as potent as ethanol and is more toxic; a single 250 mL dose of isopropanol is lethal for most adults. Following the ingestion of isopropanol, serum osmolality increases as approximately 15% of the isopropanol is metabolized to acetone. When isopropanol intake is small, acetone is found only in the urine, but it appears in both blood and urine when large amounts are ingested.

Normal Values

Normally, isopropanol is not present in the blood or urine; the blood concentrations that produce intoxication are:

>30 mg/dL	Toxic
(0.03%)	
150 mg/dL	Lethal
(0.15%)	

Methodology

Isopropanol determinations require 5 mL of venous blood collected with an oxalate anticoagulant (black-stoppered vacuum tube) or without anticoagulants (red-stoppered tube). Because alcohol or tincture of iodine at the venipuncture site may falsely elevate isopropanol test results, an aqueous germicidal solution such as benzalkonium chloride should be used to cleanse the patient's arm. Isopropanol measurements also may be performed on urine or gastric fluid specimens.

▶▶ Nursing Responsibilities and Implications

1. Cleanse the patient's arm for the venipuncture with an aqueous germicidal solution rather than the usual alcohol swab or antiseptic.

2. Record the time and amount of isopropanol ingestion on the laboratory request slip; include the patient's drug history and dosage schedule of any drugs being taken.

3. Collect the specimen following the proper precautions if the test results will be used as legal evidence (see Medicolegal Specimen Collection and Handling earlier in this chapter).

Methanol

Methyl alcohol (methanol), also known as wood alcohol, is a toxic substance that can produce metabolic acidosis and result in blindness or death when ingested. It is used frequently in antifreeze, industrial solvents, fuel, and a number of industrial processes, and often is added to bootleg liquor (moonshine). Therefore, methanol intoxication should be suspected in workers repeatedly exposed to these substances and in chronic alcoholics who exhibit symptoms of intoxication.

Methanol is oxidized slowly by the liver, causing its metabolites, formaldehyde and formic acid, to accumulate in the blood. Toxic symptoms can result after a single, large dose of methanol or repeated small, nontoxic doses. Laboratory determinations of methanol levels are used to identify and confirm the degree of methanol intoxication, investigate severe metabolic acidosis unexplained by more common causes, and guide treatment.

Signs and Symptoms

Symptoms of mild to moderate methanol intoxication include drowsiness, headaches, tinnitus, nausea, vomiting, diarrhea, abdominal distress, oliguria, optic neuritis, photophobia, blurred vision with dilated and poorly reactive pupils, and blindness. Life-threatening symptoms of methanol ingestion include stupor, cerebral edema, marked cyanosis, convulsions, coma, respiratory failure, metabolic acidosis, and cardiovascular collapse. Inhalation of methanol vapors irritates the mucosa of the eyes and respiratory tract.

Clinical Significance

Although methanol is less potent than ethanol, it is more toxic, with fatal intoxication usually occurring after the ingestion of 30–100 g. A latent period of 8–36 hours occurs between methanol ingestion and the gradual appearance of toxic symptoms. Complete oxidation and excretion of toxic doses may take several days because methanol is metabolized at approximately one-seventh the rate of ethanol.

Hemodialysis frequently is used to retard the formation of formaldehyde and formic acid, which may be detectable in blood and urine up to 48 hours following the ingestion of large doses of methanol. Treatment of methanol intoxication also may include the administration of ethanol and bicarbonate, which compete for the metabolizing enzyme alcohol dehydrogenase.

Normal Values

Normally, methanol is not present in the blood or urine; the blood concentrations that produce intoxication are:

>20 mg/dL (0.02%)	Toxic
>80 mg/dL (0.08%)	Lethal

Methodology

Methanol determinations require 5 mL of venous blood collected with oxalate or citrate anticoagulants (black- or blue-stoppered vacuum tube) or without anticoagulants (red-stoppered tube). Alcohol and tincture of iodine should not be used to cleanse the venipuncture site because they can cause falsely elevated test results.

Precautions

To ensure accurate determinations, do not use heparin or EDTA anticoagulants because they produce false-positive methanol test results.

▶▶ Nursing Responsibilities and Implications

1. Use an aqueous germicidal solution to cleanse the venipuncture site rather than alcohol or tincture of iodine. Note the substance used on the laboratory slip.

2. Collect the specimen following the proper precautions if the test results will be used as legal evidence (see Medicolegal Specimen Collection and Handling earlier in this chapter).

AMINOGLYCOSIDES

The aminoglycosides, a group of potent antimicrobial agents, are used to treat serious infections that are resistant to or cannot be treated with less toxic drugs. The most commonly used aminoglycosides are amikacin, gentamicin, kanamycin, and tobramycin. Because they are poorly absorbed from the gastrointestinal tract, aminoglycosides usually are administered intravenously or intramuscularly to treat burns, bacteremia, meningitis, osteomyelitis, peritonitis, pneumonitis, urinary tract infections, and some venereal diseases. Aminoglycosides are most active against staphylococci and gram-negative bacteria, including *Acinetobacter, Citrobacter, Proteus, Pseudomonas, Klebsiella,* and *Escherichia coli.* Aminoglycosides are ideal for cleansing the bowel of bacteria before surgery and for controlling the bacterial production of ammonia associated with hepatic coma.

Peak serum values that remain above toxic levels generally produce adverse reactions; steadily rising trough levels indicate that aminoglycosides are not being metabolized adequately from tissue stores and are potentially troublesome. A single aminoglycoside test result within the toxic range is not immediately life threatening and is less serious than persistently elevated values. Laboratory determinations of peak and trough aminoglycoside concentrations are used to maintain plasma levels within the narrow therapeutic range and prevent the development of intoxication.

Signs and Symptoms

Symptoms of aminoglycoside intoxication include hearing loss, vertigo, loss of balance, vomiting, nystagmus, weakness, blurred vision, convulsions, purpura, and anemia. Additional adverse reactions include malabsorption syndrome, neurotoxic pain, acute organic brain dysfunction, depressed cardiac function, renal failure, and abnormal liver function tests.

Clinical Significance

The most common adverse reactions to aminoglycoside therapy are ototoxicity and nephrotoxicity, which usually are reversible if the drug is discontinued at the first sign of dysfunction. Nephrotoxicity is more prevalent in patients with preexisting renal disease and occurs more frequently during the administration of gentamicin and tobramycin than amikacin and kanamycin. Symptoms of nephrotoxicity may not appear until 1−2 weeks after aminoglycoside therapy is begun (Table 7-1).

TABLE 7-1   Characteristics of Aminoglycosides

Aminoglycoside	Half-Life	Peak Concentrations	Steady-State Levels
Amikacin	2−3 hours	30−90 minutes (intramuscular) 15−30 minutes (intravenous)	10−15 hours
Gentamicin	2−3 hours	30−90 minutes (intramuscular) 15−30 minutes (intravenous)	10−15 hours
Kanamycin	2−3 hours	30−90 minutes (intramuscular) 15−30 minutes (intravenous)	10−15 hours
Tobramycin	2−3 hours	30−90 minutes (intramuscular) 15−30 minutes (intravenous)	10−15 hours

Ototoxicity and hearing damage may occur 2–3 weeks following the completion of therapy because it takes that long for various aminoglycosides to be dispersed from tissue stores. Clinical manifestations of aminoglycoside intoxication occur more readily in individuals with impaired renal function; therefore, blood concentrations must be monitored carefully in patients on dialysis to prevent adverse reactions. The risk of aminoglycoside intoxication also is increased in neonates, patients over 50 years of age, and those with dehydration, oliguria, or shock or who require diuretics or nephrotoxic drugs.

Normal Values

Normally, aminoglycosides are not present in the blood; the therapeutic and toxic concentrations are:

| | Therapeutic | Toxic Levels | |
Drug	Range	Peak	Trough
Amikacin	8–25 μg/mL	>35 μg/mL	>10 μg/mL
Gentamicin	4–12 μg/mL	>12 μg/mL	>2 μg/mL
Kanamycin	5–25 μg/mL	>35 μg/mL	>10 μg/mL
Tobramycin	4–10 μg/mL	>12 μg/mL	>2 μg/mL

Methodology

Aminoglycoside determinations require 5 mL of blood collected without anticoagulants (red-stoppered tube) from an area or extremity away from the site of intravenous infusion.

▶▶ Nursing Responsibilities and Implications

1. Collect serum specimens to measure peak levels 15–30 minutes after intravenous administration and 45–90 minutes after an intramuscular injection; trough levels should be measured 30–60 minutes before the next scheduled dose.

2. Use the same time interval between dose administration and specimen collection when comparing serial samples for initial dosage adjustment.

AMPHETAMINES

Amphetamines are powerful central nervous system stimulants, chemically related to catecholamines, that are used to increase blood pressure and decrease appetitite. Medications such as amphetamine sulfate, dextroamphetamine sulfate, methamphetamine hydrochloride, and phenmetrazine hydrochloride are used clinically to treat behavioral problems in children and narcolepsy. Known as "uppers" to members of the drug culture, amphetamines are commonly abused; prolonged use is characterized by marked tolerance, strong emotional dependence, and mild physical dependence.

Patients in methadone maintenance programs are screened routinely for amphetamines and other commonly abused drugs (see Drug Screening later in this chapter). Urine specimens currently are used to measure amphetamine concentrations because serum levels are usually too small to determine accurately. Laboratory determinations of amphetamine levels are used to monitor therapeutic administration, to detect the presence of nonprescribed amphetamines, and diagnose amphetamine intoxication.

Signs and Symptoms

Symptoms of moderate amphetamine intoxication include restlessness, agitation, irritability, tremors, dilated but reactive pupils, euphoria, palpitations, tachycardia, hyperthermia, and gastrointestinal disturbances and rarely occur with doses under 15 mg. Manifestations of acute amphetamine intoxication, including hallucinations, panic states, hyperreflexia, hypertension or hypotension, arrhythmia, rapid respirations, profuse sweating, delirium, and circulatory collapse, occur with 30 mg doses. These symptoms may persist for as long as 5 days after large doses, although prolonged use leads to tolerance, which means that high daily doses of amphetamine can be taken without ill effects. Fatal amphetamine intoxication usually is preceded by convulsions, coma, and respiratory failure.

Clinical Significance

Amphetamines are absorbed well from the gastrointestinal tract and appear in the urine about 3 hours after ingestion. Although the rate of excretion depends on urine pH (the rate of excretion is increased in acid urine and decreased in alkaline urine), 30%–40% of the amphetamine dose normally is excreted unchanged within 24 hours. Thus, the pH of the urine specimen should be measured and noted immediately after collection to allow the accurate interpretation of test results.

Normal Values

Normally, amphetamines are not present in urine or blood; the urine concentrations that produce therapeutic and toxic effects are:

Drug	Therapeutic Range	Toxic Levels
Amphetamine	2–3 μg/mL	>30 μg/mL
Dextroamphetamine	1–1.5 μg/mL	>15 μg/mL
Methamphetamine	3–5 μg/mL	>40 μg/mL
Phenmetrazine	5–30 μg/mL	>50 μg/mL

Methodology

Laboratory determinations of urine amphetamine levels require 100 mL of fresh urine collected without preservatives.

▶▶ Nursing Responsibilities and Implications

1. Measure the pH of the urine specimen promptly so that amphetamine test results can be interpreted accurately.

2. Send the specimen to the laboratory immediately in a tightly sealed container to prevent deterioration or contamination, which could alter the test results.

3. Refrigerate urine specimens that cannot be delivered or tested promptly to prevent bacterial overgrowth.

ANALGESICS

Acetaminophen

Acetaminophen is a nonprescription analgesic and antipyretic compound that is used to treat mild to moderate pain and fever. The major adverse reaction to acetaminophen, hepatotoxicity, usually occurs when large amounts are ingested but occasionally may result from chronic therapeutic doses. Although laboratory determinations of serum acetaminophen levels are helpful in predicting the probability of hepatotoxicity and guiding therapy following overdose, they have limited value in the daily monitoring of therapy.

Signs and Symptoms

Symptoms of acetaminophen intoxication may be observed within the first 12–24 hours after overdose. They include nausea, vomiting, abdominal pain, delayed reflexes, anorexia, hypoglycemia, and metabolic acidosis. Following overdose, clinical evidence of hepatic abnormalities, including a rise in AST (aspartate aminotransferase, formerly SGOT) and ALT (alanine aminotransferase, formerly SGPT) levels, occurs within 2 days but may not become evident until 4–6 days following acetaminophen ingestion.

Clinical Significance

Adult intake of 325–650 mg of acetaminophen (one to two tablets) every 3–4 hours generally produces the serum concentrations necessary to achieve analgesic response with essentially no side effects. Serious acetaminophen intoxication, with delayed but potentially fatal hepatic failure, results from the ingestion of more than 140 mg of acetaminophen per kilogram of body weight.

Establishing the acetaminophen half-life in patients with serum concentrations above 120 mg/mL helps to indicate the potential for liver damage because toxic doses prolong the drug's half-life. Hepatic necrosis may occur during an episode of acute intoxication if the half-life of acetaminophen exceeds 4 hours, and hepatic coma is very likely if the half-life exceeds 12 hours. The concurrent administration of acetaminophen and liver enzyme-inducing drugs, such as phenobarbital and alcohol, also may cause hepatotoxicity.

The elimination half-life of acetaminophen is determined by measuring serum levels in two blood samples. The first blood sample is collected at least 4 hours after drug ingestion and the second blood sample is obtained 4 hours later (Table 7-2). The difference between serum acetaminophen values in the first and second samples represents the amount of drug eliminated in 4 hours and is used to estimate its half-life. If the first postingestion sample is greater than 150 mg/mL, therapy with acetylcysteine should be started immediately. Therapy that is begun more than 12 hours after acute acetaminophen ingestion generally is less effective in preventing serious toxicity than treatment started earlier.

TABLE 7-2 Characteristics of Analgesics

Analgesic	Half-Life	Peak Concentrations	Steady-State Levels
Acetaminophen	2–4 hours	½–1 hour	10–20 hours
Salicylates	2–4½ hours (adults) 2–3 hours (children)	1–2 hours	10–22½ hours (adults) 10–15 hours (children)

Normal Values

Normally, acetaminophen is not present in the blood or urine; the serum concentrations that produce therapeutic and toxic effects are:

4.5–25 μg/mL	Therapeutic range
>120 μg/mL	Toxic symptoms but no liver damage
>200 μg/mL	Hepatotoxicity
>300 μg/mL	Hepatic necrosis

Methodology

Serum acetaminophen determinations require 3 mL of venous blood collected without anticoagulants (red-stoppered vacuum tube), although specimens collected with EDTA anticoagulant (lavender-stoppered tube) also may be used.

▶▶ Nursing Responsibilities and Implications

To ensure significant single acetaminophen determinations, note the amount of time since ingestion, quantity ingested, and patient's history of recent barbiturate use on the laboratory slip.

Acetylsalicylic Acid

Acetylsalicylic acid (aspirin) is a nonprescription analgesic drug with antipyretic, anti-inflammatory, and antirheumatic properties. It is used frequently in large therapeutic doses to control the symptoms of rheumatic fever and rheumatoid arthritis. Salicylates also are commonly used to relieve the symptoms of influenza, mild pain such as headache, muscle aches, toothaches, and dysmenorrhea, and to lower body temperature in febrile patients.

Metabolism and excretion of salicylates generally occur at a constant rate, with traces appearing in the urine about 30 minutes after absorption. However, the rate of salicylate excretion varies with the pH of the urine and may slow as the size of the ingested dose increases in acute poisoning. Very little salicylate remains in the blood 2 days after therapeutic use of the drug is discontinued in patients with normal renal function.

Laboratory measurements of salicylate concentrations in blood are used to check therapeutic levels to prevent intoxication and to diagnose salicylate poisoning. Urine salicylate screening tests are of greatest use in the differential diagnosis of coma of unknown etiology. Because glucose and salicylate appear as reducing substances in the urine, salicylate screening tests are helpful in distinguishing between diabetes and salicylate intoxication as the cause of acidosis and coma.

Signs and Symptoms

Salicylate intoxication initially stimulates and then depresses the central nervous system, causing the prognosis of salicylate intoxication to become increasingly grave as blood levels rise. Initial symptoms of mild salicylate intoxication include headache, dizziness, tinnitus, sudden weakness, drowsiness, irritability, confusion, deafness, blurred vision, vomiting, diaphoresis, thirst, and hyperventilation. The early stages of acute salicylate intoxication are evidenced by hyperpnea, gastrointestinal irritation, prolonged bleeding time, petechial hemorrhage, hypoglycemia, dehydration, and acid-base disturbances with respiratory alkalosis. The later stages of acute salicylate intoxication are characterized by metabolic acidosis and ketosis, which can progress to respiratory failure, coma, and death. Occasional bleeding episodes caused by salicylate ingestion are related to gastrointestinal irritation and capillary damage; however, these symptoms usually occur when chronic salicylate therapy is superimposed on severe liver disease or peptic ulcer.

Clinical Significance

Salicylate intake of 5–6 g/day (15–20 adult-sized aspirin tablets) generally is prescribed for treatment of rheumatoid arthritis in adults (see Table 7-2). Salicylate intoxication generally occurs following the ingestion of 10 g of aspirin within a 24-hour period; an adult dose of 20–30 g or 300 mg/kg of body weight is fatal. The easy availability of salicylate compounds makes therapeutic overdose a common occurrence, and their accessibility in the home is responsible for a high number of accidental poisonings in children. In addition, a significant number of suicide attempts in adults are associated with this drug.

Salicylate levels in the blood provide an accurate indication of the severity of the intoxication, as well as establish the general prognosis in older children and adults. Serum salicylate concentrations measured 2 hours after ingestion provide a good guide to the severity of the poisoning. Young children have a variable sensitivity to salicylate levels, although fatalities in children occur more frequently when preexisting fever or infection alters the metabolic effect of salicylates. Metabolism and excretion of salicylates generally occur at a constant rate, but the rate of excretion may slow with acute poisoning as the size of the ingested dose increases.

Initial blood levels of salicylates must be correlated carefully with the time interval since salicylate ingestion to obtain the most significant diagnostic and prognostic information. Prognosis is based on a calculated initial blood level rather than on the actual salicylate level at the time of examination, especially following the ingestion of a single large salicylate dose. For example, a moderate elevation persisting many hours after salicylate intoxication may be more serious than a higher elevation occurring shortly after the drug is taken. Salicylate levels in blood measured within 6 hours of acute ingestion and intoxication may be considered as the initial salicylate level.

Normal Values

Normally, salicylates are not present in the blood or urine; the blood concentrations that produce therapeutic and toxic effects are:

15–30 mg/dL	Maximum anti-inflammatory action*
>25 mg/dL	Tinnitus
>30 mg/dL	Mild toxicity
>35 mg/dL	Moderate toxicity, hyperventilation
>45 mg/dL	Acidosis
>50 mg/dL	Severe toxicity
>60 mg/dL	Lethal

*This level may be toxic to some children.

Methodology

Salicylate determinations require 5 mL of venous blood collected without anticoagulants (red-stoppered tube) for serum specimens or with heparin (green-stoppered tube) for plasma or whole blood specimens. The significance of therapeutic salicylate monitoring is ensured by consistently using the same time interval between sampling and dose administration when comparing serial samples.

Urine salicylate measurements require a 10 mL random urine specimen. Qualitative measurement of salicylates in urine is extremely sensitive, producing positive findings after the ingestion of as little as 300 mg of salicylate (one adult-sized aspirin tablet). However, urine assay is not recommended for monitoring therapy or detecting toxic levels because of the wide fluctuations in excretion rates.

ANTICONVULSANTS

Carbamazepine

Carbamazepine, commonly used to treat trigeminal neuralgia (tic douloureux), is also effective in controlling generalized convulsive seizures, tonic-clonic (grand mal) seizures, and complex partial seizures (psychomotor, temporal lobe). Although carbamazepine is not the drug of choice for these disorders, it may be part of a multidrug regimen when certain types of epilepsy do not respond to phenytoin, phenobarbital, or primidone therapy alone. However, the concurrent administration of carbamazepine and these other anticonvulsants significantly alters the plasma carbamazepine level required to control seizures. Thus, plasma levels of carbamazepine must be higher in patients receiving this drug alone than plasma levels in patients receiving multidrug therapy to achieve the same degree of seizure control. Laboratory monitoring of carbamazepine concentrations helps to attain and maintain therapeutic drug levels and prevent toxic side effects.

Signs and Symptoms

Ingestion of toxic carbamazepine doses produces a mild to moderate intoxication characterized by dizziness, drowsiness, ataxia, stupor, nausea, vomiting, restlessness, agitation, disorientation, tremor, abnormal reflexes, mydriasis, nystagmus, cyanosis, and urinary retention. Massive carbamazepine overdosage results in severe intoxication, which may be accompanied by convulsions, seizures, and coma. Chronic carbamazepine therapy also can lead to a generalized bone marrow depression, which is heralded by such early signs of potential hematologic problems as fever, sore throat, mouth ulcers, easy bruising, and purpura.

Clinical Significance

Carbamazepine dosage should be adjusted promptly to the minimum amount needed for effective seizure control, usually four to six tablets daily for adults and two to four tablets daily for children (Table 7-3). Prolonged carbamazepine therapy may produce serious and occasionally fatal hematologic abnormalities, including aplastic anemia, leukopenia, agranulocytosis, eosinophilia, leukocytosis, and thrombocytopenic purpura. Complete blood counts should be performed before beginning treatment and at regular intervals during the next 2–3 years of therapy to detect any evidence of bone marrow depression.

TABLE 7-3   Characteristics of Anticonvulsants

Drug	Half-Life	Peak Concentrations	Steady-State Levels
Carbamazepine	10–30 hours (adults) 8–19 hours (children)	6–24 hours	2–6 days (adults) 2–4 days (children)
Ethosuximide	40–60 hours (adults) 30–50 hours (children)	2–4 hours	8–12 days (adults) 6–10 days (children)
Phenobarbital	2–6 days (adults) 1½–3 days (children)	6–18 hours	11–25 days (adults) 8–15 days (children)
Phenytoin	18–30 hours (adults) 12–22 hours (children)	3–12 hours	4–6 days (adults) 2–5 days (children)
Primidone	4–12 hours (adults) 4–6 hours (children)	2–4 hours	16–60 hours (adults) 20–30 hours (children)
Valproic Acid	8–15 hours (adults) 6–15 hours (children)	½–1½ hours	40–75 hours (adults) 30–75 hours (children)

Test results within the following ranges indicate bone marrow depression and warrant immediate discontinuation of carbamazepine administration:

Red blood cell count	<4.0 million/mm^3
Hemoglobin	<11 g/dL
Hematocrit	$<32\%$
White blood cell count	<4000/mm^3
Platelets	$<100,000$/mm^3
Reticulocyte count	$<0.3\%$
Serum iron	<150 μg/dL

Normal Values

Toxic and therapeutic carbamazepine concentrations are:

3–9 μg/mL	Therapeutic range
>10 μg/mL	Toxic level

Methodology

Carbamazepine determinations require 5 mL of blood collected without anticoagulants (red-stoppered tube) and without hemolysis and lipemia. Serum specimens for carbamazepine measurements remain stable for 4 days at room temperature. The same time interval between dose administration and specimen collection should be used consistently when comparing results from serial samples for therapeutic drug monitoring.

▶▶ Nursing Responsibilities and Implications

1. Withhold the administration of carbamazepine if significantly abnormal test results occur in pretreatment or follow-up blood counts.

2. Caution the patient to discontinue the use of carbamazepine and consult the physician immediately at the first sign of fever, sore throat, mouth ulcerations, or abnormal bruising.

Ethosuximide

Ethosuximide, although not effective in treating the major motor seizures, is the anticonvulsant drug of choice for absence (petit mal) seizures. It significantly reduces the frequency of these seizures, particularly in children, by depressing the motor cortex of the brain and elevating the threshold of convulsive stimulation. Laboratory determinations of ethosuximide levels are used to achieve and maintain therapeutic concentrations while reducing the risk of toxic side effects.

Signs and Symptoms

Ethosuximide overdosage generally is accompanied by drug intoxication, although the relationship of serum concentrations to toxic effects has not been completely established. However, the side effects that are common with therapeutic administration appear to be dose related and include gastric distress, ataxia, diplopia, blurred vision, nystagmus, mydriasis, vertigo, anorexia, fatigue, and lethargy. Profound sedation is common during the early stages of ethosuximide therapy and generally persists for several days; however, the patient quickly adapts to this and other acute side effects.

Clinical Significance

Serum ethosuximide concentrations maintain the same degree of seizure control regardless of whether the recommended dose is administered once a day or in divided doses. Because children metabolize drugs faster than adults, they require higher doses and can tolerate higher serum ethosuximide concentrations than adults without evidence of toxic effects (see Table 7-3). Unlike several of the other anticonvulsants, ethosuximide levels are not altered by concurrent therapy with additional antiepileptic agents.

Normal Values

Therapeutic and toxic ethosuximide concentrations are:

40–100 μg/ml	Therapeutic range
>150 μg/mL	Toxic level

Methodology

Ethosuximide determinations require 5 mL of blood collected without anticoagulants (red-stoppered tube) and without hemolysis and lipemia. Serum specimens for ethosuximide determinations remain stable for 5 days at room temperature.

Phenobarbital

Phenobarbital, a long-acting barbiturate, is the least toxic and most effective anticonvulsant for the long-term treatment of tonic-clonic (grand mal) and focal seizures. It is the drug of choice for seizure control in infants and preschool children in whom phenytoin therapy produces adverse effects. Phenobarbital frequently is used in combination with phenytoin in older individuals when phenytoin therapy alone is not sufficient to completely suppress tonic-clonic seizures. It also is particularly useful in seizures caused by the withdrawal of alcohol and barbiturates but is not effective in, and may actually worsen, petit mal and psychomotor seizures. (The use of phenobarbital as a sedative and hypnotic agent is discussed under Barbiturates later in this chapter.)

Routine phenobarbital monitoring is especially important to prevent excessive plasma levels during chronic administration because recent reports suggest that prolonged therapy may impair learning in some children. In prolonged phenobarbital administration, tolerance to potentially toxic plasma levels can develop rapidly without causing noticeable signs of toxicity. Laboratory determinations of phenobarbital concentrations are helpful in initiating adequate seizure therapy, monitoring prolonged administration, and identifying toxic levels when adverse signs and symptoms appear.

Signs and Symptoms

The most common side effect of phenobarbital administration is somnolence or drowsiness, which usually disappears within several weeks as the patient develops a tolerance to therapeutic levels. The early symptoms of moderate intoxication include disorientation, lethargy, slurred speech, ataxia, headaches, and miosis. The later stages of intoxication are characterized by hallucinations and changes in the rate of respiration. Acute phenobarbital intoxication may produce nystagmus, flaccid muscles, absence of corneal reflexes, anoxia, cyanosis, hypotension, shock, deep coma, and ultimately cardiovascular collapse. Any plasma concentration of phenobarbital may cause central nervous system stimulation in the elderly, resulting in confusion and delirium; in young children phenobarbital may cause irritability and hyperactivity.

Clinical Significance

Prepubescent children metabolize phenobarbital faster than adults; therefore, the dose of phenobarbital needed to maintain adequate seizure control in children is approximately twice the dose needed in adults (see Table 7-3). These high doses must be carefully reduced to prevent the development of toxicity with the onset of puberty and change of metabolic patterns to those of adults. The sudden withdrawal of phenobarbital in patients on long-term, high-dose therapy can precipitate episodes of status epilepticus.

Normal Values

Therapeutic and toxic phenobarbital concentrations are:

10–25 μg/mL	Therapeutic range
>25 μg/mL	Toxic level
>30 μg/mL	Ataxia; slurred speech; disorientation
>40 μg/mL	Changes in respiratory rate
>50 μg/mL	Nystagmus; hallucinations; flaccid muscles
>60 μg/mL	Deep coma; cyanosis; shock
>100 μg/mL	Loss of deep tendon reflexes; cardiovascular collapse

Methodology

Phenobarbital determinations require 5 mL of blood collected without anticoagulants (red-stoppered tube) or with sodium oxalate (black-stoppered tube). It is important to use the same time interval between dose administration and the collection of blood specimens when monitoring serial samples for therapeutic phenobarbital levels. A 25 mL specimen of urine or gastric aspirate also may be used to detect the presence of phenobarbital in the system, although these specimens are not adequate for monitoring therapeutic efficacy.

Phenytoin

Phenytoin, the major anticonvulsant for treating epilepsy, is used primarily for controlling tonic-clonic (grand mal), focal sensorimotor, and psychomotor seizures. It inhibits seizure activity in the motor cortex without generalized central nervous system depression in all types of epilepsy except absence (petit mal) seizures. Phenytoin also is used to treat cardiac arrhythmias such as ventricular ectopic rhythms and paroxysmal atrial tachycardia caused by digitalis toxicity.

Phenytoin usually is administered in a single daily dose to increase patient compliance, but the same degree of seizure control is achieved with divided doses (see Table 7-3). In patients who are unable to take oral medication, phenytoin levels may be maintained within the therapeutic range through intravenous administration, although close supervision is required because of the potential for adverse cardiovascular effects. Effective anticonvulsant levels must be established for each patient by correlating individual clinical findings with the dosage regimen and repeating phenytoin assays after dosage adjustment if seizure activity or symptoms of toxicity appear. Laboratory determinations of phenytoin levels are used to monitor anticonvulsant therapy and evaluate patients with symptoms that may result from phenytoin excess due to multiple drug administration or unreliable drug intake.

Signs and Symptoms

The initial symptoms of mild phenytoin intoxication are ataxia, nystagmus, and dysarthria. The symptoms of moderate intoxication include lethargy, mental changes, and seizures. More commonly, therapeutic concentrations cause such adverse reactions as diplopia, dizziness, tremors, insomnia, slurred speech, headache, nausea, and vomiting.

Clinical Significance

Phenytoin metabolism may be altered significantly by the presence of liver disease or the concurrent use of other drugs, causing ineffective plasma concentrations or toxic manifestations. For example, chloramphenicol, coumarin anticoagulants, disulfiram, isoniazid, and phenylbutazone decrease the rate of phenytoin metabolism and cause elevated blood levels. However, other drugs, such as carbamazepine, ethanol, folate, diazepam, and clonazepam, stimulate the rate of phenytoin metabolism and lower plasma concentrations.

Concurrent phenobarbital administration has an unpredictable effect on phenytoin metabolism and may increase, decrease, or have no effect on blood levels. High doses of tricyclic antidepressants may precipitate seizures when used with phenytoin. Conversely, phenytoin administration increases phenobarbital concentrations but decreases digitoxin, dicumarol, metyrapone, cortisol, and dexamethasone levels.

Normal Values

Therapeutic and toxic phenytoin concentrations are:

10–20 µg/mL	Therapeutic range
20–30 µg/mL	Mild intoxication; ataxia; nystagmus; slurred speech
>40 µg/mL	Mental changes;* lethargy; inability to concentrate; exacerbation of seizures in some patients
>60 µg/mL	Inability to sit up in some patients

*Mental changes occur more often in elderly patients than in younger patients.

Methodology

Phenytoin determinations require approximately 5 mL of blood collected without anticoagulants (red-stoppered tube) and without hemolysis. Serum specimens for phenytoin measurements remain stable for 7 days at room temperature.

Primidone

Primidone, a phenobarbital derivative, is a potent antiepileptic agent used to control tonic-clonic (grand mal), myoclonic, complex partial (psychomotor), and focal epileptic seizures. It is especially effective in treating grand mal seizures that are refractory to other anticonvulsants and is the drug of choice, either alone or in combination with phenytoin, in temporal lobe epilepsy. Primidone is converted in the body to two metabolites, phenobarbital and phenylethylmalondiamide (PEMA), each an active anticonvulsant with the ability to elevate the seizure threshold. Laboratory tests of primidone levels generally also report phenobarbital concentrations to help assess the effectiveness of therapy and prevent the onset of adverse or toxic side effects.

Signs and Symptoms

The most frequent early reactions to therapeutic primidone administration are dose related and include drowsiness, ataxia, sedation, and vertigo, which disappear after continued therapy or reduction of the initial dose. Symptoms of intoxication such as nausea and vomiting, anorexia, fatigue, emotional disturbances, hyperirritability, impotence, diplopia, hypotension, tachycardia, and nystagmus appear when primidone levels are slightly above the therapeutic range. Prolonged primidone therapy may produce bone marrow disturbances such as a megaloblastic anemia, which responds to the administration of folic acid or vitamin B_{12}.

Clinical Significance

Administration of the recommended daily dose of primidone in three to four divided doses maintains serum concentrations within the range necessary for adequate seizure control. However, the dosage may need to be adjusted when beginning simultaneous therapy with another anticonvulsant or during stressful situations that may trigger seizures such as menstruation, holidays, or allergic reactions. It usually takes several weeks to assess the efficacy of a dosage regimen because the time required to reach steady-state levels depends on the rate of conversion of primidone to phenobarbital (see Table 7-3).

Phenobarbital normally is not produced for at least 24 hours following the ingestion of therapeutic doses of primidone, although acute ingestion of toxic primidone doses stimulates phenobarbital metabolism within 12 hours. The concurrent administration of phenytoin and primidone markedly enhances the rate of conversion of primidone to phenobarbital. Thus, significantly higher phenobarbital levels are found in patients receiving both primidone and phenytoin than in patients receiving primidone alone.

Normal Values

Therapeutic and toxic primidone levels are:

5–12 μg/mL	Therapeutic range
>15 μg/mL	Toxic level

Methodology

Primidone determinations require 5 mL of blood collected without anticoagulants (red-stoppered tube) and without hemolysis or lipemia. Serum specimens for primidone measurements remain stable for 7 days at room temperature.

Valproic Acid

Valproic acid, the newest antiepileptic agent, is indicated for the treatment of tonic-clonic (grand mal) and simple or complex absence (petit mal) seizures, especially in children. It is particularly useful in controlling absence seizures that are refractory to ethosuximide therapy and is also effective, either alone or in combination with other anticonvulsants, in controlling multiple seizure types, including absence seizures. Laboratory evaluation of valproic acid concentrations is helpful in determining appropriate dosage intervals to achieve and maintain seizure control without causing toxic side effects.

Signs and Symptoms

The most common early side effects of valproic acid therapy are transient and include nausea, vomiting, abdominal cramps, diarrhea, alopecia, fatigue, and sedation, often associated with hypersalivation. Other nonspecific symptoms such as malaise, weakness, lethargy, and anorexia, frequently accompanied by increased serum alkaline phosphatase and AST levels, may indicate hepatotoxicity caused by valproic acid therapy. Although clinical symptoms of intoxication from valproic acid overdosage are usually mild, deep coma may result from concentrations above the therapeutic range.

Clinical Significance

Valproic acid blood levels remain within the therapeutic range when the recommended dosage is administered in divided doses three to four times daily to compensate for widely fluctuating concentrations. Concurrent therapy involving valproic acid and primidone or phenobarbital causes a disproportionate increase in phenobarbital levels and results in severe central nervous system depression. Thus, the dosage of phenobarbital must be reduced by approximately one-third to keep blood levels within the therapeutic range when it is administered with valproic acid. Valproic acid also enhances the depressant effect of alcohol and has a variable effect on phenytoin concentrations, requiring that dosage adjustments be made if warranted by the clinical situation (see Table 7-3).

Because prolonged valproic acid intake may cause a serious, possibly fatal, hepatic failure within the first 6 months of therapy, liver function studies should be performed before treatment begins and frequently thereafter. Drug therapy should be discontinued immediately if symptoms of hepatotoxicity or abnormal liver function test results indicate significant hepatic dysfunction.

Normal Values
Therapeutic and toxic valproic acid levels are:

50–100 μg/mL	Therapeutic range
>125 μg/mL	Toxic level

Methodology
Valproic acid determinations require 5 mL of blood collected without anticoagulants (red-stoppered tube) or with EDTA anticoagulant (lavender-stoppered tube). Serum and plasma specimens for valproic acid measurements remain stable for 14 days at room temperature.

▶▶ **Nursing Responsibilities and Implications**

1. Collect specimens at the same time interval after each dose for accurate comparison of test results and to correlate plasma levels with clinical effects.

2. Monitor the patient's liver function studies; notify the physician of any abnormal findings.

BARBITURATES

Barbiturates are a group of central nervous system depressants that are used extensively as sedatives, hypnotics, anesthetics, and antiepileptic agents. Barbiturates are classified according to the duration of their activity as long-acting (8–16 hours), intermediate-acting (4–8 hours), short-acting (3–6 hours), and ultrashort-acting (less than 30 minutes). Ultrashort-acting barbiturates are used as intravenous anesthetics; short-acting pentobarbital or secobarbital and intermediate-acting amobarbital or butabarbital are used as sedative hypnotics; long-acting phenobarbital is used as an antiepileptic agent. (The use of phenobarbital as an antiepileptic drug is discussed in the previous section on Anticonvulsants.) Test results should include a description of barbiturates as short-, intermediate-, or long-acting when barbiturate intoxication is suspected in a seriously ill or comatose patient because this information may influence treatment.

It is difficult to diagnose barbiturate intoxication in an unconscious patient because a variety of conditions may produce coma, and a combination of drugs may be implicated in an overdosage. In addition, drug levels may not accurately reflect the patient's overall physiologic condition and prognosis, even when specific barbiturates are identified as the cause of intoxication. Patients who habitually use barbiturates, particularly individuals who are addicted to them, tolerate larger, potentially lethal doses and concentrations than patients who are not habitual users. Laboratory tests for serum barbiturate levels are used to establish the presence of a barbiturate, identify the particular agent, and indicate its concentration as an aid to therapy.

Signs and Symptoms

Barbiturate intoxication causes varying degrees of central nervous system depression, ranging from mild sedation to coma, depending on the dose, route of administration, and particular barbiturate used. The long-term intake of therapeutic barbiturate doses can produce symptoms of mild intoxication, including constipation, skin reactions, anorexia, personality changes, and impairment of liver function. Moderate intoxication is character-ized by disorientation, lethargy, slurred speech, ataxia, headaches, miosis that possibly progresses to mydriasis, and changes in respiratory rate. Acute barbiturate intake produces severe intoxication, with hallucinations, flaccid muscles, nystagmus, poor pupillary re-actions, hypotension, profound respiratory depression, absence of deep reflexes, anoxia, cyanosis, shock, deep coma, and cardiovascular collapse.

Clinical Significance

The clinical implications of any given barbiturate concentration are far more serious for short-acting compounds than for long-acting agents. Long-acting barbiturates are ab-sorbed slowly from the gastrointestinal tract, and relatively high concentrations are needed to produce coma, although their effects may persist for days (Table 7-4). On the other hand, short-acting barbiturates are absorbed more rapidly, are more toxic or potent, and much lower concentrations are needed to produce severe intoxication. However, the short-acting drugs are eliminated from the body rapidly, and their direct effect usually lasts only a few hours.

Barbiturate action in the body is enhanced by the simultaneous presence of com-pounds such as alcohol, morphine derivatives, tranquilizers, and reserpine, which greatly intensify the depressant effects of all barbiturates. The continued ingestion of large doses of barbiturates can result in cumulative toxicity, especially in patients with impaired renal or hepatic function.

TABLE 7-4 Characteristics of Barbiturates

Drug	Half-Life	Peak Concentrations	Steady-State Levels
Short-acting (secobarbital)	15–48 hours	1 hour	75–140 hours
Intermediate-acting (amobarbital)	24 hours	2 hours	120 hours
Long-acting (phenobarbital)	4–6 days	12–18 hours	20–30 days

Normal Values

Normally, no barbiturates are present in the blood or urine; the therapeutic and toxic levels of various barbiturates are:

Short-acting (secobarbital)

1–5 μg/mL	Therapeutic range
10–20 μg/mL	Mild toxicity; marked sedation
20–30 μg/mL	Moderate toxicity; comatose; reflexes present
30–40 μg/mL	Marked toxicity; comatose; reflexes absent; respiratory depression
>40 μg/mL	Acute toxicity; deep coma; cardiovascular collapse

Intermediate-acting (amobarbital)

5–15 μg/mL	Therapeutic range
15–30 μg/mL	Mild toxicity; marked sedation
30–50 μg/mL	Moderate toxicity; comatose; reflexes present
50–70 μg/mL	Marked toxicity; comatose; reflexes absent; respiratory depression
>70 μg/mL	Acute toxicity; deep coma; cardiovascular collapse

Long-acting (phenobarbital)

10–40 μg/mL	Therapeutic range
40–50 μg/mL	Mild toxicity; marked sedation
50–80 μg/mL	Moderate toxicity; comatose; reflexes present
80–110 μg/mL	Marked toxicity; comatose; reflexes absent; respiratory depression
>110 μg/mL	Acute toxicity; deep coma; cardiovascular collapse

Variations

Falsely elevated barbiturate levels may be caused by high concentrations of several drugs, including:

Antipyrine	Meperidine
Atropine	Methyprylon
Dexchlorpheniramine maleate	Nitrazepam
Glutethimide	Salicylamide
Hydantoin (therapeutic levels)	Theophylline

Methodology

Screening tests for the presence of suspected barbiturate overdose may be performed on 25 mL of fresh urine or gastric aspirate. Quantitative analysis of barbiturate levels requires 10 mL of blood collected without anticoagulants (red-stoppered tube) or with EDTA or sodium oxalate anticoagulants (lavender- or black-stoppered tube), depending on the laboratory procedure. Blood specimens collected in heparin are not satisfactory for barbiturate determinations.

▶▶ **Nursing Responsibilities and Implications**

1.   Handle the specimen gently to prevent hemolysis, which will cause falsely elevated test results.

2.   Send the specimen to the laboratory immediately or refrigerate it to ensure accurate test results.

3.   Collect the specimen following the proper precautions if the test results will be used as legal evidence (see Medicolegal Specimen Collection and Handling earlier in this chapter).

4.   Note on the laboratory slip any medications the patient has been or is receiving.

5.   Observe the patient who is unconscious because of barbiturate intoxication for signs of impending respiratory failure.

6.   Obtain serial blood specimens from the patient who is withdrawing from barbiturate dependency; convulsions and coma may result if serum barbiturate levels drop abruptly.

CARDIAC DRUGS

Digitoxin and Digoxin

Digoxin and digitoxin are highly specific digitalis glycoside drugs that strengthen heart tissue and expand cardiac output by increasing the force and velocity of myocardial contractions. They are used to produce a slower, stronger, and more regular heartbeat during the treatment of congestive heart failure and arrhythmias such as atrial fibrillation and atrial flutter. With both drugs there is a slim margin of error between safe, therapeutic levels and toxic levels (Table 7-5).

Excessively high digitalis concentrations interfere with the electrical impulses that stimulate myocardial contractions and produce dysrhythmias similar to those for which the therapy was initially prescribed. Thus, it is frequently unclear whether to increase the digitalis dose to treat a deteriorating heart problem or to withhold therapy because the patient is suffering from digitalis toxicity. Laboratory measurements of digitoxin and digoxin levels are used to diagnose digitalis intoxication, reduce the frequency of unnecessary dosage adjustments, and decrease the possibility of serious digitalis toxicity.

Signs and Symptoms

The earliest symptoms of digitalis (cardiac glycoside) intoxication include gastrointestinal manifestations such as anorexia, nausea, vomiting, and diarrhea, as well as a visual distor-

TABLE 7-5 Characteristics of Cardiac Drugs

Drug	Half-Life	Peak Concentrations	Steady-State Levels
Digitoxin	4–6 days	1–3 hours	20–30 days
Digoxin	36–51 hours (adults) 11–50 hours (children)	1–5 hours	7–11 days (adults) 2–10 days (children)
Lidocaine	1–2 hours	15–30 minutes	5–10 hours
Disopyramide	5–6 hours	½–3 hours	25–30 hours
Procainamide	2–5 hours	1–2 hours	11–24 hours
N-acetylprocainamide	6 hours	1–8 hours	30 hours
Propranolol	2–6 hours	1–3 hours	10–30 hours
Quinidine	3–9 hours	1–4 hours	20–35 hours

tion in which objects appear green and yellow. Signs of more advanced digitalis toxicity include cardiac dysrhythmias of all types, abnormal electrocardiograms, hypotension, generalized weakness, increasingly severe congestive heart failure, and alterations in cardiac rate and rhythm. Arrhythmias resulting from digitalis toxicity include extrasystole, atrioventricular dissociation, paroxysmal atrial tachycardia, and ventricular fibrillation. The final stages of digitalis intoxication are characterized by convulsions, delirium, and mental confusion, possibly followed by cardiac arrest.

Clinical Significance
Individuals vary considerably in their response to digitalis therapy and become more susceptible to intoxication with advancing age. Elderly patients develop toxicity with lower levels of digitoxin and digoxin, whereas infants can tolerate higher blood concentrations without suffering toxic effects. Other factors that may influence individual sensitivity to digitalis toxicity include anoxia, hypothyroidism, abnormal renal function, and electrolyte disturbances such as hypokalemia, hypercalcemia, hypomagnesemia, alkalosis, and acidosis. Patients with advanced heart disorders, including severe coronary artery disease, myocardial infarction, and myocarditis, or who have had recent heart surgery also are more susceptible to digitalis toxicity, even when blood concentrations are within the normal range.

The concurrent administration of cardiac glycosides with various other medications may alter digitalis metabolism; therefore, digitoxin and digoxin concentrations must be monitored closely to ensure that levels remain within the therapeutic range. For example, quinidine, propranolol, epinephrine, ephedrine, isoproterenol, reserpine, and succinylcholine increase the level of digitalis compounds in the blood and enhance the likelihood of cardiac arrhythmias. On the other hand, antacids, cholestyramine, neomycin, kaolin, pectin, sulfasalazine, and phenytoin reduce digoxin levels, and barbiturates, phenytoin, phenylbutazone, and cholestyramine decrease digitoxin concentrations.

Normal Values

Normally, digitalis glycosides are not present in the blood except during therapy. The therapeutic and toxic concentrations are:

Digitoxin

5–20 ng/mL	Therapeutic range
>25 ng/mL	Toxic level

Digoxin

0.8–1.6 ng/mL	Therapeutic range (dose of 0.25 mg/day)
1.1–1.9 ng/mL	Therapeutic range (dose of 0.50 mg/day)
>2.4 ng/mL	Toxic level

Methodology

Digitoxin and digoxin determinations require 3 mL of blood collected without anticoagulants (red-stoppered tube) or with heparin (green-stoppered tube). Specimens should be drawn 6–8 hours after the last dose so that blood levels are stable and test values correlate blood levels and cardiac effects. The differences in digitalis concentration caused by the various routes of administration are not significant because of the drug's long half-life.

Precautions

Laboratory assays of digitalis glycoside concentrations employ test reagents that are specific only to the medication being administered. However, antisera to one digitalis compound may cross-react with other cardiac glycosides, causing inaccurate test results. For example, residual digitoxin in the blood may interfere with digoxin assays for 4 days to several weeks after it has been discontinued. Thus, digitalis assays are significant only if it is known with certainty which cardiac glycoside compound is being administered to ensure measurement of the correct drug.

▶▶ Nursing Responsibilities and Implications

1. Inform the patient that there are no food or fluid restrictions.

2. Note on the laboratory slip the specific cardiac glycoside being administered and monitored.

3. Obtain the blood specimen 6 hours after the drug has been administered or before the next dose.

4. When performing serial measurements, observe the same time interval between drug administration and specimen collection.

5. Observe the patient for signs of digitalis toxicity; if toxicity is identified, withhold the drug and notify the physician.

6. Monitor the laboratory results; if toxic levels are reached, withhold the drug and notify the physician.

7. Monitor the patient's apical and radial pulses and other vital signs frequently.

Lidocaine

Lidocaine, a fast-acting drug that may be administered intravenously, intramuscularly, or topically, is used to produce local anesthesia and to control cardiac arrhythmias. Its use is indicated to convert the dysrhythmias that occur with myocardial infarction and to prevent ventricular arrhythmias during such manipulations as cardiac surgery. Because lidocaine has less of a depressant effect on cardiac conduction than other cardiac drugs, it also frequently is used to treat digitalis-induced dysrhythmias. Laboratory monitoring of lidocaine concentrations is helpful in preventing toxic accumulation, particularly in patients with heart failure or renal disease who are more prone to developing the conditions that alter normal lidocaine metabolism.

Signs and Symptoms
Mildly increased lidocaine concentrations are characterized by subtle neurotoxicity, which is difficult to observe before more severe symptoms develop. The initial symptoms of lidocaine intoxication include nonspecific manifestations such as diaphoresis, pallor, apprehension, euphoria, disorientation, lightheadedness, dizziness, drowsiness, tinnitus, and visual distortions. In the later stages of lidocaine intoxication, cardiac toxicity leads to complete atrioventricular block, decreased cardiac output, accelerated ventricular response, and bradycardia, which may progress to cardiac arrest. Acute symptoms of severe lidocaine intoxication are associated with central nervous system depression and include hypotension, tremors, grand mal seizures, unconsciousness, coma, respiratory collapse, and death.

Clinical Significance
Conversion of life-threatening ventricular dysrhythmias requires that lidocaine concentrations remain within a constant therapeutic range. Because of its rapid onset of action, however, very high and occasionally toxic lidocaine concentrations are reached shortly after a dose is administered (see Table 7-5). If initial lidocaine doses are reduced to avoid the toxic effects of high plasma concentrations, plasma levels fall very rapidly to below minimum therapeutic levels, causing dysrhythmias to recur. Therefore, lidocaine usually is administered in several intravenous loading doses given 5–10 minutes apart, along with a constant infusion to sustain concentrations between each bolus.

Lidocaine concentrations vary according to individual differences in metabolism, with toxicity related to dose administration and the overall clinical picture. Conservative dosing regimens may be necessary for lidocaine therapy because a number of factors can influence the rate of metabolism of the drug and lead to toxicity. Patients with uncompensated congestive heart failure, underlying hepatic disease, shock, or hyperkalemia are predisposed to lidocaine intoxication and are more likely to develop cardiac toxicity. Patients receiving barbiturate or phenytoin therapy also are more prone to lidocaine intoxication.

Normal Values
Lidocaine is found in the blood only during therapy; the therapeutic and toxic concentrations are:

1.5–6 μg/mL	Therapeutic range
>9 μg/mL	Toxic level

Methodology

Lidocaine determinations require 5 mL of blood collected without anticoagulants (red-stoppered tube) and delivered promptly to the laboratory. It is important when comparing clinical symptoms with lidocaine concentrations to use the same time interval between dose administration and specimen collection.

▶▶ **Nursing Responsibilities and Implications**

1. Note on the laboratory slip any medications the patient is receiving, particularly cardiac glycosides, barbiturates, or phenytoin.

2. When performing serial determinations, observe the same time interval between drug administration and specimen collection.

3. Observe the patient for signs and symptoms of lidocaine intoxication.

4. Watch for signs of hyperkalemia, which may predispose the patient to lidocaine intoxication (see Potassium in Chapter 5).

5. Monitor the patient's apical and radial pulses and other vital signs frequently.

Disopyramide

Disopyramide is a relatively new antiarrhythmic drug used to treat premature ventricular contractions (unifocal, multifocal, or paired) and ventricular tachycardia not severe enough to require electrical cardioversion. Disopyramide acts rapidly to produce a localized anesthetic effect similar to lidocaine and exerts a stabilizing effect on heart muscle similar to that exerted by quinidine and procainamide. However, the effects of disopyramide on myocardial tissue may be altered significantly in patients with heart disease, causing toxic symptoms to appear more readily than in patients with less severe cardiac abnormalities (see Table 7-5). Laboratory determinations of disopyramide concentration are used to make dosage adjustments to ensure that levels remain within the therapeutic range and to avoid cardiac toxicity.

Signs and Symptoms

The most common side effects of disopyramide therapy are dry mouth, followed much less frequently by dizziness, fatigue, muscle weakness, syncope, blurred vision, urinary retention, nausea, and constipation. Toxic symptoms are dose related and are characterized by increased congestive heart failure, a widened QRS complex, an increased QT interval, bradycardia, heart block, and hypotension.

Clinical Significance

Disopyramide must be administered carefully in patients with impaired cardiac function, hepatic insufficiency, renal failure, or hypokalemia because these conditions affect the metabolism of the drug and increase susceptibility to intoxication. Patients with urinary tract disease (especially prostatic hypertrophy), myasthenia gravis, and narrow-angle glaucoma are also at greater risk of developing toxic side effects than other patients. Concurrent use of other cardiac drugs during disopyramide therapy may enhance the drug's antiarrhythmic effect and exaggerate the myocardial depression.

Normal Values

Disopyramide appears in the blood only during therapy; the therapeutic and toxic concentrations are:

2–5 μg/mL   Therapeutic range

>7 μg/mL   Toxic level

Methodology

Disopyramide determinations require 5 mL of blood collected without anticoagulants (red-stoppered tube) or with EDTA (lavender-stoppered tube). Serum and plasma specimens for disopyramide monitoring remain stable for 7 days at room temperature.

▶▶ *Nursing Responsibilities and Implications*

1. Note on the laboratory slip any medications the patient is receiving.

2. When performing serial determinations, observe the same time interval between drug administration and specimen collection.

3. Observe the patient for signs and symptoms of disopyramide intoxication.

4. Watch for signs of hypokalemia, which may predispose the patient to disopyramide intoxication (see Potassium in Chapter 5).

5. Monitor the patient's apical and radial pulses and other vital signs frequently.

Procainamide

Procainamide and its active metabolite, N-acetylprocainamide (NAPA), are procaine derivatives used to treat various cardiac arrhythmias, except those induced by digitalis intoxication. Procainamide and NAPA are most effective in controlling ventricular tachycardia, atrial fibrillation, and paroxysmal tachycardia, particularly in patients who do not respond to the maximum tolerated dose of quinidine. However, patients who respond to one drug, for example, NAPA, do not necessarily respond favorably to the other drug when it is given alone.

Procainamide and NAPA usually are taken orally, with intramuscular and intravenous administration reserved for the treatment of life-threatening arrhythmias that do not respond to oral dosages. Intravenous infusions must be administered more slowly and cautiously than oral or intramuscular dosages because with intravenous administration the potential for these drugs to produce serious toxic effects is greatly increased. Laboratory monitoring of procainamide and NAPA concentrations is used to guide treatment because a standardized dosage regimen may not always maintain therapeutic concentrations or avoid toxicity.

Signs and Symptoms

The most common side effects of oral procainamide and NAPA administration are dose related and include nausea, anorexia, vomiting, diarrhea, psychosis, weakness, hallucinations, and a potentially fatal agranulocytosis, thrombocytopenia, or autoimmune hemolytic anemia. Long-term procainamide or NAPA administration (6 months) may produce a toxic accumulation, characterized by a lupuslike syndrome in which antinuclear antibodies appear and such symptoms as joint pain, polyarteritis, numbness, chest pain, rash, fever, and arthritis develop. Rapid intravenous administration may produce serious toxic symptoms such as asystole, myocardial depression, heart block, ventricular fibrillation and tachycardia, precipitous hypotensive reaction, convulsions, cardiac arrest, and death.

Clinical Significance
Within 1–2 days after beginning oral procainamide therapy, significant concentrations of NAPA also may accumulate in the plasma and occur in the blood of some patients at levels that equal or exceed the level of procainamide (see Table 7-5). However, the level of NAPA obtained from a given dose of procainamide is unpredictable because of individual metabolic differences, which are determined by the patient's age, sex, body size, and existing renal or hepatic diseases. Because NAPA is excreted by the kidneys and accumulates more rapidly in patients with renal dysfunction, these patients are more susceptible to procainamide intoxication. Thus, in patients receiving procainamide therapy, levels of both NAPA and procainamide should be measured because together the two drugs produce cumulative antiarrhythmic and potentially toxic effects.

Concurrent administration of procainamide and thiazide diuretics or other antiarrhythmic drugs produces a synergistic effect that causes central nervous system stimulation with myocardial depression, and requires close monitoring to prevent toxicity. The use of procainamide and NAPA increases the neuromuscular blocking effects of antibiotics (such as aminoglycosides), muscle relaxants, and magnesium salts, making the patient more susceptible to respiratory depression. In addition, the concomitant use of procaine, aminobenzoic esters, and acetazolamide increases the patient's sensitivity to procainamide and NAPA, increasing the potential for intoxication.

Normal Values
Procainamide and N-acetylprocainamide are present in the blood only during therapy; the therapeutic and toxic concentrations are:

Procainamide

4–8 μg/mL	Therapeutic range
>12 μg/mL	Toxic level

N-acetylprocainamide

2–8 μg/mL	Therapeutic range
>30 μg/mL	Toxic level

Procainamide plus N-acetylprocainamide

8–16 μg/mL	Therapeutic range
>20 μg/mL	Toxic level

Methodology
Procainamide and NAPA determinations require 5 mL of blood collected without anticoagulants (red-stoppered tube) and delivered to the laboratory immediately for prompt

testing. Test results for patients receiving oral dosages are most significant and reproducible when the specimen is collected at the trough serum level, immediately before the next dose. Peak level samples should be collected 90 minutes after an oral dose, although these values are not as important as trough levels unless toxicity or sensitivity is suspected.

Tests for procainamide concentrations in patients receiving intravenous therapy should be performed within the first 10–20 hours after administration. Negligible amounts of NAPA are formed during this period and thus produce only minimal effects on either the therapeutic efficacy or toxicity of the dose of procainamide. However, both procainamide and NAPA assays are necessary once the dosage regimen is converted from intravenous to oral maintenance, particularly in patients with renal disease.

▶▶ *Nursing Responsibilities and Implications*

1. Observe the patient for signs and symptoms of procainamide intoxication.

2. When performing serial determinations, observe the same time interval between drug administration and specimen collection; peak level samples should be obtained 90 minutes after the administration of an oral dose; trough level samples should be obtained just prior to the next dose.

3. Monitor the patient's apical and radial pulses and other vital signs frequently.

Propranolol

Propranolol, a β-adrenergic blocking agent, is a cardiac depressant and antihypertensive used to treat a number of clinical conditions, including certain cardiac arrhythmias and cardiac diseases. It is indicated for the control of atrial and ventricular premature beats, atrial flutter, atrial fibrillation, ectopic ventricular and supraventricular tachycardia, and digitalis-induced tachyarrhythmia. Propranolol also is used to alleviate angina pectoris and to manage primary hypertension associated with increased plasma renin activity. However, its use is contraindicated in patients with myocardial infarction because sudden withdrawal of the drug may aggravate this condition. Laboratory monitoring of propranolol concentrations is used to adjust the dosage regimen and helps maintain blood levels within the therapeutic range.

Signs and Symptoms
The most common side effects of propranolol therapy include nausea, vomiting, generalized weakness, lightheadedness, disorientation, visual disturbances, skin rashes, paresthesia of the hands, and hypotension. More significant adverse reactions involve hypoglycemia in diabetics, bronchospasm in asthmatics, bradycardia, asystole, dyspnea, and an intensified atrioventricular block. The most severe reaction to propranolol consists of a sudden onset of cardiac failure due to a temporary blockage of sympathetic nervous system support of a failing ventricle.

Clinical Significance
Patients receiving propranolol therapy must be monitored carefully because plasma levels vary considerably among individuals receiving the same dosage (see Table 7-5). Although test values remain relatively constant within the same individual, wide variations among patients may be due to differences in the liver's ability to extract propranolol from the

blood. Propranolol accumulates in the blood and saturates the metabolism of patients receiving large doses, with potentially toxic effects during a number of diseases that alter total protein concentrations. The most important adverse effects of propranolol therapy, as well as the beneficial effects, result from the β-blocking activity of this drug on catecholamines.

Normal Values

Propranolol appears in the blood only during therapy; the therapeutic and toxic concentrations are:

40–100 ng/mL	Therapeutic range
>150 ng/mL	Toxic level

Methodology

Propranolol determinations require 7 mL of blood collected in a syringe and promptly transferred to a tube without anticoagulants. Specimens must not be collected in vacuum tubes because substances in the stopper reduce plasma propranolol binding, causing greater than normal amounts of the drug to enter the blood cells. This redistribution of propranolol reduces the amount of drug in the circulating plasma and results in falsely low test values.

▶▶ Nursing Responsibilities and Implications

1. Observe the patient for signs and symptoms of propranolol intoxication.

2. When performing serial determinations, observe the same time interval between drug administration and specimen collection.

3. Monitor the patient's apical and radial pulses and other vital signs frequently.

Quinidine

Quinidine, an antiarrhythmic drug administered orally, intravenously, and intramuscularly, controls certain cardiac disorders by exerting a depressant effect on myocardial excitability, conduction velocity, and contractility. It is used to convert atrial fibrillation as well as to treat atrial flutter, premature atrial and ventricular contractions, and atrial or ventricular tachycardia. Laboratory monitoring of quinidine therapy is used to maintain plasma levels within the optimum range.

Signs and Symptoms

The most common side effects of quinidine therapy are nausea, vomiting, diarrhea, abdominal pain, tinnitus, vertigo, blurred vision, impaired hearing, headache, diaphoresis, and emotional disturbances. Other less common reactions to quinidine therapy include flushed skin, fever, hypotension, shock, confusion, delirium, hepatic dysfunction, thrombocytopenia, agranulocytosis, and acute hemolytic anemia. The appearance of such side effects may preclude long-term quinidine therapy in 30%–40% of the patients to whom the drug is administered. Quinidine concentrations above the therapeutic range produce toxic reactions such as drug-induced asystole, premature ventricular beats, ventricular tachycardia or fibrillation, atrioventricular block, and arterial embolism, which may cause sudden death.

Clinical Significance

Quinidine is absorbed well and exerts its maximum antiarrhythmic effects rapidly, although peak levels are delayed in patients with chronic heart failure (see Table 7-5). Simultaneous administration of quinidine and anticonvulsant drugs such as phenytoin may shorten quinidine's half-life and cause a clinically significant reduction of quinidine plasma levels. Conversely, quinidine therapy combined with antacids, sodium bicarbonate, or acetazolamide increases renal absorption of quinidine, causing elevated blood levels. Concurrent quinidine and digoxin therapy increases plasma digoxin levels.

Normal Values

Quinidine occurs in the blood only during therapy; the therapeutic and toxic concentrations are:

$2-5$ μg/mL	Therapeutic range
>10 μg/mL	Toxic level

Methodology

Quinidine determinations require 5 mL of blood collected without anticoagulants (red-stoppered tube) or with heparin (green-stoppered tube). Serum and plasma specimens should be obtained at the same time interval after drug administration so that the comparison of test results will yield useful information.

►► Nursing Responsibilities and Implications

1. Observe the patient for signs and symptoms of quinidine intoxication.

2. Note on the laboratory slip any medications the patient is receiving because certain drugs may increase or decrease serum levels.

3. When performing serial determinations, observe the same time interval between drug administration and specimen collection.

4. Monitor the patient's apical and radial pulses and other vital signs frequently.

HEMOGLOBIN DERIVATIVES

Carbon Monoxide

Carbon monoxide, a chemical asphyxiant found in the fumes of automobile exhausts, improperly functioning furnaces, and defective gas-burning appliances, is an odorless gas produced by the incomplete combustion of carbon-containing fuels. When inhaled, carbon monoxide combines with hemoglobin in red blood cells with an affinity that is 200 times greater than that of oxygen. This combination produces the hemoglobin derivative, carboxyhemoglobin, which is unable to transport or release oxygen throughout the body, depriving the tissues of oxygen and producing hypoxia.

Carbon monoxide intoxication probably is responsible for more deaths than any other poison and usually results from occupational exposure to exhaust gases in industrial plants or garages. Most individuals, including nonsmokers and city dwellers, normally have a low level of carbon monoxide in their blood from environmental exposure to tobacco smoke, traffic fumes, and industrial smoke. However, miners, urban taxi or bus drivers, and garage mechanics, as well as workers involved in blast furnaces, boiler rooms, and coke oven refinery operations, are at greater risk of exposure to high concentrations of carbon monoxide. Unsuspected chronic monoxide intoxication and fatal poisoning also may result from repeated or prolonged exposure to defective home heating units. Laboratory identification of increased amounts of carboxyhemoglobin in the blood is used to detect chronic or low-grade toxic exposure and establish the diagnosis of carbon monoxide poisoning.

Signs and Symptoms

The intensity of carbon monoxide intoxication varies with the amount of carboxyhemoglobin produced, whereas the severity of symptoms reflects the carbon dioxide concentration of the air and the length of exposure (Table 7-6). The principal early symptoms of carbon monoxide intoxication result from hypoxia and include headache, vertigo, weakness, malaise, full pulse, and throbbing temples. Carbon monoxide intoxication also produces a characteristic cherry-red blood, which imparts a bright red color to mucous membranes such as lips and oral mucosa. Prolonged exposure to carbon monoxide causes the symptoms of intoxication to progress rapidly to nausea, confusion, hypertension, mydriasis, ataxia, anoxia, convulsions, coma, respiratory paralysis, and death.

Clinical Significance

Due to the hypoxia produced by carboxyhemoglobin intoxication, carbon monoxide exposure is especially dangerous to individuals with high oxygen requirements or a precarious oxygen transport system. Thus, patients with cardiopulmonary diseases, children with their characteristically high metabolic rate, and anemic individuals with low hemoglobin concentrations are particularly susceptible to carbon monoxide toxicity. For example, although toxic symptoms of intoxication generally appear at 20% saturation and

TABLE 7-6 Carbon Monoxide Saturation of Hemoglobin

Concentration of Carbon Monoxide in Air	Time Needed to Saturate 10% of Hemoglobin With Carbon Monoxide	Time Needed to Saturate 30% of Hemoglobin With Carbon Monoxide
0.02%	3 hours	Never
0.05%	1 hour	5 hours
0.10%	30 minutes	2 hours
0.20%	10 minutes	50 minutes
0.50%	4 minutes	20 minutes
1.00%	1 minute	5 minutes

SOURCE: From Gambino, R and Galen, RS: How Carbon Monoxide Kills. *Diagnostic Medicine*, Sept/Oct 1981, p 82. Reproduced with permission.

acute poisoning occurs at 30% saturation, much lower saturation levels produce intoxication in individuals with anemia.

Inhaling a carbon monoxide concentration of 5 parts in 10,000 parts of air (0.05%) produces hemoglobin saturation of 10% within 1 hour and 30% saturation after 5 hours of exposure. However, carboxyhemoglobin gradually is replaced by normal, oxygenated hemoglobin at a rate of 15% per hour when exposure stops and the patient breathes pure air; this rate is increased when the patient breathes oxygen. Thus, although a heavy smoker may inhale smoke containing more than 0.05% carbon monoxide, hemoglobin saturation decreases between cigarettes and may return to near-normal levels after an overnight abstinence from cigarettes.

Normal Values

The normal and toxic carbon monoxide values are:

0.05%–2.5%	Normal: rural environment, non-smokers; no symptoms
2.0%–5.0%	Normal: urban environment, light or moderate smokers; slight impairment of cognitive skills
5.0%–10%	Normal: heavy smokers, taxi drivers; slight breathlessness on severe exertion
10%–20%	Mild toxicity; mild headache, breathlessness on moderate exertion
20%–30%	Moderate toxicity; throbbing headache, irritability, impaired judgment, defective memory, rapid pulse, fatigue, first signs of anoxia
30%–40%	Marked toxicity; severe headache, nausea, weakness, dimness of vision, confusion
40%–50%	Acute toxicity; disorientation, ataxia, hallucinations, hyperventilation, and collapse, occasionally fatal
50%–60%	Deep coma, possible convulsions
>60%	Lethal level

Methodology

Carbon monoxide determinations require 7 mL of blood collected with heparin (green-stoppered tube) as soon as possible after exposure. Although oxalated blood (black-stoppered tube) frequently is used, it may cause falsely low test results. Blood specimens are most suitable for carboxyhemoglobin analysis when testing is performed immediately, although specimens may be preserved for several hours if they are refrigerated in tightly stoppered, completely filled tubes.

▶▶ *Nursing Responsibilities and Implications*

1.   Obtain a health history to document exposure to carbon monoxide.

2.   Collect the specimen following the proper precautions if the test results will be used as legal evidence (see Medicolegal Specimen Collection and Handling).

3.   Observe the patient for signs of hypoxia; administer oxygen as ordered.

4.   Prevent contamination of the specimen by room air, which would cause inaccurate results; transport the specimen to the laboratory immediately.

5.   Provide for safety and rest if the patient is confused, weak, and/or lethargic.

6.   Monitor the patient's vital signs frequently.

Methemoglobin

Methemoglobin is a hemoglobin derivative produced by oxidation of iron in the hemoglobin molecule to the ferric rather than the normal ferrous form. This form of hemoglobin does not transport or release oxygen throughout the body because it binds the oxygen so closely that it cannot dissociate and is therefore unavailable for respiration. Small amounts of methemoglobin normally are formed within erythrocytes but are prevented from accumulating by an intraerythrocytic enzyme system that continuously reduces methemoglobin to hemoglobin to maintain a physiologic concentration. Accumulation of methemoglobin in amounts exceeding this normal level is always pathologic and produces **methemoglobinemia**, which is characterized by hypoxia and cyanosis.

Methemoglobinemia may be caused by a congenital defect in the erythrocyte enzyme system that normally reduces methemoglobin, although this is rare. Most cases of methemoglobinemia are toxic or acquired and occur when methemoglobin is produced in the blood faster than it can be reduced, thus overwhelming the physiologic enzyme system. Laboratory identification of methemoglobinemia is helpful in determining the cause of hypoxia and cyanosis and can guide the follow-up investigation of the source of methemoglobin intoxication.

Signs and Symptoms

The symptoms of methemoglobinemia occur in proportion to the methemoglobin concentration and are similar to the manifestations of carbon monoxide poisoning. However, because methemoglobinemia can be reversed by the administration of reducing agents and certain enzymes, methemoglobin intoxication is not as serious as carbon monoxide toxicity and the symptoms are usually not as severe.

Clinical Significance

Methemoglobin intoxication may result from the action of many chemicals and drugs that accelerate the oxidation of hemoglobin and cause abnormally large amounts of methemoglobin to accumulate in the blood. The effect of therapeutic agents such as sulfonamides, nitroglycerine, chlorates, phenacetin, acetanilid, and amyl or sodium nitrite stimulates this oxidation process. In addition, exposure to certain industrial compounds, including nitrates and nitrites, nitrobenzene-containing products, and aniline dyes or derivatives, such as marking ink and furniture polish, may cause methemoglobinemia.

However, exposure to these toxic agents, particularly nitrates and nitrites, is not always obvious. For example, certain foods, such as spinach and some sausage products, are rich in nitrates that can be converted into potentially dangerous nitrites. Likewise, well water with a high nitrate content from surface contaminants can cause methemoglobinemia when the nitrate is converted to nitrite by intestinal bacteria. Large amounts of nitrites also are absorbed during severe bacterial enteritis, and the treatment of extensive burns with silver nitrate may cause methemoglobinemia from nitrate absorption.

Infants are more susceptible to methemoglobinemia than older children or adults. The potential for methemoglobin formation and accumulation is greater in infants during the first 3 months because they have high concentrations of fetal hemoglobin, which is oxidized more readily than adult hemoglobin. The erythrocytes of newborn infants also are relatively deficient in methemoglobin-reducing enzymes, which slows the rate at which methemoglobin is converted to hemoglobin.

Normal Values

The normal and toxic methemoglobin values are:

0.3%–3.1%	Normal range
2.2%	Premature infants
1.0%–1.5%	Infants (<1 year)
<1.0%	Children and adults
15%–30%	Cyanosis
35%–45%	Dyspnea
60%	Symptoms of hypoxia; lethargy, semistupor
60%–70%	Lethal level; vascular collapse, death

Methodology

Methemoglobin determinations require 5 mL of blood collected with heparin (green-stoppered tube) and delivered to the laboratory immediately for prompt analysis. Delay in processing the specimen allows the erythrocyte enzyme system to continue reducing methemoglobin to hemoglobin and produces falsely decreased test results.

▶▶ Nursing Responsibilities and Implications

1. Obtain a health history to document exposure to toxic chemicals or medications that promote the oxidation of hemoglobin to methemoglobin.

2. Observe the patient for signs of hypoxia; administer oxygen as ordered.

3. Note on the laboratory slip any medications the patient has been or is receiving.

4. Send the specimen to the laboratory immediately for prompt analysis since delay can cause falsely decreased test results.

5. Monitor the patient's vital signs frequently.

Sulfhemoglobin

Sulfhemoglobin, an intraerythrocytic hemoglobin derivative that often accompanies methemoglobinemia, is a stable compound resulting from the irreversible linkage of sulfur and hemoglobin. It is produced by the toxic effects of certain drugs and chemicals, which cause a structural change within the hemoglobin molecule and results in the clinical condition **sulfhemoglobinemia**. Like methemoglobin and carboxyhemoglobin, sulfhemoglobin is unable to transport and release oxygen throughout the body and produces symptoms of oxygen deprivation when present in significant concentrations. Laboratory determinations of sulfhemoglobin concentrations often are performed with methemoglobin measurements to help identify the cause of hypoxia and monitor the effects of treatment.

Signs and Symptoms
The symptoms of sulfhemoglobin intoxication progress from those that characterize hypoxia to those associated with anoxia as concentrations increase and include dizziness, weakness, headache, intense cyanosis, hypertension, convulsions, and coma.

Clinical Significance
Sulfhemoglobinemia may occur with the administration of various drugs, including acetanilid, nitrates and nitrites, phenacetin, sulfonamides, and sulfur-containing cathartics. Exposure to certain industrial chemicals such as aniline dyes, nitrobenzene, hydrogen sulfide, trinitrotoluene, and zinc ethylene bisdithiocarbamate also induces sulfhemoglobin formation. Sulfhemoglobin is so stable that it does not disappear from the bloodstream until the erythrocytes containing it complete their life cycle and are completely destroyed. Thus, because sulfhemoglobin formation cannot be reversed and resists treatment, therapy usually is directed toward the accompanying methemoglobinemia and the sulfhemoglobinemia is allowed to resolve itself.

Normal Values
The normal and toxic sulfhemoglobin values are:

0%−2.0%	Normal range
>2.2%	Toxic level

Methodology
Sulfhemoglobin determinations require 5 mL of blood collected with heparin (green-stoppered tube) and delivered to the laboratory shortly after collection so that analysis can be performed within 4 hours.

▶▶ Nursing Responsibilities and Implications

1. Obtain a health history to document exposure to toxic chemicals or medications that promote sulfhemoglobin formation.

2. Observe the patient for signs of sulfhemoglobinemia such as hypoxia; administer oxygen as ordered.

3. Note on the laboratory slip any medications the patient has been or is receiving.

4. Send the specimen to the laboratory immediately because the test should be performed within 4 hours of specimen collection.

5. Monitor the patient's vital signs frequently, particularly the pulse, respirations, and blood pressure; notify the physician if hypertension occurs.

6. Provide safety measures and promote rest if the patient is dizzy or weak.

HEAVY METALS

Arsenic

Arsenic, a highly toxic heavy metal, is a common ingredient in herbicides, insecticides, and rodenticides, as well as paints, dyes, glass alloys, cosmetics, and antiprotozoal medications. Arsenic enters the body through the mouth, lungs, or skin and causes varying degrees of toxicity, depending on the amount and duration of exposure. Thus, prolonged exposure to small doses of arsenic-containing preparations produces chronic intoxication, whereas the ingestion of large doses results in acute poisoning. Laboratory determinations of arsenic concentrations are used to investigate the cause of toxicity and are performed during the treatment of arsenic poisoning to monitor the effectiveness of therapy.

Signs and Symptoms
Chronic arsenic poisoning has an insidious onset, manifested in the early stages by such nonspecific symptoms as diarrhea, fatigue, muscular weakness, weight loss, nausea, bleeding gums, and dermatitis. As poisoning continues, toxic symptoms progress to include hyperkeratosis, skin pigmentation, motor paralysis, peripheral neuritis, respiratory tract inflammation, gastrointestinal distress, progressive liver disorders with hepatomegaly, renal tubular damage, and encephalopathy.

Acute arsenic poisoning causes a sudden onset of gastrointestinal symptoms such as severe nausea, vomiting, and gastric pain, along with profuse diarrhea and thirst. Later symptoms include dehydration, electrolyte imbalance, metallic taste, garlicky breath, hematuria, jaundice, hypoxia, irritability, convulsions, coma, cardiovascular collapse, and death.

Clinical Significance
Minute quantities of arsenic are ingested routinely with common foods, such as seafood or fruits and vegetables contaminated by insecticidal spray residues, but are present in such small amounts that the individual remains asymptomatic. However, taxidermists, enamelers, painters, metal refiners, landscape gardeners, or workers involved in the manufacture of brass, bronze, and ceramics are exposed routinely to higher arsenic concentrations and are at risk for arsenic intoxication. Arsenic is absorbed well from the gastrointestinal tract and accumulates, within 30 hours after ingestion, in the cells of bone, hair, and nails as they form. Carefully selected and measured hair or nail specimens may be used to detect chronic arsenic exposure and pinpoint the time of exposure. Acute arsenic poisoning may be diagnosed by detecting large concentrations of the substance in the urine, stomach contents, vomitus, or gastric washings.

Normal Values

The normal and toxic arsenic values are:

Normal range—no known exposure

Blood	<1 μg/dL
Gastric contents	None detected
Hair	20–60 μg/100 g
Nails	20–60 μg/100 g
Urine	<100 μg/L

Acceptable level—industrial exposure

Blood	3–7 μg/dL
Hair	<65 μg/100 g
Nails	90–180 μg/100 g
Urine	<200 μg/L

Toxic level

Hair	>100 μg/100 g
Urine	>850 μg/L

Methodology

The specimen of choice for the measurement of arsenic concentrations is a 24-hour urine specimen collected without preservatives and sent to the laboratory in its entirety. When this is not possible, the urine specimen should be mixed well and a 100 mL aliquot sent to the laboratory; the total 24-hour urine volume should be noted on the request slip so that test results can be interpreted properly. Arsenic determinations also may be performed on 0.5 g of hair or nails, 50 mL of gastric washings, or 20 mL of blood collected with sodium or potassium oxalate (black-stoppered tube). However, blood usually is not recommended for the detection of arsenic intoxication because blood concentrations are very low except in acute arsenic poisoning.

▶▶ Nursing Responsibilities and Implications

1. Obtain a health history to document exposure to toxic chemicals that may have precipitated arsenic intoxication.

2. Obtain the specimen following the proper precautions if the test results will be used as legal evidence (see Medicolegal Specimen Collection and Handling earlier in this chapter).

3. Observe the patient for signs of acute and chronic arsenic poisoning.

4. Collect nail, hair, urine, and gastric specimens as indicated.

Iron

Iron, an inorganic element essential to the formation of hemoglobin and various cellular enzymes, is contained in many foods but frequently is administered in therapeutic doses to supplement dietary intake. However, although large iron dosages may be tolerated well by adults, the ingestion of relatively small amounts of iron causes toxicity in children and results in a serious medical emergency. Laboratory measurement of serum iron levels may be used to detect acute iron intoxication following accidental overdose, determine its severity, and monitor the course of therapy. (Serum iron levels are discussed further in Chapter 3.)

Signs and Symptoms

Significant iron intoxication produces gastrointestinal irritation, which is characterized by repeated vomiting, upper abdominal pain, and black, tarry, or bloody diarrhea within 30 minutes to several hours after ingestion. Iron poisoning also may cause cyanosis, drowsiness, lethargy, convulsions, acidosis, cardiovascular collapse, coma, and death within 4−6 hours.

Clinical Significance

Acute ingestion of large amounts of iron damages the gastric and intestinal mucosa, producing severe ulceration and occasionally massive hemorrhage. Depending on the size of the child, a single iron dose of 150 mg/kg or a total of 3 g or more may be fatal. If death does not occur within the first few hours following iron poisoning, the patient usually enters an asymptomatic phase in which improvement occurs either spontaneously or in response to treatment. Such improvement may progress to complete recovery or may be disrupted within 18−24 hours by a progressive cardiovascular collapse that often leads to death. Individuals who survive iron poisoning experience a phase of gastrointestinal obstruction several weeks or months later due to severe scarring of the intestinal mucosa caused by the corrosive injury.

Normal Values

The normal and toxic iron values are:

60−200 μg/dL	Normal range
<350 μg/dL	No significant toxicity
>500 μg/dL	Toxic level
>600 μg/dL	Serious iron poisoning
>700 μg/dL	Shock, coma, death

Methodology

Iron measurements require 3 mL of blood collected without anticoagulants (red-stoppered tube) and without hemolysis. Test results are most significant if the specimen is collected after iron absorption is complete but before protein binding and tissue distribution cause peak serum concentrations to fall. Thus, a serum specimen should be obtained within 1−2 hours of ingestion and a second serum sample collected several hours later.

▶▶ Nursing Responsibilities and Implications

1. Obtain a health history to document the recent ingestion of iron.

2. Observe the patient for signs of iron intoxication or poisoning.

3. Monitor fluid intake and output if the patient has diarrhea and/or vomiting.
4. Provide safety measures if the patient is weak, drowsy, or lethargic; institute seizure precautions if serum iron values are above 600 μg/dL.

Lead

Lead, a toxic metal that interferes with heme synthesis, commonly is used in the manufacture of storage batteries, rubber, some paints and enamels, unglazed pottery, and gasoline. It enters the body through the gastrointestinal and respiratory tracts, accumulates slowly, especially in bone, and is excreted even more slowly in the urine, causing a cumulative effect. Toxic lead accumulations can produce both chronic and acute forms of poisoning, which are characterized by increased blood and urine lead levels and elevated erythrocyte protoporphyrin values. (Free erythrocyte protoporphyrin is discussed in Chapter 3.)

Chronic intoxication is the most frequently encountered form of lead poisoning and results from repeated exposure to small amounts of lead compounds. However, chronic lead intoxication can coexist with normal blood and urine levels due to the deposition of lead in bone and body tissues. Conversely, acute lead poisoning usually follows a single exposure to large amounts of lead compounds but also may occur after prolonged chronic exposure with the abrupt release of large lead stores from the bones. Laboratory measurements of blood and urine lead concentrations are used to verify lead poisoning and can identify an acute episode superimposed on chronic lead intoxication. Determinations of erythrocyte protoporphyrin levels provide a sensitive index of lead toxicity and confirm chronic lead exposure in individuals with increased blood lead concentrations.

Signs and Symptoms

The early symptoms of chronic lead poisoning are nonspecific and include facial pallor, anorexia, lethargy, malaise, weight loss, abdominal colic, constipation, vomiting, headaches, weakness, apathy, and muscle pains. In prolonged lead exposure, lead compounds may be deposited in a bluish-black line (lead line) at the gingival margin.

Severe lead intoxication affects the hematopoietic system, producing basophilic stippling and anemia, and often causes neurologic manifestations, which may resemble the symptoms of a brain tumor. Acute neurologic toxicity, which may develop without previous symptoms, frequently produces irreversible damage such as mental retardation, seizure disorders, behavior abnormalities, and occasionally blindness, aphasia, and hemiparesis. The resulting lead encephalopathy is characterized by a sudden onset of cerebral edema, clumsiness, irritability, delirium, neuromuscular excitement, convulsions, and coma.

Clinical Significance

Lead is a common environmental constituent, with trace amounts found normally in plant and animal foodstuffs and larger amounts used in many industrial processes. The blood levels at which lead intoxication is manifested vary depending on the individual's age and nutritional status. The detection and treatment of lead intoxication before symptoms become obvious are important because poisoning may be fatal. Thus, potential lead toxicity should be investigated in workers in high-risk occupations and in any anemic child with a history of eating dirt or other nonfood materials.

Lead intoxication probably is most common in children who chew lead-based paint, which contains as much as 10,000 μg of lead in each chip, from the flaking surfaces of toys, furniture, and walls. Clinical lead intoxication also may occur in plumbers, solderers, painters, and individuals involved in the manufacture of lubricants, ceramics, and insecticides. In addition, workers routinely exposed to automobile emissions or fumes from burning storage batteries and individuals who remove old paint in poorly ventilated areas are susceptible to lead intoxication. Toxic blood and urine lead levels also are observed in persons who drank whiskey that was distilled in lead-contaminated equipment and those who prepared or ate food in unglazed pottery.

Normal Values

The normal and toxic lead values are:

Blood

<30 μg/dL	Normal
30−50 μg/dL	Acceptable industrial exposure; mildly elevated
50−80 μg/dL	Excessive exposure; toxicity
>80 μg/dL	Poisoning
>100 μg/dL	Lead encephalopathy in children

Urine

<80 μg/L	Normal
80−120 μg/L	Acceptable industrial exposure; mildly elevated
>120 μg/L	Excessive exposure; toxicity
>150 μg/L	Poisoning

Free erythrocyte protoporphyrin

<60 μg/dL	Normal
60−100 μg/dL	Acceptable industrial exposure; mildly elevated
100−150 μg/dL	Excessive exposure; toxicity
>190 μg/dL	Poisoning

Methodology

Measurements of lead or erythrocyte protoporphyrin values require 5 mL of blood collected in heparin, oxalate, or EDTA anticoagulant (green-, black-, or lavender-stoppered tube). Although specimens for erythrocyte protoporphyrin determinations are not affected by exposure to environmental lead, specimens for blood lead analysis must be handled scrupulously to avoid such contamination. Therefore, some laboratories prefer to collect specimens for blood lead determinations in specially treated lead-free tubes (brown-stoppered tube).

Measurement of urinary lead excretion requires a 24-hour urine specimen collected without preservatives in a special large, lead-free glass bottle. Makeshift containers, such as bottles or jars with metallic lids, are not suitable containers for collecting or transporting urine specimens for lead determinations because contamination could produce falsely elevated test results. A diagnosis of lead poisoning cannot be excluded on the basis of normal urine lead content alone. Lead is a general systemic poison that affects renal function, causing urine lead concentrations that may not correlate with the symptoms or the blood or erythrocyte protoporphyrin levels.

Precautions

To ensure accurate test results, the following precautions should be observed:

1. Maintain the patient on a low-calcium diet for at least 3 days prior to urine lead analysis to mobilize lead stores from bone and prevent false-negative test results.

2. Use lead-free containers to collect blood and urine specimens.

▶▶ Nursing Responsibilities and Implications

1. Obtain a health history to document acute or chronic exposure to lead; determine whether there is any evidence of pica.

2. Observe the patient for signs of lead intoxication.

3. Provide adequate hydration to prevent hemoconcentration.

4. Monitor the patient's fluid intake and output because increased serum lead levels may interfere with renal function.

5. Prepare the patient for chelation therapy, which involves several painful injections; calcium disodium edetate (EDTA) and dimercaprol (BAL) are commonly used.

6. Provide safety measures, including seizure precautions.

7. Provide teaching to prevent a recurrence; teaching may include the identification and removal of lead from the home, precautions for limiting exposure in lead-related occupations, measures to prevent pica, and the need for continued medical supervision.

Mercury

Mercury, a metallic element also known as quicksilver, formerly was used widely in purgatives, antisyphilitics, disinfectants, astringents, intestinal antiseptics, and as an alternative treatment for chronic inflammation. It currently is used in the manufacture of many agricultural and industrial products, including scientific instruments, electric lamps, agricultural poisons, germicides, herbicides, and dyes. However, because mercury produces a variety of chronic and acute toxic manifestations when ingested, inhaled, or absorbed through the skin, the therapeutic use of mercurial agents is diminishing.

Mercury intoxication results from prolonged or excessive exposure to inorganic mercury salts, such as mercury chloride, or organic mercury compounds. The most toxic of the environmental mercury contaminants are organic ethyl and methyl mercurials, which are several hundred times more toxic than inorganic mercury compounds. The most reliable way to assess inorganic mercury exposure is the measurement of urinary mercury excretion; exposure to organic mercury compounds is analyzed best with whole blood. Laboratory determination of mercury concentrations cannot positively diagnose mercury poisoning but does indicate the degree of exposure to help prevent the development of toxicity in industrially exposed individuals.

Signs and Symptoms

Acute mercury ingestion immediately produces local symptoms such as a metallic taste, burning throat, severe abdominal pain, and laryngeal edema, which usually persist for 24–48 hours. Early symptoms of acute poisoning occur during the first few hours after mercury absorption and include salivation, excitement, restlessness, disorientation, stupor, and coma. The later symptoms of acute poisoning are marked vomiting, bloody diarrhea, oliguria, rapid, weak pulse, fluid and electrolyte imbalance, slow respirations, shock, circulatory collapse, and death.

The early symptoms of chronic mercury intoxication include stomatitis, metallic taste, a blue line on the gingival margin, sore gums that bleed easily, gingivitis, loosening of the teeth, headache, and corneal opacity. Continued chronic exposure is characterized by later symptoms such as generalized edema, colitis, progressive renal damage, peripheral neuritis, irritability, behavioral changes, tremors, bleeding stools, shock, and circulatory collapse. Chronic poisoning with organic mercury compounds produces central nervous system symptoms, including ataxia, grotesque movements, paralysis, inability to concentrate, apathy, and fatigue, and progresses with severe intoxication to coma and death. Chronic inhalation of mercury vapors causes pneumonitis, bronchitis, fever, cough, chest pain, and other symptoms of pulmonary irritation.

Clinical Significance

Acute mercury poisoning may result from organic mercury exposure but usually is caused by the ingestion of inorganic mercury salts, which accumulate in all tissues, particularly the kidneys, brain, and lungs. Chronic mercury poisoning occurs following prolonged absorption or ingestion of low concentrations of mercury salts or continued exposure and inhalation of mercury vapors and fine dust. Inhalation of mercury vapors causes elemental mercury to pass into the bloodstream, penetrate the blood-brain barrier, and accumulate in the central nervous system.

Hazardous mercury exposure and the excretion of larger than normal urinary concentrations may occur in jewelers, photographers, taxidermists, and workers involved in the manufacture of paper, caustic soda, batteries, and dental amalgams. Industrial contamination of waterways with organic mercury compounds causes high concentrations to occur in fish, gradually accumulate in humans, and produce symptoms of chronic toxicity. However, although mercury excretion continues for months after exposure has stopped, the quantity of urinary mercury excretion is not related to the severity of the clinical symptoms of intoxication.

Normal Values

The normal and toxic mercury values are:

Blood

<3.0 μg/dL	Normal environmental exposure; nonindustrial population
>10.0 μg/dL	Increased exposure; not necessarily toxic

Urine

<20 μg/L	Normal environmental exposure; nonindustrial population
<150 μg/L	Acceptable industrial exposure; not necessarily toxic
>150 μg/L	Toxic level

Methodology

Mercury determinations require 5 mL of blood collected with heparin (green-stoppered tube) or a 24-hour urine specimen collected without preservatives. Because urine mercury excretion rates vary considerably within a single patient, as well as among symptomatic patients, a 24-hour urine specimen should be collected for quantitation, with the total volume noted on the laboratory request slip.

Precautions

Test values for mercury concentrations may be falsely decreased in patients receiving iodine-containing medications.

▶▶ Nursing Responsibilities and Implications

1. Obtain a health history to document acute or chronic exposure to mercury.

2. Note on the laboratory slip if the patient is receiving iodine-containing medications, which may falsely decrease serum mercury concentrations.

3. Observe the patient for signs of acute or chronic mercury intoxication.

MISCELLANEOUS SUBSTANCES

Bromide

Bromide, a central nervous system depressant, is a common constituent of a variety of patent medicine preparations used as sedatives and anticonvulsive agents. Bromide-containing drugs formerly enjoyed widespread medical endorsement, but their use has diminished because of their toxicity and the increasing availability of less toxic hypnotic agents and sedatives. However, chronic bromide intoxication is not uncommon, especially in individuals who are prone to treating themselves with over-the-counter preparations such as Bromo-Seltzer, which have a cumulative effect.

Bromide also is used extensively in photography and the chemical industry, and chronic exposure occurs among petroleum refinery workers, chemists, dye makers, and photographers. Bromide is absorbed rapidly from the large and small intestines following ingestion but is eliminated slowly through all excretory routes, including urine, sweat, tears, and nasal excretions. Laboratory determination of bromide concentration is used to diagnose excess bromide ingestion and toxicity as the cause of psychotic behavior or inexplicable neurologic disorders.

Signs and Symptoms

Mild bromide intoxication can result from chronic bromide ingestion and produces a variety of nonspecific symptoms, including fever, anorexia, irritability, agitation, skin rash (ulceration, delayed healing), nausea, and vomiting. Severe bromide intoxication is characterized by neurologic disturbances such as tremors and motor incoordination, delirium, hypothermia, impaired intellectual function, emotional instability, shallow respirations, and coma. In general, toxic symptoms become increasingly severe as bromide levels increase, although some patients may show signs of severe intoxication when the drug is present in relatively low concentrations.

Clinical Significance

The response to increased bromide concentrations varies considerably from person to person, but in general alcoholics are especially susceptible to bromide intoxication. Large doses of bromide preparations irritate the gastrointestinal tract, which usually discourages massive ingestion, although rare fatalities may occur when children accidentally ingest bromide preparations. Bromide excretion is rapid in the early stages after ingestion but subsequently slows down, and it may take as long as 3 weeks for the bromide to be excreted completely once ingestion has stopped.

Normal Values

Normally, bromide levels in the blood are low; therapeutic and toxic levels are:

<20 mg/dL	Normal level
20–90 mg/dL	Therapeutic range
>100 mg/dL	Toxic level
>250 mg/dL	Psychotic behavior

Methodology

Bromide determinations require 5 mL of blood collected without anticoagulants (red-stoppered tube) or with heparin (green-stoppered tube).

▶▶ Nursing Responsibilities and Implications

1. Obtain a health history to document exposure to bromide; include both over-the-counter and prescribed medications because many drugs contain bromide compounds.

2. Observe the patient for signs of chronic bromide ingestion.

3. Provide adequate fluids and monitor the patient's urinary output because bromide compounds are excreted primarily by the kidneys.

Methotrexate

Methotrexate, a folic acid antagonist with immunosuppressive and antitumor activity, inhibits the ability of cells to produce the purine and nucleic acid required for DNA synthesis and cell replication. Methotrexate has long been used in chronic low-dose oral therapy for severe psoriasis, and more recently has been administered in high-dose intravenous infusions for the treatment of various cancers. Methotrexate therapy is indicated for bone marrow transplantation, breast carcinoma, acute lymphocytic and childhood leukemias, brain tumors, choriocarcinoma, osteogenic sarcoma, sarcoidosis, non-Hodgkin's lymphoma, and other highly malignant tumors. However, methotrexate is quite toxic when administered in high doses over an extended period of time, causing severe intoxication, which may be fatal. Laboratory monitoring of methotrexate concentrations in patients receiving massive intravenous infusions is helpful in evaluating the efficacy of treatment and adjusting the dosage to achieve the maximum chemotherapeutic effects with the fewest toxic effects.

Signs and Symptoms

Low- to medium-dose methotrexate therapy may produce toxic side effects such as ulcerations of the mouth, hepatotoxicity with hepatitis, leukopenia, and gastrointestinal mucositis with nausea, vomiting, and diarrhea. Patients receiving high-dose methotrexate therapy are at high risk of developing serious toxicity, including hematologic reactions characterized by anemia, B-lymphocyte dysfunction, and thrombocytopenia, along with nephrotoxicity and acute dermatitis. Intrathecal methotrexate therapy causes acute neurotoxicity, which is characterized by headaches, dizziness, backaches, fever, and convulsions; a less acute form of neurotoxicity that produces motor dysfunction may develop several weeks after therapy begins.

Clinical Significance

Because methotrexate is excreted primarily through the kidneys, clearance of the drug from the body depends on the effectiveness of renal function. Thus, any potential decrease in methotrexate clearance is signaled and accompanied by an equal decrease in the rate of creatinine clearance. Therefore, a patient's ability to accommodate high-dose methotrexate infusions may be predicted by carefully monitoring creatinine clearance values prior to and during therapy to help interpret serum drug levels.

Because methotrexate is a relatively insoluble compound, toxic blood levels cause the drug to precipitate and be deposited in the renal tubules when the urine pH is below 5.5. In addition, the incidence of methotrexate toxicity increases when salicylate is administered concurrently. Methotrexate therapy produces falsely elevated cerebrospinal fluid protein values, which must be considered when interpreting cerebrospinal fluid protein values during intrathecal methotrexate therapy for such malignancies as meningeal leukemias and lymphomas.

Normal Values

Methotrexate appears in the blood only during therapy; the range of therapeutic values depends on the dosage regimen employed. Toxic methotrexate levels obtained 48 hours after dose administration are:

<21 μg/mL	Severe toxicity unlikely
>41 μg/mL	Toxic level; myelosuppressive and nephrotoxic complications

---

Methodology

Methotrexate determinations require 5 mL of blood collected without anticoagulants (red-stoppered tube). Specimens should be drawn 24, 48, and 72 hours after the start of intravenous methotrexate therapy to obtain good predictive information regarding the potential degree of toxicity that may be associated with a particular dosage.

▶▶ Nursing Responsibilities and Implications

1. Obtain blood specimens 24, 48, and 72 hours after the start of intravenous methotrexate therapy.

2. Obtain blood and urine specimens prior to and during therapy so that creatinine clearance values can be determined; methotrexate is nephrotoxic and the glomerular

filtration rate is an indicator of the individual's ability to tolerate high-dose metho-trexate therapy; monitor the patient's fluid intake and output.

3. Monitor urinary pH; maintain urine pH above 5.5 to limit nephrotoxicity; encourage an acid ash diet, if necessary.

4. Observe the patient for signs of methotrexate intoxication, particularly if the patient is receiving concomitant salicylate therapy.

5. Monitor the patient's blood values for anemia, leukopenia, and thrombocytopenia because methotrexate depresses bone marrow activity; observe the patient for bleed-ing tendencies if the number of platelets is decreased, institute protective isolation if the number of white blood cells is severely depressed, and encourage bedrest if the number of red blood cells is decreased.

Theophylline

Theophylline, a potent smooth muscle relaxant and cardiac stimulant, commonly is used as a bronchodilator in the treatment of bronchial asthma, emphysema, and the reversible bronchspasms of obstructive pulmonary diseases. It may be administered intravenously to stimulate respiration during acute bronchial asthma or orally in a long-term therapeutic regimen to control chronic asthma. However, because theophylline has a narrow thera-peutic range, dosage adjustments based on clinical response alone can result in the abrupt onset of serious toxic reactions. Laboratory monitoring of theophylline concentrations helps to maintain serum values within the optimum range and prevent the accumulation of toxic levels.

Signs and Symptoms

Side effects of chronic theophylline ingestion are related to its stimulatory action on the central nervous system and include irritability, anorexia, headaches, insomnia, and anxi-ety. Because theophylline also enhances gastric secretion, its use may produce nausea, vomiting, and gastric irritation even at levels well within the therapeutic range. As blood concentrations increase above the toxic level, symptoms of theophylline toxicity progress from hematuria, tremors, delirium, and fever to palpitations, tachycardia, convulsions, respiratory failure, and cardiac arrest.

Clinical Significance

Theophylline degradation and half-life are significantly prolonged by the concurrent use of certain antibiotics, compromised cardiac or hepatic status, and the effects of growth and maturation on the metabolic rate. Thus patients receiving troleandomycin or erythro-mycin, elderly patients, and individuals with ventricular failure, acute pulmonary edema, liver dysfunction, or chronic obstructive pulmonary disease require lower theophylline dosages to maintain therapeutic levels and avoid intoxication. For example, patients with congestive heart failure or liver dysfunction frequently require only half the normal the-ophylline dose, whereas dosages may be reduced by approximately one-third in patients over 50 years of age.

Conversely, theophylline's half-life is significantly shorter in young smokers, and higher doses are needed for bronchodilation in these individuals than in patients who do not smoke. In addition, theophylline potentiates the effect of catecholamines and has a synergistic effect when combined with ephedrine.

Normal Values

Theophylline is not normally present in the blood; the therapeutic and toxic values are:

<2 μg/mL	Dietary xanthine intake
5–10 μg/mL	Slight therapeutic effect
10–20 μg/mL	Optimum therapeutic range
15–20 μg/mL	Some adverse effects
>20 μg/mL	Toxic level; anorexia, nausea, vomiting, abdominal discomfort
30–60 μg/mL	Severe toxicity; cardiac arrhythmias, seizures, respiratory failure, cardiac arrest

---

Methodology

Theophylline determinations require 3 mL of blood collected without anticoagulants (red-stoppered tube). Once steady-state levels are reached, specimens should be obtained approximately 3 hours after drug administration as well as immediately prior to the next dose. Consistent use of the same time interval between dose administration and sampling is important when comparing test results for possible dosage adjustment.

Precautions

To ensure accurate test results; the following precautions should be observed:

1. Avoid the concurrent use of furosemide, barbiturates, phenylbutazone, sulfonamides, or xanthines such as caffeine and theobromine because these substances interfere with certain methods for measuring theophylline and may alter the test results.

2. Instruct the patient not to drink tea, coffee, cocoa, chocolate, or cola for at least 12 hours before testing because these substances contain xanthine, which will increase the theophylline values.

▶▶ Nursing Responsibilities and Implications

1. Begin therapeutic monitoring only after the patient has been receiving theophylline for 72 hours.

2. When performing serial determinations, observe the same time interval between drug administration and specimen collection. To monitor peak levels, the blood sample should be obtained about 2 hours after drug administration; to monitor trough levels, the blood sample should be obtained just prior to the next dose.

3. Note on the laboratory slip any medications the patient is receiving.

4. Instruct the patient to avoid substances that contain xanthine, such as tea, coffee, cocoa, cola, and chocolate, for 12 hours before the test.

5. Observe the patient for signs of theophylline intoxication.

6. Monitor the patient's vital signs frequently.

PSYCHOTHERAPEUTIC DRUGS

Lithium

Lithium, usually administered as a carbonate salt, is widely used to control manic-depressive disorders and also is an important supplement to or alternative for the treatment of other psychologic disturbances. Lithium therapy limits the depressive phase and lowers the excitement phase of acute mania by normalizing the increased psychomotor activity and emotional lability without producing the drugged feelings associated with other antipsychotic agents. In general, approximately two-thirds of the lithium concentration necessary to attain remission of mania is required to maintain the mania-free state without undesirable side effects.

However, the range between therapeutic and toxic lithium levels is quite narrow, and results in toxic side effects involving the central nervous system and kidneys when lithium concentrations exceed the therapeutic level. Thus, regular monitoring is required in patients receiving lithium therapy to maintain effective nontoxic concentrations and prevent the irreversible, fatal toxic effects that result when concentrations are four to six times higher than therapeutic levels (Table 7-7). Laboratory determinations of lithium concentrations are the most effective means of monitoring a dosage regimen to maintain appropriate therapeutic levels and avoid lithium intoxication.

Signs and Symptoms

Undesirable, but expected, side effects of lithium administration may occur at any plasma concentration and include gastric irritation, fatigue, drowsiness, and fine muscle tremors, which generally subside when the drug is reduced to therapeutic levels. Toxic manifestations of lithium therapy progress from mild to severe as serum levels increase above the therapeutic range. Symptoms of mild to moderate lithium intoxication include gastrointestinal disturbances such as anorexia, vomiting, diarrhea, and abdominal pain, together with neuromuscular irritation characterized by slurred speech, coarse tremors, muscle weakness and twitching, unsteady gait, sedation, and ataxia. Acute lithium intoxication is associated with aphasia, confusion, delirium, hyperreflexia, clonic contractions, stupor, chorea, athetosis, coma, cardiac arrhythmias, circulatory failure, and death due to central nervous system depression and cardiovascular collapse.

Toxic lithium levels also produce irreversible renal damage, which frequently leads to oliguria, anuria, and glycosuria. Miscellaneous side effects of lithium toxicity include

TABLE 7-7   Characteristics of Psychotherapeutic Agents

Drug	Half-Life	Peak Concentrations	Steady-State Levels
Lithium	8–35 hours	1–3 days	2–7 days
Amitriptyline	17–40 hours	2–8 hours	4–8 days
Nortriptyline	18–93 hours	2–8 hours	4–19 days
Imipramine	9–24 hours	1–2 hours	2–5 days
Desipramine	14–54 hours	2–6 hours	3–11 days
Doxepin	17 hours	2–6 hours	4 days
Protriptyline	54–198 hours	6–12 hours	10–40 days

acne, exacerbation of psoriasis, alopecia, vertigo, headache, blurred vision, increased serum calcium, magnesium, glucose, and parathormone levels, and decreased thyroid function tests. The nurse should caution the patient and family to stop taking the medication immediately and notify the physician if any symptoms of lithium toxicity develop.

Clinical Significance

Regular monitoring of lithium concentrations is necessary in any patient receiving lithium therapy, but it is essential in the elderly and patients with diabetes, epilepsy, poor general health, or a diminished renal capacity. Lithium is cleared from the body by the kidneys, and major toxic side effects occur in patients with impaired renal function or fluid and electrolyte imbalance. Lithium therapy therefore is contraindicated in patients with renal disease, as well as those with cardiac disease and women of childbearing age.

Lithium toxicity occurs in patients in whom lithium retention is increased because of a sodium deficiency, either due to a salt-restricted diet or loss of sodium from diarrhea or dehydration. The potential for lithium toxicity also is increased by methyldopa and the concomitant use of thiazide diuretics, which cause the body to lose sodium and therefore to retain lithium. For this reason, cardiac patients are more susceptible to lithium toxicity because they often are given salt-depleting diuretic medications, which may cause lithium-related arrhythmias.

Conversely, lithium excretion is enhanced by increased sodium intake and conditions associated with salt retention, lowering plasma levels below the therapeutic range. Lithium increases the toxic potential of supplemental psychotherapeutic drugs, which frequently are used in the management of acutely psychotic patients being treated with high doses of lithium. Thus, the concomitant use of haloperidol, phenothiazines, tricyclic antidepressants, diazepam, and oxazepam produces an additive antidepressant effect that may necessitate a reduction in the lithium dosage.

Normal Values

Lithium normally appears in the blood only during therapy; the therapeutic and toxic lithium values are:

<0.1 mEq/L	Reference levels; nontherapeutic
0.6–1.4 mEq/L	Therapeutic range; nontoxic side effects
1.5–2.5 mEq/L	Mild toxicity; drowsiness, diarrhea, vomiting, polyuria, neuromuscular symptomatology
2.5–3.5 mEq/L	Marked toxicity; tremors, myoclonic jerks, cogwheel rigidity
3.5–4.5 mEq/L	Life-threatening toxicity; pulmonary complications
>4.5 mEq/L	Lethal level

Methodology

Accurate lithium measurements require 3 mL of blood collected without anticoagulants (red-stoppered tube) 8–12 hours after the last oral dose. The most effective guide to therapy is obtained when levels are monitored 2 and 5 days after therapy begins, followed by weekly monitoring and dosage adjustments for the first month. Thereafter, chronic lithium therapy should be monitored monthly or as clinically indicated by toxic symptoms.

▶▶ *Nursing Responsibilities and Implications*

1. Begin therapeutic monitoring only after the patient has been receiving lithium for 2−5 days; lithium blood levels should be obtained weekly for 1 month and then monthly; a lithium blood level should be performed whenever the patient exhibits signs of toxicity.

2. Obtain blood samples 8−12 hours after the last oral dose; when performing serial determinations, observe the same time interval between drug administration and specimen collection.

3. Observe all patients for signs of intoxication, particularly those who are elderly, receiving other medications, or have concomitant illnesses; withhold the medication and notify the physician if toxicity occurs.

4. Encourage the patient to ingest adequate fluids and sodium because lithium limits antidiuretic hormone (ADH) secretion, thus promoting fluid excretion; observe the patient for signs of dehydration; diuretics should be avoided.

5. Teach the patient and family the signs and symptoms of toxicity; instruct the patient to stop the medication and notify the physician if toxicity occurs.

Phenothiazines

The phenothiazines generally are used as antipsychotic tranquilizing drugs, although they also have antihistaminic, antipruritic, and antiemetic properties. This widely distributed and frequently prescribed group of medications includes chlorpromazine, promazine hydrochloride, prochlorperazine, promethazine hydrochloride, thioridazine, and trifluoperazine, among others. Phenothiazines have a high therapeutic index and rarely cause severe intoxication because extremely large amounts are needed to produce toxicity in adults. However, phenothiazines may cause marked intoxication in infants, young adults, and febrile or dehydrated patients and, although fatalities are exceedingly rare, these drugs often are used in suicide attempts. Laboratory screening for phenothiazines occasionally is helpful in emergency situations to determine if a patient has taken any of these drugs.

Signs and Symptoms

Each phenothiazine medication exerts its own characteristic normal and toxic side effects, but many reactions are common to the entire group of compounds. In general, the side effects accompanying therapeutic phenothiazine administration include drowsiness, disorientation, restlessness, weakness, anxiety, palpitations, visual disturbances, nasal congestion, dry mucosa, and dermatologic reactions. In addition, phenothiazines are hepatotoxic, producing characteristic jaundice and abnormal liver function tests in susceptible patients. Following severe overdose, symptoms of phenothiazine intoxication include tremors, rigidity, motor disorders, salivation, spasms, muscle twitching, postural hypotension, chills, convulsions, cardiovascular depression, shock, coma, and cardiac arrhythmias.

Clinical Significance

The presence of phenothiazine drugs in the system greatly prolongs the depressant effects of alcohol, barbiturates, morphine, and meperidine, all of which may be used in suicide attempts. Phenothiazine levels in the blood generally are very low because these compounds are bound rapidly in the tissues. However, they are excreted very slowly by the kidneys, so their presence may be demonstrated in urine specimens for prolonged periods after administration. In fact, traces of unchanged phenothiazines and their derivatives can persist in the urine for many months and in tissues for up to 1 year after discontinuing a long-term therapeutic drug regimen.

Normal Values

Normally, phenothiazine compounds are not present in the body; therapeutic and toxic values vary depending on the particular phenothiazine used. Phenothiazine determinations usually are performed as qualitative screening tests on urine or gastric fluid, with the results reported only as positive or negative for the presence of these drugs in the body.

Methodology

Tests for phenothiazine drugs require a 100 mL random urine sample collected in a routine specimen container. The detection of phenothiazines in stomach contents requires 20 mL of gastric secretions or washings.

Tricyclic Antidepressants

The tricyclic antidepressants are used to treat endogenous depression, enuresis, bipolar disorder—depressed phase, minimal brain damage, hyperactivity, and cataleptic attacks associated with narcolepsy. The group of tricyclic antidepressants includes amitriptyline and its metabolite nortriptyline, imipramine and its metabolite desipramine, doxepin, and protriptyline. The sedative and anticholinergic effects produced by these drugs block the reuptake of norepinephrine and serotonin to help control the genetic biochemical abnormality that causes many incapacitating endogenous depressions. These primary depressions affect the ability of an individual to cope with the environment and disrupt body rhythms such as sleep, appetite, sexual drive, and motor activity. Laboratory measurement of tricyclic antidepressant levels is used to assess therapeutic response, evaluate suspected symptoms of toxicity, establish evidence of overdose, and monitor dissipation of the drug during clinical recovery.

Signs and Symptoms

The adverse reactions associated with tricyclic antidepressant therapy are comparatively minor and include autonomic nervous system, metabolic, and psychiatric or neurologic effects, along with cardiovascular disturbances. The most frequent side effects are attributed to anticholinergic action and include dry mouth, dizziness, blurred vision, palpitations, severe sweating, paralytic ileus; constipation, delayed ejaculation, and urinary retention. Additional side effects of therapeutic tricyclic antidepressant therapy include confusional states, tremors, headaches, epigastric distress, ataxia, tachycardia, and orthostatic hypotension.

Acute intoxication resulting from tricyclic antidepressant overdose produces seizures, convulsions, hyperpyrexia, neuromuscular irritability, bowel or bladder paralysis, blood pressure changes, respiratory depression, cyanosis, shock, delirium, and coma. Cardiac disturbances are the most life threatening of the toxic symptoms and include supraventricular arrhythmia and electrocardiographic abnormalities such as prolonged PR and QRS intervals and T-wave changes. Untreated tricyclic antidepressant intoxication progresses to respiratory depression, which is characterized by irregular, weak, and rapid breathing, hypoxia, and subsequent respiratory arrest.

Clinical Significance

The therapeutic range reported for the tricyclic antidepressants represents the combined value resulting from the cumulative effect of a parent drug and its active metabolite. For example, when amitriptyline or imipramine is administered as the parent drug, the action of their respective derivatives, nortriptyline and desipramine, also must be considered in determining the plasma concentration and evaluating the total therapeutic effect. Because many side effects of tricyclic antidepressant therapy resemble symptoms of depression, plasma concentrations both above and below the therapeutic range may be associated with a lack of clinical improvement. Thus, routine monitoring of tricyclic antidepressant levels during therapy is used to determine if the clinical increase in the patient's depression results from poor dosage compliance or concentrations above the therapeutic range.

When the liver's capacity to metabolize tricyclic antidepressant derivatives becomes saturated by overdose, any further increase in the level of the parent drug or metabolite causes a disproportionate increase in plasma concentrations and keeps levels high. For this reason, plasma concentrations may remain at toxic levels for 5−6 days following acute tricyclic antidepressant ingestion and serious overdose. This sustained elevation in drug levels may be a contributing factor in cardiac death occurring 3−6 days after the overdose, and continuous cardiac monitoring is needed if serious overdose is suspected (see Table 7-7).

The concomitant administration of enzyme-inducer drugs such as phenobarbital accelerates the rate of metabolism of tricyclic antidepressants and lowers the effective plasma level, whereas methylphenidate, neuroleptic, and corticosteroid therapy increase tricyclic antidepressant levels. On the other hand, the tricyclic antidepressants enhance the cardiotoxic effects of quinidine, procainamide, and thioridazine but reverse the antihypertensive effects of guanethidine, methyldopa, and clonidine. The concurrent use of tricyclic antidepressants and sedatives or alcohol produces an additive effect.

Normal Values

Tricyclic antidepressants are present in the blood and urine only during therapy; the therapeutic and toxic levels in the blood are:

Amitriptyline plus nortriptyline

120−250 ng/mL	Therapeutic range
>500 ng/mL	Toxic level

(continued)

Normal Values (Continued)

Nortriptyline (taken as the parent drug)

50–150 ng/mL	Therapeutic range
>500 ng/mL	Toxic level

Imipramine plus desipramine

150–300 ng/mL	Therapeutic range
>1000 ng/mL	Toxic level

Desipramine (taken as the parent drug)

20–160 ng/mL	Therapeutic range
>1000 ng/mL	Toxic level

Doxepin

100–240 ng/mL	Therapeutic range
>1000 ng/mL	Toxic level

Protriptyline

50–150 ng/mL	Therapeutic range
?	Toxic level not established

Methodology

Tricyclic antidepressant determinations require 10 mL of urine for qualitative measurements or 5 mL of blood collected without anticoagulants for quantitative measurements. Blood specimens should be drawn into a syringe and transferred carefully to a clean tube to avoid contact with the rubber stopper of vacuum tubes, which may alter drug levels.

▶▶ **Nursing Responsibilities and Implications**

1. Note on the laboratory slip the specific tricyclic antidepressant the patient is receiving.

2. Observe the patient carefully as the depression lifts because the patient will begin to have enough energy to act on suicidal ideation.

MINOR TRANQUILIZING AGENTS

Benzodiazepines

Benzodiazepines, the most commonly prescribed drugs in the United States, are a group of sedative-hypnotic tranquilizers used for the management of anxiety disorders and the short-term relief of tension. These antianxiety agents also are indicated for the treatment of insomnia, status epilepticus, symptoms of acute alcohol withdrawal, and the induction of amnesia during minor surgical procedures such as colonoscopy. Benzodiazepine compounds such as chlordiazepoxide, clonazepam, clorazepate, diazepam, and flurazepam cause significant toxicity with overdosage and frequently produce adverse reactions in elderly or debilitated individuals at therapeutic doses. Laboratory detection and measurement of benzodiazepine compounds may be included in the investigation of coma resulting from drug overdose and the screening for drug abuse.

Signs and Symptoms

Each benzodiazepine compound produces a unique pattern of adverse reactions, although many side effects and toxic symptoms are common to all benzodiazepines. Initial reactions to benzodiazepine administration may include drowsiness, lethargy, vertigo, ataxia, nystagmus, nausea, blurred vision, and tinnitus, which gradually subside as tolerance develops with continued therapy. The manifestations of toxic overdosage progress as concentrations increase from profound sedation, somnolence, mental confusion, slurred speech, diminished reflexes, and stupor to convulsions, cyanosis, respiratory depression, shock, and coma.

Clinical Significance

Benzodiazepines, particularly chlordiazepoxide, are among the most commonly used agents, either alone or combined with other drugs, in attempted suicides. For example, the concomitant use of barbiturates, tricyclic antidepressants, or alcohol produces an additive central nervous system depressant effect by increasing benzodiazepine levels significantly higher than if the drug were ingested alone (Table 7-8). Thus, multiple drug intake or simultaneous alcohol use must be suspected and investigated in comatose patients following sedative overdose regardless of the benzodiazepine concentrations.

Normal Values

Benzodiazepines normally are not present in the blood; the therapeutic and toxic blood levels are:

Chlordiazepoxide

0.1–3.0 μg/mL	Therapeutic range
>3.0 μg/mL	Toxic level

Clonazepam

5–50 ng/mL	Therapeutic range
?	Toxic level not established

Clorazepate

123–2175 ng/mL	Therapeutic range
>1000 ng/mL	Toxic level

Diazepam

105–1540 ng/mL	Therapeutic range
>3000 ng/mL	Toxic level

Flurazepam

10–140 ng/mL	Therapeutic range (measured as n-desalkylflurazepam metabolite)
4–17 ng/mL	Therapeutic range (measured as hydroxyethylflurazepam metabolite)
>2000 ng/mL	Toxic level (measured as flurazepam)

Methodology

Benzodiazepine determinations require 5 mL of blood collected without anticoagulants (red-stoppered tube) or with sodium or potassium oxalate (black-stoppered tube).

TABLE 7-8 Characteristics of Sedative/Tranquilizing Agents

Drugs	Half-Life	Peak Concentrations	Steady-State Levels
Chlordiazepoxide	16−27 hours	2−4 hours	3½−6 days
Clonazepam	18−39 hours	1−2 hours	4−7½ days
Diazepam	21−46 hours	1−1½ hours	5−10 days
Flurazepam	47−100 hours	1−2 hours	7−20 days
Ethchlorvynol	24 hours	1 hour	5 days
Glutethimide	8−18 hours	1−6 hours	2−4 days
Meprobamate	6−17 hours	2 hours	1½−4 days
Methaqualone	33−38 hours	2 hours	7−8 days

▶▶ *Nursing Responsibilities and Implications*

1. Note on the laboratory slip the specific benzodiazepine the patient is receiving.

2. Collect the specimen following the proper precautions if the test results will be used as legal evidence (see Medicolegal Specimen Collection and Handling earlier in this chapter).

3. Observe the patient for side effects; inform the patient that these initial side effects gradually subside as therapy continues.

4. Provide safety measures if the patient is experiencing weakness, lethargy, dizziness, vertigo, ataxia, and/or blurred vision.

5. Observe for and teach the patient and family the signs of toxicity; notify the physician if they occur.

Other Sedative/Tranquilizing Agents

A number of central nervous system depressant compounds belonging to a variety of drug families are used for the short-term therapy of insomnia or anxiety and tension. Medications in this category include ethchlorvynol, glutethimide, meprobamate, methaqualone, and methyprylon, all of which have been implicated in suicide attempts and drug abuse. Long-term administration of these hypnotic agents is not recommended because prolonged use frequently produces tolerance, which can progress to physical and psychologic dependence. Laboratory detection and measurement of drugs in the sedative/tranquilizer group are important to the investigation of toxic symptoms or coma resulting from chronic and acute overdosage or multiple drug ingestion.

Signs and Symptoms

Each sedative and tranquilizing agent produces its own pattern of reactions to therapeutic use as well as chronic and acute overdose, although there are many similarities. Adverse side effects of therapeutic administration result from central nervous system depression and gastrointestinal disturbances and include drowsiness, dizziness, anorexia, nausea, vomiting, blurred vision, hangover, headache, and numbness of the extremities. In general, chronic overdosage is characterized by ataxia, tremors, impaired memory and inability to concentrate, diminished reflexes, muscle weakness, slurred speech, lowered pulse and blood pressure, somnolence, constricted pupils, and confusion. Manifestations of acute overdosage include cyanosis, anoxia, respiratory depression and collapse, shock, severe hypotension, occasional convulsions, profound coma, tachycardia, arrhythmia, hypothermia, pulmonary edema, and occasionally cardiac arrest.

Clinical Significance

Sedative/tranquilizing drugs, particularly glutethimide, are sequestered in fat deposits in concentrations several times higher than blood, causing the drug to enter the blood and continue its activity after therapy is discontinued. Thus, the extent of intoxication may not be accurately reflected by a single test result, and serial determinations are mandatory to properly evaluate clinical recovery following acute overdosage. The concurrent use of additional central nervous system depressants or tranquilizing agents such as alcohol and barbiturates may produce an additive or exaggerated sedative effect.

Abrupt discontinuation after prolonged and excessive use of these drugs may precipitate a recurrence of preexisting anxiety symptoms or cause severe withdrawal symptoms similar to those observed during alcohol and barbiturate detoxification. These symptoms usually appear within 12–48 hours after discontinuing therapy but may occur up to 9 days later with certain drugs (see Table 7-8).

Normal Values

Sedative and tranquilizing drugs are not normally found in the blood or urine; the therapeutic and toxic blood levels are:

Ethchlorvynol

0.5–6.5 μg/mL	Therapeutic range
>20 μg/mL	Toxic level

Glutethimide

2–6 μg/mL	Therapeutic range
>10 μg/mL	Toxic level
>30 μg/mL	Deep unconsciousness or coma
30–200 μg/mL	Death

Meprobamate

16–27 μg/mL	Therapeutic range
>35 μg/mL	Toxic level
30–100 μg/mL	Mild to moderate toxicity; stupor, light coma
100–200 μg/mL	Deep coma; some fatalities

Methaqualone

0.9–8.0 μg/mL	Therapeutic range
>5.0 μg/mL	Toxic level

Methyprylon

<10 μg/mL	Therapeutic range
>30 μg/mL	Toxic level

Methodology

Quantitative measurement of ethchlorvynol, glutethimide, meprobamate, or methaqualone levels requires 7–10 mL of blood collected without anticoagulants (red-stoppered tube) or with sodium oxalate or EDTA (black- or lavender-stoppered tube); specimens for methyprylon determinations must be collected without anticoagulants. Qualitative detection of these drugs may be performed on a 50 mL random urine specimen collected without preservatives.

▶▶ ### Nursing Responsibilities and Implications

1. Note on the laboratory slip the specific sedative/tranquilizing agent the patient is receiving.

2. Collect the specimen following the proper precautions if the test results will be used as legal evidence (see Medicolegal Specimen Collection and Handling earlier in this chapter).

3. Provide safety measures if the patient is experiencing drowsiness, dizziness, blurred vision, ataxia, diminished reflexes, weakness, low blood pressure, and/or confusion.

4. Observe for and teach the patient and family the signs of toxicity; notify the physician if they occur.

DRUG ABUSE

A variety of therapeutic and illicit drugs are ingested, injected, or inhaled to deliberately produce an unnatural state of euphoria. Abused substances generally are classified as central nervous system stimulants and depressants, narcotic analgesics, cannabinoids, and psychedelics or hallucinogens. These substances frequently are combined to enhance or prolong the intoxication. Therapeutic agents such as amphetamines, barbiturates, glutethimide, and methaqualone are among the central nervous system stimulants and depressants that are commonly abused by unnecessary use or intentional overdose.

Narcotic analgesics are highly addictive substances with limited therapeutic usefulness that are derived from opium or coca or have properties similar to those of morphine. The most commonly abused opiate is heroin, although other narcotic drugs such as morphine, methadone, codeine, cocaine, meperidine, propoxyphene, and oxycodone also are widely abused. Quinine is a non-narcotic substance that often is used as a diluent for heroin and may be detected by tests for drug abuse. Whereas heroin and its metabolite, morphine, generally are eliminated from the body within 2 days, quinine may be detected in the urine for up to 5 days following its use.

Psychotogenic or hallucinogenic drugs have very limited, if any, clinical or medical applications and are used primarily by cults or individuals for religious or "mind-expanding" experiences. They are mainly derived from plant sources and include psilocybin, peyote, mescaline, lysergic acid diethylamine (LSD), and cannabinoids such as hashish and marijuana. Laboratory detection of narcotics, hallucinogens, and other abused substances provides a practical means of diagnosing intoxication and monitoring therapeutic maintenance programs and is more clinically important than quantitative measurement (see the following section on Drug Screening).

Signs and Symptoms

Narcotic intoxication produces central nervous system depression, which is characterized by drowsiness, euphoria, mental clouding, hypothermic shock, urinary retention, cyanosis, coma, and marked respiratory depression that may cause death. Although cocaine is classified as a narcotic, its systemic effect is central nervous system stimulation, which produces symptoms that generally are opposite to those associated with opiates. Symptoms of cocaine intoxication include excitement, restlessness, garrulousness, anxiety, confusion, hyperreflexia, headache, tachycardia, hyperthermia, mydriasis, Cheyne-Stokes respiration, and convulsions.

Hallucinogenic intoxication produces euphoria, hallucinations of time, space, color, and form, visual and auditory disorientation, extroversion, altered states of consciousness, palpitations, increased respirations, hyperreflexia, and circulatory collapse. Although hallucinogens are not typically lethal, fatalities may result from accidents that occur while an individual is under the influence of the drug. The psychotic states produced by hallucinogen abuse are occasionally irreversible and may occur up to 3 weeks after the original use.

Clinical Significance

Methadone maintenance programs are currently the preferred method of rehabilitation for the narcotic addict because a single oral dose of methadone produces a consistent state of euphoria for 24 hours. Urine tests are an important aid to therapeutic monitoring of these programs because they can confirm that the patient has taken the methadone dose and indicate the presence of other abused drugs. Combined use of narcotic drugs and any sedatives, particularly phenothiazines and barbiturates, enhances the analgesia, respiratory depression, and hypotension produced by the narcotic.

Normal Values

Central nervous system stimulants and depressants, narcotics, and hallucinogenic drugs are not normally found in the blood or urine. Under certain clinical conditions, therapeutic levels of any drugs are beneficial, although overdosage or abuse of these agents is never desirable.

Methodology

Tests to detect drug abuse or monitor patients on methadone maintenance programs require a 50 mL random urine specimen collected without preservatives and under supervision. Although most abused substances may be detected by urine screening procedures, confirmatory tests frequently are necessary to overcome the effects of certain interfering substances and metabolites. Such quantitative determinations require 5 mL of blood collected without anticoagulants (red-stoppered tube). Current test methods on urine or blood are not sensitive enough to detect the presence of the minuscule amounts of LSD that produce psychosis.

Precautions

False-positive results for heroin and morphine abuse may occur if the patient has ingested 20 mg of codeine in cough syrup or consumed 5–15 g of poppy seeds 24 hours prior to testing. False-positive results for the presence of quinine (frequently used to cut heroin) may occur if the patient has ingested quinine water or used quinidine (an antiarrhythmic) within 5 days of testing.

▶▶ *Nursing Responsibilities and Implications*

1. Supervise the patient while the urine specimen is being collected.

2. Handle the specimen following the proper precautions if the results will be used as legal evidence (see Medicolegal Specimen Collection and Handling earlier in this chapter).

DRUG SCREENING

Drug screening is designed to aid the investigation and treatment of coma, hallucinations, somnolence, excitation, and aberrant behavior in patients who may have overdosed with unidentified drugs. In general, these procedures can detect a broad spectrum of abused and nonabused drugs simultaneously, as well as a single drug or group of drugs (see also the previous section on Drug Abuse). The compounds commonly included in drug screening procedures are those with the potential to produce severe or life-threatening toxicity and those frequently involved in attempted suicide or drug abuse. Laboratory screening of body fluids can qualitatively identify the presence of barbiturate and non-barbiturate hypnotics, narcotic and non-narcotic analgesics, tranquilizers, and central nervous system stimulants and depressants, including:

Acetaminophen	Glutethimide	Phenmetrazine
Amphetamines	Heroin	Phenothiazines
Barbiturates	Meperidine	Phentermine
Benzodiazepines	Meprobamate	Phenylpropanolamine
Brompheniramine	Mescaline	Phenytoin
Chlorpheniramine	Methadone	Propoxyphene
Cocaine	Methamphetamines	Quinine
Codeine	Methapyrilene	Salicylates
Dextromethorphan	Methaqualone	Tricyclic antidepressants
Diphenhydramine	Methyprylon	Volatiles (acetone,
Ephedrine	Morphine	alcohol)
Ethchlorvynol	Phencyclidine (PCP)	

Clinical Significance

Drug screening procedures usually are performed to detect the presence of unprescribed substances or misuse of toxic agents, although they also are used to determine the degree of compliance with drug therapy. Their use also is indicated for persons such as pilots and competitive athletes whose safety and performance may be significantly altered or com-promised by drugs. In addition, routine testing by proper authorities is helpful in control-ling drug abuse in penal institutions, the military, and schools and among persons on pro-bation or enrollees of drug clinics. Broad-spectrum screening is used in the forensic laboratory to detect and identify drugs in the victim or perpetrator of a crime and to determine their presence in material from the scene of a crime.

Methodology
Broad-spectrum drug screening requires 20 mL of blood collected without anticoagulants (red-stoppered tube) or with sodium or potassium oxalate (black-stoppered tube) plus 100 mL of urine collected without preservatives.

▶▶ **Nursing Responsibilities and Implications**

1. Supervise the patient while the urine specimen is being collected.

2. Handle the specimen following the proper precautions if the results will be used as legal evidence, to monitor drug levels to assess compliance, or to monitor methadone maintenance programs (see Medicolegal Specimen Collection and Handling earlier in this chapter).

REFERENCES

American Association for Clinical Chemistry. 1980. *Therapeutic drug monitoring data.* Washington, D.C.: American Association for Clinical Chemistry.

Bauer, J. D. 1982. *Clinical laboratory medicine.* 9th ed. St. Louis: The C. V. Mosby Co.

Berman, E. 1981. Heavy metals. *Lab. Med.* 12(11):677.

Byers, J. M. 1980. What is a therapeutic range? *Lab. Med.* 11(12):784.

Cavanaugh, A. L., and Mancini, R. E. 1980. Drug interactions and digitalis toxicity. *Am. J. Nurs.* (Dec.):2170.

Clinical Assays, Inc. 1981. *Digoxin RIA test kit.* Cambridge, Mass.: Clinical Assays, Inc.

Dito, W. R. 1979. Therapeutic drug monitoring: tricyclic antidepressants. *Diagn. Med.* 2(5):2.

———. 1979. Therapeutic drug monitoring: procainamide and N-acetylprocainamide. *Diagn. Med.* 2(6):23.

———. 1980. Therapeutic drug monitoring: lithium. *Diagn. Med.* 3(1):39.

———. 1980. Therapeutic drug monitoring: aminoglycoside antibiotics. *Diagn. Med.* 3(2):77.

———. 1980. Therapeutic drug monitoring in your laboratory. *Diagn. Med.* 3(4):21.

Froede, R. C., and Sachs, J. L. 1980. The law and therapeutic drug monitoring. *Diagn. Med.* 3(4):27.

Gambino, R., and Galen, R. 1981. How carbon monoxide kills. *Diagn. Med.* 4(5):8.

Garb, S. 1976. *Laboratory tests in common use.* 6th ed. New York: Springer Publishing Co.

Henry, J. B. 1984. *Clinical diagnosis and management by laboratory methods.* 17th ed. Philadelphia: W. B. Saunders Co.

Hoevet, M. J., and Baer, D. M. 1980. Emergency toxicology: what does the community hospital physician need? *Lab. Med.* 11(5):301.

Jones, D. 1981. *Concepts in broad-spectrum drug detection.* Laguna Hills, Calif.: Analytical Systems, Inc.

Larson, F. C. 1982. *Clinical significance of tests available on the DuPont Automatic Clinical Analyzer.* Wilmington, Del.: DuPont Industries.

Medical Economics Company. 1984. *Physicians' desk reference*. 38th ed. Oradell, N.J.: Litton Industries, Inc.

Merck, Sharp, and Dohme Research Laboratories. 1982. *The Merck manual*. 14th ed. Rahway, N.J.: Merck, Sharp, and Dohme Research Laboratories.

Miale, J. B. 1982. *Laboratory medicine—hematology*. 6th ed. St. Louis: The C. V. Mosby Co.

Monitor Science Corporation. 1978. *Amikacin RIA test*. Newport Beach, Calif.: Monitor Science Corporation.

————. 1979. *The physician's guide to therapeutic aminoglycoside drug monitoring*. Newport Beach, Calif.: Monitor Science Corporation.

Nuclear Medical Laboratories, Inc. 1977. *Serum digoxin levels—necessity for interpretation in the full clinical context*. Dallas, Tex.: Nuclear Medical Laboratories, Inc.

Orynch, R. E., and Weissman, N. 1979. *The BioScience handbook of clinical and industrial toxicology*. Van Nuys, Calif.: BioScience Laboratories.

Syva Company. 1980. *Therapeutic monitoring for antimicrobial drugs*. Palo Alto, Calif.: Syva Co.

Tilkian, S. M., Conover, M. H., and Tilkian, A. G. 1983. *Clinical implications of laboratory tests*. 3rd ed. St. Louis: The C. V. Mosby Co.

Werner, M. 1980. Management of apparently inappropriate therapeutic drug monitoring data. *Lab. Med.* 11(12):818.

Widmann, F. K. 1983. *Clinical interpretation of laboratory tests*. 9th ed. Philadelphia: F. A. Davis Co.

8

Chemistry: Body Fluid Analysis

AMNIOTIC FLUID ANALYSIS   424
Specimen Collection and Handling   ·   Physical Examination
· α-Fetoprotein   ·   Bilirubin   ·   Creatinine
·   Lecithin/Sphingomyelin Ratio

CEREBROSPINAL FLUID ANALYSIS   434
Specimen Collection and Handling   ·   Physical Examination
·   Cell Counts   ·   Glucose   ·   Lactic Acid   ·   Protein   ·   Microbiologic
Examination   ·   Tests for Syphilis

FECAL ANALYSIS   449
Specimen Collection and Handling   ·   Physical Examination
·   Fecal Fat   ·   Occult Blood   ·   Trypsin   ·   Urobilinogen
·   Microbiologic Examination

GASTRIC ANALYSIS   458
Specimen Collection and Handling   ·   Physical Examination
·   Gastric Acidity

PLEURAL FLUID ANALYSIS   464
Specimen Collection and Handling   ·   Physical Examination
·   Cell Counts   ·   Glucose   ·   pH   ·   Specific Gravity and Total
Protein   ·   Microbiologic Examination

SYNOVIAL FLUID ANALYSIS   469
Specimen Collection and Handling   ·   Physical Examination
·   Cell Counts   ·   Crystals   ·   Glucose   ·   Microbiologic Examination

AMNIOTIC FLUID ANALYSIS

Amniotic fluid is a substance similar to extracellular fluid that contains undissolved material from the fetal urinary and respiratory tracts plus secretions from placental membranes. Many of the constituents of amniotic fluid are clinically useful for predicting genetic defects and evaluating fetal distress because they are produced by the fetus and reflect its gestational development. Prompt delivery may be desirable when clinical and technical monitoring detect fetal distress due to hemolytic disease of the newborn or pregnancies complicated by placenta previa, maternal diabetes, preeclampsia, or eclampsia.

Analysis of the biochemical, physical, and cytologic characteristics of amniotic fluid helps to balance the risks of premature delivery against continued exposure to the progressive problems associated with deteriorating intrauterine conditions. Amniotic fluid studies may be indicated for a variety of reasons, including:

- To assess fetal jeopardy resulting from Rh sensitization, diabetes mellitus, preeclampsia, and eclampsia.
- To detect structural malformations such as neural tube closure defects.
- To determine fetal sex in fetuses at risk for sex-linked diseases.
- To determine fetal pulmonary maturity when early delivery is indicated.
- To diagnose genetic or chromosomal disorders in offspring of high-risk parents, including Tay-Sach's disease, Down's syndrome, congenital hemoglobinopathies, and hemophilia.
- To document biochemical deficiencies or abnormalities.
- To evaluate fetal well-being.
- To predict the spontaneous onset of labor.

Amniotic fluid analysis usually is performed between 15 and 18 weeks of gestation, when samples can be obtained without difficulty, although the timing of amniocentesis varies according to the clinical circumstances. For example, tests to identify chromosomal abnormalities should be performed early in the second trimester in older mothers or if genetic defects are suspected. Studies to detect hemolytic disease and neural tube defects also should be performed during the second trimester. Although pulmonary and renal development may be evaluated during the late second and third trimesters, tests for fetal maturity usually are performed during or after the thirty-fifth week of gestation.

Many amniotic fluid assays are helpful in evaluating the degree of fetal jeopardy and maturity, although only those related to bile pigment concentrations, fetal weight, and pulmonary development are clinically useful. The most significant biochemical examinations of amniotic fluid include bilirubin analysis for Rh sensitization, creatinine determinations for fetal weight and renal development, and the L/S (lecithin/sphingomyelin) ratio for fetal pulmonary maturity. A variety of other biochemical determinations also may be performed on amniotic fluid, but these assays do not provide any additional diagnostic information. (Miscellaneous normal amniotic fluid values are summarized in Table 8-1.)

Specimen Collection and Handling

Amniotic fluid must be obtained by an experienced physician after the placenta and all fetal parts have been located by ultrasound examination. This procedure, known as **am-**

TABLE 8-1   Miscellaneous Normal Amniotic Fluid Values

Parameter	Level
Fluid volume	450–1500 mL
Calcium	4 mEq/L
Chloride	102 mEq/L
Carbon dioxide	16 mEq/L
Estriol	
Early gestation	<10 μg/dL
Term	<60 μg/dL
Glucose	29.8 mg/dL
pH	
Early gestation	7.12–7.38
Term	6.91–7.43
Potassium	4.9 mEq/L
Sodium	133 mEq/L
Total protein	2.5 g/dL
Albumin	1.42 g/dL (56.5%)
α_1-Globulin	0.19 g/dL (7.3%)
α_2-Globulin	0.17 g/dL (6.5%)
β-Globulin	0.40 g/dL (15.5%)
γ-Globulin	0.32 g/dL (12.2%)
Urea	
Early gestation	12–24 mg/dL
Term	19–42 mg/dL
Uric acid	
Early gestation	2.76–4.68 mg/dL
Term	7.67–12.13 mg/dL

niocentesis, is performed in an outpatient setting. Specimens must be aspirated under strict aseptic conditions using a syringe with a 22-gauge, 5-inch spinal needle, which is inserted through the abdominal wall into an intrauterine pool of amniotic fluid. Amniocentesis is contraindicated during pregnancies complicated by abruptio placentae, placenta previa, incompetent cervix, or a history of premature labor (before 34 weeks' gestation) unless the patient is receiving antilabor medications.

Immediately after amniocentesis, a 10–15 mL amniotic fluid specimen should be transferred from the collecting syringe into an appropriate sterile, siliconized sample container. Specimens for all types of culture and genetic studies, however, should be placed into polystyrene transport containers because cells may adhere to glass and affect test results. Specimens for bilirubin analysis should be placed in an amber-colored container or otherwise protected from light by wrapping the container in aluminum foil or placing it in an opaque bag.

▶▶ *Nursing Responsibilities and Implications*

1. Explain the purpose of amniotic fluid testing to the patient and describe the 20- to 30-minute amniocentesis procedure.

2. Obtain a signed consent form from the mother before the amniocentesis is begun.

3. Assure the mother that the procedure causes only mild discomfort associated with a slight cramping or pulling sensation as the needle enters the uterus and the fluid is withdrawn.

4. Have the patient void prior to the procedure to decrease the possibility of bladder puncture if the amniocentesis is performed after 20 weeks of gestation; prior to 20 weeks' gestation the bladder is left full to support the uterus.

5. Place the patient in a supine position and prepare the skin overlying the chosen site.

6. Monitor the mother's vital signs as well as the fetal heart rate before and after amniocentesis to detect any adverse effects of the procedure. Inform the physician of any change in fetal heart tones so that fetal distress can be detected promptly.

7. Assess the mother for nausea and dizziness during and after the procedure; encourage her to rest on her right side for several minutes before leaving the examining room.

8. Deliver amniotic fluid specimens to the laboratory immediately or keep them refrigerated to maintain the viability of cells for culture.

9. Instruct the mother to report to her physician any fluid loss, fever, bleeding, cramping, or dizziness that occur following the amniocentesis.

10. If the mother is Rh negative, have RhoGAM available because many physicians administer anti-D globulin to these women following amniocentesis if they are not already sensitized.

Physical Examination

Visual examination of amniotic fluid to evaluate color, transparency, and the presence of blood should be performed as soon as possible after the specimen is collected.

Normal Values
Normal amniotic fluid is a colorless to light straw-colored liquid that may appear turbid or milky because of the presence of vernix caseosa and squamous debris.

Color

Abnormal amniotic fluid color, including various shades of yellow, green, brown, or red, reflects fetal distress states, and further investigation is warranted to establish the cause.

Yellow amniotic fluid, ranging from pale yellow to bright yellow-orange, results from fetal bilirubin and bile pigments released during increased red blood cell hemolysis, which is associated with erythroblastosis fetalis or inherited erythrocyte disorders.

Green amniotic fluid, including green-brown and green-black specimens, usually is caused by biliverdin, which is released by meconium expelled from the lower gastro-intestinal tract during fetal distress. Meconium contamination of amniotic fluid prevents accurate spectral analysis of bilirubin and interferes with the evaluation of fetal lung maturity by certain methods.

Green amniotic fluid may occur with:

Breech presentation	Fetal hypoxia, acute or chronic
Fetal death	Intrauterine growth retardation
Fetal defecation, spontaneous	Postmaturity
Fetal distress or damage	Vagal stimulation, reflex

Red amniotic fluid indicates recent hemolysis or the presence of intact erythrocytes due to intrauterine hemorrhage, usually of maternal origin. Specimens may exhibit a characteristic port wine color due to extravasation of blood into the amniotic cavity in acute fetal distress such as abruptio placentae.

Brown amniotic fluid, ranging from deep amber or chocolate brown to brown-black, usually indicates the presence of oxidized hemoglobin from deteriorating erythrocytes, most frequently due to maternal tissue trauma. Brown amniotic fluid may result from fetal death, fetal maceration, and severe hemolysis.

α-Fetoprotein

α-Fetoprotein (AFP), a globulin produced by the fetal liver between the sixth and thirty-second weeks of gestation, reaches maximum concentrations in the fetal blood-stream during the second trimester. Large amounts of AFP normally enter the amniotic fluid as a result of fetal urination and are present in smaller amounts in the mother's bloodstream during the first trimester. Although normal AFP values in maternal serum and amniotic fluid vary with the length of gestation, the concentration in fetal blood remains 100–150 times greater than either maternal serum or amniotic fluid levels throughout the entire pregnancy.

Enormous amounts of AFP enter the amniotic fluid, however, if the neural tube of the fetus fails to close properly; therefore, excessive amounts of AFP in amniotic fluid are an important indicator of open neural tube lesions. Although laboratory determination of AFP levels in amniotic fluid is useful in the diagnosis of neural tube closure defects, negative results do not guarantee the absence of neural tube malformations. Measurement of AFP in maternal serum between 16 and 20 weeks of gestation, on the other hand, sometimes is performed along with ultrasound to screen for possible neural tube closure defects. Evaluation of AFP in maternal serum is a less reliable indicator of neural tube defects than amniotic fluid values because AFP levels in maternal serum vary widely and may be elevated substantially by fetomaternal transfusion. (The significance of α-fetoprotein as a tumor marker is discussed in Chapter 4.)

Normal Values

The normal values for α-fetoprotein in the amniotic fluid and serum of pregnant women are:

Amniotic fluid

12 weeks gestation	<43 μg/mL
14 weeks gestation	<36 μg/mL
16 weeks gestation	<30 μg/mL
18 weeks gestation	<21 μg/mL
20 weeks gestation	<19 μg/mL
22 weeks gestation	<15 μg/mL
30 weeks gestation	3 μg/mL
35 weeks gestation	2 μg/mL
40 weeks gestation	0.8 μg/mL

Maternal serum

8 weeks gestation	<75 ng/mL
12 weeks gestation	<130 ng/mL
16 weeks gestation	<210 ng/mL
20 weeks gestation	<300 ng/mL
24 weeks gestation	<400 ng/mL
28 weeks gestation	<450 ng/mL
32 weeks gestation	<450 ng/mL
36 weeks gestation	<400 ng/mL
40 weeks gestation	<375 ng/mL

Variations

Elevated amniotic fluid α-fetoprotein levels may occur with:

Esophageal atresia

Fetal death

Nephrosis, congenital

Neural tube defects

  Anencephaly

Meningomyelocele

Spina bifida

Omphalocele, severe

Twin pregnancies

Elevated α-fetoprotein levels in maternal serum may occur with:

Complications of pregnancy

  Diabetes mellitus

  Fetal death

  Toxemia

Duodenal atresia

Esophageal atresia

Hydrocephalus

Nephrosis, congenital

Turner's syndrome

Twin pregnancies

Methodology

α-Fetoprotein determinations require an amniotic fluid specimen that has not been contaminated by fetal blood, which contains extremely high concentrations of AFP.

Precautions

To ensure an accurate analysis of AFP in amniotic fluid, the following precautions should be observed:

1. Do not submit specimens that were contaminated with fetal blood during amniocentesis because a very small puncture or hemorrhage can cause falsely elevated values and confuse test results.

2. Record the accurate gestational age of the fetus because incorrect dating of the pregnancy can interfere with the interpretation of test results.

▶▶ Nursing Responsibilities and Implications

See Specimen Collection and Handling (amniocentesis)—Nursing Responsibilities and Implications.

Bilirubin

Bilirubin, the metabolic by-product of hemoglobin breakdown, appears in amniotic fluid after 14–20 weeks of gestation because of the physiologic hemolysis of fetal erythrocytes and reaches peak concentrations after 26 weeks of gestation. Amniotic fluid bilirubin levels gradually decrease after the second trimester and disappear entirely after 36 weeks of gestation because the fetal liver is able to clear bile pigments from the bloodstream by this time. However, rapid destruction of fetal red blood cells by maternal antibodies that cross the placenta increases bilirubin concentrations and can cause the fetus to become dangerously anemic.

Although the actual presence of bile pigment does not endanger the fetus, amniotic fluid bilirubin levels provide an index to the degree of fetal red blood cell involvement and the severity of anemia. Laboratory analysis of amniotic fluid for bilirubin levels routinely is performed to detect and evaluate hemolytic disease of the newborn in women with antibodies against red blood cell antigens such as Rh factor. Bilirubin concentrations in amniotic fluid are no longer measured routinely to evaluate fetal maturity, however, because levels indicating maturity may appear earlier in an Rh-sensitized pregnancy. (The formation and significance of bilirubin also are discussed in Chapters 1 and 3.)

Normal Values

The normal and clinically significant values for amniotic fluid bilirubin are:

Normal	
Early gestation	<0.075 mg/dL
Term	<0.025 mg/dL
Fetal involvement	0.10–0.28 mg/dL
Fetal distress	>0.47 mg/dL
Fetal death	>0.95 mg/dL

Interpretation

<0.28 mg/dL	1+ Freda's classification (fetus normal or slightly affected but in no imminent danger of death)
0.28−0.46 mg/dL	2+ Freda's classification (fetus affected but not in danger for at least 7−10 days; possible indication for transfusion)
0.47−0.95 mg/dL	3+ Freda's classification (fetus greatly affected and in jeopardy of death within 3 weeks; transfusion or delivery as soon as possible)
>0.95 mg/dL	4+ Freda's classification (fetal death imminent; immediate delivery or transfusion)

Bilirubin levels at different gestational ages after the twenty-sixth week can be correlated with the degree of fetal danger and need for early intrauterine transfusion in Rh-sensitized women. Thus, amniotic fluid bile pigment concentrations and gestational age plotted on a Liley graph fall into one of three critical zones and reflect the risk of fetal hemolytic disease as follows:

Zone I	Fetus not anemic or only mildly affected; delivery may be at term
Zone II	Fetus affected with slight to moderate anemia; may require intrauterine transfusion or delivery prior to due date
Zone III	Fetus severely affected with marked anemia; may require intrauterine transfusions, immediate delivery, and exchange transfusions

Variations

Elevated amniotic fluid bilirubin levels may occur with:

Anencephaly
Hemolytic disease
Hydrops fetalis

Obstruction, intestinal
Rh sensitization

Methodology

Amniotic fluid specimens for the evaluation of Rh-sensitization and hemolytic disease of the newborn should be obtained at 24−28 weeks of gestation.

Precautions

To ensure accurate interpretation of amniotic fluid bilirubin concentrations, the following precautions should be observed:

1. Minimize the inclusion of maternal and fetal blood in amniotic fluid specimens during amniocentesis.

2. Protect amniotic fluid from light by performing amniocentesis in a darkened room and placing specimens in a lightproof amber collection container or immediately covering the container with aluminum foil.

▶▶ *Nursing Responsibilities and Implications*
See Specimen Collection and Handling (amniocentesis)—Nursing Responsibilities and Implications.

Creatinine

Creatinine, the metabolic end product of protein metabolism, enters the amniotic fluid with fetal urine in concentrations that rise sharply between 34 and 36 weeks of gestation. Amniotic fluid creatinine values reflect the gestational age of the fetus and are influenced by such factors as fetal muscle mass and renal maturity as well as maternal serum creatinine levels. However, although rising creatinine concentrations reflect increasing fetal muscle mass, amniotic fluid values may not rise with abnormal fetal growth to values appropriate for a specific level of fetal maturation.

Laboratory determinations of amniotic fluid creatinine are used to assess fetal maturity, muscle mass, and renal function, although concentrations are a less reliable index of fetal development than evaluation of pulmonary function using the L/S ratio. Because renal and pulmonary function do not always mature at the same rate, measurement of the L/S ratio is a more significant indicator of fetal maturity than creatinine levels (see the section on the Lecithin/Sphingomyelin [L/S] Ratio later in this chapter). Creatinine determinations also may be used to verify that amniotic fluid is not contaminated with maternal urine because specimens normally contain no impurities that would react with creatinine methods. (Creatinine is discussed in Chapters 1 and 4.)

Normal Values
The normal and clinically significant values for amniotic fluid creatinine are:

<28 weeks gestation	0.8–1.1 mg/dL
30–34 weeks gestation	1.1–1.8 mg/dL
35–40 weeks gestation (maturity)	1.8–4.0 mg/dL
Large muscle mass (diabetes)	>2 mg/dL
Low birthweight	<2 mg/dL
Contamination with maternal urine	>4 mg/dL

Interpretation
Accurate interpretation of amniotic fluid creatinine levels requires adequate renal function and creatinine clearance in the mother and a maternal serum to amniotic fluid ratio of approximately 2:1.

▶▶ *Nursing Responsibilities and Implications*
See Specimen Collection and Handling (amniocentesis)—Nursing Responsibilities and Implications.

Lecithin/Sphingomyelin Ratio

The **lecithin/sphingomyelin (L/S) ratio** is a phospholipid profile that measures the concentration of surfactant produced by the fetal lungs and secreted into the amniotic fluid. Surfactant is a generic term for an important phospholipid-protein complex that lowers the surface tension of the water lining the alveoli of the lungs and is necessary for alveolar stability. Thus, if the fetal lungs contain sufficient amounts of surfactant, adequate pulmonary ventilation is assured to prevent the lungs from collapsing after delivery.

The concentration of lecithin, the most important phospholipid in surfactant, rises slowly in the lungs and amniotic fluid during the first two trimesters of pregnancy and increases rapidly after 35 weeks of gestation. Sphingomyelin secretion by the immature fetal lungs, on the other hand, remains fairly constant throughout pregnancy and is present in the amniotic fluid in greater concentrations than lecithin. The absolute values of lecithin and sphingomyelin are less important, however, than the ratio between them, which indicates whether sufficient surfactant is present to permit normal respiration after delivery.

Because premature birth frequently is associated with breathing difficulty due to alveolar instability, an index of pulmonary maturity is necessary to evaluate the potential for normal respiration. The L/S ratio therefore provides a reliable indicator of susceptibility to respiratory distress syndrome, including its severity and the potential for extrauterine survival if premature delivery is necessary. Laboratory determination of the L/S ratio is used to evaluate fetal maturity, assess alveolar development in the fetal lungs, and predict whether respiratory distress will occur after delivery.

Clinical Significance

Analysis of the L/S ratio during normal pregnancy indicates whether the fetal lungs are sufficiently mature to function properly if premature delivery is necessary because of diabetes, erythroblastosis fetalis, or other complications of pregnancy. The L/S ratio indicates maturity earlier in the gestation, however (before pulmonary stability), during pregnancies complicated by severe preeclampsia, severe diabetes, major hemoglobinopathies, or prolonged rupture of the membranes. Conversely, a mature L/S ratio is attained later than expected in pregnancies complicated by less severe diabetes, collagen diseases, hepatitis, renal disease, and hemolytic disease of the newborn.

Thus, the L/S ratio is not an absolute index of pulmonary maturity and should be interpreted along with significant clinical and laboratory findings because it does not guarantee that respiratory distress syndrome will or will not occur. However, phospholipid studies such as phosphatidylinositol (PI) and phosphatidylglycerol (PG) tests are more accurate than the L/S ratio in pregnancies complicated by diabetes and may be included in the fetal lung profile. The **foam stability test**, also known as the shake test, is a screening procedure that bypasses the need for tedious quantitation in the indication of fetal lung maturity. When an aliquot of amniotic fluid is added to 95% ethyl alcohol with saline and shaken vigorously, the persistence of bubbles for 15 minutes indicates that lecithin and the L/S ratio are adequate. Complete quantitative analysis is necessary if the shake test is negative to differentiate fetal immaturity from false-negative results.

Normal Values

The normal and clinically significant values for amniotic fluid phospholipids are:

Lecithin

<35 weeks gestation	6−9 mg/dL
>35 weeks gestation	15−20 mg/dL

Sphingomyelin	4−6 mg/dL

L/S ratio

Immature	<1.5
Borderline	1.5−1.9
Mature	2.0−4.0
Postmature	>4.0

Interpretation

>2.0	Fetal lung maturity sufficient for extra-uterine survival; respiratory distress syndrome not expected
1.5−1.9	Fetal lungs in transition between immaturity and maturity; mild to moderate respiratory distress syndrome anticipated; pulmonary maturity expected in 14 days; repeat amniocentesis in 1 week
1.0−1.5	Fetal lungs immature; moderate to severe respiratory distress syndrome anticipated; pulmonary maturity expected within 2−3 weeks; repeat amniocentesis in 2 weeks
<1.0	Fetal lungs markedly immature; severe respiratory distress syndrome anticipated; associated with hyaline membrane disease; repeat amniocentesis no sooner than 2 weeks

Methodology

Measurement of the L/S ratio requires 10 mL of amniotic fluid that is not contaminated with blood or meconium.

Precautions

To ensure accurate interpretation of the L/S ratio, the following precautions should be observed:

1. Minimize the presence of fetal blood, maternal blood, or meconium in test specimens because they may seriously interfere with the test results.

2. Note the exact time of gestation on both the specimen container and the laboratory request slip.

▶▶ *Nursing Responsibilities*
See Specimen Collection and Handling (amniocentesis)—Nursing Responsibilities and Implications.

CEREBROSPINAL FLUID ANALYSIS

Cerebrospinal fluid (CSF) is normally a clear, colorless, sterile fluid produced by cellular secretions and plasma filtration within the highly vascular choroid plexus of the brain. Approximately 400–600 mL of CSF is continuously produced and reabsorbed into the bloodstream to maintain a total CSF volume of 100–160 mL in adults. A normal spinal fluid volume is required to provide optimum intracranial pressure and act as a fluid buffer to protect the brain and spinal cord from trauma or compression injuries. Spinal fluid also helps to supply oxygen and other nutrients to brain cells, remove waste products of cerebral metabolism, and prevent harmful effects of certain drugs and plasma pigments.

Cerebrospinal fluid studies are useful in the diagnosis of many central nervous system diseases because spinal fluid is readily accessible and reflects many biochemical and cell-shedding alterations of the brain and spinal cord. Spinal fluid examinations should be included in the diagnosis of patients with suspected meningitis, encephalitis, brain abscess, subarachnoid hemorrhage, multiple sclerosis, leukemia involving the central nervous system, and spinal cord tumors. Laboratory analysis of spinal fluid generally includes a description of the gross appearance, cell counts, glucose and protein determinations, various microbiologic studies, and serologic tests for syphilis.

A variety of other determinations also may be performed on CSF, although they are not clinically significant and provide no additional diagnostic information. (Miscellaneous normal spinal fluid values are summarized in Table 8-2.)

Specimen Collection and Handling

Spinal fluid specimens must be obtained under aseptic conditions by a physician who is experienced in the procedure and aware of its indications and potential complications. Cerebrospinal fluid is collected by introducing a needle into the spinal canal, usually in the lumbar area, although it also may be obtained directly from the ventricles of the brain during radiologic or surgical procedures. Fluid should be dripped into a series of small, sterile test tubes, allowing 3–5 mL of fluid to collect in each of three or more tubes that are numbered sequentially.

Although no trauma is apparent during spinal puncture, it is possible to rupture a minute blood vessel in the process and contaminate the fluid with a small amount of blood. Thus, fluid collected in the first tube is used to flush the needle and may have to be discarded because blood from a traumatic spinal tap alters the level of normal CSF constituents. The uncontaminated fluid collected in the second tube should be used for microscopic analysis such as cell counts, chemical determinations, including glucose, protein, or enzyme studies, and serologic studies. The third tube should be reserved for microbiologic studies such as culture and smears because earlier tubes may be contaminated with organisms from the patient's skin.

TABLE 8-2   Miscellaneous Normal Spinal Fluid Values

Parameter	Level
Total volume	
Infants	10–60 mL
Children	60–100 mL
Adults	100–160 mL
Specific gravity	1.006–1.008
Acid-base balance	
pH	7.30–7.40
P_{CO_2}	42–52 mm Hg
Bicarbonate	22.9 mEq/L
Cholesterol	0.2–0.6 mg/dL
Creatinine	0.4–1.5 mg/dL
Electrolytes	
Calcium	2.0–2.7 mEq/L
Chloride	113–133 mEq/L
Magnesium	2.0–3.1 mEq/L
Phosphorus	1.2–2.1 mg/dL
Potassium	2.7–3.9 mEq/L
Sodium	138–154 mEq/L
Glutamine	6–16 mg/dL
Aspartate aminotransferase (GOT)	0–19 units
5-Hydroxyindoleacetic acid	1.5–4.5 mg/dL
Iron	1–2 mg/dL
Lactate	10–18 mg/dL
Lactic dehydrogenase	6–50 units
Urea	6–28 mg/dL
Uric acid	0.5–4.5 mg/dL

When tuberculous meningitis is suspected, a fourth tube should be collected and refrigerated without shaking to observe clot formation. In addition, if spinal fluid is highly colored or very cloudy, one specimen should be collected in 0.5 mL of sterile sodium citrate per 5 mL of CSF to prevent clotting. All CSF specimen tubes must be delivered to the laboratory immediately for prompt examination because delays may cause erroneous cell counts or chemical and microbiologic results.

Precautions
To prevent contamination of staff members and ensure clinically significant test results, the following precautions should be observed when collecting spinal fluid specimens:

1. Handle the spinal fluid specimens cautiously because they may contain extremely contagious organisms.

TABLE 8-3   Cerebrospinal Fluid Values in Selected Disorders

Condition	Appearance	Cells/μL and Type	Glucose (mg/dL)	Protein (mg/dL)
Normal	Clear, colorless	0–10 lymphocytes	45–80	15–45
Brain abscess	Normal to slightly turbid	10–60 neutrophils	Slight decrease	Normal to moderate increase
Encephalitis	Normal	50–100 lymphocytes	Slight decrease	Slight increase
Hemorrhage				
Subarachnoid	Red, cloudy, xanthochromic	Many red blood cells	Normal	Marked increase
Subdural	Normal to xanthochromic	10–60 lymphocytes	Normal	Normal to slight increase
Meningitis				
Acute pyogenic	Turbid to purulent	>1000 neutrophils	Decreased	Marked increase
Aseptic	Normal to slightly turbid	10–60 lymphocytes	Slight decrease	Slight increase
Fungal	Normal to hazy	10–60 lymphocytes	Decreased	Slight increase
Tuberculous	Slightly turbid, opalescent	50–100 lymphocytes	Decreased	Moderate increase
Viral	Normal	100–500 lymphocytes	Normal	Slight increase
Multiple sclerosis	Normal	10–60 lymphocytes	Normal	Slight increase
Neurosyphilis	Normal	10–60 lymphocytes	Normal	Normal to slight increase
Polyneuritis	Normal to xanthochromic	10–60 lymphocytes	Normal	Normal to marked increase
Thrombosis	Normal	10–60 lymphocytes	Normal	Normal to slight increase

2. Refrigerate CSF specimen tubes when it is not possible to deliver them to the laboratory immediately for prompt analysis to delay cell lysis and disintegration.

▶▶ *Nursing Responsibilities and Implications*

1. Describe the procedure for collecting spinal fluid to reassure the patient before lumbar puncture; secure an informed consent.

2. Instruct the patient to lie on the side on the examining table or bed, with the spine parallel to and hips perpendicular to the surface.

3. Instruct the patient to clasp the knees to the chest and flex the chin toward the knees to bow the back into a convex position.

4. Stand in front of the patient to provide support behind the knees and neck during the lumbar puncture.

5. Encourage the patient to breathe slowly and naturally.

6. Maintain sterile conditions during the collection and handling of the CSF specimen, particularly if the spinal tap was performed because of suspected infection.

7. Number the specimen tubes in the order of collection to help differentiate traumatic tap from preexisting intracranial hemorrhage.

8. Observe the patient for any untoward reactions to lumbar puncture such as elevated pulse rate, moist, clammy skin, and pallor.

9. Caution the patient to lie flat for several hours after lumbar puncture to prevent or lessen the occurrence of postpuncture headache, nausea, dizziness, and neck pain until spinal fluid volume can be replaced; administer analgesics for headache if ordered.

10. Transport the CSF specimens to the laboratory immediately because bacteria and cells continue glycolysis, and undue delays will affect test values.

11. Continue to observe the patient for complications such as bleeding into the spinal canal, neurologic injury, or infection (alterations in vital signs, numbness or tingling of the lower extremities, neck rigidity, and changes in the level of consciousness).

Physical Examination

Laboratory reports of CSF analysis contain a description of the overall appearance of the spinal fluid, including color, transparency or clarity, and the presence of blood. Cerebrospinal fluid values in various disorders are summarized in Table 8-3.

> ### Normal Values
> Normal cerebrospinal fluid is a crystal clear, colorless liquid that looks like water.

Clarity
Decreased CSF clarity or transparency, which can range from slight cloudiness to marked turbidity, indicates a significant increase in the number of cells as the result of an infectious process (acute or purulent meningitis, meningoencephalitis). Thus, CSF turbidity

may be caused by the presence of leukocytes (usually neutrophils), erythrocytes, or microorganisms such as bacteria, fungi, and amebas. Cerebrospinal fluid turbidity may be graded from 0 to 4+, as follows:

0   = crystal clear.

1+ = faintly cloudy, smoky, or hazy, with slight (barely visible) turbidity.

2+ = turbidity clearly present, but newsprint can be read easily through the test tube.

3+ = newsprint cannot be read easily through the test tube.

4+ = newsprint cannot be seen through the test tube.

Erythrocyte counts above 400 cells/μL are required to produce slight turbidity, whereas visible CSF clouding occurs with leukocyte counts above 200 white blood cells/μL. Cerebrospinal fluid containing 200–500 white blood cells/μL appears hazy or smoky, and marked turbidity results from counts greater than 500 white blood cells/μL. However, clear CSF does not eliminate the diagnosis of central nervous system disorders such as encephalitis, intracranial hemorrhage, and tuberculous meningitis.

Color

The supernatant fluid of centrifuged CSF may be abnormally colored because of the presence of bile, pus, or red, brown, and yellow pigments, which reflect a mixture of bilirubin and other hemoglobin derivatives. The supernatant appears **red** 4–10 hours after subarachnoid hemorrhage if hemoglobin has been released into the fluid as a result of erythrocytic lysis. A **brown** supernatant results from methemoglobin, an oxidation product of hemoglobin found in fluids aspirated from subdural and intracerebral hematomas.

A **yellow** or **orange** (xanthochromic) supernatant results from old blood or extremely elevated protein levels that may appear in the central nervous system following pathologic bleeding or brain tissue destruction. The presence of xanthochromia indicates past subarachnoid or intracerebral hemorrhage and results from the degradation of released hemoglobin and subsequent formation of bilirubin and other hemoglobin metabolites. Xanthochromic supernatant also may occur in patients with severe or chronic icterus associated with liver disease when the serum bilirubin level exceeds 6 mg/dL or the total protein level exceeds 150 mg/dL.

Xanthochromia results from disintegrated blood in CSF following cerebral hemorrhage or previous lumbar puncture provided that erythrocytes were present in the CSF long enough to cause lysis. Thus, a pale pink to pale orange CSF discoloration begins 2–5 hours after subarachnoid hemorrhage, reaches a peak in 24–36 hours, and gradually disappears in 4–8 days. Yellow xanthochromia due to bilirubin formation appears in the CSF about 12 hours after subarachnoid hemorrhage, reaches peak levels in 2–4 days, and gradually disappears within 2–4 weeks.

Blood

The appearance of blood in CSF specimens may result from traumatic spinal puncture or may be associated with pathologic bleeding due to subarachnoid hemorrhage, intracerebral hemorrhage (ruptured aneurysm, cerebral arteriosclerosis, hypertension), or trauma. Cerebrospinal fluid specimens collected after subarachnoid or cerebral hemorrhage contain blood cells distributed evenly among all three specimen tubes and a yellowish supernatant fluid due to hemolysis and bilirubin formation. An intracranial hemorrhage also may be identified by the presence of crenated red blood cells, which indicate that blood has been in contact with the CSF for an extended period of time.

Conversely, traumatic spinal puncture produces blood that is distributed unevenly throughout the CSF specimen, appearing in the first tube and diminishing to little or none in the last. Although visual clearing of blood in consecutive CSF specimen tubes denotes traumatic spinal tap, comparison of red blood cell counts performed on serial specimens is a more exact way of making the distinction. Likewise, supernatant fluid is clear in bloody CSF specimens resulting from traumatic spinal puncture, although this does not rule out intracranial hemorrhage because fewer than 360 red blood cells/μL are not visible. In addition, CSF specimens containing more than 200,000 red blood cells/μL due to traumatic spinal tap will clot on standing, whereas specimens associated with subarachnoid bleeding will not clot on standing.

▶▶ *Nursing Responsibilities and Implications*
See Specimen Collection and Handling (CSF)—Nursing Responsibilities and Implications.

Cell Counts

The CSF cell count includes an actual enumeration of erythrocytes and leukocytes present in 1 μL of CSF and a classification of the different types of white blood cells. The distribution of the white blood cells present in CSF is determined by performing a differential count and reporting the relative percentages of segmented cells (mostly neutrophils) and mononuclear cells (mainly lymphocytes). Differential classification of white blood cells generally is not significant when the total cell count is within the normal range but may have important diagnostic values when the number of cells is increased. Laboratory determinations of total and differential CSF cell counts may be used in the diagnosis and treatment of central nervous system disorders such as meningitis, poliomyelitis, and encephalitis.

Clinical Significance
A variety of neurologic disorders produce elevated CSF cell counts (**pleocytosis**) and cause abnormal leukocyte counts, which vary depending on the nature and duration of the disease involved. For example, moderate pleocytosis generally indicates a viral infection such as poliomyelitis, tuberculous meningitis, neurosyphilis, and encephalitis, whereas marked pleocytosis occurs in most types of meningitis, especially pyogenic or bacterial meningitis. There is no relationship, however, between the white blood cell count and the prognosis of the condition. Likewise, a normal CSF cell count does not necessarily exclude a central nervous system disorder because values may remain within normal limits in individuals with multiple sclerosis, epilepsy, and brain tumors.

Cellular reactions in CSF are identified according to the predominant cell type encountered and are classified as neutrophilic, mixed (neutrophils, lymphocytes, and monocytes), or mononuclear (lymphocytes and monocytes). Lymphocytes predominate in most conditions that produce markedly elevated CSF cell counts such as acute inflammation and purulent infections. (The function and significance of each type of leukocyte are discussed in Chapter 2.)

Erythrocyte counts on CSF occasionally are used to correct the leukocyte count or protein measurement of CSF contaminated with peripheral blood due to a traumatic spinal tap. A rough rule for discounting the presence of blood introduced accidentally into the CSF is to allow 1–2 leukocytes for every 1000 erythrocytes. For example, bloody fluid containing 20,000 red blood cells/μL should contain no more than 30–40 white blood cells/μL derived solely from the blood introduced during the traumatic spinal puncture.

Thus, the presence of more than 45 white blood cells/μL indicates preexisting pleocytosis unless the blood introduced by local injury during lumbar puncture has an unusually high leukocyte count.

Normal Values

The normal and clinically significant values for cerebrospinal fluid cells are:

Erythrocytes

Neonates	0−675/μL
Adults	0−10/μL

Leukocytes

Children

<1 year	0−30/μL
1−4 years	0−20/μL
5 years to puberty	0−10/μL
Adults	0−10/μL

Leukocyte differential

Lymphocytes	63%−99%
B-lymphocytes	0%−4%
T-lymphocytes	89%−97%
Monocytes	3%−37%
Neutrophils	0%
Eosinophils	<5%

Pleocytosis

Mild	20−100 white blood cells/μL
Moderate	100−500 white blood cells/μL
Marked	>500 white blood cells/μL

Variations

Increased cerebrospinal fluid cell counts (pleocytosis) may occur with:

Bacterial meningitis	Neurosyphilis	Syphilis, latent
Encephalitis	Poliomyelitis	Viral meningitis

Increased cerebrospinal fluid neutrophil counts may occur with:

Amebic encephalomyelitis	Bacterial meningitis, acute
Aseptic meningitis	Epidemic meningitis
Cerebral abscess	Granulocytic leukemia involving the central nervous system
Osteomyelitis of the spine or skull	
Phlebitis of the dural sinuses	Hemorrhagic central nervous system infarct
Subdural empyema	

Injection into the subarachnoid space
  Contrast media
  Lidocaine
  Methotrexate
Intracerebral hematoma
Meningovascular syphilis, early
Mycotic meningitis
Pneumoencephalogram (post)
Poliomyelitis (early stages)
Pyogenic meningitis

Coliform
Hemophilus influenzae
Neisseria meningiditis
Pneumococci
Staphylococci
Streptococci
Subarachnoid hemorrhage
Syphilitic meningitis (early stages)
Tuberculous meningitis
Viral meningoencephalitis, early

Increased cerebrospinal fluid lymphocyte counts may occur with:

Aseptic meningitis
  Cerebral abscess
  Osteomyelitis of the spine or skull
  Phlebitis of the dural sinuses
  Subdural empyema
Bacterial meningitis, partially treated
Cerebral thrombosis
Disseminated encephalomyelitis, acute
Encephalopathy due to drug abuse
Epidemic encephalitis
Fungal meningitis
  Coccidioides
  Cryptococcus neoformans
Guillain-Barré syndrome
Herpetic infection of the central nervous system
Leptospiral meningitis
Leukemia of the central nervous system

Lymphocytic choriomeningitis
Multiple sclerosis
Neurosyphilis, late
Parasitic disease
  Cysticercus (cysticercosis)
  Toxoplasma gondii (toxoplasmosis)
  Trichinella spiralis (trichinosis)
Periarteritis involving the central nervous system
Poliomyelitis, anterior
Polyneuritis
Postinfectious meningitis (communicable diseases)
Sarcoidosis of the meninges
Syphilitic meningoencephalitis, acute
Tuberculous meningitis
Viral meningoencephalitis

Increased cerebrospinal fluid eosinophil counts (>5%) may occur with:

Bronchial asthma, allergic
Coccidioidomycosal meningitis
Drug reactions
Food allergies
Intracranial shunt
Lymphocytic leukemia with central nervous system involvement
Parasitic infestation

Polyneuritis, acute
Pneumococcal meningitis
Rabies vaccination
Syphilitic meningoencephalitis
Tuberculous meningitis
Urticaria
Viral meningoencephalitis

Methodology

Cerebrospinal fluid cell counts usually are performed on the second or third tube in the CSF collection series because they are less likely to contain minute amounts of red blood cells introduced accidentally during spinal puncture. Cell counts should be performed promptly after the specimen is collected because cells begin to deteriorate and disintegrate within 1 hour.

►► Nursing Responsibilities and Implications

See Specimen Collection and Handling (CSF)—Nursing Responsibilities and Implications.

Glucose

Cerebrospinal fluid glucose concentrations are related directly to the rate of glucose diffusion from the blood and increase or decrease in proportion to physiologic alterations in plasma concentrations. However, any change in blood glucose content precedes a corresponding increase or decrease in CSF glucose levels by 2–4 hours. Thus, CSF glucose values must be compared with postprandial serum glucose concentrations to determine whether abnormal levels reflect significant variation in blood glucose levels or result from a pathologic process within the cerebrospinal canal. Laboratory measurements of CSF glucose are useful in diagnosing viral and tuberculous meningitis because they alone can differentiate these central nervous system disorders.

Clinical Significance

Although high CSF glucose levels have no diagnostic significance, low CSF fluid glucose values may result from increased glucose utilization due to the presence of erythrocytes, leukocytes, microorganisms, or metastatic cancer cells. The most dramatic drop in CSF glucose levels occurs with purulent meningitis when the combination of pyogenic bacteria and leukocyte activity may reduce the CSF glucose concentration to zero. However, low CSF glucose values are nonspecific and have little value in the diagnosis of bacterial meningitis (including tuberculous meningitis) unless pleocytosis is present.

Normal Values

The normal and clinically significant cerebrospinal fluid glucose values are:

Adults	
Normal	40–80 mg/dL
	50%–80% of serum glucose
Hyperglycemia (>800 mg/dL)	240–320 mg/dL
	30%–40% of serum glucose
Children	35–75 mg/dL
Premature infants	24–63 mg/dL
Full-term infants	34–119 mg/dL

Variations
Decreased cerebrospinal fluid glucose levels ($<$ 40 mg/dL) may occur with:

Bacterial meningitis

Brain abscess

Fungal meningitis

Hypoglycemia, systemic

Leukemic infiltration

Lymphocytic meningitis

Lymphomas

Melanomatosis

Meningeal carcinomatosis

Neurosyphilis

Pyogenic meningitis, acute

Sarcoidosis of the central nervous system

Subarachnoid hemorrhage

Toxoplasmosis

Tuberculous meningitis

Tumors of the brain and choroid plexus

Elevated cerebrospinal fluid glucose levels ($>$80 mg/dL) may occur with:

Cerebral hemorrhage

Diabetes

Increased intracranial pressure

Brain tumors

Cerebral trauma

Hypothalamic lesions

Postinfectious encephalitis (mumps)

Normal cerebrospinal fluid glucose levels may accompany viral meningitis.

Methodology
Measurement of CSF glucose must be performed promptly to prevent the utilization and decomposition of glucose by bacteria and leukocytes, which continues even after the specimen is collected. When testing must be delayed, particularly in specimens suspected of containing leukocytes or microorganisms, the breakdown of CSF glucose can be prevented by adding 1 mg of sodium fluoride for each milliliter of spinal fluid.

▶▶ *Nursing Responsibilities and Implications*
In addition to the nursing responsibilities listed under Specimen Collection and Handling (CSF), the nurse should proceed as follows:

1. Instruct the patient to fast for at least 4 hours before the spinal puncture so that the blood and CSF glucose will equilibrate fully.

2. Discontinue any intravenous infusion of glucose and replace it with saline at least 1–2 hours before the lumbar puncture.

3. Obtain a blood specimen for glucose determination immediately before the spinal puncture is performed.

4. Transport the CSF specimens to the laboratory immediately so that analysis can occur within 1 hour of spinal puncture because cells in the fluid may continue glycolysis, causing falsely low test results.

Lactic Acid

Lactic acid in CSF results from the anaerobic metabolism of glucose within the central nervous system and accurately reflects increased glucose utilization in the CSF. Elevated

CSF lactic acid values indicate low CSF glucose levels that accompany conditions associated with reduced cerebral blood flow or oxygenation of the brain and increased intracranial pressure. Thus, increased CSF lactic acid levels appear in patients with bacterial and tuberculous meningitis but not in those with viral infections; CSF lactic acid levels decrease during effective treatment of such purulent conditions. Laboratory measurement of CSF lactic acid may be used to detect central nervous system disease, differentiate bacterial or fungal meningitis from viral meningitis, and monitor the effectiveness of therapy in CSF infections.

Normal Values

The normal and clinically significant values for lactic acid in cerebrospinal fluid are:

Normal	10–22 mg/dL
Bacterial meningitis	>35 mg/dL
Viral meningitis	<25 mg/dL

Variations

Elevated cerebrospinal fluid lactic acid levels may occur with:

Alkalosis, respiratory

Bacterial meningitis

Brain abscess

Carcinoma involving the central nervous system (primary or metastatic)

Cerebral infarct

Cerebral ischemia due to arteriosclerosis

Fungal meningitis

Hydrocephalus

Hypotension

Intracranial hemorrhage

Multiple sclerosis

Seizures, idiopathic

Traumatic brain injury

Tuberculous meningitis

Methodology

Measurement of CSF lactic acid should be performed on the second or third tube of the specimen collection sequence to minimize contamination of the specimen by blood.

▶▶ **Nursing Responsibilities and Implications**

See Specimen Collection and Handling (CSF)—Nursing Responsibilities and Implications.

Protein

Cerebrospinal fluid protein normally is derived from small quantities of serum protein that diffuse from the blood in addition to the protein that is synthesized within the central nervous system by immunocompetent cells. Elevated CSF protein concentrations are the most frequently noted abnormality in CSF analysis and provide a nonspecific but reliable indication of central nervous system pathology. Evaluation of total CSF protein, demonstration of IgG and oligoclonal bands by electrophoresis, and analysis of myelin basic protein provide the most significant information used to diagnose many central nervous system disorders. Laboratory determinations of CSF protein concentrations therefore may be useful in the diagnosis of meningeal inflammation, viral diseases, demyelinating disorders, central nervous system syphilis, and spinal block caused by tumor. (Total protein, immunoglobins, and protein electrophoresis determinations are discussed in Chapter 4.)

Clinical Significance

Elevated CSF protein values may indicate serious pathologic conditions such as disorders characterized by the disintegration of nonblood cells or by increased leakage of plasma proteins through diseased capillary walls. Elevated CSF protein values may provide little additional diagnostic information, however, because the increase often results from intracellular proteins released when previously identified erythrocytes and leukocytes disintegrate. Thus, the appearance of blood associated with traumatic spinal tap increases CSF protein values by 1 mg/dL for every 1000–1200 red blood cells present if hematocrit and serum protein values are normal.

Analysis of CSF protein fractions through CSF protein electrophoresis aids the differential diagnosis and evaluation of central nervous system diseases characterized by similar clinical features and common total CSF protein values. For example, CSF protein electrophoresis is particularly valuable in the diagnosis of multiple sclerosis and other inflammatory central nervous system diseases that produce quantitative and qualitative changes in the α-globulin fraction. Such changes can be demonstrated in the electrophoretic pattern by the appearance of γ-globulin that does not migrate as a homogeneous unit but breaks into several discrete bands. These **oligoclonal bands** represent the presence of antibodies produced only in the central nervous system but not seen in vascular diseases, brain tumors, or other nonimmunologic brain disorders.

The primary immunoglobulin demonstrated by protein electrophoresis is IgG, which enters the CSF from plasma but also can be synthesized by immunocompetent cells of the central nervous system. IgG values may be expressed as a percentage of total CSF protein or as an IgG/albumin index, which is helpful in distinguishing between exudation of serum IgG and synthesis in the central nervous system. This ratio increases in diseases associated with increased IgG production, such as multiple sclerosis, and decreases in conditions characterized by elevated CSF albumin concentrations such as neoplastic infiltration of the spinal cord. Thus, the IgG/albumin index can be used to distinguish demyelinating or inflammatory diseases, which increase immunoglobulin and IgG synthesis, from meningitis, cerebral infarction, and central nervous system tumors, which affect CSF permeability.

Myelin basic protein is a constituent of myelin, the insulating material necessary for the proper conduction of nerve impulses, that is released into the spinal fluid only during active demyelinating diseases. Thus, elevated myelin basic protein levels appear in the CSF during the acute phase of multiple sclerosis but do not occur in patients with normal CSF. Myelin basic protein determinations therefore are used to differentiate and monitor the clinical stages of multiple sclerosis because patients with chronic progressive demyelinating disorders exhibit intermediate values; negligible values are seen in patients in remission.

Normal Values

The normal and clinically significant values for spinal fluid proteins are:

Total protein

Normal

Premature infants	<400 mg/dL
Full-term infants	20–170 mg/dL
6–30 days	30–150 mg/dL
1 month–3 months	20–100 mg/dL
3 months–6 months	15–50 mg/dL
6 months–10 years	10–30 mg/dL
10–40 years	15–45 mg/dL
40–50 years	20–50 mg/dL
50–60 years	20–55 mg/dL
>60 years	30–60 mg/dL
Slight increase	60–75 mg/dL
Moderate increase	75–150 mg/dL
Marked increase	150–500 mg/dL

Protein electrophoresis

Prealbumin	2%–7%
Albumin	45%–83.5%
α_1-Globulin	1.1%–7%
α_2-Globulin	3%–12.6%
β-Globulin	7.3%–18%
γ-Globulin	3%–13%
IgG	1–4 mg/dL
IgA	0–0.2 mg/dL
IgM	0–0.06 mg/dL
IgG/albumin index	0.34–0.58
Albumin/globulin (A/G) ratio	4:1

Myelin basic protein

Negative	<4 ng/mL
Weakly positive	4–8 ng/mL
Positive	>9 ng/mL

Variations

Elevated cerebrospinal fluid total protein levels may occur with:

Ascending polyneuritis	Bacterial meningoencephalitis
Aseptic meningeal reaction	Brain abscess

Brain tumor

Cerebral arteriosclerosis

Cerebral thrombosis

Degenerative diseases

Diabetic neuropathy

Encephalitis

Froin's syndrome

Guillain-Barré syndrome

Hyperproteinemia

Intracerebral hemorrhage

Local anesthetics, in spinal canal

Meningitis

  Bacterial

  Fungal

Tubercular

Viral

Multiple sclerosis

Mycotic meningoencephalitis

Myxedema

Neurosyphilis

Poliomyelitis

Subarachnoid hemorrhage

Toxic conditions

  Ethanol

  Isopropanol

  Heavy metals

  Phenytoin

Vascular malformations

Falsely elevated cerebrospinal fluid total protein levels may occur with:

Drug therapy

  Analgesics, some

  Aspirin

  Chlorpromazine

  Phenacetin

Salicylates

Streptomycin

Sulfonamides

Traumatic spinal puncture

Elevated cerebrospinal fluid β-globulin levels may occur with cerebral vascular diseases, acute meningitis, and neoplasms.

Elevated cerebrospinal fluid γ-globulin levels may occur with multiple sclerosis, neurosyphilis, and subacute sclerosing leukoencephalitis.

Oligoclonal bands may occur with:

Multiple sclerosis

Neurosyphilis

Polyneuropathy

Rubella panencephalitis, progressive

Subacute sclerosing panencephalitis

Elevated cerebrospinal fluid IgG levels may occur with:

Guillain-Barré syndrome

Multiple sclerosis

Neurosyphilis

Subacute sclerosing panencephalitis

Systemic lupus erythematosus involving the central nervous system

Viral meningoencephalitis

Elevated cerebrospinal fluid myelin basic protein levels may occur with cerebral infarcts, demyelinating diseases, and acute multiple sclerosis.

Methodology

Cerebrospinal fluid protein determinations should be performed on the second or third tube of the CSF collection sequence to minimize contamination with blood from the spinal puncture.

▶▶ *Nursing Responsibilities and Implications*
See Specimen Collection and Handling (CSF)—Nursing Responsibilities and Implications.

Microbiologic Examination

Microbiologic examination of CSF is essential for identifying bacteria, fungi, myco-bacteria, protozoa, or viruses in patients with suspected meningitis or central nervous sys-tem infections. Cerebrospinal fluid cultures and smears must be performed as quickly as possible so that treatment may be instituted without delay. (Microbiologic examination and culture of CSF specimens are discussed in Chapter 9.)

Methodology
Microbiologic examination of CSF should be performed on the third tube in the CSF col-lection sequence to minimize contamination of the specimen from organisms on the skin. However, when very small amounts of fluid are collected from patients with suspected meningitis such as neonates, the entire specimen should be sent directly to the micro-biology laboratory so that it can be handled aseptically. Although very small amounts of CSF are needed to detect most microorganisms, relative large (5 – 10 mL) fluid specimens are required to identify fungi and mycobacteria; the larger the specimen, the greater the chance of a positive culture.

Precautions
Special care should be taken to avoid self-contamination with CSF specimens because meningitic infections are usually produced by highly virulent organisms.

▶▶ *Nursing Responsibilities and Implications*
See Specimen Collection and Handling (CSF)—Nursing Responsibilities and Implications.

Tests for Syphilis

Serologic tests for syphilis, such as the Venereal Disease Research Laboratories (VDRL) test and the fluorescent treponemal antibody absorption (FTA-ABS) test, may be performed on CSF to detect the presence of neurosyphilis. A positive serologic test of the CSF usually indicates central nervous system involvement by the causative organism (*Treponema pal-lidum*). Positive test results, however, do not necessarily indicate active syphilis because CSF tests for syphilis may remain elevated even after the patient has been adequately treated. Conversely, tests for syphilis may be negative in 40%–50% of patients with neuro-syphilis. (Serologic tests for syphilis are discussed in Chapter 11.)

Normal Values
Cerebrospinal fluid tests for syphilis are normally nonreactive.

Variations
Biologic false-positive VDRL reactions may occur with:

Encephalitis	Meningitis, acute
Hemorrhage	Traumatic spinal puncture

Methodology
Serologic tests for syphilis must not be performed on bloody CSF specimens because results may be falsely positive or reactive.

►► Nursing Responsibilities and Implications
See Specimen Collection and Handling (CSF)—Nursing Responsibilities and Implications.

FECAL ANALYSIS

Examination of fecal material, the waste product of the intestinal digestion and absorption of foodstuffs, frequently is performed during the investigation and evaluation of gastrointestinal tract disorders. Fecal material normally is composed of water, vegetable residue, small amounts of fat, intestinal secretions, and desquamated cells, along with enteric bacteria and their waste products. Fecal analysis provides a valuable guide to the diagnosis of obstructive jaundice, gastrointestinal tract bleeding, dysentery, ulcerative colitis, steatorrhea, and gastrointestinal obstruction and may aid in the detection and identification of parasitic infestation. Laboratory analysis of feces generally includes an evaluation of gross appearance, an assessment of occult blood, fecal fat, trypsin, and urobilinogen, and microbiologic examination for pathogenic organisms as well as ova and parasites.

Specimen Collection and Handling

Random stool specimens generally are acceptable for most fecal analyses, although screening tests occasionally suggest conditions that must be confirmed by a quantitative determination on total or timed specimens. Plastic, cardboard, or glass containers with screw caps or tight-fitting lids generally are used to collect and transport stool specimens because they are odor-free and leakproof. A small sample of fecal material removed with a gloved finger during rectal examination and transferred to a piece of filter paper also may serve to identify unsuspected occult bleeding or to evaluate striking abnormalities of stool color or consistency.

Precautions
To ensure accurate analysis of stool specimens, the following precautions should be observed:

1. Do not administer laxatives, purgatives, or enemas to the patient before specimen collection because they interfere with intestinal motility and alter the test results.

2. Do not schedule the patient for diagnostic procedures requiring the use of barium before specimen collection because this substance interferes with the examination of the stool.

3. Do not submit specimens for fecal analysis that are contaminated with urine or toilet water containing chemicals such as soap and cleansers, which may alter the test results.

4. Do not submit specimens that have been mixed with toilet paper because this can interfere with the stool analysis.

▶▶ *Nursing Responsibilities and Implications*

1.   Explain the purpose and procedure for stool collection to the patient.

2.   Provide the patient with a clean, dry bedpan or a plastic or cardboard container suitable for collecting and transporting stool specimens.

3.   Instruct the patient to defecate directly into the specimen container or the clean, dry bedpan.

4.   Give the patient tongue blades to transfer stool from the bedpan to the specimen container. Specimens collected on cloth or disposable diapers also should be transferred to the specimen container.

5.   Instruct the patient to collect diarrheal stools as well as formed specimens.

6.   Caution the patient not to overfill the specimen container and not to contaminate the outside of the container.

7.   Label all specimens with the patient's name and room number and send them to the laboratory as soon as they are collected. Make sure that the outer surface of the container has been well cleaned to prevent the contamination of hospital personnel.

Physical Examination

Examination of the physical characteristics of stool should include an evaluation of the color and consistency of the fecal material, as well as the presence of blood, pus, mucus, fat, tissue fragments, food residue, and parasites. However, the appearance of muscle fibers and undigested food particles in stool is not diagnostic because they may occur in diarrhea, due to the rapid transit time, as well as in malabsorption and steatorrhea.

> **Normal Values**
> The average normal adult excretes 100–300 g/day of brown stool that is neither fluid, mushy, nor hard but has a somewhat firm consistency.

Color

The normal brown fecal color is due to the presence of stercobilinogen (urobilin), which results from the action of bacteria on bilirubin in the intestinal tract. Abnormal fecal color may have diagnostic significance but also may reflect normal darkening following prolonged exposure to the air or the influence of certain foods, food dyes, and drugs. An adequate patient history generally helps to distinguish natural color changes from significant or pathologic abnormalities.

   Yellow to yellow-green stools occur in breast-fed infants because of the lack of stimulation of normal intestinal flora. Sterilization of the bowel by antibotics and severe diarrhea with rapid intestinal transit also reduce bacterial breakdown of bile pigments and produce yellowish stools. Yellow stools may occur with large amounts of dietary rhubarb and santonin therapy.

   Green stools may be due to severe diarrhea; the dark green meconium passed by newborn infants is due to the excretion of biliverdin and porphyrins. Green stools may result from:

Antibiotic therapy (due to impaired digestion)

Calomel administration

Dithiazanine iodide

Green vegetables (spinach), large quantities in the diet

Mercurous chloride administration

Tan or clay-colored stools are characteristic of obstructive jaundice and suggest the reduction or absence of bile due either to blockage of the common bile duct or intrinsic liver disease. A pale, greasy, acholic stool is the result of excessive fat excretion and suggests malabsorption syndrome or pancreatic insufficiency. Light-colored stools may result from:

Antacids	Deficiency of meat products in the diet
Barium sulfate	Milk, large amounts in the diet

Black stools may be caused by bleeding from upper gastrointestinal tract abnormalities such as malignant tumors or peptic ulcers and gives stools a tarry consistency. Black stools may result from:

Anticoagulants, excess dosage (due to gastrointestinal bleeding)	Iron salts (ferrous sulfate)
	Meat, large amounts in the diet
Bismuth	Phenylbutazone (due to gastro-intestinal bleeding)
Charcoal	
Cherries in the diet	Salicylates (due to gastrointestinal bleeding)
Indomethacin (due to gastrointestinal bleeding)	

Red stools may result from bleeding into the lower intestinal tract (lower colon, rectum, or anus), which generally appears as a red streaking on the surface only. Blood streaks on the outer surface of a stool specimen usually suggest a minor pathology of the lower colon such as hemorrhoids or an anal fissure. Red stools may result from:

Anticoagulants, excess dosage (due to gastrointestinal bleeding)	Phenolphthalein dye
	Phenylbutazone (due to gastro-intestinal bleeding)
Beets in the diet	
Bromsulphthalein (BSP) dye	Pyrvinium pamote
Carmine	Salicylates (due to gastrointestinal bleeding)
Indomethacin (due to gastrointestinal bleeding)	
	Tetracyclines (in glucosamine-potentiated syrup form)
Phenazopyridine hydrochloride	

Consistency

The appearance of blood, mucus, or pus, either mixed in or on the surface of feces, is never normal and may be due to a variety of gastrointestinal tract disorders. For example, pus usually results from ulcerating or fungating lesions other than amebic colitis but is seldom recognized unless a draining rectal infection is present. Mucus associated with blood and pus is found in the stool of patients with bacillary dysentery (shigellosis, salmonellosis), carcinoma of the colon, ulcerative colitis, acute ulcerating diverticulitis, or intestinal tuberculosis. Bloody mucus clinging to the fecal mass suggests a neoplasm or inflammatory process in the rectal canal.

Large quantities of mucus in the stool may occur with:

Amebiasis	Tumors, mucus-producing
Cholera	Typhoid
Constipation, spastic	Typhus
Irritable bowel syndrome (mucous colitis)	

Large quantities of pus in the stool may occur with:

Abscess, localized	Inflammation, acute
Bacillary dysentery, chronic	Salmonellosis
Enteritis, regional	Shigellosis
Fistulas (sigmoid colon, rectum, or anus)	Ulcerative colitis, chronic

Pasty, putty-like stools due to high fat content may occur with:

Celiac disease	Sprue, tropical
Fibrocystic disease of the pancreas	Steatorrhea, idiopathic
Jaundice, obstructive	Surgical resection of the small bowel or stomach
Pancreatitis, chronic	

▶▶ *Nursing Responsibilities and Implications*
See Specimen Collection and Handling (fecal)—Nursing Responsibilities and Implications.

Fecal Fat

Fat usually is excreted in the feces in relatively small amounts because most dietary lipids are hydrolyzed to fatty acids by the pancreatic enzyme lipase and absorbed into the bloodstream. Conversely, large amounts of neutral fat appear in the feces of patients with pancreatic disorders that decrease lipase activity, prevent hydrolysis of ingested fats, and impair fat absorption. A patient history of characteristically large, greasy, foul-smelling, light-colored, floating stools, a condition referred to as steatorrhea, indicates malabsorption and impaired assimilation of nutrients from the small intestine. Laboratory determinations of fecal fat may be used to evaluate the overall malabsorption syndrome, confirm the presence of steatorrhea, aid the diagnosis of pancreatic disorders, and monitor the effects of therapy.

Clinical Significance
Diagnosis of pathologic fat excretion may be confirmed by the microscopic screening of stained fecal smears for large neutral fat globules and by the measurement of total fat content. Because fecal smears with normal fat content exhibit many small fatty acid globules and occasional large neutral fat globules, the presence of many large globules indicates significant fat loss. Thus, patients with pancreatic steatorrhea frequently exhibit many large fatty acid globules and an increase in large neutral fat globules that can be confirmed

by measurement of total fecal fat. The amount of total fat excreted in feces generally is expressed as the percentage of ingested fat retained and absorbed or as the weight of fat excreted in 24 hours. The most significant expression of fecal fat content is the weight excreted in 24 hours based on an analysis of a 3- to 5-day collection following the ingestion of a standard fat diet.

Normal Views

The normal and clinically significant values for fecal fat excretion are:

Qualitative

Normal	<50 small (1−4 μm) fatty acid globules per high-power field
	Few large neutral fat globules
Steatorrhea	>50 large (6−75 μm) fatty acid globules per high-power field
	Significant increase in neutral fat globules

Quantitative

Normal	1−7 g/24 hours
	15%−25% of weight of total specimen
	1%−9% of fat intake
	>95% fat retention
Steatorrhea	>10% of fat intake
	<90% fat retention

Variations

Increased fat excretion (steatorrhea) may occur with:

Altered intestinal flora

Amyloidosis

Biliary tract obstruction

Blind loop syndrome

Carcinoma of the pancreas

Celiac disease

Cystic fibrosis

Deficiency of β-lipoprotein

Deficiency of bile salts

Deficiency of pancreatic enzymes

Diverticulosis

Fibrocystic disease of the pancreas (mucoviscidosis)

Fistulas

Hypogammaglobulinemia

Intestinal lipodystrophy (Whipple's disease)

Intestinal hypermotility

Lymphangiectasis

Lymphoma

Pancreatitis, chronic

Sprue

Surgery (loss of bowel function following resection)

Methodology

Qualitative screening tests for fat excretion that detect the presence of increased fatty acid globules on stained fecal smears may be performed on a single random stool specimen. Quantitative measurement of total fat excretion on random specimens has little significance, however, and a timed stool collection is required along with a known dietary fat intake for several days before testing. Fecal fat may be evaluated in infants, children, and adults who are unable to eat a standard fat diet by expressing the difference between fat ingestion and fat excretion as the percentage of fat retained.

Precautions

To ensure accurate test results, when collecting specimens for fecal fat analysis, prevent the contamination of feces with mineral oil, either from oral ingestion or local application to the rectal area, which gives false-positive reactions for fecal fat and invalidates the test results.

▶▶ *Nursing Responsibilities and Implications*

In addition to the nursing responsibilities listed under Specimen Collection and Handling (fecal), the nurse should proceed as follows:

1.   Provide the patient with a standard diet containing approximately 100 g of fat daily for 2–3 days before and during the specimen collection period.

2.   Instruct the patient in the proper procedure for collecting a satisfactory stool specimen (see Specimen Collection and Handling).

3.   Provide the patient with a specimen container suitable for collecting material for fecal fat analysis. Consult the laboratory for recommendations regarding satisfactory specimen containers because waxed cartons may alter the fat content of stool and should not be used.

4.   Collect all stool passed during a 3- to 5-day test period to eliminate daily variations in the amount of fat excretion.

5.   Refrigerate the entire specimen as it is collected to minimize the hydrolysis of fatty acids.

Occult Blood

The occult blood test is an important fecal screening procedure used to detect small, grossly invisible quantities of blood that do not alter the appearance of the stool. Whereas loss of more than 50 mL of blood into the gastrointestinal tract usually darkens the feces to the characteristic black color known as **melena**, lesser amounts are invisible and must be identified by the occult blood test. Laboratory determination of occult blood helps to confirm the presence of blood in black stools and may be useful in the diagnosis of serious gastrointestinal tract lesions.

Clinical Significance

Occult blood tests may remain positive for several weeks after a single bleeding episode and usually indicate the need for further investigation. The presence of hemoglobin breakdown products in feces, however, produces a false-positive reaction with guaiac or benzidine, the occult blood test reagents. On the other hand, a negative test for occult blood in a patient with an otherwise unexplained hypochromic anemia should not exclude the possibility of an undiagnosed gastrointestinal tract malignancy.

Normal Values
The occult blood test on feces is normally negative.

Variations
Positive occult blood tests may occur with:

Drug therapy	Thiazide diuretics	Upper gastrointestinal bleeding
Colchicine	Lower gastrointestinal bleeding	Bleeding varices
Indomethacin		Gastric carcinoma
Rauwolfia derivatives	Colitis	Gastritis
Salicylates	Colon carcinoma	Peptic ulcer
Steroids	Diverticulitis	

False-positive occult blood tests may occur with:

Heme compounds from meat, poultry, or fish in the diet

Iron salts (ferrous sulfate)

Toothbrushing, vigorous (with gum disease)

Vegetables (leafy green) in the diet

Vegetable peroxidase (horseradish) in the diet

False-negative occult blood tests may occur in patients receiving large doses of ascorbic acid (2–4 g/day).

Methodology
Occult blood tests may be performed on a single random stool specimen or on the small amount of fecal material remaining on a glove after rectal examination. Two to three separate samples from stool specimen collected on each of 3 consecutive days are needed to screen high-risk populations or individuals above 50 years of age.

Precautions
To ensure accurate results, the following precautions should be observed when collecting specimens for occult blood tests:

1. Instruct the patient to abstain from meat, poultry, and fish for 3 days before testing to eliminate false-positive reactions from the hemoglobin in these foodstuffs.

2. Withhold interfering substances such as vitamin C, bromides, iodines, potassium permanganate, and iron-containing medications that may interfere with test reactions for at least 3 days before testing.

▶▶ Nursing Responsibilities and Implications
In addition to the nursing responsibilities listed under Specimen Collection and Handling, the nurse should proceed as follows:

1. Describe the procedure to the patient and explain that two to three samples from different parts of a stool specimen collected on 3 consecutive days will be required.

2. Instruct the patient to collect stool specimens according to the procedure described under Specimen Collection and Handling (fecal).

Trypsin

Trypsin, the main proteolytic enzyme produced by the pancreas, is excreted into the duodenum with the pancreatic fluid and appears in large amounts in the stools of young children. Trypsin activity decreases, however, in the stools of older children and adults because the enzyme is destroyed by bacteria within the gastrointestinal tract. Trypsin activity usually is measured by testing the ability of the enzyme in a test solution of the patient's stool to digest and remove the opaque gelatin emulsion on x-ray film. Laboratory determinations of fecal trypsin usually are included in the investigation of malabsorption syndrome and cystic fibrosis in infants or children under 4 years of age and chronic pancreatic insufficiency in adults.

Clinical Significance

Fecal trypsin activity provides an unreliable indicator of pancreatic function in older children and adults and usually is undetectable in constipated stools due to their prolonged exposure to intestinal bacteria. Trypsin activity may be detected more readily, however, in stools with a rapid gastrointestinal transit time and may be used to evaluate diarrhea and steatorrhea of unknown etiology.

Normal Values

The normal values for fecal trypsin are:

Quantitative screening	Positive
Digestion of gelatin	2+ to 4+

Variations

Diminished or absent fecal trypsin may occur with severe constipation, cystic fibrosis, and chronic pancreatitis.

Methodology

Screening tests for fecal trypsin require only a small amount of stool from a random specimen.

▶▶ **Nursing Responsibilities and Implications**

See Specimen Collection and Handling (fecal)—Nursing Responsibilities and Implications.

Urobilinogen

Urobilinogen, the end product of bilirubin metabolism, is normally present in the stool because of the bacterial degradation of bile pigments in the intestinal tract. The amount of urobilinogen in the stool depends on the amount of bilirubin reaching the intestine via the bile ducts. It appears in somewhat decreased amounts in infants. A portion of the urobilinogen formed is reabsorbed from the intestine and excreted in the urine, and the remainder appears in the feces. Laboratory determinations of fecal urobilinogen levels are used to diagnose obstructive jaundice but have little diagnostic significance in patients receiving antibiotic therapy, which may decrease the activity of intestinal bacteria on bile pigments. (The significance and interpretation of urobilinogen values are discussed in Chapters 1 and 3.)

Clinical Significance

The concentration of fecal urobilinogen is influenced by the amount of bilirubin formed, the rate of flow through the common bile duct, and the rate of red blood cell destruction. Urobilinogen excretion is diminished in proportion to the degree of obstruction to bile flow, with the total absence of fecal urobilinogen or its derivative, urobilin, indicating complete obstruction. Fecal urobilinogen concentrations are increased in a number of conditions related to excessive red blood cell hemolysis, although urine urobilinogen procedures generally are performed to diagnose these disorders because they are less complicated.

Normal Values

The normal values for fecal urobilinogen are:

Qualitative	Positive
Quantitative	40–250 mg/24 hours
	75–350 mg/100 g of stool

Variations

Decreased fecal urobilinogen levels may occur with:

Antibiotic therapy	Diminished red blood cell production
Aplastic anemia	Obstructive jaundice
Bile duct obstruction	

Increased fecal urobilinogen levels may occur with hemolytic anemia, hemolytic jaundice, and excessive red blood cell hemolysis.

Methodology

Qualitative screening tests for fecal urobilinogen may be performed on a single random stool specimen collected in a standard specimen container. Quantitative determinations of fecal urobilinogen concentrations require a 3- to 4-day total stool specimen, which must be kept refrigerated during the entire collection period.

Precautions

To ensure accurate results, the following precautions should be observed when collecting specimens for fecal urobilinogen determinations:

1. Withhold antibiotic therapy, whenever possible, for at least 1 week before and during the specimen collection period to promote normal activity of intestinal bacteria.

2. Protect stool specimens from light during the entire collection period to prevent urobilinogen from being converted to urobilin, which will interfere with the test results.

▶▶ *Nursing Responsibilities and Implications*

In addition to the nursing responsibilities listed under Specimen Collection and Handling, the nurse should proceed as follows:

1. Describe the procedure for fecal urobilinogen to the patient and explain that a 3- to 4-day total stool specimen will be required.

2. Provide the patient with a suitable container and instruct the patient to collect stool specimens as described in Specimen Collection and Handling (fecal).

3. Refrigerate the entire stool specimen during the collection period.

Microbiologic Examination

Tests for specific pathogenic fecal microorganisms such as those responsible for typhoid, dysentery, brucellosis, and amebiasis are discussed in Chapter 9.

GASTRIC ANALYSIS

Secretions continuously produced by parietal cells of the stomach may be collected by gastric intubation to determine the amount of acid present during the resting state and following stimulation. Gastric secretions consist of mucus, hydrochloric acid, and electrolytes, along with enzymes that are vital to the digestion of food and absorption of vitamin B_{12}, folic acid, and iron. Analysis of the acidity and total volume of the gastric contents may be used to determine the following:

1. The location and type of ulcer.

2. The presence of the Zollinger-Ellison syndrome.

3. The type of surgical procedure to be performed in patients with peptic ulcers.

4. The success of surgical or medical therapy for peptic ulcer.

Laboratory analysis of gastric contents is essential to the diagnosis of peptic ulcers (including the Zollinger-Ellison syndrome), gastric neoplasms, atrophic gastritis, and pernicious anemia and guides their treatment. Because the normal values of gastric secretions are poorly defined, only the extremes of anacidity or marked hypersecretion are considered to indicate a problem. Therefore, gastric analysis alone is seldom diagnostically significant and must be evaluated along with the patient's history and other pertinent clinical, radiographic, and laboratory studies.

Specimen Collection and Handling

Gastric secretions are aspirated with a syringe attached to a nasogastric tube, which is passed through the mouth or nasopharynx with the patient in a sitting position. Many tubes used for gastric intubation have distance markers to aid in proper positioning in the most dependent portion of the stomach; the tube may be positioned fluoroscopically to ensure good intragastric placement. The distance from the tip of a properly positioned tube to the teeth is about 60 cm.

The most significant information regarding gastric contents is obtained by a two-part test that measures the basal acid output (BAO) and the histamine-augmented maximal acid output (MAO). The entire fasting gastric contents usually are aspirated and discarded before the test begins but may be examined for residual volume, gross composition, and the presence of bacteria, particularly *Mycobacterium tuberculosis*. Four samples of basal gastric secretion are then aspirated at 15-minute intervals during the first portion of the test, placed in clean specimen containers, numbered, and sent to the laboratory for analysis.

The appropriate histamine or betazole (Histalog) dose is then administered to the patient to stimulate maximal acid production in the stomach, and an additional four or eight specimens are aspirated at 15-minute intervals. The entire procedure requires about 3 hours and, except for the initial gagging associated with the insertion of the nasogastric tube, is not uncomfortable. A more complete volume of gastric secretion is recovered by applying continuous manual suction with the syringe rather than removing accumulated secretions intermittently. It is essential that basal physiologic and stable environmental conditions be maintained during testing to avoid extraneous stimulation of gastric mucosal cells.

Gastric intubation usually is contraindicated for patients with suspected esophageal varices, diverticula, esophageal stenosis, malignant esophageal tumors, aortic aneurysms, recent severe gastric hemorrhage, carcinoid syndrome, congestive heart failure, myocardial infarction, or pregnancy. The histamine-augmented measurement of maximal acid secretion is contraindicated in patients with a history of allergies, bronchial asthma, urticaria, hypertension, and severe cardiac, pulmonary, or renal disease.

Precautions
To ensure the clinical validity of gastric analysis, the following precautions should be observed:

1.   Protect the patient from stressful situations that may evoke physiologic reactions such as fear, anger, or depression.

2.   Instruct the patient not to smoke on the morning of testing until after the gastric analysis is completed because smoking stimulates gastric acid secretion.

3.   Withhold any medications that may influence the test results for the 24 hours prior to the test, including anticholinergic drugs, which inhibit histamine stimulation of gastric acid secretions and produce falsely decreased acid measurements. Gastric stimulants such as adrenocorticosteroids, alcohol, and reserpine also should be withheld.

4.   Instruct the patient to expectorate all saliva and nasorespiratory secretions while the gastric contents are being aspirated.

▶▶ Nursing Responsibilities and Implications

1.   Instruct the patient to fast after the evening meal on the day before testing because food and fluid will alter gastric secretion. Water is permitted until midnight or 8 hours before intubation.

2.   Explain the general intubation procedure required for gastric analysis so that the patient will be cooperative.

3. Provide emotional support to help reduce the patient's apprehension about the procedure.

4. Instruct the patient to avoid the sight or smell of food during the collection of stomach contents to prevent the stimulation of gastric secretions.

5. Position the patient in a high Fowler's position or on the left side with the head elevated approximately 45 degrees. Instruct the patient to breathe deeply through the mouth during intubation.

6. Insert the lubricated tip of a Levin nasogastric tube (#14, #16, or #18) into the floor of the patient's nose and gradually advance it into the stomach. Carefully position the tip of the tube in the dependent portion of the stomach to ensure complete aspiration of gastric contents. (The tip of the Levin tube usually is well within the stomach when the second marker is at the nares.)

7. Tape the nasogastric tube securely to the patient's nose or cheek, making sure that the tube does not press or pull against the nares.

8. Position the patient on the back and slightly to the left to promote relaxation before the residual fasting gastric contents are collected.

9. Attach a 50 mL syringe to the nasogastric tube and aspirate the residual fasting gastric contents. This specimen may be discarded or sent to the laboratory for analysis of volume and composition. The collection of basal acid secretion begins after the fasting contents have been removed.

10. Begin the continuous aspiration of gastric contents and separate the aspirate into 15-minute samples. Disregard the first one or two 15-minute samples following initial aspiration to allow the patient to recover from the intubation procedure.

11. Collect four 15-minute samples of gastric contents. If the basal secretion study is to be followed by the augmented histamine test, administer a suitable dose of parenteral antihistamine 30 minutes after beginning the collection of the basal specimen.

12. Administer a test dose of 0.4 mg of histamine acid phosphate, 0.5 mg of betazole (Histalog), or 6 μg of pentagastrin per kilogram of body weight as soon as the collection of basal secretion is completed. When Histalog is used to stimulate gastric secretions, the prior administration of the parenteral antihistamine may be omitted, but eight rather than four 15-minute samples must be collected.

13. Monitor the patient following the administration of histamine for adverse side effects, including increased pulse, decreased blood pressure, flushing, intense headache, dyspnea, vomiting, diarrhea, and shock.

14. Continue to collect gastric contents in 15-minute samples for 1 hour if histamine acid phosphate has been used or for 2 hours if Histalog has been administered.

15. Clamp and withdraw the tube when all test specimens have been obtained.

16. Send all basal and maximal acid secretion samples to the laboratory for analysis. Make certain that each sample is correctly labeled with the collection time and whether the sample is basal or stimulated.

Physical Examination

Laboratory examination of the secretions collected during gastric analysis frequently includes an evaluation of the fasting stomach contents for residual volume, color, mucus, blood, and the presence of bacteria. Gastric secretions usually separate into three distinct layers after aspiration, with mucus at the top, an opalescent fluid in the center, and sediment at the bottom. The presence of food particles following a 12-hour fast is abnormal and often occurs in pyloric obstruction, which delays the emptying of the stomach.

Normal Values

A normal fasting stomach contains 50–80 mL of pale gray, clear, or translucent, slightly viscous fluid, which should be free of undigested food particles, blood, or bile.

Volume

Decreased fasting volume (<50 mL) may occur with:

Gastric atrophy   Gastric hypermotility

Gastric carcinoma   Pernicious anemia

Increased fasting volume (>80 mL) may occur with:

Duodenal ulcers   Pyloric obstruction

Gastric hypomotility   Zollinger-Ellison syndrome

Mucus

Mucus is a normal constituent of gastric secretions and is largely responsible for the viscosity of the gastric contents. Additional mucus may result from swallowed saliva or nasorespiratory secretions, as well as small amounts of reflux from the duodenal contents. **Increased gastric mucus** may occur with gastritis and pyloric obstruction.

Color

Abnormally colored gastric secretions may have a **red-brown** appearance similar to coffee grounds because of the presence of blood or may exhibit a **yellow-green** color because of the presence of bile. Bile is not usually present in gastric contents but frequently accompanies excessive retching or gagging during intubation. The presence of marked amounts of bile indicates the possibility of an obstructing lesion high in the small intestine.

Blood

Blood may appear in gastric secretions as flecks or streaks resulting from minor trauma during intubation or the excessively vigorous aspiration of stomach contents. The presence of old, semidigested blood or larger amounts of blood produces a red-brown appearance similar to coffee grounds and indicates that the tube should be removed immediately. Significant quantities of blood in gastric contents should be confirmed by the Hematest or guaiac test.

Marked amounts of blood may result from:

Esophageal varices   Hiatal hernia, accompanied by
                                    esophagitis
Gastric carcinoma

Gastritis   Mallory-Weiss syndrome

                                    Peptic ulcer

Nursing Responsibilities and Implications

See Specimen Collection and Handling (gastric)—Nursing Responsibilities and Implications.

Gastric Acidity

The complete role of gastric acidity in normal and pathologic processes is complex, but secretion of hydrochloric acid is important to the initiation of protein digestion. Gastric acid output during the unstimulated or fasting state is correlated to some degree with body weight and therefore is usually somewhat higher in men than in women. However, although small amounts of acid are normally secreted under resting or unstimulated conditions, emotional stimuli and the sight or smell of food induce gastric secretion and increase acid production. Laboratory measurement of gastric acidity is used to diagnose peptic ulcer disease, including Zollinger-Ellison syndrome, and often can be correlated with clinical findings and prognosis.

Clinical Significance

Analysis of gastric acidity provides the most clinically significant information when values for basal or maximal acid output are at either the extreme upper or lower limit of acid secretion. **Basal acid output** (BAO) is the amount of gastric acid secreted during 1 hour following an overnight fast without any external stimulation. Basal acid secretion represents the response of the stomach to physiologic stimuli such as vagal and hormonal influences, which continually act on the gastric mucosa during the interdigestive state. The total gastric output during 1 hour of basal secretion is collected in four separate samples at 15-minute intervals, with the acid content of each combined and reported as milliequivalents per hour.

   Maximal acid output (MAO) is the total amount of gastric acid secreted during 1 hour following intense stimulation of the gastric mucosal cells by the parenteral administration of histamine or betazole (Histalog). The acidity of four specimens collected at 15-minute intervals following pharmacologic stimulation is measured separately and reported as milliequivalents per hour or as the percentage of increase over basal acid output. The term **peak acid output** (PAO) refers to the sum of the two highest consecutive 15-minute specimen values and is reported as milliequivalents per 30 minutes.

   Laboratory reports of gastric analysis generally record three measurements on each basal sample of gastric contents collected: volume in milliliters, titratable acidity expressed in milliequivalents, and pH measured electrometrically. Test reports also may include the calculated acid output for each individual sample as well as total acid output and total volume obtained by adding individual sample values. The distinction between free acid, total acid, and combined acid, which formerly was used, is no longer significant because previous concepts regarding gastric secretion have been found to lack physiochemical validity.

   Although many individuals lose some basal acidity with advancing age, failure to secrete gastric acid after physiologic stimulation indicates a loss of parietal cell mass and strongly suggests atrophic gastritis. Thus, the principal diagnostic value of tests for MAO is to demonstrate anacidity or the failure of gastric acid to fall below pH 6.0 at any time. Measurement of gastric acid secretion is also helpful in the diagnosis of hematologic disorders characterized by impaired absorption of vitamin B_{12}, folic acid, or iron.

Normal Values

The normal and clinically significant values for gastric acidity are:

Basal Acid Output

Normal

Men	2−5 mEq/hr
Women	1−4 mEq/hr

Duodenal ulcer

Men	5−10 mEq/hr
Women	3−8 mEq/hr

Gastric carcinoma	0−3 mEq/hr

Gastric ulcer

Men	1−5 mEq/hr
Women	1−3 mEq/hr
Zollinger-Ellison syndrome	>20 mEq/hr

Maximal Acid Output

Normal

Men	5−26 mEq/hr
Women	7−15 mEq/hr

Duodenal ulcer

Men	15−35 mEq/hr
Women	10−20 mEq/hr

Gastric carcinoma

Men	0−20 mEq/hr
Women	0−5 mEq/hr

Gastric ulcer

Men	10−20 mEq/hr
Women	5−15 mEq/hr
Gastritis, pernicious anemia	0 mEq/hr
Zollinger-Ellison syndrome	35−60 mEq/hr
pH	1.6−1.8

BAO/MAO Ratio

Normal	0.3−0.6
	1 : 2.5−1 : 5
	20% of maximal
Duodenal ulcer	20%−40% of maximal
Gastric carcinoma	20% of maximal
Gastric ulcer	20%−40% of maximal
Zollinger-Ellison syndrome	>60% of maximal

Variations

Increased hydrochloric acid production (hyperchlorhydria) occurs with peptic ulcers, particularly those in the duodenal or pyloric areas.

Diminished hydrochloric acid production (hypochlorhydria) frequently accompanies gastric atrophy.

Absence of hydrochloric acid production (anacidity, achlorhydria) may indicate gastric carcinoma and is characteristic of pernicious anemia.

Measurement

Analysis of stomach secretions and evaluation of gastric acidity require numerous specimens collected following intubation according to the procedure described in Specimen Collection and Handling (gastric).

Precautions

Measurement of MAO following gastric stimulation with histamine frequently requires increased attention and care from the nursing staff for the duration of the test. Administration of 0.04 mg of histamine per kilogram of body weight in a sensitive individual may result in severe allergic reactions, including facial flushing, headache, a drop in blood pressure, and loss of consciousness. Thus, the use of 50–100 mg of betazole (Histalog) is preferred because it produces minimal side effects while providing gastric stimulation and test results comparable to those of histamine.

▶▶ **Nursing Responsibilities and Implications**

See Specimen Collection and Handling (gastric)—Nursing Responsibilities and Implications.

PLEURAL FLUID ANALYSIS

Pleural fluid is a serous effusion produced by plasma ultrafiltration within the slitlike compartment surrounding the lungs that lubricates the parietal and visceral tissues. Abnormal accumulation of fluid in the pleural cavity occurs in various primary and secondary lung diseases and is classified as transudate or exudate. A **pleural transudate** is an effusion produced by the factors, including increased venous pressure or decreased plasma albumin, that accompany congestive heart failure, hepatic cirrhosis, or hypoproteinemia resulting from nephrotic syndrome. A **pleural exudate** is an effusion caused by damage to the mesothelial lining of the pleural cavity resulting from conditions such as pneumonia, tuberculosis, neoplasms, trauma, rheumatoid disease, or pulmonary infarcts.

Clinical indications for pleural fluid aspiration include effusion of unknown etiology, dyspnea caused by fluid accumulation, hemothorax, or empyema, and intrapleural treatment of infection or malignancy. Laboratory tests of pleural effusions often provide valuable diagnostic information about the disorders that cause their formation and guide further therapy. The collection of pleural fluid also relieves symptoms produced by the effusion, provides lifesaving lung decompression, and allows drugs to be instilled into the pleural cavity. Analysis of pleural effusions generally includes a physical evaluation of gross appearance, total and differential leukocyte counts, microbiologic examination, and determination of glucose, specific gravity, and total protein.

Specimen Collection and Handling

Pleural fluid must be obtained aseptically through aspiration of the pleural cavity (**thoracocentesis**) by a physican who is skilled in the procedure and aware of its potential complications. At least 20–50 mL of effusion should be collected with a sterile syringe and needle and transferred to a sterile flask containing 2 mL of sterile 4% sodium citrate or a few drops of sterile heparin. A small amount of the specimen also should be transferred to a flask without citrate or heparin so that clot formation can be observed.

Because most pleural effusions produce at least 100 mL of fluid, sufficient fluid is readily available to perform all necessary diagnostic tests on a single specimen to avoid repeating the procedure. Specimens should be delivered to the laboratory immediately for analysis within 1 hour of collection to prevent bacterial overgrowth and alteration of cellular constituents or chemical composition. When prompt delivery to the laboratory is not possible, pleural fluid specimens should be refrigerated to help ensure accurate cellular, chemical, and microbiologic test results.

▶▶ *Nursing Responsibilities and Implications*

1. Explain the purpose and procedure of thoracocentesis to the patient to reinforce the physician's discussion.

2. Determine the patient's understanding of the procedure and obtain an informed consent.

3. Instruct the patient not to move during the procedure to prevent additional damage to the pleura and lung; inform the patient to expect some discomfort and pain when the pleura is entered.

4. Place the patient in the high Fowler's position or on the unaffected side with the arm on the affected side raised over the head.

5. Monitor the patient's vital signs before, during, and after the procedure; observe for changes in color, respirations, and amount of diaphoresis.

6. Observe the patient for bleeding at the insertion site or hemoptysis following the procedure.

Physical Examination

The physical characteristics of pleural fluid may be diagnostically significant and generally include an assessment of the volume, color, clarity, and clot formation.

Normal Values
The pleural cavity normally contains less than 20 mL of clear, transparent, or pale yellow to amber, sterile fluid that does not produce a clot.

Volume
Increased pleural fluid volume may occur with:

Bacterial pneumonia	Congestive heart failure	Lymphoma
Bronchogenic carcinoma	Hypoproteinemia	Metastatic carcinoma
	Liver disease, chronic	Neoplasms

Nephrotic syndrome	Systemic lupus	Tuberculosis
Pulmonary infarcts	erythematosus	Viral pneumonia
Rheumatoid disease	Trauma	

Color

Abnormal pleural fluid may be pink, red, yellow, or white. Pleural fluid appears **pink** when the red blood cell count reaches 5000–10,000 cells/μL; **red** fluid usually is due to the presence of at least 100,000 red blood cells/μL. **Yellow** pleural fluid may be due to xanthochromia, although this can be difficult to assess because normal fluid is straw-colored; **white** fluid usually is caused by the presence of fat.

Clarity

Abnormal pleural fluid may appear turbid, milky, creamy, or bloody. **Turbid** pleural fluid may be caused by the presence of increased leukocytes associated with septic or nonseptic inflammations. **Milky** fluid usually is caused by the presence of cholesterol and is characteristic of true chylous effusions, due to the leakage of thoracic duct contents, or pseudochylous effusions, due to the breakdown of cellular lipids. **Creamy** fluid may result from damage to the thoracic duct. **Bloody** specimens may result from bleeding induced by thoracocentesis or may indicate the presence of a hemorrhagic effusion, reflecting either underlying disease or a ruptured blood vessel in the pleural cavity.

Turbid or cloudy pleural fluid may occur with:

Bacterial infection	Rheumatoid disease
Rheumatic fever	Tuberculosis

Bloody pleural fluid may occur with:

Congestive heart failure	Pneumonia	Pulmonary infarcts
Hepatic cirrhosis	Postmyocardial infarction	Trauma, closed chest
Pancreatitis	syndrome	Tumors, intrapleural

Cell Counts

Pleural fluid cell counts enumerate the leukocytes present in 1 μL of the effusion and should be performed on turbid fluid whenever an inflammatory process is suspected. A differential white blood cell count usually is performed on pleural fluid with elevated leukocyte counts to determine the relative percentage of specific cell types. Red blood cells normally are not found in pleural fluid, and their presence indicates either trauma or a malignant process.

Normal Values

The normal pleural fluid cell counts are:

Leukocytes	<1000/μL
Eosinophils	<10%
Lymphocytes	<50%
Neutrophils	<50%

Variations
Elevated pleural fluid leukocyte levels ($>1000/\mu$L) may occur with:

Carcinoma

Chylothorax

Inflammatory processes

Lymphatic leukemia, chronic

Lymphoma involving the pleural cavity

Parapneumonic effusions

Postpneumonic effusions

Tuberculosis

Tuberculous empyema

Uremia

Glucose

Normal pleural fluid glucose concentrations are essentially the same as serum glucose levels and reflect changes in blood values after a lag of 2−4 hours. Thus, systemic hyperglycemia or hypoglycemia may be associated with falsely increased or decreased pleural fluid test results. Determination of pleural fluid glucose levels is used to diagnose bacterial infections and malignancies and may be helpful in differentiating rheumatoid effusions from those produced during systemic lupus erythematosus.

Normal Values
The normal and clinically significant values for pleural fluid glucose are:

Normal	>60 mg/dL
	<40 mg/dL below the plasma glucose level
Rheumatoid disease	<60 mg/dL
	>40 mg/dL below the plasma glucose level

Variations
Decreased pleural fluid glucose levels may occur with:

Bacterial infections

Malignancies

Neoplastic effusions

Rheumatoid effusions

Septic effusions

Tuberculous effusions

Methodology
Pleural fluid glucose measurements require 5 mL of pleural effusion obtained several hours after serum glucose analysis to aid in the interpretation of test results.

pH

Pleural fluid pH measurements may be used to guide the evaluation and treatment of pleural effusions and are valuable in the diagnosis of esophageal rupture.

Normal Values

Normal pleural fluid has a pH of 7.4.

Variations

Decreased pleural fluid pH may occur with:

Empyema ($<$7.3)	Parapneumonic effusions ($<$7.2)
Esophageal rupture ($<$6.0)	Tuberculous effusions ($<$7.3)
Loculated effusions ($<$7.3)	

Methodology

Pleural fluid pH determinations require 3 mL of pleural effusion collected anaerobically in a heparinized syringe. Specimens should be placed in an ice bath, with the tip of the needle or syringe sealed, and delivered to the laboratory immediately for analysis within 20 minutes. However, markedly acidic pleural effusions associated with esophageal perforation may be evaluated immediately after collection with pH reagent paper.

Specific Gravity and Total Protein

Determination of the specific gravity and total protein level of pleural fluid is used to identify the effusion as a transudate or an exudate. For example, most transudates exhibit normal total protein levels, whereas exudates are characterized by elevated protein values. In addition, the increased total protein concentrations resulting from disease and damage to the mesothelial lining of the pleural cavity elevates the specific gravity of exudates. Individual pleural fluid protein fractions may be analyzed by protein electrophoresis on the fluid. (The significance of total protein and protein fractions is discussed in Chapter 4.)

Normal Values

The normal and clinically significant values for specific gravity and total protein are:

Normal	
Specific gravity	1.015
Total protein	1−2 g/dL
Transudate	
Specific gravity	1.010−1.020
Total protein	$<$3 g/dL
Exudate	
Specific gravity	$>$1.020
Total protein	$>$3 g/dL

Microbiologic Examination

Microbiologic examination of pleural fluid may be performed to detect the presence of bacteria, mycobacteria, fungi, viruses, or parasites and to help determine the cause of inflammatory and noninflammatory disease processes. Microbiologic evaluations of pleural fluid routinely includes an examination of Gram-stained and acid-fast stained smears along with aerobic and anaerobic cultures. (The purpose and significance of various microbiologic procedures are discussed in Chapter 9.)

Methodology

Routine microbiologic examination requires 3–5 mL of pleural fluid collected in a sterile screw-capped container containing sterile sodium heparin or EDTA to prevent the formation of clots, which may trap microorganisms. Detection of suspected mycobacterial and mycologic infections requires 5–10 ml of pleural fluid submitted separately in a sterile anticoagulated tube. Pleural fluid specimens for anaerobic culture should be collected in an evacuated syringe, inoculated into an oxygen-free transport tube, and delivered to the laboratory within 30 minutes.

SYNOVIAL FLUID ANALYSIS

Synovial fluid is a modified connective tissue fluid produced in joint and tendon spaces by ultrafiltration of plasma and secretion of a mucoid hyaluronic acid-protein complex by synovial membranes. Synovial fluid provides nourishment for joint cartilage and acts as a lubricant for joint surfaces to minimize friction between bones during movement or weight bearing. The need for synovial fluid analysis is indicated by greatly increased joint effusion and may prove useful in the diagnosis of suspected infections and the differential diagnosis of arthritis.

Laboratory analysis of synovial fluid normally includes an evaluation of physical appearance, volume, viscosity, and clotting ability, along with microscopic examination for cells and crystals, microbiologic studies, and various chemistry determinations. The results of synovial fluid studies usually do not indicate a specific diagnosis but often are useful in categorizing a joint disease into one of the arthritides disease groups. Thus, synovial fluid may be assigned, according to its physical, microscopic, and chemical characteristics, to one of five pathologic groups, each of which overlaps with a number of disease states. In many cases, however, the specific diagnosis within these disease groups must be made on the basis of the patient's clinical history, physical examination, and radiographic results.

Joint disease may be divided into several arthritides groups, which are categorized as Group I (noninflammatory), Group II (inflammatory), Group III (infectious), Group IV (crystal-induced), and Group V (hemorrhagic), as follows:

Group I (noninflam-
matory)

  Osteoarthritis

  Osteochronditis
dissecans

  Osteochrondromatosis

  Neuroarthropathy

Traumatic arthritis

Group II (inflammatory)

  Ankylosing spondylitis

  Reiter's disease

  Rheumatic fever

  Rheumatoid arthritis

  Scleroderma

Systemic lupus erythe-
matosus

Group III (infectious/
septic)

  Bacterial infections

  Fungal infections

  Tuberculous infections

Group IV (crystal-induced)	Group V (hemorrhagic)	Pigmented villonodular synovitis
Gout	Hemophilia	Synovioma
Pseudogout	Neuropathic osteoar-thropathy	Trauma

Specimen Collection and Handling

Aspiration of a joint effusion (**arthrocentesis**) must be performed by a physician skilled in the procedure using sterile technique under strict aseptic conditions. Although synovial fluid may be obtained from any joint, it usually is aspirated from the knee to aid in the diagnosis of joint disease and relieve symptoms. Synovial fluid specimens should be collected with a disposable needle and plastic syringe and distributed into three sterile test tubes for chemical analysis, microscopic examination, and microbiologic culture.

▶▶ *Nursing Responsibilities and Implications*

1. Describe the procedure for arthrocentesis and reassure the patient; obtain an informed consent.
2. Instruct the patient not to eat anything for at least 4–6 hours (preferably 12 hours) before arthrocentesis to allow equilibration between synovial fluid and blood glucose.
3. Transfer 2–5 mL of the specimen to two sterile test tubes containing 25 units of sterile heparin per milliliter of synovial fluid for chemical analysis, cell count, differential, and examination of crystals.
4. Transfer 2–5 mL of the specimen to the third tube, which should be free of anticoagulants, for microbiologic culture and observation of spontaneous clot formation.
5. Apply an elastic bandage to the joint to provide support and limit edema.
6. Apply cold packs to the joint as ordered to reduce pain and edema.
7. Advise the patient to avoid excessive use of the joint for several days.

Physical Examination

Laboratory evaluation of synovial fluid normally includes a measurement of the volume along with a description of the overall appearance, including clarity, color, the presence of blood, viscosity, and mucin clot formation (Table 8-4).

Normal Values
Normal joints produce 0.13–3.5 mL of crystal clear, transparent, or pale yellow, slightly viscous synovial fluid.

Volume
The relatively small amount of synovial fluid generally encountered during aspiration of a normal knee or other uninflamed joint is reflected by a "dry tap." The presence of arthri-

tides or other joint disease produces synovial fluid effusion several times greater than normal, with the volume of fluid aspirated proportional to the severity of joint involvement. Although there is no absolute correlation between synovial fluid volume and the cause, severity, or duration of joint disease, the greatest amount of effusion is present during acute inflammation. Because the amount of effusion decreases as the severity of the inflammation subsides, the volume of synovial fluid removed during aspiration may help to monitor the course of joint disease.

Clarity

Decreased synovial fluid clarity or transparency, ranging from slight cloudiness to marked turbidity, indicates a significant increase in the number of inflammatory cells resulting from septic and noninfectious joint diseases. The degree of synovial fluid turbidity correlates directly with a number of factors, including the presence of leukocytes, erythrocytes, crystals, and microorganisms. Thus, synovial fluid becomes cloudy to purulent in septic joint disease but may remain clear or become slightly turbid to cloudy in inflammatory and noninflammatory arthritides.

Synovial fluid turbidity may be assessed by the ability to read newsprint through a glass tube, but the specimen may appear falsely turbid if viewed through a plastic collecting syringe. Synovial fluid clarity may be graded from 0 to 4+ according to the following:

0   = crystal clear fluid.

1+ = faintly cloudy, smoky, or hazy fluid with slight (barely visible) turbidity.

2+ = turbidity clearly present, but newsprint can be read easily through the tube.

3+ = newsprint not easily read through the tube.

4+ = newsprint cannot be seen through the tube.

Turbid synovial fluid may occur with:

Cartilage fragments, floating	Leukocytes, increased
Crystals, suspended	Synovial fragments, floating
Inflammatory cells	

Milky synovial fluid may occur with:

Gouty arthritis, acute	Systemic lupus erythematosus
Lymphatic drainage into the joint	Tuberculosis arthritis
Rheumatoid arthritis, chronic	

Grossly purulent synovial fluid may occur during the later stages of acute septic arthritis.

Color

The appearance of abnormally colored synovial fluid indicates the presence of joint disease, hemorrhage, inflammation, or trauma and must be noted on the laboratory report form. **Dark yellow-orange**, **pink**, **red**, or **dark red-brown** supernatant fluid, especially when associated with bloody specimens, suggests that hemarthrosis occurred at least 1–2 hours before arthrocentesis. The significance of **yellow** (xanthochromic) specimens may be difficult to interpret, however, because normal synovial fluid appears pale yellow; **gray-green** specimens indicate joint disease or inflammation.

TABLE 8-4 Synovial Fluid Characteristics in Selected Disorders

Condition	Appearance	Viscosity/ Mucin Clot	White Blood Cells/μL (percentage of neutrophils)	Glucose (mg/dL below serum)	Culture
Normal	Clear/straw-colored	High/good	<180 (<25%)	<10	Sterile
Group I	Slightly turbid/ yellow	High/good	200–5000 (<30%)	<20	Sterile
Group II	Turbid/yellow-white	Decreased/fair to poor	3000–100,000 (>50%)	>25	Sterile
Group III	Opaque/gray-green	Decreased/poor	5000–200,000 (>80%)	>40	Often positive
Group IV	Turbid/opalescent	Decreased/poor	1000–100,000 (>70%)	<10	Sterile
Group V	Bloody/red-brown	Decreased/poor	>5000 (>25%)	<10	Sterile
Gout	Cloudy to milky/ yellow	Decreased/fair to poor	100–100,000 (<90%)	<80	Sterile

	Appearance	Viscosity/mucin clot	WBC count (%PMN)		Culture
Osteoarthritis	Clear/yellow	Variable/good to fair	50–5000 (<30%)	<10	Sterile
Pseudogout	Clear to slightly turbid/yellow	Decreased/fair to poor	50–75,000 (<90%)	<20	Sterile
Rheumatic fever	Slightly turbid	Variable/good to fair	50–50,000 (<60%)	<20	Sterile
Rheumatoid arthritis	Turbid to milky/yellow-green	Decreased/fair to poor	200–80,000 (<90%)	<60	Sterile
Septic arthritis	Turbid to purulent/gray	Decreased/poor	200–200,000 (>50%)	>40	Often positive
Systemic lupus erythematosus	Clear to slightly turbid/yellow	Variable/good to fair	50–10,000 (<40%)	<30	Sterile
Traumatic arthritis	Clear/yellow (occasionally bloody)	Variable/good to fair	50–10,000 (<30%)	<20	Sterile
Tuberculous arthritis	Turbid/yellow	Decreased/poor	2000–100,000 (<95%)	<100	Often positive

Greenish synovial fluid may occur with:

Crystal-induced arthritis, acute	Pseudogout, acute
Gout, acute	Rheumatoid arthritis, chronic
Hemophilus influenzae septic arthritis	

Blood

The presence of relatively small amounts of blood in synovial fluid specimens due to a traumatic aspiration may be visually indistinguishable from the blood produced by frank bleeding in the joint (**hemarthrosis**). However, bright red blood incurred during a traumatic tap is streaked unevenly throughout the specimen and decreases as aspiration proceeds or appears toward the end of the procedure. Blood from a traumatic tap may clot spontaneously during or shortly after synovial fluid collection because of the presence of fibrinogen and other clotting factors. Conversely, blood in synovial fluid prior to aspiration, particularly blood resulting from hemophilia, appears red-brown and is distributed evenly throughout the syringe. Blood from hemarthrosis caused by fracture, tumor, or hemophilia will clot only when the hemorrhage immediately precedes or coincides with the arthrocentesis.

Bloody synovial fluid may occur with:

Fracture through the joint surface	Osteoarthritis	Septic arthritis
Hemophilic arthritis	Pigmented villonodular synovitis	Traumatic arthritis
Neurogenic arthropathy	Rheumatoid arthritis	Traumatic tap
		Tumor involving the joint

Viscosity

Synovial fluid viscosity, normally high because of the hyaluronic acid content, is markedly decreased in all effusions associated with inflammatory joint disease, indicated by a thin, watery fluid containing degraded hyaluronidase molecules. The viscosity of freshly drawn synovial fluid may be evaluated qualitatively by measuring how far a drop of fluid will stretch before breaking when expressed slowly from the collecting syringe. Normal synovial fluid viscosity produces a string 5 cm or more in length; in abnormally low synovial fluid viscosity, the length of the string is 4 cm or less.

Decreased synovial fluid viscosity may occur with:

Gout	Rheumatic fever	Septic arthritis
Inflammatory joint disease, chronic	Rheumatoid arthritis	Trauma
	Sepsis	

Mucin Clot Formation

Synovial fluid normally clots firmly when mixed with diluted acetic acid (the mucin clot test) but clots poorly in essentially all inflammatory joint diseases. Mucin clot formation may be evaluated by adding one part of synovial fluid to four parts of 2%–5% acetic acid and observing the quality of the clot produced after 1 minute. The quality of the clot produced is a measure of the hyaluronic acid content of synovial fluid and reflects the nature or degree of polymerization of the hyaluronoprotein. Mucin clot formation may be evaluated as follows:

Good = firm, compact clot surrounded by clear solution; does not break up when agitated.

Fair = soft clot surrounded by a slightly turbid solution.

Poor = friable clot surrounded by a turbid solution; breaks up readily when agitated.

Very poor = cloudy suspension without a true clot.

Decreased mucin clot formation may occur with:

Gout

Inflammatory conditions, active (fair mucin clot)

Rheumatoid arthritis (fair mucin clot)

Septic arthritis (poor mucin clot)

Cell Counts

Synovial fluid cell counts enumerate the leukocytes present in 1 μL of fluid and differentiate the type of leukocytes to aid in the diagnosis of joint disease. An evaluation of erythrocytes is purely academic, however, because red blood cells are not normally found in synovial fluid, although they may appear following local trauma during aspiration. Therefore, it is important to determine whether red blood cells are due to a traumatic tap or result from hemorrhagic effusion in the joint cavity during hemarthrosis in a hemophilic patient (see the previous section on Physical Examination).

Normal Values
The normal and clinically significant cell counts in synovial fluid are:

Erythrocytes	0–2000 cells/μL
Leukocytes	13–180 cells/μL
Neutrophils	0%–25%
Lymphocytes	0%–78%
Monocytes	0%–71%
Macrophages	0%–26%
Synovial cells	0%–12%
Group I arthritides	200–300 white blood cells/μL
	<30% neutrophils
Group II arthritides	3000–100,000 white blood cells/μL
	>50% neutrophils
Group III arthritides	10,000–>100,000 white blood cells/μL
	>80% neutrophils
Group IV arthritides	1000–10,000 white blood cells/μL
	>70% neutrophils
Group V arthritides	>5000 white blood cells/μL
	>25% neutrophils

Variations
Group I (noninflammatory) joint effusions may occur with:

Amyloidosis

Aseptic necrosis

Charcot's joint

Degenerative joint diseases

Epiphyseal dysplasia

Hemochromatosis

Hypertrophic pulmonary osteoarthropathy

Mechanical derangement

Osteoarthritis

Osteochondritis dissecans

Paget's disease

Sickle cell disease

Traumatic arthritis

Villonodular synovitis

Group II (inflammatory) joint effusions may occur with:

Connective tissue diseases

Crystal-induced arthritis

Enteritis, regional

Gout

Polymyositis

Psoriasis

Reiter's disease

Rheumatic fever

Rheumatoid arthritis

Sarcoidosis

Scleroderma

Subacute bacterial endocarditis

Systemic lupus erythematosus

Ulcerative colitis

Group III (infectious/septic) joint effusions may occur with advanced bacterial infections and fungal infections.

Methodology
Synovial fluid cell counts usually require 3–5 mL of joint fluid collected in heparin, although they may be performed on the few drops of fluid remaining in the needle after arthrocentesis.

Crystals

Crystals are not normally found in synovial fluid but frequently occur in acutely inflamed joints associated with Group IV arthritides. The synovial fluid crystals of greatest clinical significance include the following:

Monosodium urate crystals appear most characteristically in patients with acute gout and chronic gouty arthritis.

Calcium pyrophosphate dihydrate crystals may be found in patients with chondrocalcinosis (pseudogout) and must be distinguished from monosodium urate crystals because these patients have symptoms that mimic gout.

Cholesterol crystals are associated with chronic joint inflammation and may occur in patients with familial hypercholesterolemia, osteoarthritis, and rheumatoid arthritis.

Corticosteroid crystals may be present following therapeutic intra-articular injection of steroids.

Hypoxyapatite crystals may occur in some joint inflammations and also may induce an acute inflammatory reaction.

Methodology
Microscopic examination of synovial fluid for crystals requires 3−5 mL of fluid collected in heparin.

Glucose

Synovial fluid glucose levels are equal to or slightly less than serum glucose levels in normal joint fluid and degenerative joint diseases. Glucose concentrations in synovial fluid decrease to about 60% of plasma levels during inflammatory joint diseases such as rheumatoid arthritis and drop to 40% in septic arthritis. Thus, for accurate interpretation, the synovial fluid glucose level should be compared with a simultaneously obtained serum glucose level, although simultaneous collection is usually impractical and not absolutely necessary.

Normal Values
The normal and clinically significant values for synovial fluid glucose are:

Normal	
Fasting	65−120 mg/dL
Nonfasting	<10 mg/dL lower than the serum glucose level
Decreased, nonfasting	<40 mg/dL
Group I arthritides	<20 mg/dL lower than the serum glucose level
Group II arthritides	>25 mg/dL lower than the serum glucose level
Group III arthritides	>40 mg/dL lower than the serum glucose level
Group IV arthritides	<10 mg/dL lower than the serum glucose level
Group V arthritides	<10 mg/dL lower than the serum glucose level

---

Variations
Decreased synovial fluid glucose levels may occur with:

Inflammatory arthritis, severe	Septic arthritis
Noninflammatory arthritis	Tuberculous arthritis
Rheumatoid arthritis	

Methodology

Synovial fluid glucose determinations require 3–5 mL of fluid collected in a tube containing fluoride anticoagulant following a 6- to 10-hour fast to allow glucose to equilibrate between plasma and joint fluid. Synovial fluid glucose levels should be determined at the same time as the serum glucose level so that the two specimens can be compared.

Microbiologic Examination

Microbiologic examination of synovial fluid specimens should routinely be included in the differential diagnosis of inflamed joints because bacterial arthritis may be superimposed on preexisting noninfectious joint disease. Microbiologic cultures of synovial fluid are normally sterile and are positive only in Group III arthritides. The bacteria most often involved in synovial fluid and joint infections are *Staphylococcus aureus, Hemophilus influenzae, Neisseria,* β-hemolytic streptococci, pneumococci, and mycobacteria. Other predisposing factors for bacterial arthritis include corticosteroid administration, diabetes mellitus, systemic infection, and trauma. (Microbiologic examination of synovial fluid is discussed in Chapter 9.)

Methodology

Microbiologic examination of synovial fluid requires 3–5 mL of fluid collected in a sterile tube containing heparin. The more fluid submitted for microbiologic examination, the greater the likelihood of a positive culture if bacteria are present.

REFERENCES

Bailey, W. R., and Scott, E. G. 1982. *Diagnostic microbiology.* 6th ed. St. Louis: The C. V. Mosby Co.

Bauer, J. D. 1982. *Clinical laboratory methods.* 9th ed. St. Louis: The C. V. Mosby Co.

BioScience Laboratories. 1982. *Directory of services.* Van Nuys, Calif.: BioScience Laboratories.

———. 1982. *The BioScience handbook.* 13th ed. Van Nuys, Calif.: BioScience Laboratories.

Bologna, C. V. 1971. *Understanding laboratory medicine.* St. Louis: The C. V. Mosby Co.

Bradley, G. M. 1980. Fecal analysis: much more than an unpleasant necessity. *Diagn. Med.* 3(2):64.

Collins, R. D. 1975. *Illustrated manual of laboratory diagnosis.* 2nd ed. Philadelphia: J. B. Lippincott Co.

Dito, W. R., Patrick, C. W., and Shelly, J. 1975. *Clinical pathologic correlations in amniotic fluid.* Chicago: American Society of Clinical Pathologists.

Doucet, L. D. 1981. *Medical technology review.* Philadelphia: J. B. Lippincott Co.

Freeman, J. A., and Beehler, M. F. 1983. *Laboratory medicine—clinical microscopy.* 2nd ed. Philadelphia: Lea & Febiger.

French, R. M. 1980. *Guide to diagnostic procedures.* 5th ed. New York: McGraw-Hill Book Co.

Garb, S. 1976. *Laboratory tests in common use.* 6th ed. New York: Springer Publishing Co.

Glasser, L. 1980. Reading the signs in synovia. *Diagn. Med.* 3(6):35.

———. 1981. Cells in cerebrospinal fluid. *Diagn. Med.* 4(2):33.

——— 1981. Tapping the wealth of information in CSF. *Diagn. Med.* 4(1):23.

Glasser, L., and Finley, P. 1981. Body fluids: amniotic fluid and the quality of life. *Diagn. Med.* 4(5):31.

Henry, J. B. 1984. *Clinical diagnosis and management by laboratory methods.* 17th ed. Philadelphia: W. B. Saunders Co.

Killingsworth, L. M., et al. 1980. Protein analysis: deciphering cerebrospinal fluid patterns. *Diagn. Med.* 3(2):23.

MetPath. 1983. *Reference manual.* Teterboro, N.J.: MetPath.

Pagana, K. D., and Pagana, T. J. 1982. *Diagnostic testing and nursing implications.* St. Louis: The C. V. Mosby Co.

Raphael, S. S., et al. 1983. *Medical laboratory technology.* 4th ed. Philadelphia: W. B. Saunders Co.

Rippey, J. H. 1979. Synovial fluid analysis. *Lab. Med.* 10(3):140.

Seivard, C. 1983. *Hematology for medical technologists.* 5th ed. Philadelphia: Lea & Febiger.

Slockbower, J. M., and Blumenfeld, T. A. 1983. *Collection and handling of laboratory specimens.* Philadelphia: J. B. Lippincott Co.

Strand, M. M., and Elmer, L. A. 1983. *Clinical laboratory tests.* 3rd ed. St. Louis: The C. V. Mosby Co.

Tilkian, S. M., Conover, M. B., and Tilkian, A. G. 1983. *Clinical implications of laboratory tests.* 3rd ed. St. Louis: The C. V. Mosby Co.

Velander, R., and Pickering, N. 1981. Fetal maturity—clinical biochemical evaluation. *Lab. Med.* 12(10):604.

White, W. L., Erickson, M. M., and Stevens, S. C. 1976. *Chemistry for the clinical laboratory.* 4th ed. St. Louis: The C. V. Mosby Co.

Widmann, F. K. 1983. *Clinical interpretation of laboratory tests.* 9th ed. Philadelphia: F. A. Davis Co.

9

Microbiology

SPECIMEN COLLECTION AND HANDLING   482
Specimens for General Examination   ·   Specimens for the Examination of
Stained Smears   ·   Specimens for Anaerobic Examination   ·   Specimens
for Fungus Examination   ·   Specimens for Virus Examination

MICROSCOPIC EXAMINATION OF STAINED SMEARS   486
Gram's Stain   ·   Acid-Fast Stain

CULTURES   488
Anaerobic Cultures   ·   Fungus Cultures

SPECIMENS FOR MICROBIOLOGIC EXAMINATION   489
Blood   ·   Cerebrospinal Fluid   ·   Ear   ·   Eye   ·   Genitourinary Tract
Secretions and Discharges   ·   Hair, Skin, and Nails   ·   Nasopharynx and
Throat Secretions and Discharges   ·   Sputum   ·   Stool   ·   Synovial
Fluid   ·   Urine   ·   Wound Exudates and Drainage

ANTIBIOTIC SUSCEPTIBILITY TESTS   528
Antibiotic Activity   ·   Disk Diffusion Tests   ·   Quantitative Dilution Tests

The field of clinical microbiology is concerned with the rapid isolation and precise identification of pathologic organisms as an aid to the diagnosis and management of infectious diseases. Infectious diseases can be caused by a variety of microorganisms, including bacteria, fungi, parasites, rickettsiae, and viruses, and can involve any body surface, system, or organ. Laboratory classification of microorganisms based on their morphologic, cultural, and biochemical characteristics, as well as their antimicrobial susceptibility patterns, is usually sufficient to permit prompt treatment of infections. However, although most clinical microbiology laboratories have the ability to isolate and identify bacteria, fungi, and parasites, few perform the specialized techniques required for viral and rickettsial cultivation.

Clinical bacteriology studies the ability of certain bacteria to produce disease according to their toxicity, virulence, and invasiveness, as well as the resistance and immunity of the affected individual. However, not all bacteria are consistently pathogenic because the same organism can produce disease in one site while growing harmlessly in another. Thus, identification of significant pathogens requires a knowledge of the normal organisms common to each body area and the type of specimen to be examined.

Clinical mycology studies the pathogenic fungi, including yeasts and molds, that commonly cause infections. Fungal infections can range from minor, transient skin conditions (superficial mycoses) to insidious, chronic, fatal internal diseases (systemic mycoses). The virulence of systemic infections may be increased in debilitated patients, producing a severe progressive infection as the initial disease spreads to visceral organs, bones, skin, and subcutaneous tissues. Because pathogenic fungi can coexist with bacteria that may or may not produce disease, systemic fungal infections may mimic bacterial disease and may go undetected unless special tests are performed. Diagnosis of fungal infections requires culture of all clinical material on appropriate media, as well as direct microscopic examination to identify morphologic characteristics, including hyphae (vegetative portion) and spores (reproductive body). Laboratory investigation of fungal diseases also includes skin tests, serologic studies, and biochemical analyses, although these studies are not designed to replace culture procedures. (See Serologic Tests for Fungal Infections in Chapter 11.)

Clinical parasitology studies detect and identify pathogenic parasitic organisms such as amebas, flagellates, flukes, roundworms, tapeworms, and hookworms from urine, stool, sputum, blood, duodenal contents, and tissue biopsies. Parasitic diseases generally are diagnosed by demonstration of the ova (eggs), larvae (immature stage), or adults of helminths and the cysts (inactive stage) or trophozoites (motile forms) of protozoa. A basic knowledge of the disease cycle aids prompt diagnosis because parasites may cause clinical disease before diagnostic forms are present at the expected site. Precise laboratory identification of significant parasites is vital to treatment because specific therapy is governed by the type of invading organism and the site of the infestation. (See Serologic Tests for Parasitic Infections in Chapter 11.)

Clinical virology laboratories normally perform the specialized morphologic examinations and cultures required to study the infectious, ultramicroscopic, intracellular microorganisms that commonly cause disease. Viruses penetrate tissue cells, causing cellular damage, and genetically alter cellular metabolism to produce abnormal viral products that cause the clinical manifestations of viral disease. Laboratory identification of viral diseases includes morphologic study of a direct smear of the specimen, isolation of the causative agent by specialized culture procedures, and examination of tissues for characteristic pathologic changes. Viral diseases also may be identified by demonstrating a rise in the specific serologic antibody titer during the course of the disease. (See Serologic Tests for Viral Infections in Chapter 11.)

The final identification of most clinical pathogens and documentation of their reactions to chemotherapeutic agents are determined by isolating and classifying the microorganism according to routine culture procedures and antibiotic susceptibility tests. However, certain microorganisms are difficult to culture, and definitive identification requires additional laboratory studies, including stained smears, cultures on special media, biochemical tests, and serologic analyses based on their morphologic, physiologic, biochemical, and immunologic characteristics. Microbiology reports require at least 24 hours (longer when subculture, drug sensitivities, biochemical tests, and viral, rickettsial, or fungal studies are necessary) and must be interpreted in light of the patient's clinical symptoms and history.

SPECIMEN COLLECTION AND HANDLING

Proper collection and transportation of material for microbiologic examinations are extremely important and govern the diagnostic significance of laboratory results. Therefore, selection of a clinical specimen that is most representative of the disease process is a critical but often neglected component of the diagnostic process. The site for specimen collection is obvious when symptoms are localized, as in meningitis, abscesses, wound infections, or purulent pneumonias. However, greater selectivity is required in more diffuse processes such as respiratory tract symptoms where the choice must be made among nasopharyngeal, throat, or sputum specimens to be tested or in the investigation of dysuria where the choice is between urinary or genital tract specimens.

Specimens for General Examination

Selection and handling of clinical material for examination are simpler in theory than in fact. Thus, failure to isolate the causative organism of an infectious process is not necessarily due to faulty laboratory techniques but frequently may be the result of faulty specimen selection and collection. Therefore, all nursing, medical, and allied health personnel handling material for microbiologic examination must be familiar with the procedures and precautions needed to ensure clinically significant laboratory reports.

▶▶ *Nursing Responsibilities and Implications*
Requirements for the collection and handling of specific specimens are included in the discussion of procedures performed on each type of material. However, the nurse also should keep in mind the following general considerations regarding the material for microbiologic examination and culture:

1. Obtain specimens for culture before administering any antibiotics or instituting any other antimicrobial therapy. When this is not possible or if the patient has taken medication before admission, notify the laboratory of the type and amount of medication so that appropriate counteractive measures can be taken.

2. Collect biologic specimens at the most active stage of the disease to help ensure the successful isolation and identification of the causative agent. For example, cerebro-

spinal fluid obtained during the onset of the disease is more likely to contain pathogens than if it is collected after the acute symptoms have subsided. Likewise, enteric pathogens are present in much greater numbers and are more easily demonstrated during the acute or diarrheal phase of intestinal infections.

3. Request and encourage the active cooperation of the patient in the collection of such specimens as clean-catch urine and morning sputum samples. Make certain the patient has adequate instructions and the proper equipment to provide a satisfactory specimen.

4. Collect material for culture from the body area, lesion, exudate, or drainage most likely to contain the suspected pathogenic organism. Obtain material that is truly representative of the infectious process by using the aseptic technique to avoid contamination with organisms from the surrounding area.

5. Collect material for microbiologic examination in sterile specimen containers without external contamination. Use only the standard equipment recommended by the laboratory; do not substitute makeshift containers, bottles, or tubes for those specified by the laboratory. Do not use specimen containers that are cracked or broken or that cannot be sealed completely.

6. Collect a sufficient quantity of the specimen to ensure an adequate sample for a complete microbiologic examination.

7. Obtain material from the throat, nose, eye, ear, rectum, urogenital orifices, wounds, or operative sites on sterile cotton- or polyester-tipped swabs.

8. Submit swabs to the laboratory in a tube containing a small amount of transport or holding media such as thioglycolate or Transgrow to prevent the specimen from drying out and to maintain viability of the organisms. A sterile disposable culture unit (Culturette) is available commercially. This unit consists of a plastic tube, a sterile swab, and a small ampule of Stuart holding medium, which provides sufficient moisture for storage for up to 72 hours at room temperature. When using the Culturette unit, the nurse should be sure to crush the ampule and force the swab into the transport medium as stated in the directions supplied with the package.

9. Collect specimens for anaerobic culture as directed (see Specimens for Anaerobic Examination later in this chapter). Specimens such as pus from any deep wound or abscess, necrotic tissue from areas where gas gangrene is suspected, and material from brain or lung abscess are most likely to contain clinically significant anaerobes.

10. Discard any specimen, container, applicator, swab, test tube, or stopper that comes in contact with an unsterile surface.

11. Prevent subsequent contamination of patients and hospital personnel by cleaning any infectious material from the outside of the specimen container. Containers that leak or are contaminated on their outer surface present a hazard to those who handle the specimen and may contribute to the spread of infection, with potentially serious consequences.

12. Label all specimens carefully with the patient's name and identification number, type of specimen, and the date and time of specimen collection.

13. Deliver all specimens to the laboratory promptly so that microbiologic procedures can be performed while pathogens remain viable and can still be isolated. When it is impossible for specimens to reach the laboratory within 30 minutes, they should be

refrigerated to prevent overgrowth with insignificant or nonpathogenic organisms that may interfere with the isolation of the pathogens. The exceptions are cerebrospinal fluid specimens, which should be placed in a bacteriologic incubator or left for short periods at room temperature rather than refrigerated because they may contain organisms that are sensitive to cold.

14. Protect all specimens from extremes of heat and cold or other damaging factors during transport.

15. Provide the laboratory with sufficient clinical information to guide the selection of suitable culture media and appropriate microbiologic techniques. Specimens should be accompanied by a requisition slip listing the following information:

    • Patient's full name, age, identification number, and room number.
    • Nature and exact anatomic source of the specimen.
    • Type of examination requested.
    • Patient's current therapy and antibiotic history.
    • Patient's clinical diagnosis and type of infection suspected.
    • Any traveling the patient has done in the past year.

Specimens for the Examination of Stained Smears

A properly prepared and stained smear can provide sufficient tentative information concerning the nature of an infection to permit a presumptive diagnosis and allow preliminary therapy to be started without delay. Rapid examination of direct smears also may provide an excellent guide to the selection of an appropriate culture medium and indicate the need for additional microbiologic procedures.

▶▶ *Nursing Responsibilities and Implications*
Although smears from the material on a swab usually are prepared by the laboratory, it occasionally may be necessary for the nurse to prepare a smear for microbiologic examination. To prepare a smear properly, the nurse should proceed as follows:

1. Use only clean, nongreasy slides. Although new slides are preferred, used slides may be employed if they are not scratched and have been cleaned with a mild detergent.

2. Mark the underside of the slide with a glass-marking pencil, outlining the area near the center that will contain the material for staining.

3. Spread the material evenly over the designated area using either an inoculating loop or swab. Do not make the smear too thick or too thin and do not spread it over a wide area when the material is sparse. When preparing a smear for gonococci, roll rather than rub the swab on the slide and do not go over the same area twice.

4. Allow the smear to air dry.

5. Spray the dried smear with a fixative solution or pass it rapidly through a flame to fix the material to the slide.

6. Mark the slide adequately for patient identification and identify the source of the smear.

Specimens for Anaerobic Examination

Special anoxic specimen collection and culture techniques are needed to isolate and identify anaerobic organisms in the laboratory. Thus, several special precautions must be observed, in addition to the general specimen collection procedures listed in the previous section, to reduce exposure of the specimen to oxygen.

Needle and syringe aspiration is recommended whenever possible to minimize contamination and protect certain organisms from contact with the lethal effects of atmospheric oxygen.

The **two-tube swab system**, although the least desirable procedure, may be used to collect specimens for anaerobic examination when the amount of available material is insufficient for aspiration.

▶▶ *Nursing Responsibilities and Implications*

When obtaining an anaerobic specimen by needle and syringe aspiration, the nurse should proceed as follows:

1. Expel all the air from a sterile syringe by pushing the plunger until it touches the hub of the needle.

2. Aspirate pus, exudates, and other body fluids directly into the syringe.

3. Immediately inject the specimen into a sterile "gassed-out" tube that has been flushed with oxygen-free carbon dioxide or nitrogen gas to provide an anaerobic environment. Tubes, such as the anaerobic Culturette system, which have a double stopper (a recessed rubber stopper along with a screw cap), should be used to avoid the introduction of air when injecting the specimen.

4. If anaerobic transport tubes are not available, the collection needle should be capped or embedded in a sterile rubber stopper to prevent exposing the specimen to the atmosphere.

5. Maintain all specimens for anaerobic culture at room temperature and deliver them to the laboratory within 30 minutes for immediate processing.

When obtaining an anaerobic specimen using the two-tube swab system, the nurse should proceed as follows:

1. Collect the specimen on a sterile swab that has been prepared and stored in an oxygen-free carbon dioxide tube, exposing the swab to the atmosphere as briefly as possible.

2. Quickly place the swab in a second tube containing a prereduced transport medium with a methylene blue indicator. Transport tubes should be held in an upright position as the swab is introduced to prevent the loss of carbon dioxide. The tube should not be used if the blue color extends beyond a ring across the surface because this indicates that the transport media is not oxygen-free.

Specimens for Fungus Examination

The success or failure of laboratory procedures to recover and isolate the etiologic agent of mycotic infections depends on proper collection and processing of suitable tissue or fluid specimens. For example, small bits of tissue such as nails, skin, hair, or material obtained from within the lesion are needed to diagnose superficial mycoses, depending on the location of the infection. On the other hand, a variety of materials, including pus or exudate from draining lesions, material aspirated from unopened abscesses or sinus tracts, and biopsied tissue, may be used to diagnose subcutaneous mycoses. Likewise, specimens from any internal organ, including blood, bone, bone marrow, bronchial secretions, and cerebrospinal fluid; draining lesions or sinuses; pus or exudates from abscesses; sputum; and skin or subcutaneous tissues may be used to investigate systemic mycoses.

▶▶ *Nursing Responsibilities and Implications*

1. Follow the guidelines for the collection and handling of specimens under Specimens for General Examination earlier in this chapter.

2. Collect specimens for fungus examinations that are as free from bacterial contamination as possible because it takes less time to collect a specimen properly than to identify a contaminant.

3. Collect and examine the specimen for yeast investigation at the patient's bedside whenever possible, or place the specimen in a sterile container and deliver it promptly to the laboratory.

4. Indicate the source of the specimen and the suspected disease on the laboratory request slip to aid the laboratory in selecting the proper culture media and test procedures.

Specimens for Virus Examination

Extra precautions are required during the collection of material for virus studies to obtain adequate specimens for accurate test results. Test material such as stool or rectal swabs, cerebrospinal or pleural fluid, throat swabs, clotted blood, tissue specimens, urine, and skin scrapings should be collected when the patient is admitted. Similar specimens also should be collected for comparison about 2 weeks after the onset of symptoms of viral disease.

Swabs and other samples that may become less virulent during transport to the laboratory should be placed in virus transport media to prevent them from drying out. A screw-capped tube or vial containing 2 mL of veal infusion broth or 1% bovine serum albumin are viable alternatives for nutrient transport media. In addition, a buffered saline solution with protein as a stabilizer and added antibiotics such as penicillin, gentamicin, and amphotericin B to suppress bacterial and fungal overgrowth, also is commonly used.

All material for virus studies, even if contaminated, should be collected in sterile containers using the sterile technique and either flash-frozen as soon as possible or maintained at 4° C, depending on the specimen, shipment time, and laboratory preferences. Shipments should be protected from fluctuations in temperature to prevent alternate freezing and thawing of the specimen.

MICROSCOPIC EXAMINATION OF STAINED SMEARS

Microscopic examination of a direct smear prepared from the original biologic specimen can classify organisms according to their shape, relative size, growth configuration, and staining characteristics, as well as estimate their quantity and predominance. Although cultivation of organisms on culture media gives the most accurate microbiologic information, successful cultures require time for bacterial growth and depend on the presence of viable organisms. Therefore, direct microscopic examination of the biologic material permits a rapid presumptive diagnosis of bacterial infection if time is short or if the organisms are not viable.

Because bacteria are usually transparent and difficult to examine in their natural state, chemical staining is needed for morphologic study to enhance their visibility. Bacteria may be classified into three general morphologic types: cocci, which are oval or round; bacilli, which are rod shaped; and spirochetes, which are curved or spiral shaped. Slight variations in the chemical composition of bacteria result in typical staining characteristics, allowing the various bacterial types to be differentiated according to their morphologic details and individual staining reactions. The two most widely used stains are Gram's stain, which classifies organisms as positive or negative according to their color reaction, and the acid-fast stain, which is useful in the diagnosis of tuberculosis.

Gram's Stain

Gram's stain differentiates between various bacteria with similar morphologic features. When bacteria are exposed to a purple-blue crystal violet and iodine dye complex and then washed with alcohol or acetone, certain organisms retain the stain, whereas others are decolorized. Those organisms that retain the purple color are called gram-positive, and those that lose their color when washed with alcohol or acetone are called gram-negative. A contrasting dye, usually safranin, is used to counterstain and color the gram-negative organisms red, making them visible.

Microscopic examination of a gram-stained smear containing a mixed bacterial flora is used to observe the size, shape, and other morphologic characteristics of the bacteria to aid subsequent diagnostic procedures. Identification and differentiation of organisms as, for example, gram-negative or gram-positive bacilli or cocci are important in the selection of culture media and permit a presumptive diagnosis of bacterial infection. A gram-stained smear of sputum, cerebrospinal fluid, urine, exudates, and other clinical material also may be used to confirm the purity of the culture and check on culture results. Any discrepancy between the morphologic features and staining reaction of the organisms identified from the original direct smear and those taken from the laboratory culture requires further investigation.

Acid-Fast Stain

Acid-fast stains are used for the direct examination of clinical material, culture colonies, and fixed tissue sections to detect tubercle bacilli or other mycobacteria. Although mycobacteria usually are sought with acid-fast staining procedures, certain species of *Nocardia* and *Brucella* are variably acid-fast and sometimes can be identified in tissue section by an appropriately modified acid-fast technique.

Acid-fast organisms are difficult to stain with ordinary dye but can be stained with carbolfuchsin and acid when they are applied with heat. Once stained, acid-fast organisms resist decolorization during subsequent treatment with an acid-alcohol wash, whereas most other organisms do not resist decolorization. Organisms that are not acid-fast lose their color after an acid-alcohol wash and may be studied only when counterstained.

CULTURES

Laboratory cultivation of clinical material on appropriate nutrient media is essential for the isolation, growth, and accurate identification of pathogenic organisms in the diagnosis of infectious diseases. The use of different culture media and special anaerobic techniques, which promote or discourage the growth of individual organisms, is governed by the type of specimen and organism suspected. Therefore, the nature and source of material to be cultured, as well as information concerning the patient's clinical condition, must be designated to guide the selection of suitable laboratory procedures.

Anaerobic Cultures

Anaerobic organisms, bacteria that grow best in the absence of oxygen, are part of the normal microflora of the body and are constantly present in the intestinal and genitourinary tracts and oral cavity. Thus, anaerobes may be present in tissue from nearby normal microflora or as secondary invaders introduced in tissues damaged by other microbes or trauma. The organism may spread by direct invasion or by bloodborne routes and may cause severe, often fatal, infections in any organ or tissue. The need for anaerobic cultures is indicated by the following characteristic clinical findings:

1. Pus in a deep wound or aspirated abscess.
2. Discharge with a foul or putrid odor.
3. Discharge containing sulfur granules.
4. Necrotic tissue in a patient with suspected gas gangrene.
5. Endocarditis in the presence of negative blood cultures.
6. Abscess in the brain, lung, or liver.
7. Intra-abdominal, perirectal, or subphrenic infections.
8. Infected fluids from sites such as the amniotic sac and the peritoneal, pleural, or synovial areas that normally contain sterile fluid.
9. Infected uterine secretions associated with postabortal sepsis.
10. Infections following human or other bites.
11. Infections following gastrointestinal surgery.
12. Gas in tissues or discharges.

Anaerobic organisms are frequently the predominant pathogens in bacteremia, brain abscess, lung or liver abscess, aspiration pneumonia, chronic sinusitis, peritonitis, appendicitis, puerperal sepsis, and gynecologic infections. Anaerobes are the causative agent in other conditions, including botulism, tetanus, gas gangrene, gas-forming cellulitis, infected vascular gangrene, wound infections following surgery or trauma, diverticulitis, otogenic meningitis, subdural empyema, and thoracic empyema. However, the isolation of anaerobic organisms from culture material does not prove their pathogenic significance as the agent of disease.

Fungus Cultures

The purpose of mycologic culture media is to support the growth of medically important fungi and to suppress accompanying bacterial flora and harmless fungi. Occasionally, however, opportunistic fungi originally thought to be nonpathogenic may be pathogenic in the presence of diabetes, lymphoproliferative disorders, or immunosuppression caused by corticosteroids and other drugs, congenital immunodeficiency, or acquired immuno-deficiency syndrome (AIDS). The specific culture medium used for laboratory cultivation and identification of fungus depends on the type of biologic specimen submitted and the degree of bacterial contamination expected.

SPECIMENS FOR MICROBIOLOGIC EXAMINATION

Blood

Microbiologic procedures to isolate pathogenic organisms from blood and determine their susceptibilities are used to identify the etiologic agents of septicemia and select the appro-priate antimicrobial regimen. The presence of living microorganisms in the blood may be due to a variety of conditions or diseases and generally indicates an active systemic infec-tion. Positive blood cultures do not necessarily indicate severe pathologic septicemia be-cause many organisms may produce a temporary bloodstream infection during the early stages of their invasion. A mild transient bacteremia also may occur during the course of many infectious diseases or as a complication of other disorders; however, persistent, con-tinuous, or recurrent bacteremia indicates a more serious condition.

The transient phases of bacteremia that develop during many bacterial infections per-sist in some diseases and become the dominant clinical feature, even though the organisms involved are not generally pathogenic. Although the urinary tract is usually the primary infecting site, the lungs, hepatobiliary tract, endocardium, central nervous system, perito-neal cavity or infected wound sites (especially decubiti) also may be the site from which or-ganisms enter the bloodstream. Therefore, persistent, unexplained fever of more than several days' duration in patients with urinary tract infections, infected burns, wound infections, indwelling venous catheters, or heart murmurs also warrants immediate blood cultures.

Because patients with impaired immunity are more susceptible to infection, it may be rash to consider any organism nonpathogenic in patients who are debilitated or receiving immunosuppressive therapies. Therefore, blood cultures should be performed on patients who exhibit a sudden relative increase in pulse rate, temperature, and malaise along with the onset of chills and prostration. Blood cultures also should be performed on debilitated patients who develop chills and fever during prolonged hyperalimentation or antibiotic therapy and all patients with postoperative shock. Although positive blood cultures may result from contamination during faulty blood collection techniques, organisms isolated from several cultures collected at different times are generally significant.

Clinical Significance

Bacteremia frequently is associated with pneumonia, cardiac anomalies, meningitis, trau-matic and contaminated surgical wounds, burns, septic abortion, osteomyelitis, brain abscess, cellulitis, lung abscess, empyema, peritonitis, intestinal or biliary infections, car-cinoma, urinary obstruction, and nephropathies. Positive cultures also may accompany conditions such as arteriosclerosis, chronic debility, diabetic acidosis, hematologic disorders, hepatic insufficiencies, and malignancies, as well as immunosuppressive, cytotoxic, and x-ray therapy. Positive blood cultures therefore aid the definitive diagnosis of bacterial endocarditis, salmonellosis, typhoid fever, chronic meningitis, brucellosis, gonococcemia, and tularemia, although a single negative specimen does not eliminate the possibility of these diseases or bacteremia (Table 9-1).

The time of blood collection is not critical in the diagnosis of conditions in which bacteremia is continuous such as endocarditis or endarteritis, uncontrolled infections, typhoid fever, and brucellosis. However, bacteremia is intermittent in many other conditions and can precede the onset of characteristic fever and chills by as much as 1 hour. Thus, the probability of obtaining a positive blood culture is increased if the blood is drawn immediately before the expected rise in temperature (if a pattern of elevations has been established) or during the actual temperature elevation.

Normal Flora
Normal blood should be sterile and free from organisms.

Pathogens
The pathogenic organisms most likely to be found in blood include:

Bacteria
- *Acinetobacter* species
- *Bacteroides* species
- *Brucella* species
- *Citrobacter* species
- *Clostridium perfringens*
- *Enterobacter* species
- *Escherichia coli*
- *Francisella tularensis*
- *Hemophilus influenzae*
- *Klebsiella* species
- *Leptospira* species
- *Listeria monocytogenes*
- *Mycobacterium tuberculosis*
- *Neisseria meningitidis*
- *Nocardia* species
- *Pseudomonas* species
- *Salmonella* species
- *Serratia marcescens*
- *Staphylococcus albus*
- *Staphylococcus aureus*
- *Streptobacillus moniliformis*
- *Streptococcus* species (α- and β-hemolytic and anaerobic)
- *Streptococcus faecalis*
- *Streptococcus pneumoniae*
- *Streptococcus pyogenes*
- *Streptococcus viridans*
- *Vibrio* species

Fungi
- *Blastomyces dermatitidis*
- *Candida albicans*
- *Cryptococcus neoformans*
- *Histoplasma capsulatum*
- *Torulopsis glabrata*

Parasites
- *Leishmania* species
- *Plasmodium* species
- *Trypanosoma* species

Methodology
Specimens for blood culture require 10–15 mL of blood collected using the aseptic technique to prevent the introduction of contaminating organisms during venipuncture and

subsequent handling. A total of three to four sets of cultures collected at least 1 hour apart during a 24-hour period should be adequate to isolate the causative agent of bacteremia. Each set of blood cultures consists of one aerobic and one anaerobic culture bottle containing trypticase soy or thioglycolate broth with sodium citrate or heparin anticoagulant. If bacterial growth appears, a preliminary report such as "gram-negative or gram-positive rods" generally is available within 36–48 hours, although final identification of organisms may take up to 10 days or longer.

Microbiologic procedures to identify blood parasites require 5 mL of blood collected with EDTA anticoagulant (lavender-stoppered tube) or blood smears prepared according to the directions under Specimens for the Examination of Stained Smears earlier in this chapter.

Precautions

To ensure accurate test results, specimens for blood cultures should be collected before antibiotic therapy is instituted because antimicrobial agents may interfere with the isolation and identification of organisms. Therefore, the number of cultures collected should be doubled in patients who have already received antibiotics so that an adequate sample will be obtained to establish a diagnosis.

▶▶ Nursing Responsibilities and Implications

The proper preparation of the venipuncture site and careful collection of blood specimens are critical to the isolation of pathogenic organisms. To obtain specimens that will yield clinically significant blood culture results, the nurse should proceed as follows:

1. Prepare the intended venipuncture site by thoroughly cleansing the skin with 70% alcohol followed by a benzalkonium chloride or iodine swab. The benzalkonium chloride or iodine should be allowed to remain on the skin for at least 1 minute before venipuncture. If these products cannot be used, a 2-minute alcohol prep is acceptable.

2. Do not touch the venipuncture site again with the fingers to check the position of the vein once the entire area has been disinfected.

3. Collect 10 mL of blood directly into commercially prepared sterile, rubber-capped culture bottles or special vacuum tubes containing a suitable medium. (From infants and young children it may be possible to obtain only 2 mL or less.) Blood also can be collected using a sterile needle and syringe and transferring the sample to the blood culture bottles.

4. Deliver the culture bottles to the laboratory immediately so that incubation can be started within 60 minutes.

Cerebrospinal Fluid

Microbiologic examination of purulent and clear cerebrospinal fluid (CSF) is essential to the diagnosis of suspected meningitis or other diseases of the central nervous system. Because a variety of microorganisms may produce a bacterial infection of the meninges, prompt identification of the etiologic agent is necessary to select the most suitable antimicrobial agent. Cerebrospinal fluid specimens are routinely cultured for aerobic, anaerobic, and acid-fast organisms to determine the exact cause of the meningitis. Microscopic examination of gram-stained CSF smears can detect the presence of organisms and pro-

TABLE 9-1 Diseases Associated With the Cardiovascular and Lymphatic Systems

Disease	Causative Agent	Mode of Transmission	Treatment
Bacterial diseases			
Puerperal sepsis and infections related to abortions	Primarily *Streptococcus pyogenes*; *Clostridium* and *Bacteroides* species often cause post-abortion infections	Unsanitary conditions in childbirth and abortions	Penicillin and erythromycin for *S. pyogenes*; chloramphenicol and penicillin for *Bacteroides* and *Clostridium* species
Endocarditis			
Subacute bacterial	Many organisms, especially α-hemolytic streptococci	Bacteremia localizing in the heart	Varies with agent; penicillin and erythromycin for α-hemolytic streptococci
Acute bacterial	*Staphylococcus aureus*, *Streptococcus pneumoniae*	Bacteremia localizing in the heart	Semisynthetic penicillin derivatives such as methicillin or oxacillin for *S. aureus* and penicillin for *S. pneumoniae*
Pericarditis	*Streptococcus pneumoniae*	Bacteremia localizing in the heart	Penicillin
Rheumatic fever	Group A β-hemolytic streptococci	Inhalation leading to streptococcal sore throat	Penicillin (for sore throat)
Tularemia	*Francisella tularensis*	Animal reservoir (rabbits); skin abrasions, ingestion, inhalation, bites	Streptomycin, tetracycline
Brucellosis	*Brucella* species	Animal reservoir (cows); ingestion in milk, direct contact with skin abrasions	Streptomycin, tetracycline

Anthrax	*Bacillus anthracis*	Soil or animal reservoir; skin abrasions, inhalation or ingestion of heavy spore concentrations	Penicillin, tetracycline, erythromycin, chloramphenicol
Listeriosis	*Listeria monocytogenes*	Animal reservoir; ingestion	Tetracycline or penicillin
Viral diseases			
Myocarditis	Several agents, especially coxsackievirus (enterovirus)	Coxsackievirus: inhalation and ingestion	None
Pericarditis	Same as above	Complication of viral myocarditis	None
Infectious mononucleosis	Epstein-Barr virus	Oral secretions, kissing	None
Hepatitis B (serum hepatitis)	Hepatitis B virus	Predominantly parenteral (transfusions, syringes, etc.); also by close contact	None
Protozoan and helminthic diseases			
Toxoplasmosis	*Toxoplasma gondii*	Animal reservoir (cats); inhalation and ingestion	Pyrimethamine in combination with either trisulfapyrimidines or sulfadiazine
American trypanosomiasis	*Trypanosoma cruzi*	Bite of reduviid bug	Lampit in early stages
Schistosomiasis	*Schistosoma* species	Contaminated water; cercariae enter the body through the skin	Praziquantel

Source: From Tortora, G. J., Funke, B. R., and Case, C. L. 1982. *Microbiology*. Menlo Park, Calif.: The Benjamin/Cummings Publishing Co., Inc.

TABLE 9-2   Diseases Associated With the Nervous System

Disease	Causative Agent	Mode of Transmission	Treatment
Meningococcal meningitis	*Neisseria meningitidis*	Contact with a healthy carrier via the respiratory tract	Penicillin, chloramphenicol, rifampin
Hemophilus influenzae meningitis	*Hemophilus influenzae*	Via the respiratory tract in individuals with viral respiratory infections	Ampicillin in combination with chloramphenicol
Cryptococcosis	*Cryptococcus neoformans*	Inhalation of dried infected pigeon droppings	Amphotericin B
Leprosy	*Mycobacterium leprae*	Transfer of exudates from lesions or inanimate objects	Sulfone drugs (dapsone), rifampin
Poliomyelitis	Poliovirus	Ingestion of virus	None
Rabies	Rabiesvirus	Bite of a rabid animal	Rabies immune globulin and Human diploid cell vaccine or Duck embryo vaccine after exposure

Source: Tortora, G. J., Funke, B. R., and Case, C. L. 1982. *Microbiology.* Menlo Park, Calif.: The Benjamin/Cummings Publishing Co., Inc.

vide presumptive diagnosis to guide preliminary treatment before confirmation by culture. Because a delay of 24 hours for primary culturing occasionally may be fatal, the physician should be informed of the preliminary findings immediately so that treatment can be started without delay if the Gram's stain shows any organisms.

Cerebrospinal fluid examination and culture should be performed if meningeal infection is suspected in adults who demonstrate such typical signs as fever, headache, vomiting, nuchal rigidity, and hyperreflexia. However, these manifestations may be absent in infants and neonates, who may exhibit only vague, nonspecific symptoms of meningitis. Therefore, CSF cultures also should be performed when infants have an unexplained fever and are excessively irritable.

Clinical Significance

Microorganisms may occur in CSF as a result of trauma, cranial and spinal epidural abscesses, infectious complications of surgery, brain abscesses, and septic thrombophlebitis of the venous sinuses. However, systemic infectious diseases, including severe pneumonia, tuberculosis, salmonellosis, listerosis, generalized candidiasis, and advanced septicemia with gram-negative bacilli, also can affect the meninges.

Positive CSF cultures most frequently indicate acute bacterial meningitis but also may occur secondarily in various conditions or infections in other parts of the body. The organisms that commonly cause meningitis are *Hemophilus influenzae*, *Neisseria meningitidis*, and *Streptococcus pneumoniae*. Therefore, a stained smear report of small gram-negative bacilli, especially in children, indicates infection with *Hemophilus influenzae*, whereas large gram-negative bacilli suggest the presence of *Escherichia* or *Enterobacter* species. The appearance of gram-negative, bean-shaped intracellular or extracellular diplococci generally indicates *Neisseria meningitidis*, but gram-positive cocci may be streptococci or staphylococci (Table 9-2).

Normal Flora

Cerebrospinal fluid is normally sterile.

Pathogens

The pathogenic organisms most likely to be found in CSF include:

Bacteria	*Listeria monocytogenes*	*Streptococcus faecalis*
Acinetobacter species	*Mycobacterium tuber-*	*Streptococcus pneumoniae*
Bacteroides species	*culosis*	Fungi
Enterobacter species	*Neisseria meningitidis*	*Candida albicans*
Escherichia coli	*Proteus* species	*Coccidioides immitis*
Hemophilus species	*Pseudomonas* species	*Cryptococcus laurentii*
Klebsiella species	*Salmonella* species	*Cryptococcus neoformans*
Leptospira species	*Staphylococcus aureus*	*Histoplasma capsulatum*

Methodology

Cerebrospinal fluid specimens must be collected under sterile conditions, transported to the laboratory in two or three capped, sterile tubes without delay, and examined immediately. (See Cerebrospinal Fluid—Specimen Collection and Handling in Chapter 8.) When a delay before culturing is unavoidable, CSF specimens must be stored in a bacteriologic incubator rather than a refrigerator to prevent deterioration of meningococci, which are sensitive to cold. If viral meningitis is suspected, a portion of the CSF specimen should be frozen and maintained at −20 C to allow isolation of the virus.

Precautions
To ensure accurate test results, whenever possible, specimens for CSF cultures should be collected before initiating antibiotic therapy so that bacteriologic reports will be accurate.

▶▶ Nursing Responsibilities and Implications
The nurse should be aware that material for CSF culture must be handled carefully to avoid self-contamination and spread of the highly virulent organisms responsible for meningeal infections. To obtain an adequate specimen for CSF examination, the nurse should proceed as follows:

1. Prepare the patient for a spinal tap. (See Cerebrospinal Fluid—Specimen Collection and Handling in Chapter 8.)

2. Assist the physician to collect the CSF specimen in two to three sterile tubes approved for the purpose.

3. Deliver the specimen to the laboratory immediately, designating the third specimen tube for microbiologic procedures and culture.

Ear

Microbiologic examination of material from the ear is important in the diagnosis and treatment of various localized lesions and abscesses. Organisms in the outer ear generally reflect the microbial flora of the surrounding area; therefore, diseases of the external auditory canal frequently are associated with skin disorders. However, other parts of the auditory canal, including the middle and inner ear, are affected only by pathogenic organisms that may develop as a result of localized or systemic infections.

Normal Flora
The middle and inner ear are normally sterile; organisms normally found in the external ear include:

Bacteria

  Bacillus species

  Diphtheroids (coryne forms)

  Gaffyka tetragena

  Lactobacillus species

  Klebsiella species

  Propionibacterium acnes

Staphylococcus species (coagulase-negative)

Streptococcus mitis

Streptococcus pneumoniae

Fungus

  non-albicans *Candida* species

Pathogens

The pathogenic organisms most likely to be found in the ear include:

Bacteria
Branhamella catarrhalis
Chlamydia trachomatis
Diphtheroids
Enterobacter species
Escherichia coli
Hemophilus influenzae
Klebsiella pneumoniae
Mycobacterium tuberculosis
Mycoplasma pneumoniae
Proteus species
Pseudomonas aeruginosa
Staphylococcus aureus

Streptococcus species (anaerobic and β-hemolytic)
Streptococcus pneumoniae
Streptococcus pyogenes

Fungi
Aspergillus species
Candida albicans
Candida parapsilosis
Mucor species
Penicillium species
Rhizopus species
Sporothrix schenckii

Methodology

Discharges from the ear are best collected using the sterile technique and a sterile cotton- or polyester-tipped swab. The external ear should be cleansed with a 1:1000 aqueous solution of benzalkonium chloride or similar detergent before the culture material is collected to remove contaminating bacterial flora on the surface. Swabs containing exudate from the ear should be placed immediately in a suitable transport or holding medium and delivered to the laboratory promptly.

▶▶ Nursing Responsibilities and Implications

1. Thoroughly cleanse the area surrounding the culture site with benzalkonium chloride solution on sterile cotton swabs.

2. Firmly swab but do not rub the culture site with several sterile cotton- or polyester-tipped swabs approved for bacterial use to collect the discharge. (Q-tips or similar swabs are not suitable for cultures because they may be treated with bacteriostatic solutions.)

3. Insert the swabs in transport media immediately and deliver them to the laboratory as soon as possible for prompt testing.

4. State the specific test requested on the laboratory request slip.

Eye

Microbiologic examination of eye secretions from patients with conjunctivitis or other eye infections is essential to establish the presence of pathogenic microorganisms and evaluate the nature of the disease. The healthy conjunctiva should be relatively free of microorganisms but may harbor a small number of the normal organisms found in the surrounding area. When there is the possibility of gonococcal infection in a newborn infant's

TABLE 9-3 Diseases Associated With the Eyes

Disease	Causative Agent	Treatment
Bacterial diseases		
Contagious conjunctivitis (pinkeye)	*Hemophilus aegyptii*	Sulfonamides
Neonatal gonorrheal ophthalmia	*Neisseria gonorrhoeae*	Silver nitrate, tetracycline, or erythromycin for prevention; penicillin for treatment
Trachoma	*Chlamydia trachomatis*	Sulfonamide, tetracycline
Inclusion conjunctivitis	*Chlamydia trachomatis*	Sulfonamide, tetracycline
Viral diseases		
Epidemic keratoconjunctivitis	Adenovirus	None
Herpetic keratitis	Herpesvirus (herpes simplex type 1)	Idoxuridine, vidarabine

Source: Tortora, G. J., Funke, B. R., and Case, C. L. 1982. *Microbiology.* Menlo Park, Calif.: The Benjamin/Cummings Publishing Co., Inc.

eyes, specimens should be collected for the identification of *Neisseria gonorrhoeae* as well as for routine culture. Material for culture and smears (Gram's stain) should be collected before the local application of antibiotics, irrigating solutions, and anesthetics that demonstrate antimicrobial activity and interfere with the isolation of pathogens (Table 9-3).

Normal Flora

The following organisms in small quantities may be considered normal in the eye:

Diphtheroids	*Streptococcus pyogenes*
Staphylococcus epidermidis	*Streptococcus viridans*
Streptococcus pneumoniae	

Pathogens

The pathogenic organisms most likely to be found in the eye include:

Bacteria	*Staphylococcus aureus*	*Cryptococcus neoformans*
Acinetobacter species	*Streptococcus pneumoniae*	*Histoplasma capsulatum*
Corynebacterium xerosis	*Streptococcus* species	*Mucor* species
Klebsiella pneumoniae	(β-hemolytic)	*Penicillium* species
Hemophilus influenzae	Fungi	*Rhizopus* species
Moraxella lacunata	*Candida* species	*Rhodotorula* species
Neisseria gonorrhoeae	*Cladosporium* species	*Sporothrix schenckii*
Pseudomonas aeruginosa	*Cryptococcus albidus*	

Methodology

Purulent material from infected eyes should be collected with sterile cotton- or polyester-tipped swabs from the inflamed surface of the cul-de-sac or inner canthus of the eye. Swabs for culture should be placed into a Transgrow bottle when gonococcus is suspected and into a standard transport or holding medium for routine examinations. All specimens should be delivered to the laboratory without delay for immediate processing.

▶▶ Nursing Responsibilities and Implications

1. Use the sterile technique and sterile swabs approved for microbiologic use. (Q-tips and similar swabs are not appropriate for cultures because they may be treated with bacteriostatic solutions.)

2. Firmly swab but do not rub the inner canthus or infected area to collect material for eye cultures.

3. Place the swab in the appropriate holding or transport medium to prevent the specimen from drying out before it can be cultured.

4. Indicate the specific test desired on the laboratory request slip.

5. Deliver the specimen to the laboratory immediately for prompt testing.

Genitourinary Tract Secretions and Discharges

Microbiologic examination of genitourinary tract lesions and exudates is essential to detect *Neisseria gonorrhoeae* and establish a clinical diagnosis of gonorrhea. Demonstration of characteristic gram-negative organisms within or surrounding pus cells on a stained smear of vaginal or urethral exudate provides presumptive evidence of gonorrhea. Stained smear results, however, offer no diagnostic information and usually will be reported only as intracellular and/or extracellular gram-negative diplococci morphologically resembling *Neisseria*. Therefore, reliable laboratory evaluation of gonococcal infection and definitive diagnosis of gonorrhea should be based on the isolation and identification of *N. gonorrhoeae* by standard culture techniques and gram-stained smears.

Clinical Significance

The appearance of characteristic organisms in gram-stained smears of purulent urethral discharge, particularly from males, is usually sufficient to confirm a diagnosis of an acute gonorrheal infection. However, during chronic infections, particularly in females, smears of vaginal discharge cannot be relied on to demonstrate the presence of gonococci, and cultures are generally necessary. Occasionally, material from other sites, including throat swabs, anal swabs, freshly voided urine, joint fluid, and eye swabs, also may be submitted for gonococcal culture and examination (Table 9-4).

Normal Flora

The vagina and its secretions and the prostate and its secretions are normally sterile at birth. However, small quantities of the following organisms may be considered normal in the urethral and vaginal areas:

Bacteria

Bacteroides species (premenopausal)

Clostridium species (premenopausal)

Enterobacter species (prepubertal and postmenopausal)

Escherichia coli

Gardnerella vaginalis

Lactobacillus species (Döderlein's bacillus)

Mycobacterium species

Peptostreptococcus species (premenopausal)

Propionibacterium species (premenopausal)

Selenomonas species (premenopausal)

Staphylococcus epidermidis

Streptococcus aureus

Streptococcus species (prepubertal and postmenopausal)

Veillonella species

Fungus

Candida albicans

Pathogens

The pathogenic organisms most commonly found in the genitourinary tract include:

Bacteria	*Bacteroides* species	*Escherichia coli*
Alcaligenes species	*Chlamydia trachomatis*	*Gardnerella vaginalis*

Hemophilus ducreyi	*Staphylococcus aureus*	*Geotrichum* species
Hemophilus species	*Streptococcus* species	*Histoplasma capsulatum*
Lactobacillus species (large numbers)	(anaerobic and β-hemolytic, groups B and D)	*Rhodotorula* species
Mycobacterium tuberculosis	*Streptococcus faecalis*	*Saccharomyces* species
	Treponema pallidum	*Torulopsis glabrata*
Mycoplasma species	Fungi	Parasites
Neisseria gonorrhoeae	*Candida* species	*Trichomonas vaginalis*
Proteus species	*Cephalosporium* species	Viruses
		Herpesviruses

Methodology

The best specimens for the detection of *Neisseria gonorrhoeae* and other genitourinary tract pathogens are obtained from the anterior urethral mucosa in men and the cervix or inflamed perineal areas in women. Any exudate or purulent material should be collected on a sterile polyester-tipped swab and delivered immediately to the laboratory in a suitable transport medium such as Transgrow or Stuart medium. All specimens should be handled cautiously to prevent hospital personnel from being contaminated with viable infectious material.

▶▶ Nursing Responsibilities and Implications

To obtain an adequate specimen for the diagnosis of urethritis and detection of *N. gonorrhoeae*, the nurse should proceed as follows:

1. Obtain material for urethral culture by passing a nasopharyngeal swab or small platinum loop into the anterior urethra and inoculate a modified Thayer-Martin or Transgrow medium immediately.

2. Collect vaginal material on a polyester-tipped swab approved for microbiologic procedures and insert the swab into a tube containing transport medium.

3. Obtain material for endocervical culture and isolation of *N. gonorrhoeae* from females by direct spectroscopic examination, passing a polyester- or cotton-tipped swab into the endocervical canal after wiping excess mucus from the cervical os. Immediately place the swab into the appropriate transport medium.

4. Deliver the specimens to the laboratory immediately for prompt processing.

Hair, Skin, and Nails

Microbiologic examination of hair stubs, skin scales, or nail scrapings is used to diagnose superficial or cutaneous fungal infections, which are probably the most common mycotic diseases of humans. Direct slide preparations of infected specimens frequently reveal characteristic hyphae or, occasionally, budding yeast forms, whereas cultural identification is made from growth on specialized agar incubated at room temperature. Fungus culture medium often includes antibiotics to suppress unwanted contaminants because skin and hair often harbor both saprophytic and pathogenic organisms (Table 9-5).

TABLE 9-4 Diseases Associated With the Urinary and Genital Systems

Disease	Causative Agent	Mode of Transmission	Treatment
Urinary system			
Bacterial diseases			
Cystitis (bladder infection)	*Escherichia coli, Proteus vulgaris, Pseudomonas aeruginosa,* and others	Opportunistic infections	Sulfonamides, chloramphenicol, kanamycin, penicillin G, or polymyxin
Pyelonephritis (kidney infection)	*Escherichia coli* is most frequently implicated; other agents include *Enterobacter aerogenes, Proteus* species, *Pseudomonas aeruginosa, Streptococcus pyogenes,* and staphylococci	From systemic bacterial infections or infections of the lower urinary tract	Depending on the agent, antibiotics include chloramphenicol, gentamicin, kanamycin, polymyxin, methicillin, penicillin, vancomycin, and tetracycline
Leptospirosis (kidney infection)	*Leptospira interrogans*	Direct contact with infected animals, urine of infected animals, or contaminated water	Penicillin
Glomerulonephritis (kidney infection)	Certain strains of *Streptococcus pyogenes*	Sequel to infection by certain strains of *S. pyogenes* in another part of the body	Chloramphenicol, erythromycin, lincomycin, penicillin, or vancomycin for the initial infection
Genital system			
Bacterial diseases			
Gonorrhea	*Neisseria gonorrhoeae*	Direct contact, especially sexual contact	Penicillin for nonresistant strains; spectinomycin for resistant strains

Disease	Causative agent	Mode of transmission	Treatment
Syphilis	*Treponema pallidum*	Direct contact, especially sexual contact	Penicillin, erythromycin, tetracycline
Nongonococcal urethritis (NGU)	Chlamydias or other bacteria, including *Mycoplasma hominis*, and hemolytic staphylococci and streptococci	Sexual contact or opportunistic infections	Tetracycline, erythromycin, or other antibiotics
Lymphogranuloma venereum (LVG)	*Chlamydia trachomatis*	Direct contact, especially sexual contact	Tetracycline, cycloserine antibiotics, and sulfonamides
Chancroid (soft chancre)	*Hemophilus ducreyi*	Direct contact, especially sexual contact	Tetracycline and sulfonamides
Granuloma inguinale	*Calymmatobacterium granulomatis*	Probably sexual contact	Gentamicin, chloramphenicol, tetracycline, streptomycin
Viral disease			
Genital herpes	Herpes simplex virus type 2 and occasionally type 1	Direct contact, especially sexual contact	Acyclovir
Fungal disease			
Vulvovaginal candidiasis (occasionally urethritis)	*Candida albicans*	Opportunistic pathogen, may be transmitted by sexual contact	Nystatin and amphotericin B
Protozoan disease			
Trichomoniasis (usually vaginal infection)	*Trichomonas vaginalis*	Opportunistic infection, may be transmitted by sexual contact or contact with fomites	Metronidazole

Source: Tortora, G. J., Funke, B. R., and Case, C. L. 1982. *Microbiology*. Menlo Park, Calif.: The Benjamin/Cummings Publishing Co., Inc.

TABLE 9-5 Diseases Associated With the Skin

Disease	Causative Agent	Treatment
Bacterial diseases		
Impetigo	*Staphylococcus aureus*; occasionally *Streptococcus pyogenes*	Penicillin, vancomycin, cephalothin, erythromycin, lincomycin
Erysipelas	*Streptococcus pyogenes*	Penicillin, erythromycin
Otitis externa and burn infections	*Pseudomonas aeruginosa*	Polymyxin, gentamicin
Acne	*Propionibacterium acnes*	Benzoyl peroxide, tetracycline
Viral diseases		
Warts	Papovavirus	May be removed by liquid nitrogen cryotherapy, cantharidin, salicyclic acid, dinitrochlorobenzene, bleomycin sulfate, surgical excision
Smallpox (variola)	Poxvirus (smallpox virus)	None
Chickenpox (varicella)	Herpesvirus (herpes zoster virus)	None

Measles (rubeola)	Paramyxovirus (measles virus)	None
German measles (rubella)	Togavirus (rubella virus)	None
Cold sores (herpes simplex)	Herpesvirus (herpes simplex virus)	None
Fungal diseases		
Tinea nigra	*Cladosporium wernecki*	3% sulfur and 2% salicyclic acid, tincture of iodine, griseofulvin
Ringworm (tinea)	*Microsporum, Trichophyton, Epidermophyton* species	Griseofulvin, miconazole, amphotericin B
Chromomycosis	*Phialophore verruscosa, Fonsecaea pedrosoi*	Flucytosine and bendazole
Maduromycosis	*Allescheria boydii*	Poleynes might be useful and surgical drainage
Candidiasis	*Candida albicans*	Nystatin, flucytosine, and amphotericin B in combination

Source: From Tortora, G. J., Funke, B. R., and Case, C. L. 1982. *Microbiology*. Menlo Park, Calif.: The Benjamin/Cummings Publishing Co., Inc.

> **Normal Flora**
> Hair, skin, and nails usually contain only normal, nonpathogenic surface contaminants.

Pathogens

Pathogenic organisms most commonly found on **hair** include:

Blastomyces species	*Microsporum* species	*Sporotrichum* species
Coccidioides species	*Monilia* species	*Trichophyton* species
Epidermophyton species		

Pathogenic organisms most commonly found on **skin** include:

Aspergillus species	*Cryptococcus* species	*Rhizopus* species
Blastomyces dermatitidis	*Epidermophyton* species	*Rhodotorula* species
Candida species	*Histoplasma capsulatum*	*Sporothrix schenckii*
Cladosporium species	*Microsporum* species	*Trichophyton* species
Coccidioides immitis	*Penicillium* species	

Pathogenic organisms most commonly found on the **nails** include:

Alternaria species	*Cephalosporium* species	*Epidermophyton floccosum*
Candida species	*Cladosporium* species	*Trichophyton* species

Methodology

Diagnosis of superficial or cutaneous mycoses requires hair, skin, or nail specimens obtained from infected areas. Hair stubs or scrapings from areas showing hair loss should be obtained without cleansing the scalp unless a fungicide has been applied, although gentle wiping with 70% isopropanol reduces contamination. Both the shaft and root of infected or suspicious hairs should be clipped or plucked with sterile forceps and sent to the laboratory in a sterile Petrie dish. Infected hairs often break off easily and have a twisted, grayish appearance in normal light but exhibit a bright yellow-green fluorescence when examined under ultraviolet light (Wood's light).

Specimens of skin or nails for fungal examination and culture should be obtained only after the affected site is washed carefully with 70% isopropanol and sterile water. After drying, several sites of the spreading edge of the lesion should be scraped with a sterile scalpel or thin-edged spatula and the specimens placed in a sterile, disposable Petrie dish or clean paper envelope. The most superficial scrapings of the infected nail surface should be discarded and only deeper shavings submitted for fungal examinations, although small nail clippings may be obtained with sterile scissors if necessary.

Nasopharynx and Throat Secretions and Discharges

Microbiologic examination of the upper respiratory tract with nasopharyngeal and throat cultures is important in the diagnosis of various localized and systemic infectious diseases.

Upper respiratory tract cultures must be interpreted cautiously because the nose, oral cavity, nasopharynx, and throat normally harbor a number of potentially pathogenic organisms. Thus, although an unusual predominance of any normal bacteria may be clinically significant, its presence in a nasopharyngeal culture does not necessarily implicate it as the cause of a respiratory disease. The relationship between many organisms and various infections may be evaluated only after clinical findings and related laboratory reports have been correlated. The isolation of certain organisms, such as *Mycobacterium tuberculosis*, *Corynebacterium diphtheriae*, and *Bordetella pertussis*, is always abnormal.

Clinical Significance

Upper respiratory tract cultures can aid the diagnosis of infections such as streptococcal sore throat, thrush, and diphtheria. They also can help determine the cause of certain systemic diseases, including scarlet fever, rheumatic fever, and acute glomerulonephritis. Throat cultures usually are requested to detect streptococcal pharyngitis and less frequently to investigate pertussis or viral pharyngitis. On the other hand, nasopharyngeal swabs are obtained to identify the presence of pneumococci, meningococci, or *Hemophilus influenzae* in suspected carriers because these organisms occur more commonly in the nasopharynx than in the throat.

Nasopharyngeal cultures also should be performed to aid in the diagnosis of whooping cough, croup, and pneumonia in infants and small children, in whom sputum specimens are not easily obtained. The presence of many pathogenic organisms in the throat is clinically significant and, especially in the absence of a sputum specimen, may reflect a lower respiratory tract infection. Examination of a gram-stained smear of material from nasopharyngeal swabs also can provide a preliminary indication of pulmonary infection when one type of organism is predominant (Table 9-6).

Normal Flora

Organisms normally found in the nasopharynx and throat include:

Bacteria

 Actinomyces naeslundii

 Bacillus species

 Bacteroides species

 Borrelia species

 Clostridium species

 Corynebacterium diphtheriae

 Enterobacter species

 Escherichia coli

 Fusobacterium species

 Hemophilus hemolyticus

 Hemophilus influenzae
 (in small numbers)

 Klebsiella species

 Mycobacterium species

 Neisseria catarrhalis

 Proteus species

 Staphylococcus albus

 Staphylococcus epidermidis

 Streptococcus species (α- and β-hemolytic)

 Streptococcus faecalis

 Streptococcus pyogenes
 (in small numbers)

 Streptococcus viridans

Fungus

 Candida albicans (in small numbers)

TABLE 9-6 Diseases Associated With the Respiratory System

Disease	Causative Agent	Mode of Transmission	Treatment
Upper respiratory system			
Bacterial diseases			
Streptococcal sore throat ("strep" throat)	Streptococci, especially *Streptococcus pyogenes*	Respiratory secretions	Penicillin and erythromycin
Scarlet fever	Erythrogenic toxin-producing strains of *Streptococcus pyogenes*	Respiratory secretions	Penicillin and erythromycin
Diphtheria	*Corynebacterium diphtheriae*	Respiratory secretions, healthy carriers	Antitoxin and penicillin, tetracyclines, erythromycin
Cutaneous diphtheria	*Corynebacterium diphtheriae*	Respiratory secretions, healthy carriers, direct contact	Antitoxin and penicillin, tetracyclines, erythromycin
Otitis media	Several agents, especially *Staphylococcus aureus*, *Streptococcus pneumoniae*, β-hemolytic streptococci, and *Hemophilus influenzae*	Complication of sore throat	Penicillin or erythromycin
Viral disease			
Common cold	Coronaviruses (rhinoviruses)	Respiratory secretions	None
Lower respiratory system			
Bacterial diseases			
Whooping cough	*Bordetella pertussis*	Respiratory secretions	Erythromycin, tetracyclines, chloramphenicol in severe cases; none in mild cases

Tuberculosis	*Mycobacterium tuberculosis*	Respiratory secretions; infrequently by food, especially milk	Isoniazid and rifampin
Pneumococcal pneumonia	*Streptococcus pneumoniae*	Healthy carriers; primarily a disease following viral respiratory infection or other stress	Penicillin
Klebsiella pneumonia	*Klebsiella pneumoniae*	Primarily a disease in debilitated hosts, e.g., alcoholics	Cephalosporins or gentamicin
Mycoplasmal pneumonia	*Mycoplasma pneumoniae*	Respiratory secretions (probably)	Tetracycline, erythromycin
Legionnaires' disease	*Legionella pneumophila*	Unknown; thought to be aerosols from contaminated air-conditioning cooling tower water	Erythromycin, rifampin
Psittacosis (ornithosis)	*Chlamydia psittaci*	Animal reservoir; aerosols of dried droppings and other exudates of birds; person-to-person transmission is rare	Tetracyclines
Q fever	*Coxiella burnetii*	Animal reservoir; aerosols in dairy barns and similar places; unpasteurized milk	Tetracyclines
Acute epiglottitis	*Hemophilus influenzae*	Complication of sore throat	Ampicillin in combination with chloramphenicol started immediately
Other bacterial pneumonias	*Proteus, Serratia,* and *Pseudomonas* species; *Escherichia coli,* and other bacteria	Bacteria are opportunistic	Varies with agent

(continued)

TABLE 9-6   Diseases Associated With the Respiratory System (*continued*)

Disease	Causative Agent	Mode of Transmission	Treatment
Viral diseases			
Viral pneumonia	Several viruses	Aerosols; complication of other viral diseases	None
Influenza	Influenza viral strains; many serotypes	Respiratory secretions	Amantadine (Influenza A only)
Fungal diseases			
Histoplasmosis	*Histoplasma capsulatum*	Animal reservoir; aerosols of dried bird droppings; person-to-person transmission is rare	Amphotericin B, ketoconazole
Coccidioidomycosis	*Coccidioides immitis*	Soil organism; aerosols of dust	Amphotericin B
Blastomycosis	*Blastomyces dermatitidis*	Soil organism; aerosols of dust	Amphotericin B
Other fungal pneumonias	Species of *Aspergillus, Rhizopus, Mucor,* and other genera	Aerosols of dust containing opportunistic fungi	Amphotericin B
Protozoan and helminthic diseases			
Pneumocystis pneumonia	*Pneumocystis carinii*	Direct contact (?)	Pentamidine, trimethoprim-sulfamethoxazole
Hydatidosis	*Echinococcus granulosis*	Direct contact with dogs	Surgical removal of cysts
Paragonimiasis	*Paragonimus westermani*	Ingestion of crayfish	Chloroquine

Source: Tortora, G. J., Funke, B. R., and Case, C. L. 1982. *Microbiology.* Menlo Park, Calif.: The Benjamin/Cummings Publishing Co., Inc.

Pathogens

Pathogenic organisms commonly found in the nasopharnyx and throat include:

Bacteria

Actinomyces israelii

Bordetella pertussis

Borrelia vincentii

Corynebacterium diphtheriae

Hemophilus influenzae (in large numbers)

Klebsiella pneumoniae

Mycobacterium tuberculosis

Neisseria gonorrhoeae

Neisseria meningitidis

Pseudomonas aeruginosa

Staphylococcus aureus (in large numbers)

Streptococcus species (β-hemolytic, groups A, B, C, and G)

Streptococcus pneumoniae

Streptococcus pyogenes (in large numbers)

Fungi

Candida albicans

Coccidioides immitis

Histoplasma capsulatum

Methodology

Material from the throat and nasopharnyx should be obtained on sterile polyester or calcium alginate swabs before the patient has received antibiotic or antimicrobial therapy. A flexible wire swab suspended in Carey-Blair or Amies transport medium or a Culturette tube containing a disposable applicator and capsule of Stuart transport medium are most suitable for collecting upper respiratory tract specimens. A long, curved wire swab is recommended for reaching the posterior pharyngeal wall via the nares when whooping cough is suspected. Nasopharyngeal cultures, however, have little advantage over throat cultures in the diagnosis of upper respiratory tract infections and often should be limited to cases where adequate throat cultures are difficult to obtain. Culture material should be collected on two separate swabs for inoculation in separate media when diphtheria is suspected.

▶▶ Nursing Responsibilities and Implications

To obtain an adequate **nasopharyngeal** culture specimen, the nurse should proceed as follows:

1. Elevate the tip of the nose and pass the curved wire swab along the floor of the nasal cavity under the middle turbinate until it reaches the posterior pharyngeal wall.

2. Leave the swab in place for 5–10 seconds to allow the fibers to become saturated with nasal secretions.

3. Remove the swab quickly, taking care to avoid touching the nares.

4. Place the swab into Stuart, Carey-Blair, or Amies transport medium. It is imperative that the swab remain moist until it is cultured in the laboratory.

5. Specify the suspected infection whenever possible on the request slip so that laboratory personnel will perform the appropriate procedures to isolate the etiologic agent.

6. Deliver the swab to the laboratory as soon as possible for prompt processing.

To obtain an adequate **throat** culture specimen, the nurse should proceed as follows:

1. Tilt the patient's head back, illuminate the throat, depress the tongue, and have the patient say "ah" to elevate the uvula.

2. Insert a sterile swab through the mouth, taking care to avoid touching the tongue, lips, cheek, or other oral surface.

3. Rub the swab firmly with a side-to-side motion over the posterior pharynx, tonsils, and any area of inflammation, ulceration, or exudation. Any obvious lesions, such as abscesses, follicles, or plaques in the throat or on the tonsillar surface, should be rubbed with the swab. When no obvious throat lesions are present, obtain material from the nasopharyngeal area above and behind the uvula.

4. Remove the swab deftly, again taking care to avoid touching the teeth, tongue, or lips.

5. Replace the swab in the Culturette tube, crush the ampule of holding medium, and force the swab into the liquid. When a wire swab is used, replace it in the tube of broth with the wire portion bent over the rim of the tube and screw the lid on as tightly as possible. It is imperative that the swab remain moist until it is cultured in the laboratory.

6. Deliver the swab to the laboratory immediately for prompt processing. When the swab cannot be delivered to the laboratory within 1 hour, it should be refrigerated at 4 C.

Sputum

Microbiologic examination of sputum, material raised from the lungs and bronchi during deep coughing, is important in the evaluation and diagnosis of lung disease. Sputum is a thick, sticky pulmonary exudate and must be distinguished from the saliva or postnasal discharge that may accompany it. Although sputum itself generally is relatively free of microorganisms, sputum specimens are commonly contaminated with the microbial flora encountered during passage through the throat and nasopharynx.

An early presumptive diagnosis of bacterial pneumonia or tuberculosis often can be made by careful examination of an acid-fast or gram-stained smear of sputum. The appearance of many encapsulated, lancet-shaped cocci accompanied by pus cells usually indicates pneumococcal infection, whereas acid-fast bacilli strongly suggest infection with *Mycobacterium tuberculosis*. However, definitive diagnosis and confirmation of such subjective impressions requires the actual isolation and identification of pneumococci, staphylococci, klebsiellae, or tubercle bacilli from sputum cultures.

Clinical Significance

Clear-cut diagnostic results of sputum cultures are seldom obtained because at present no completely satisfactory method for identifying the etiologic agent of pulmonary infections is available. Accurate evaluation of the significance of many potential pathogens in sputum cultures may be subject to error because expectorated sputum frequently contains upper respiratory tract contaminants. Isolation of several colonies of normally nonpathogenic organisms is most likely insignificant, although a heavy or predominant growth may be diagnostic. However, the presence of *M. tuberculosis* and *Corynebacterium diphtheriae* in sputum is always significant and may be presumed to be responsible for the respiratory tract disease (Table 9-6).

Normal Flora

Organisms normally found in small amounts in expectorated sputum include:

Bacteria

  Bacteroides species

  Borrelia species

  Corynebacterium diphtheriae

  Fusobacterium species

  Hemophilus influenzae

  Neisseria catarrhalis

Staphylococcus aureus

Staphylococcus epidermidis

Streptococcus species (group A, B, D)

Streptococcus pneumoniae

Streptococcus viridans

Fungus

  Candida albicans

Pathogens

Pathogenic organisms most frequently found in sputum and associated with upper respiratory tract infections include:

Bacteria

  Acinetobacter calcoaceticus

  Actinomyces species

  Bacteroides species

  Bordetella bronchiseptica

  Corynebacterium diphtheriae

  Enterobacter species

  Escherichia species

  Hemophilus influenzae

  Klebsiella pneumoniae

  Legionnella species

  Mycobacterium tuberculosis

  Mycoplasma pneumoniae

Neisseria species

Nocardia asteroides

Pasteurella bronchosepticus

Peptostreptococcus species

Proteus species

Pseudomonas aeruginosa

Serratia species

Staphylococcus aureus

Streptococcus pneumoniae

Streptococcus pyogenes

Fungi

  Alternaria species

  Aspergillus species

  Blastomyces dermatitidis

  Candida species

Coccidioides immitis

Cryptococcus species

Histoplasma capsulatum

Monilia species

Mucor species

Penicillium species

Rhizopus species

Scopulariopsis species

Sporothrix schenckii

Parasites

  Ascaris lumbricoides

  Pneumocystis carinii

  Strongyloides stercoralis

  Toxoplasma gondii

  Trichomonas hominis

Methodology

Routine culture and microbiologic examination of sputum require 1–3 mL of purulent or cheesy material, although special procedures to identify acid-fast tuberculosis organisms require 5–10 mL of material. Sputum specimens should be collected as soon as possible after the patient awakens because a first-morning expectorated sputum provides the most accurate culture results. Acceptable sputum specimens must not contain saliva or postnasal secretions. They should be obtained after the patient has brushed the teeth and thoroughly rinsed the mouth and throat to reduce contamination with oropharyngeal flora.

The patient should be instructed to collect material, raised by several deep coughs, in a sterile wide-mouthed container with a tightly fitting lid. The patient should be cautioned strongly to avoid contaminating the outside of the specimen container and surrounding area with the sputum to help prevent the spread of infection. Contaminated specimen cups present a health hazard to everyone who handles the material.

For optimum recovery and identification of *Mycobacterium tuberculosis,* a series of three to five single early morning specimens should be obtained on successive days. Collection of 24- to 72-hour pooled sputum specimens frequently reduces the rate of positive isolations and increases the incidence of contaminated cultures. Thus, the practice of extending specimen collection over a prolonged period or pooling sputum accumulated over several days when tuberculosis is present or suspected is not recommended. Sputum specimens for routine and tuberculosis culturing should be delivered promptly to the laboratory or refrigerated to avoid an overgrowth of nonpathogenic organisms.

▶▶ *Nursing Responsibilities and Implications*

1. Provide the patient with a sterile wide-mouthed container with a tightly fitting lid.

2. Coach the patient to take several deep breaths before coughing deeply to raise material from the lungs. It is often necessary for patients who do not have a productive cough to use a nebulizer early in the morning to induce coughing and bring up pooled overnight bronchial secretions.

3. Assist the patient to collect a sufficient amount of the first-morning sputum specimen to allow a thorough examination.

4. Label the container with the patient's name and identification number, time of specimen collection, and examinations desired.

5. Deliver the specimen container to the laboratory within 1 hour.

Stool

Microbiologic examination of feces is an important aid to the detection and identification of pathologic bacteria, fungi, and parasites responsible for intestinal diseases such as typhoid, dysentery, and amebiasis. Stool normally contains about 50 different organisms, composed mainly of anaerobic gram-negative bacilli, including several varieties that are potentially pathogenic in large numbers. Isolation and diagnosis of these pathogenic intestinal organisms require a variety of specialized culture media and biochemical procedures, as well as techniques to identify parasites and their ova. Stained stool smears, although not useful in identifying specific bacteria through morphologic and staining characteristics, demonstrate the presence of significant gram-positive cocci or yeastlike cells and indicate their ratio to gram-negative organisms.

Clinical Significance
Laboratory procedures to isolate and identify the etiologic agent of infectious intestinal disorders are most significant when stool cultures are performed during the acute phase of diarrheal disease. The laboratory should be notified of the suspected disease to speed the selection of the appropriate culture medium and identification of the responsible organism. Demonstration of enteric pathogens, particularly *Salmonella* and *Shigella*, is most likely during the first 3 days of an intestinal infection because organisms generally are present in appreciable numbers during this period. Therefore, repeated examinations and cultures of at least three stool specimens collected on successive or alternate days are necessary to diagnose or rule out the presence of intestinal infection (Table 9-7).

Following confirmation of salmonellosis or shigellosis, microbiologic surveillance of convalescent individuals and all possible carriers should be performed until at least three negative specimens have been obtained. A single negative culture is not sufficient evidence to confirm the absence of pathogens, especially when the clinical picture suggests bacterial involvement. In addition, the patient's recent dietary and travel history is required so that stool cultures and test results can be interpreted accurately.

The number of stool specimens required for the detection and identification of ova and parasites varies with the severity of the infestation and the quality of the specimens obtained. Most helminth ova are shed at a fairly uniform rate from day to day; however, protozoa, as well as certain helminth ova and segments, are shed irregularly. Therefore, three normally passed stool specimens collected with a day or two in between, together with one specimen obtained after the patient has received buffered sodium bisulfate, are generally examined.

Stool specimens should be examined immediately after they are collected to detect living trophozoites because many protozoa become nonmotile and degenerate within 30 minutes. Loose, fluid stools are more likely to contain the trophozoite form of intestinal ameba and flagellates, whereas semiformed or well-formed specimens contain the cysts, ova, and larvae of parasites. Older stools can be examined for cysts, ova, and larvae because these forms of the organisms retain their viability and morphology for longer periods of time.

Stool specimens are not suitable for microbiologic examination if they are obtained after the administration of antibiotics, such as tetracycline, that are absorbed in the gastrointestinal tract, antidiarrheals, antacids, oils, bismuth, or barium. Therefore, fecal specimens should be collected before the administration of any of these substances or delayed for 7–10 days to minimize their effects. Because antihelminthics, laxatives, and soap or hypotonic salt enemas suppress parasites, the initiation of therapy also should be postponed until the specific organism is identified.

Normal Flora

The human gastrointestinal tract usually does not harbor parasites, but a number of organisms normally are present within 24–48 hours after birth, including:

Bacteria

Acinetobacter species

Alcaligenes faecalis

Bacteroides species

Clostridium perfringens

Citrobacter species

Corynebacterium species

Enterobacter species

Escherichia coli

Klebsiella species

Lactobacillus species

Proteus species

Pseudomonas species

Serratia species

Staphylococcus aureus

Staphylococcus epidermidis

Staphylococcus pyogenes

Streptococcus faecalis

Streptococcus viridans

Vibrio species

Fungus

Candida albicans

Parasites

Entamoeba coli

Flagellates (some)

TABLE 9-7 Diseases Associated With the Mouth and Gastrointestinal System

Disease	Causative Agent	Mode of Transmission	Prevention or Treatment
Mouth			
Bacterial diseases			
Dental caries	*Streptococcus mutans*, lactobacilli, *Veillonella, Actinomyces*	Bacteria use sucrose to form plaque; bacteria produce acids	Restrict the ingestion of sucrose; brushing, flossing, and professional cleaning to remove plaque; fluoridation
Periodontal disease	*Actinomyces, Nocardia, Corynebacterium*	Plaque initiates an inflammatory response	Same as above plus antibiotics such as penicillin and tetracycline
Gastrointestinal system			
Bacterial diseases			
Botulism	*Clostridium botulinum*	Ingestion of exotoxin in food, usually improperly preserved	Antitoxin
Staphylococcal food poisoning (enterotoxicosis)	*Staphylococcus aureus*	Ingestion of exotoxin in food, usually improperly refrigerated	Replace lost water and electrolytes
Salmonellosis	*Salmonella* species	Ingestion of contaminated food and drink	Replace lost water and electrolytes
Typhoid fever	*Salmonella typhi*	Ingestion of contaminated food and drink	Ampicillin and trimethoprim-sulfamethoxazole, chloramphenicol
Bacillary dysentery (shigellosis)	*Shigella* species	Ingestion of contaminated food and drink	Replace lost water and electrolytes; ampicillin, chloramphenicol, or trimethoprim-sulfamethoxazole
Asiatic cholera	*Vibrio cholerae*	Ingestion of contaminated food and drink	Replace lost water and electrolytes
Vibrio parahaemolyticus gastroenteritis	*Vibrio parahaemolyticus*	Ingestion of contaminated shellfish	Tetracycline, chloramphenicol, or penicillin in severe cases

Disease	Causative agent	Mode of transmission	Treatment/Prevention
Escherichia coli gastroenteritis	Enterotoxigenic, enteroinvasive, and enteropathogenic strains of *Escherichia coli*	Ingestion of contaminated food and drink	None usually, but doxycycline has been used in some cases for traveler's diarrhea
Clostridium perfringens gastroenteritis	*Clostridium perfringens*	Ingestion of contaminated food and drink	Replace lost water and electrolytes
Viral diseases			
Mumps	Mumps virus	Saliva and respiratory secretions	None, but a vaccine is available (MMR)
Cytomegalovirus (CMV) inclusion disease	Cytomegalovirus (CMV)	Placental transfer and multiple blood transfusions	None
Hepatitis A	Hepatitis A virus	Ingestion of contaminated food and drink	None, but passive immunization is available
Protozoan diseases			
Giardiasis	*Giardia lamblia*	Ingestion of contaminated water	Metronidazole and quinacrine hydrochloride
Balantidiasis (balantidial dysentery)	*Balantidium coli*	Ingestion of contaminated food and water	Antibiotics (chlortetracycline, oxytetracycline) and diiodohydroxyquin
Amebic dysentery (amebiasis)	*Entamoeba histolytica*	Ingestion of contaminated food and water	Metronidazole
Helminthic diseases			
Tapeworm infestation	*Taenia saginata* (beef tapeworm), *T. solium* (pork tapeworm), *Diphyllobothrium latum* (fish tapeworm)	Ingestion of contaminated food and water	Quinacrine hydrochloride, niciosamide, and paramomycin
Trichinosis	*Trichinella spiralis*	Ingestion of contaminated food, especially improperly cooked pork	Thiabendazole and corticosteroids

Source: From Tortora, G. J., Funke, B. R., and Case, C. L. 1982. *Microbiology.* Menlo Park, Calif.: The Benjamin/Cummings Publishing Co., Inc.

Pathogens

Pathogenic organisms most commonly found in stool include:

Bacteria

Aeromonas species

Arizona species

Bacteroides species (in large numbers)

Campylobacter fetus, jejuni

Citrobacter species (in large numbers)

Clostridium species (in large numbers)

Enterobacter species (in large numbers)

Escherichia coli (in large numbers)

Klebsiella species (in large numbers)

Proteus mirabilis

Pseudomonas aeruginosa

Salmonella typhi

Serratia species (in large numbers)

Shigella species

Staphylococcus species (in large numbers)

Vibrio cholerae

Yersinia enterocolitica

Fungi

Aspergillus fumigatus

Candida albicans (in large numbers)

Candida tropicalis

Cryptococcus laurentii

Geotrichum species

Rhodotorula species

Torulopsis glabrata

Parasites

Ancylostoma duodenale (Old World hookworm)

Ascaris lumbricoides (roundworm)

Balantidium coli

Chilomastix mesnili

Clonorchis sinensis (Chinese liver fluke)

Dientamoeba fragilis

Diphyllobothrium latum (fish tapeworm)

Endolimax nana

Entamoeba coli

Entamoeba histolytica

Enterobius vermicularis (pinworm)

Fasciola hepatica (intestinal fluke)

Giardia lamblia

Hymenolepis nana (dwarf tapeworm)

Iodamoeba buetschlii

Necator americanus (New World hookworm)

Paragonimus westermani (long fluke)

Schistosoma japonicum (Oriental blood fluke)

Schistosoma mansoni (blood fluke)

Strongyloides stercoralis (threadworm)

Taenia saginata (beef tapeworm)

Taenia solium (pork tapeworm)

Trichomonas hominis

Trichuris trichiura (whipworm)

Methodology

Stool specimens should be collected directly in a sterile, wide-mouthed, waxed cardboard or plastic carton with a tight-fitting lid but also may be collected in a clean, preferably sterile bedpan and transferred to a suitable container. It is not necessary to submit the entire stool specimen to the laboratory because stool cultures and other microbiologic procedures require only a small amount of feces. A walnut-sized portion, about 1 inch in diameter, is usually satisfactory, particularly if it contains bits of bloody mucus or purulent material, which frequently harbor the organisms responsible for enteric disease. However, the entire amount of stool passed following treatment for tapeworm infestation should be sent to the laboratory for identification of the tapeworm head (scolex) to ensure that the worm has been dislodged. (See Chapter 8 for Procedure.)

Stool specimens should be delivered to the laboratory immediately after collection but may be refrigerated for a limited period of time to prevent overgrowth of non-pathogenic organisms and ensure accurate culture results. When culture of fresh specimens is not possible, stool preservatives such as phosphate buffer mixed with equal volumes of glycerol may be added during collection to promote the survival of many pathogens. Specimens for ova and parasite procedures that are delayed in reaching the laboratory should not be refrigerated but should be preserved with formalin or polyvinyl alcohol (PVA) fixative. One part of fresh feces mixed with three parts of PVA fixative solution or 5% formalin is sufficient for most routine examinations.

If stool specimens for microbiologic examination are not readily obtainable, as with children or debilitated patients, fecal material may be collected with a Culturette swab and placed into a transport medium or buffered glycerol. However, rectal swabs are less valuable than actual stool specimens in the evaluation of convalescent patients or known typhoid carriers and should not be relied on for the isolation of many pathogens. On the other hand, rectal swabs are recommended for the diagnosis of diarrheal disease when *Shigella* infection is suspected.

A proctoscopic aspiration or scraping may be used to identify protozoan trophozoites, whereas an intestinal biopsy, obtained through proctoscopic examination, serves to identify *Schistosoma* ova. Specimens collected from the anal margin on special adhesive swabs or cellophane tape preparations may be used to test for *Enterobius vermicularis* ova and detect pinworm infestation. Specimens are best obtained a few hours after the patient has retired, perhaps at 10–11 PM, or first thing in the morning before bathing, defecating, or urinating (females). Specimens may have to be repeated six times on six different days before pinworm infestation can be ruled out.

Precautions
To ensure accurate test results, the following precautions should be observed:

1. Do not fill specimen containers to the top and properly seal containers to prevent leakage and contamination because fecal material from individuals with infectious intestinal diseases or parasitic infestations is extremely hazardous.

2. Collect stool specimens before the patient has received barium or mineral oil, which can inhibit bacterial growth.

3. Keep specimens free of paper, soap, disinfectant, water, or urine, which may speed the deterioration of ova and make adequate stool examination impossible.

▶▶ Nursing Responsibilities and Implications
To obtain an adequate **stool specimen** for microbiologic examination, culture, or ova and parasite procedures, the nurse should proceed as follows:

1. Provide an appropriate specimen container and instruct the patient in the proper collection technique.

2. Caution the patient not to include paper or urine in the specimen or to contaminate the outside of the container with fecal material.

3. Deliver the specimen to the laboratory within 30 minutes for prompt examination.

4. Alert laboratory personnel to the possibility of infestation with parasites common to other geographic areas by noting on the laboratory request slip if the patient has recently traveled out of the country.

To collect an adequate **cellophane tape specimen** for the detection and identification of *Enterobius vermicularis* (pinworm) ova, the nurse should proceed as follows:

1. Apply a 3-inch long strip of ¾-inch transparent cellophane tape to a glass slide so that the tape is wrapped around one end of the slide. (Frosted or opaque tape is not satisfactory.) Fold a small portion of the end on itself to provide a nonsticky surface for handling the tape.

2. To obtain a sample, pull the folded tab so that the sticky side of the tape is freed, still leaving some of it stuck to the back of the slide.

3. Hold the slide against a tongue depressor, 1 inch from the end, and loop the freed tape over one end of the tongue blade so that the gummed surface is exposed.

4. Spread the anal folds apart and firmly touch all four quadrants of the mucocutaneous junction with the sticky surface of the tape but do not insert the blade into the rectum.

5. Replace the sticky surface of the tape onto the slide and deliver the slide to the laboratory for microscopic examination for *Enterobius* ova.

Synovial Fluid

Microbiologic culture and examination of synovial fluid are used to categorize septic joint disease and establish the diagnosis of infectious arthritis. Synovial fluid, a substance normally present in joints, lubricates the surfaces between bones and minimizes friction during movement, especially in joints bearing heavy loads. Synovial fluid normally is present in small quantities, although the amount is greatly increased in joint disease when the inflammation is most severe but decreases as the inflammation subsides. However, there is no absolute correlation between the volume of synovial fluid and the cause, severity, or duration of microbiologic infection and septic joint disease. (Synovial fluid studies also are discussed in Chapter 8.)

Clinical Significance

Infectious arthritis may result from the circulatory dissemination of infection to joint spaces, local extension of infected bone or soft tissue, or direct injection of microorganisms into joint capsules through trauma or surgery. Septic arthritis resulting from bacterial, tubercular, or fungal infections usually produces a rapid, irreversible destruction of the joints, most often involving the knees and hips. Bacterial arthritis frequently is superimposed on preexisting noninfectious joint disease but also may be caused by predisposing factors such as corticosteroid administration, diabetes mellitus, trauma, or extra-articular infection.

Normal Flora
Synovial fluid normally is sterile.

Pathogens

Pathogenic organisms most commonly found in the synovial fluid include:

Bacteria

Hemophilus influenzae

Moraxella osloensis

Mycobacterium tuberculosis

Neisseria gonorrhoeae

Neisseria meningitidis

Staphylococcus aureus

Streptobacillus moniliformis

Streptococcus species (β-hemolytic)

Fungi

Actinomyces species

Candida species

Cryptococcus neoformans

Nocardia species

Sporothrix species

Viruses

Adenovirus

Cytomegalovirus

Hepatitis B virus

Herpes simplex virus

Influenza virus

Mumps virus

Rubella virus

Varicella virus

Methodology

Microbiologic examination and standard bacterial culture require at least 1 mL of synovial fluid obtained by arthrocentesis under aseptic conditions by an individual skilled in the procedure. However, a 3–5 mL sample is preferred because the likelihood of positive culture increases if more fluid is submitted. Specimens should be aspirated with a disposable plastic needle and syringe and submitted in a tightly sealed syringe or sterile screw-capped container without an anticoagulant. Synovial fluid specimens should not be refrigerated to ensure the survival of pathogenic organisms but may be stored at 30 C if delays in processing are unavoidable.

▶▶ Nursing Responsibilities and Implications

1. Obtain the synovial fluid specimen before the administration of antibiotics.

2. Collect an acute-phase specimen immediately after the appearance of clinical illness when viral arthritis is suspected because the shedding of viruses into body fluids decreases rapidly after the onset of viral disease.

3. Deliver the specimen to the laboratory as soon as possible because proper treatment of septic joint infection may depend on the prompt results of microbiologic examination.

4. Record the patient's history of drug therapy on the laboratory request slip if antibiotics were administered. Any previous joint surgery or arthrocentesis also should be noted because these may have resulted in bacterial contamination of the joint space.

Urine

Microbiologic examination and culture of urine are essential to the diagnosis and evaluation of urinary tract infections from the kidneys to the urethra but most often are used to detect bladder infections. Although bacteriuria (bacteria in the urine) generally is caused by the predominance of a single type of bacteria, urine may contain a variety of different organisms. However, the presence of two or more distinct species of organisms in fairly equal proportions, especially in relatively small numbers, suggests that the urine specimen was contaminated during collection.

A single urine specimen obtained before the initiation of therapy is frequently sufficient to diagnose bacteriuria in individuals with symptoms such as pyuria, hematuria, and fever. Urine cultures repeated 48−72 hours after antimicrobial administration are helpful in evaluating their effectiveness because the patient's symptomatic response may be a poor indicator of successful therapy. The presence or absence of pyuria is unreliable as an index of urinary tract infections because it does not always accompany bacteriuria.

Clinical Significance

Isolation of bacteria, even known pathogens, from urine cultures does not necessarily establish a diagnosis of urinary tract infection because urine specimens frequently are contaminated by organisms from the urethra and external genitals. The number of organisms in 1 mL of urine, estimated by a quantitative culture technique known as the **colony count**, must be evaluated carefully to differentiate true bacteriuria from contamination. The colony count is performed by inoculating several culture plates with different urine dilutions and, after incubation, counting the number of colonies growing on the plate with the greatest dilution. This number is multiplied by the appropriate dilution factor to determine the approximate number of organisms per milliliter of urine.

A bacterial concentration of 100,000 or more per milliliter represents significant bacteriuria and indicates definite urinary tract infection, although lower counts may occur in patients receiving antibacterial therapy or with a urine specific gravity below 1.003. Bacterial counts between 10,000 and 100,000 per milliliter of urine are highly suggestive of infection and should be confirmed by a repeat culture of a fresh specimen. Fewer than 1000 bacteria per milliliter of urine are insignificant and probably represent transurethral or external contamination.

Any organism responsible for urinary tract infection must be identified and subjected to antibiotic susceptibility testing before the laboratory report is released. However, a single negative urine culture does not necessarily eliminate the possibility of an infection such as a low-grade pyelonephritis, and several specimens occasionally are required to demonstrate bacteriuria in asymptomatic individuals. Culture results of sterile urine are reported as "no growth," although there is always the possibility of infection with an organism that does not grow on routine culture media.

Normal Flora

Urine normally is sterile within the bladder. However, noninfected voided urine commonly contains small quantities of the following organisms as contaminants:

Bacteria	Staphylococcus albus
Bacillus species	Staphylococcus aureus
Corynebacterium diphtheriae	Streptococcus faecalis
Enterobacter species	Streptococcus species (α- and
Escherichia coli	β-hemolytic and group D)
Lactobacillus species	Fungus
Propionibacterium species	Candida albicans
Proteus species	Pityrosporum species

Pathogens
Pathogenic organisms most commonly found in infected urine include:

Bacteria		
Acinetobacter calcoaceticus	*Hemophilus* species	*Serratia* species
Alcaligenes faecalis	*Herellea* species	*Shigella* species
Citrobacter species	*Klebsiella* species	*Staphylococcus aureus*
Corynebacterium vaginalis	*Mycobacterium* species (in large numbers)	*Staphylococcus saprophyticus*
Enterobacter species (in large numbers)	*Neisseria gonorrhoeae*	*Streptococcus faecalis*
Enterococcus species	*Proteus mirabilis*	*Streptococcus pyogenes*
Escherichia coli (in large numbers)	*Proteus* species	*Streptococcus* species (β-hemolytic, groups B, C, and D)
	Providencia species	
	Pseudomonas aeruginosa	Fungus
	Pseudomonas species	*Candida albicans* (in large numbers)
	Salmonella species	

Methodology
Urine specimens for microbiologic examination should be collected using the clean-catch midstream technique to reduce contamination with organisms from the perianal area. (The procedures for collecting urine specimens are discussed in Chapter 1.) The nurse must assist the patient during specimen collection or provide complete instruction regarding thorough cleansing of the periurethral area (glans penis or labial folds). The cleansing procedure must remove contaminating organisms from the urethral meatus so that bacteria found in the urine specimen can be assumed to come only from the bladder and urethra. Urine specimens obtained from a bedpan, break in the catheter drainage system, or catheter drainage bag are unsuitable for culture.

It is not recommended that specimens for urine culture be collected by urethral catheterization because, despite all precautions, insertion of a catheter often introduces organisms into the bladder and may actually produce infection. Thus, although the clean-catch method may contaminate the urine specimen, it is preferable to introducing contaminants into the bladder. For accurate evaluation of urine culture results, a notation on the laboratory requisition slip is required stating whether the specimen was obtained by the clean-catch method or catheterization.

Specimens for urine culture and microbiologic examinations must be submitted to the laboratory within 30 minutes after collection or refrigerated at 4 C for no more than 24 hours to retard bacterial growth. Because urine supports the growth of most urinary pathogens, a small or insignificant number of bacteria can multiply rapidly at room temperature and invalidate the significance of quantitative culture results.

▶▶ Nursing Responsibilities and Implications

1. Provide the patient with a wide-mouthed, sterile plastic or glass container with a tightly fitting lid.

2. Encourage the patient to wash the hands before beginning the procedure.

3. Offer to help the patient during the cleansing and collection process. Female patients, especially those who are bedfast, often require assistance.

4. Instruct the patient to cleanse the labia or penis with several sterile gauze pads soaked

with a liquid antiseptic solution, beginning with outer areas and working in to the urinary meatus. Two separate washes with the antiseptic solution provide sufficient cleansing for reliable culture results.

5. Instruct the patient to void the first few milliliters of urine into the toilet bowl, stop, and then begin voiding directly into the sterile urine collection container until the cup is approximately half full.

6. Carefully seal the cap of the container so that it is tight and does not leak.

7. Label the container, not the lid, with the patient's identification information, including the time of specimen collection. Make sure the label will adhere to the container if the specimen is refrigerated.

Wound Exudates and Drainage

Microbiologic examination of material from wounds (traumatic or surgical incisions) can document the presence of infection and identify the causative agent as aids to appropriate therapy. Microorganisms isolated from these lesions reflect their anatomic site, the manner and environment in which they were inflicted, and the degree of microbial contamination in the adjacent areas. However, although all wounds are usually contaminated with organisms from the skin, only a few actually become infected with potential pathogens. Special specimen handling and culture techniques are required with deep or penetrating wounds to detect the presence of anaerobic organisms, which present a more serious threat.

Clinical Significance
The significance of wound or postoperative infections may vary according to the clinical condition of the patient as well as the organism isolated from the culture material. Exudate from a previously undrained abscess normally contains the invading organism, whereas repeated cultures of open or draining wounds frequently yield a variety of organisms whose significance is uncertain. Pathogenic organisms are more consistently isolated from infected wounds when the culture material is obtained from an area as close as possible to normal tissue (Table 9-8). Aerobes, including normal skin flora, usually are recovered from the outer edges of an ulcerated area, whereas the deeper folds and base usually reveal anaerobic organisms.

Normal Flora
The skin surrounding a wound or surgical incision is normally contaminated with a variety of potential pathogens, including:

Bacteria	
Acinetobacter species	*Proteus vulgaris*
Bacillus subtilis	*Staphylococcus aureus*
Corynebacterium diphtheriae	*Staphylococcus epidermidis*
Escherichia coli	*Streptococcus pyogenes*
Mycobacterium species	*Streptococcus viridans*
Propionibacterium acnes	Fungus
	Candida albicans

Pathogens
Pathogenic organisms isolated from infected wounds may include:

Bacteria

Bacillus anthracis

Bacillus subtilis

Bacteroides species

Clostridium species

Citrobacter species

Corynebacterium diphtheriae

Escherichia coli

Klebsiella species

Mycobacterium tuberculosis

Nocardia species

Pasteurella tularensis

Proteus species

Providencia species

Pseudomonas species

Serratia species

Staphylococcus aureus

Staphylococcus pyogenes

Streptococcus faecalis

Streptococcus species (anaerobic)

Fungi

Aspergillus species

Blastomyces dermatitidis

Candida species

Cladosporium species

Coccidioides immitis

Cryptococcus species

Histoplasma capsulatum

Microsporum species

Penicillium species

Rhizopus species

Rhodotorula species

Sporothrix schenckii

Methodology
Pus from superficial wounds should be collected on at least two separate sterile Culturette swabs to provide sufficient material to identify pathogenic organisms. Swabs must be placed in a tube with a suitable transport medium to prevent drying and should be delivered to the laboratory promptly. Material from deep wounds or surgical incisions should be aspirated into a sterile syringe before the abscess ruptures and immediately inoculated into oxygen-free transport tubes when anaerobic infection is suspected. Although anaerobic transport media must be used if a prolonged delay in processing is anticipated, the syringe used to aspirate material from deep wounds also can be used as a short-term transport container.

▶▶ Nursing Responsibilities and Implications

1. Remove superficial debris adjacent to the lesion and decontaminate the wound by gently wiping the surface with a 70% isopropanol or povidone-iodine disinfectant.

2. Aspirate or assist the physician to aspirate pus and suppurative material from unopened deep wounds, particularly fluctuant abscesses, by using a sterile needle and syringe. Immediately place the material collected into an anaerobic transport tube.

3. Collect as much pus as possible from a draining lesion by aspirating with a sterile pipette and immediately inoculating a tube of transport media. Gentle pressure or massage over the open sinus of the lesion (when not contraindicated) may be helpful in obtaining material for microbiologic studies. More material is needed for mycologic studies than for bacteriologic examination.

4. Collect material from the active site of superficial wounds, not normal skin areas,

TABLE 9-8 Summary of Diseases Associated With Wounds and Bites

Disease	Causative Agent	Mode of Transmission	Treatment
Wounds:			
Gangrene	*Clostridium perfringens*	Contamination of open wound by clostridial endospores	Debridement, amputation, hyperbaric chamber, penicillin, clindamycin, chloramphenicol
Tetanus	*Clostridium tetani*	Contamination of open wound by clostridial endospores	Penicillin before neurotoxin reaches nerves
Animal bites and scratches:			
Pasteurellosis	*Pasteurella multocida*	Animal bites from domestic animals such as cats and dogs	Penicillin and tetracycline
Rat bite fever	*Spirillum minor* or *Streptobacillus moniliformis*	Rat bite	Penicillin or tetracycline
Cat scratch fever	Unknown	Cat scratch or bite	Tetracycline

Disease	Causative agent	Vector	Treatment
Arthropod bites:			
Malaria	*Plasmodium species*	*Anopheles* mosquito	Quinine and its derivatives
African trypanosomiasis	*Trypanosoma brucei*	*Glossina* species (tsetse fly)	Bayer 205 (sodium suramin) and pentamidine isethionate
Yellow fever	Arbovirus (yellow fever virus)	*Aedes aegypti* mosquito	None
Dengue	Arbovirus (dengue fever virus)	*Aedes aegypti* mosquito	None
Arthropod-borne encephalitis	Arbovirus (encephalitis virus)	*Culex* mosquito	None
Epidemic typhus	*Rickettsia prowazekii*	*Pediculus vestimenti* (louse)	Tetracycline and chloramphenicol
Endemic murine typhus	*Rickettsia typhi*	*Xenopsylla cheopis* (rat flea)	Tetracycline and chloramphenicol
Rocky Mountain spotted fever	*Rickettsia rickettsii*	*Dermacentor andersoni* and other species (tick)	Tetracycline and chloramphenicol
Plague	*Yersinia pestis*	*Xenopsylla cheopis* (rat flea)	Tetracycline and streptomycin
Relapsing fever	*Borrelia* species	*Ornithodorus* species (soft ticks)	Tetracycline

Source: Tortora, G. J., Funke, B. R., and Case, C. L. 1982. *Microbiology.* Menlo Park, Calif.: The Benjamin/Cummings Publishing Co., Inc.

using two or more approved sterile polyester-tipped swabs and placing them in transport media. (Specimens collected on cotton swabs are seldom satisfactory for microbiologic examinations because they may be treated with bactericidal or bacteriostatic solutions.)

5. Deliver specimens to the laboratory immediately so that processing can take place within 60 minutes after collection.

ANTIBIOTIC SUSCEPTIBILITY TESTS

Antibiotic susceptibility tests measure the ability of various antimicrobial agents to slow or stop the growth of a particular microorganism. Susceptibility implies that an organism will be killed or inhibited by therapeutic blood levels of a particular antibiotic and indicates which drug is most effective against the organism responsible for a patient's illness. Therefore, antibiotic susceptibility tests can guide the selection of an appropriate antimicrobial agent.

Susceptibility tests are not indicated, however, when laboratory cultures isolate organisms whose relationship to the clinical picture is doubtful or when the organisms identified are known to have predictable susceptibility patterns. For example, organisms such as *Streptococcus pyogenes*, *Streptococcus pneumoniae*, *Clostridium perfringens*, and *Corynebacterium diphtheriae* as well as various *Hemophilus*, *Neisseria*, *Actinomyces*, and *Brucella* species consistently respond to adequate therapy with penicillin G, cephalothin, or tetracycline. However, resistant strains have emerged among some species that for many years were uniformly susceptible to the antibiotics of choice; thus, the need for routine susceptibility testing of particular organisms is increased.

Laboratory tests of antibiotic susceptibility are necessary under the following conditions:

- When cultures isolate organisms that frequently are resistant to antibiotics or that demonstrate a variable susceptibility pattern. Such organisms include the gram-negative enteric bacteria *Escherichia coli*, various *Enterobacteriaceae*, *Klebsiella*, *Salmonella*, *Shigella*, *Listeria*, *Proteus*, and *Pseudomonas* species, as well as *Staphylococcus* species and *Streptococcus faecalis*.

- When the clinical picture of bacterial meningitis, endocarditis, or osteomyelitis indicates that rapid bactericidal drugs should be used rather than bacteriostatic agents.

- When bacteria develop varying degrees of resistance to certain drugs during therapy or to the therapeutic dosage administered.

- When the patient's defense system is impaired by such conditions as hypogammaglobulinemia and lymphoproliferative disorders.

Susceptibility tests, however, may be equivocal or misleading in some cases and do not always ensure clinical efficacy of the antimicrobial regimen. For example, laboratory procedures do not interpret the patient's resistance to an organism, the type of infection, or the antibiotic concentration in the patient's tissues or at the site of infection. Thus, accurate antimicrobial therapy requires that a connection be established between the minimum quantity of drug necessary to inhibit growth of a pathogen and the achievable drug level. The lowest concentration of an antibiotic that prevents visible growth of a cultured organism is known as the **minimum inhibitory concentration** (MIC).

Antibiotic Activity

Antibiotic activity may be divided into five general groups:

1. Antibiotics that act primarily against gram-positive bacteria, including ampicillin, bacitracin, cephalothin, chloramphenicol, clindamycin, erythromycin, gentamicin, kanamycin, lincomycin, methicillin, penicillin G, oleandomycin, streptomycin, tetracycline, and vancomycin.

2. Antibiotics that act primarily against gram-negative bacteria and enterococci, including amikacin, ampicillin, carbenicillin, cefoxitin, cephalothin, chloramphenicol, colistin, gentamicin, kanamycin, nitrofurantoin (urine only), novobiocin, polymyxin B, streptomycin, sulfonamides, tetracycline, and tobramycin.

3. Antibiotics that act against gram-positive and gram-negative bacteria (broad-spectrum antibiotics), including ampicillin, cephalothin, chloramphenicol, kanamycin, neomycin, penicillin, streptomycin, and tetracycline.

4. Antibiotics that are particularly active against fungi, including amphotericin, griseofulvin, and nystatin.

5. Antibiotics that act primarily against the tubercle bacilli, including isoniazid (INH) and para-aminosalicylic acid (PAS), and rifampin.

The use of two or more antimicrobial agents for treating patients with serious infections may be recommended for a variety of reasons. The effect of two or more antimicrobial agents used together may be:

*   More effective than their individual effects (synergy);
*   Equal to their individual effects (additive);
*   No more effective than the more active antibiotic used alone;
*   Less effective than either antibiotic used alone (antagonistic).

It is highly desirable that antibiotic combinations selected to treat a serious infection be synergistic, and it is essential that their total effect not be antagonistic. Thus, laboratory procedures to evaluate the effectiveness of an antibiotic combination are an important part of susceptibility testing. Laboratory tests such as the checkerboard titration procedure evaluate not only synergy but also the degree to which the combination of the two drugs is more effective than either drug alone.

Disk Diffusion Tests

The most common method of susceptibility testing is the disk diffusion test, which uses small segments of filter paper impregnated with an antibiotic solution. When a variety of disks are placed on a culture plate streaked with a single bacteria, a zone of growth inhibition surrounds the antibiotic disk to which the organism is sensitive. The size of the inhibition zone is indirectly proportional to the MIC of the drug, determines the susceptibility of the organism to the drug, and indirectly indicates the clinical response. Conversely, bacterial growth surrounds those antibiotic disks to which the organism is resistant.

Quantitative Dilution Tests

Quantitative dilution tests are used to determine the minimum concentration of an antimicrobial agent that is required to inhibit or kill a particular organism (minimum inhibitory concentration, or MIC). The test is performed by inoculating various dilutions of antimicrobial agents in a culture medium with a suspension of the patient's infecting organism, incubating the mixture for 16–20 hours, and examining the mixture for turbidity. A lack of turbidity indicates a lack of microbial growth.

Quantitative dilution susceptibility tests are more advantageous than qualitative disk diffusion tests because the procedure can be performed on virtually any antibiotic or organism, whereas disk diffusion tests have more limited applications. In addition, dilution tests can detect varying degrees of organism sensitivity and resistance and, within broad limits, can be used to determine antibiotic dosages. The use of dilution susceptibility testing is becoming more widespread with the introduction of prediluted microdilution trays and inoculation equipment. Trays of serially diluted antibiotics are available for gram-positive and gram-negative organisms and for urinary pathogens, and several antibiotic determinations can be performed on an 80-well disposable tray.

Microdilution test reports are very helpful because they include information concerning the antibiotic level expected in the various physiologic compartments of the body such as the blood, tissue, urine, and bile. This information helps the physician to select the best antibiotic for the patient, including the dosage and route of administration. However, although the simplicity of the microdilution test is intellectually satisfying, reports do not provide an absolute value that reflects in vivo conditions with substantial precision and pose many difficulties of interpretation in clinical situations.

REFERENCES

Bailey, W., and Scott, G. 1982. *Diagnostic microbiology*. 6th ed. St. Louis: The C. V. Mosby Co.

Bauer, J. D. 1982. *Clinical laboratory methods*. 9th ed. St. Louis: The C. V. Mosby Co.

Collins, R. D. 1975. *Illustrated manual of laboratory diagnosis*. 2nd ed. Philadelphia: J. B. Lippincott Co.

Delaat, A. 1984. *Microbiology for the allied health professions*. 3rd ed. Philadelphia: Lea & Febiger.

Doucet, L. D. 1981. *Medical technology review*. Philadelphia: J. B. Lippincott Co.

French, R. M. 1980. *Guide to diagnostic procedures*. 5th ed. New York: McGraw-Hill Book Co.

Garb, S. 1976. *Laboratory tests in common use*. 6th ed. New York: Springer Publishing Co.

Glasser, L. 1980. Reading the signs in synovia. *Lab. Med.* 3(6) : 35.

Hargiss, C. O., and Larson, E. 1981. How to collect specimens and evaluate results. *Am. J. Nurs.* (Dec.) : 2166.

Heggers, J. P. 1980. Medically important yeasts. *J. Am. Med. Technol.* 42(2) : 73.

Henry, J. B. 1984. *Clinical diagnosis and management by laboratory methods*. 17th ed. Philadelphia: W. B. Saunders Co.

Koneman, E. W., and Truell, J. E. 1983. Microbiology for low-volume laboratories. *Lab. Med.* 14(1):26.

Lenette, E. H., Spaulding, E. H., and Truant, J. P. 1980. *Manual of microbiology.* 3rd ed. Washington, D.C.: American Society of Microbiology.

Marymont, J. H., and Marymont, J. 1980. Laboratory evaluation of antibiotic combinations. *Lab. Med.* 12(1):47.

Murray, P. R. 1983. Antibiotic susceptibility testing. *Lab. Med.* 14(6):345.

Raphael, S. S., et al., editors. 1983. *Medical laboratory technology.* 4th ed. Philadelphia: W. B. Saunders Co.

Rippey, J. H. 1979. Synovial fluid analysis. *Lab. Med.* 10(3):140.

Schoenknecht, F. D., and Sherris, J. C. 1980. Recent trends in antimicrobial susceptibility testing. *Lab. Med.* 11(12):824.

Stockblower, J. M., and Blumenfeld, T. A., editors. 1983. *Collection and handling of laboratory specimens.* Philadelphia: J. B. Lippincott Co.

Strand, M. M., and Elmer, L. A. 1983. *Clinical laboratory tests.* 3rd ed. St. Louis: The C. V. Mosby Co.

Tilkian, S. M., Conover, M. B., and Tilkian, A. G. 1983. *Clinical implications of laboratory tests.* 3rd ed. St. Louis: The C. V. Mosby Co.

Tortora, G. J., Funke, B. R., and Case, C. L. 1982. *Microbiology.* Menlo Park, Calif.: The Benjamin/Cummings Publishing Co., Inc.

Wertz, R. K. 1981. Relationship of MIC to drug level. *Diagn. Med.* 4(5):99.

Widmann, F. K. 1983. *Clinical interpretation of laboratory tests.* 9th ed. Philadelphia: F. A. Davis Co.

10

Hemostasis and Coagulation

HEMOSTASIS   533

COAGULATION   534
Stage I   ·   Stage II   ·   Stage III   ·   Stage IV

COAGULATION FACTORS   537
Factor I (Fibrinogen)   ·   Factor II (Prothrombin)   ·   Factor III
(Thromboplastin)   ·   Factor IV (Calcium)   ·   Factor V
(Proaccelerin)   ·   Factor VII (Proconvertin)   ·   Factor VIII
(Antihemophilic Factor)   ·   Factor IX (Plasma Thromboplastin
Component)   ·   Factor X (Stuart-Prower Factor)   ·   Factor XI (Plasma
Thromboplastin Antecedent)   ·   Factor XII (Hageman Factor)   ·   Factor
XIII (Fibrin Stabilizing Factor)   ·   Fletcher Factor (Prekallikrein)

COAGULATION PROFILE   543

SPECIMEN COLLECTION AND HANDLING   543

TESTS OF VASCULAR AND PLATELET FUNCTION   544
Bleeding Time   ·   Tourniquet Test   ·   Clot Retraction   ·   Platelet
Count   ·   Platelet Adhesion and Aggregation

TESTS OF OVERALL COAGULATION   553
Whole Blood Clotting Time   ·   Circulating Anticoagulants   ·   Partial
Thromboplastin Time   ·   Plasma Recalcification Time

TESTS TO EVALUATE STAGE I COAGULATION   558
Prothrombin Consumption Time   ·   Thromboplastin Generation Time

TESTS TO EVALUATE STAGE II AND III COAGULATION   561
Prothrombin Time   ·   Stypven Time   ·   Thrombin Time
·   Antithrombin III   ·   Fibrinogen Assay

TESTS TO EVALUATE STAGE IV COAGULATION   568
Fibrin-Fibrinogen Degradation Products   ·   Euglobulin Lysis
Time   ·   Paracoagulation Tests   ·   Plasminogen

ANTICOAGULANT THERAPY AND ASSOCIATED TESTS   573
Heparin   ·   Coumarin Derivatives

HEMOSTASIS

Hemostasis is a delicately balanced physiologic mechanism that controls the ability of the blood to coagulate (form a fibrin clot), thus preventing spontaneous bleeding and controlling hemorrhage. Normally, blood remains in a fluid state, circulating under pressure through a closed system until coagulation becomes necessary. Any injury to the vascular system or defect in a vessel wall usually sets in motion a complex sequence of physical and biochemical reactions that result in clot formation.

Hemostasis is achieved and maintained through the interaction of a number of vascular and intravascular processes, including constriction of blood vessels, platelet aggregation and adhesion, plasma factor activity, clot retraction, tissue repair, and fibrinolysis. The orderly progression of these processes transforms fluid blood into a fibrin clot that effectively closes and seals the damaged lining of an injured vessel.

Blood vessels provide the first line of defense against bleeding and generally prevent loss of blood unless actual injury to the vessel occurs. Following injury, muscle cells in the blood vessel walls contract immediately (a neural reflex reaction known as vasoconstriction) to decrease blood flow through the traumatized area. Vascular defects that affect structure, permeability, contractility, or ability to resist trauma more often cause inadequate hemostasis and bleeding tendencies than coagulation factor deficiencies or circulating anticoagulants.

Platelets are small fragments of cytoplasm from large megakaryocytes that have a variety of functions and play a vital role in maintaining hemostasis. Platelets help preserve normal vascular integrity by occluding small gaps in vessel walls and providing structural support to the endothelial lining of the walls. Following vascular injury, platelets adhere to exposed collagen fibrils and aggregate at the site of trauma to form an emergency hemostatic plug that slows blood flow. Platelets also release several substances (such as platelet factor 3) that prolong local vasoconstriction and interact with certain coagulation factors to reinforce and stabilize the platelet plug. Thus, effective coagulation and hemostasis require an adequate number of morphologically and functionally normal platelets. (See Tests of Vascular and Platelet Function later in this chapter.)

Plasma coagulation factors, also known as procoagulants, are a group of at least ten interdependent enzymes that are necessary for the formation of a firm, stable fibrin clot. A normal response to trauma requires the presence of adequate concentrations of each coagulation factor; these coagulation factors must remain inactive until the clotting sequence is initiated. A deficiency of any one of these coagulation factors may be inherited or acquired and generally results in excessive blood loss following injury. However, an increased concentration of some of these factors, due to a change in the rate of blood flow, may lead to thrombus formation. (See Tests of Overall Coagulation, later in this chapter).

Clot retraction is essential to the effectiveness of the hemostatic plug. Retraction results from rearrangement of fibrin strands within the clot, which causes the clot to decrease in size. An adequate number of intact, functionally normal platelets are needed to firmly secure the clot to a vessel wall until it is overgrown by epithelium and gradually disappears. (See Clot Retraction later in this chapter.)

Fibrinolysis and clot dissolution begin almost as soon as hemostasis is achieved to confine the clot to the damaged portion of the blood vessel. Because the body normally maintains a delicate balance between clot formation and dissolution, any deficiency of vital fibrinolytic enzymes allows undissolved fibrin to remain within the bloodstream. Conversely, increased fibrinolytic activity can deplete the supply of essential clotting proteins, causing excessive bleeding during obstetric complications, liver disease, or use of the heart-lung pump. (See Tests to Evaluate Stage IV Coagulation later in this chapter.)

Dysfunction of any one or more of these processes may produce clinical evidence of a bleeding tendency. On the other hand, overstimulation of the clotting mechanism in individuals with thromboembolic disorders may result in excessive clot formation and thrombosis.

COAGULATION

The complex interaction of the numerous tissue, platelet, and plasma factors involved in coagulation have as their ultimate aim the formation of a stable fibrin clot. The coagulation sequence occurs in four progressive stages, which are difficult to describe or illustrate adequately because several stages frequently occur simultaneously (Figure 10-1). Greatly simplified, these stages may be summarized as follows:

Stage I—activation of thromboplastin activity through intrinsic and extrinsic pathways

Stage II—conversion of prothrombin to thrombin by thromboplastin activity

Stage III—conversion of fibrinogen to fibrin by thrombin

Stage IV—fibrinolysis

Stage I

The coagulation sequence can be activated by external trauma such as a cut (extrinsic pathway) or by trauma within the circulatory system that exposes vascular endothelium (intrinsic pathway). Thus, an event within the blood itself or injury to blood vessels and their surrounding tissues provides a site for platelet accumulation and exposes the coagulation factors to a foreign surface.

The **extrinsic pathway** is triggered when blood escapes from the vascular system and contacts damaged tissues, which release tissue thromboplastin, a clot-promoting substance not present in blood. The thromboplastin contained in tissue fluid forms a complex with plasma factor VII, which, in the presence of platelets and calcium, activates factor X to continue the clotting process. Plasma factor VII participates only in the extrinsic pathway of the coagulation mechanism and is essential for the activation of tissue thromboplastin.

The **intrinsic pathway** is a progressive activation sequence that is best visualized as a cascade or waterfall because the stimulation of each plasma factor initiates the next reaction. The intrinsic clotting system employs only those coagulation factors normally present in blood to generate plasma thromboplastin, which has the same final activity as tissue thromboplastin. Plasma thromboplastin is not found in the bloodstream but is formed at the site of injury as a result of the progressive activation of specific coagulation factors in the presence of several cofactors.

The intrinsic pathway is initiated when blood comes in contact with an unfamiliar substance such as collagen, elastin, microfibrils, or vascular endothelium from an injured blood vessel wall. Thus, surface contact triggers the initial activity of factor XII, which then stimulates factor XI and converts prekallikrein (Fletcher factor) to the enzyme kal-

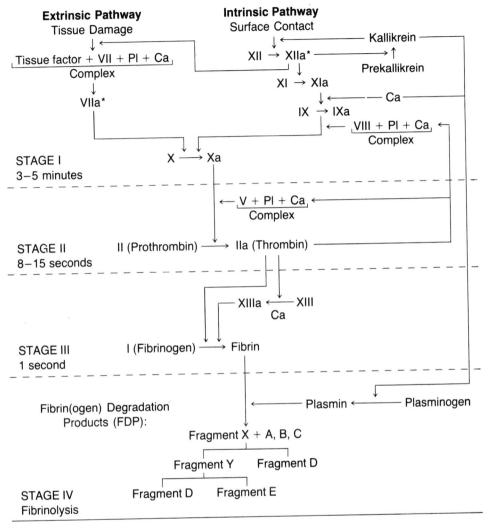

Figure 10-1 Progression of the coagulation sequence.

likrein (activated Fletcher factor). The conversion of prekallikrein to kallikrein has a feed-back effect that is necessary for factor XII activation to proceed more rapidly. Stimulation of factor XI in turn converts factor IX to its active form to initiate factor X activity in the presence of calcium, activated factor VIII, and platelet phospholipids (platelet factor 3). Factors XII, XI, IX, VIII, and the Fletcher factor participate only in the intrinsic pathway, whereas factor X participates in both the extrinsic and intrinsic pathways. (See Tests to Evaluate Stage I Coagulation later in this chapter.)

Stage II

The plasma and tissue thromboplastin formed or released during stage I converts prothrombin to thrombin with the aid of factors X and V in the presence of calcium and platelets. Thrombin, a powerful proteolytic agent required to split fibrinogen molecules in stage III, is derived from the inactive precursor prothrombin normally found in the bloodstream. Adequate concentrations of thrombin are also essential to platelet aggregation (during formation of the hemostatic plug), activation of factor XIII, and initiation of fibrinolysis. (See Tests to Evaluate Stage II and III Coagulation later in this chapter.)

Thrombin formation is prevented at inappropriate times and controlled during coagulation by several inhibitors that limit the rate of clotting and stop it entirely when hemostasis is achieved. These natural coagulation inhibitors include α_1-antitrypsin, α_2-macroglobulin, and antithrombin III (the most clinically significant substance) and constitute an important feedback system that progressively and irreversibly inactivates the thrombin that has been formed. Although an excess of thrombin inhibitors does not appear to be responsible for an increased tendency to bleed, a decrease in these substances may cause hypercoagulability and produce thrombosis during a number of conditions. (See Antithrombin III later in this chapter.)

Stage III

Circulating fibrinogen is split by the enzymelike action of thrombin to produce a network of fibrin strands that combine end-to-end and side-by-side to form a soluble clot. The loosely joined fibrin strands assume a stronger configuration through the stabilizing action of factor XIII, resulting in a firm, insoluble clot. (See Tests to Evaluate Stage II and III Coagulation later in this chapter.)

Stage IV

The fibrinolytic system, activated by fibrin formation, restricts clotting to the area of injury by slowly removing unnecessary fibrin through digestion. Plasminogen, a substance incorporated into the clot, is converted by activators present in the blood and vascular epithelium to plasmin, a fibrin-dissolving enzyme. Plasminogen activators generally are released when the vascular lining has been repaired. They also may be produced by emotional stress, anxiety, physical exercise, trauma, surgery, or anoxia.

Fibrinolysis results in the formation of partially digested fragments, referred to as fibrin degradation products (FDP), which are identified by the letters X, Y, D, E, A, B, and C. Some of these degradation products, which also are released by the digestion of fibrinogen, have an anticoagulant action and inhibit clotting when their presence in the bloodstream is excessive. Thus, because of increased FDP production and plasma factor depletion, abnormally active fibrinolysis is a potential danger to effective hemostasis in pathologic conditions such as disseminated intravascular coagulation syndrome (DIC), thromboembolic disorders, and renal diseases. (See Tests to Evaluate Stage IV Coagulation later in this chapter.)

COAGULATION FACTORS

Coagulation factors currently are identified by Roman numerals to avoid confusion because a variety of synonyms previously have been used. Factors have been assigned numerals according to their sequence of discovery rather than the order in which they act during clot formation. However, fibrinogen (I), prothrombin (II), thromboplastin (III), and calcium (IV) are regularly referred to by name because of their key roles in the clotting mechanism. The numeral VI is not used at present because the original factor VI was discovered to be the activated form of factor V rather than a separate substance.

Adequate concentrations of all coagulation factors are necessary to maintain normal hemostasis, but all factors do not produce recognizable clinical symptoms if they are absent or deficient. Hemorrhagic syndromes are not associated with deficiencies of factors III, IV, or XII. However, a deficiency of any of the remaining factors may produce a bleeding tendency. Defective coagulation may be due to an inherited deficiency of one or more factors or may be an acquired disorder accompanying liver disease or numerous other conditions.

Factor I (Fibrinogen)

Factor I (fibrinogen) is an essential plasma protein that is split by thrombin during stage III of the coagulation sequence to produce fibrin strands that combine and form a solid clot. A congenital form of fibrinogen deficiency may result in bleeding episodes, which are usually mild. However, low levels of fibrinogen may be life threatening in emergency situations such as the intravascular clotting syndrome following obstetric complications. Fibrinogen deficiencies, either congenital or acquired, may be detected by markedly prolonged prothrombin time, coagulation time, partial thromboplastin time, and thrombin time tests. Basal fibrinogen concentrations can only be measured in individuals who are not actively bleeding and who have not received a blood transfusion within the previous 3–4 weeks.

Decreased fibrinogen may occur in:

Acquired deficiencies (liver disease, especially severe biliary cirrhosis, severe cachectic states, especially terminal carcinomatosis, severe chronic tuberculosis)

Circulating fibrinogen inhibitors

Congenital deficiencies (afibrinogenemia, hypofibrinogenemia, dysfibrinogenemia)

Normal and premature newborn infants

Excessive utilization (obstetric complications, fibrinolysis, disseminated intravascular coagulation [DIC], severe shock during surgery or following trauma, metastatic carcinoma of the prostate)

Increased fibrinogen may occur with:

Acute infections

Burns

Collagen diseases (rheumatoid arthritis, rheumatic carditis)

Hepatitis without severe liver damage

Nephrosis

Normal menstruation

Surgery, developing 5–10 days postoperatively

X-ray therapy or irradiation

Factor II (Prothrombin)

Factor II (prothrombin) is an inactive plasma protein that is converted to the proteolytic enzyme thrombin by the action of extrinsic and intrinsic thromboplastin during stage II of the coagulation sequence. Congenital prothrombin deficiencies are rare. Acquired deficiencies are more common and may result from a number of conditions or agents. Acquired prothrombin deficiency is almost always accompanied by a decreased concentration of one or more of the other clotting factors, mainly factors VII, IX, and X. Prothrombin deficiencies may be detected by prolonged prothrombin time and partial thromboplastin time tests.

Decreased prothrombin levels may occur with:

Congenital deficiencies

Drug therapy (excessive salicylate therapy, prolonged antibiotic administration, coumarin drugs, phenylbutazone therapy)

Liver disease (cirrhosis, obstructive jaundice, acute liver necrosis, severe

hepatitis, reactions to hepatotoxic drugs)

Vitamin K deficiency (due to insufficient dietary intake or faulty intestinal absorption such as sprue, celiac disease, idiopathic steatorrhea, intestinal obstruction, ulcerative colitis, prolonged diarrhea)

Factor III (Thromboplastin)

Factor III (thromboplastin) is an enzymelike protein, not normally present in plasma, that is capable of converting prothrombin to thrombin during stage II of the coagulation sequence. Two separate types of thromboplastin generally are available for use in the coagulation sequence, extrinsic tissue thromboplastin and intrinsic plasma thromboplastin. Most connective tissues and cells throughout the body, particularly the lungs, brain, and placenta, contain tissue thromboplastin. This substance is released immediately and acts within seconds following injury. Plasma thromboplastin, on the other hand, is generated during stage I of the coagulation sequence from the interaction of Fletcher factor, factors XII, IX, XI, VIII, and X, platelets, and calcium and requires several minutes for its production.

Although a complete lack of tissue thromboplastin is impossible, the amount of plasma thromboplastin can be insufficient because of an absence or deficiency of one or more of the coagulation factors. Tissue thromboplastin may be inappropriately released into the bloodstream, resulting in the stimulation of intravascular coagulation following amniotic embolism, other obstetric accidents, tissue necrosis, trauma, and severe shock.

Factor IV (Calcium)

Factor IV (calcium) is an inorganic ion, normally present in the blood and tissues, that is essential to more than one reaction in the coagulation sequence, although the exact mechanisms are not known. Calcium is required for thromboplastin generation in stage I, for the enzymatic conversion of prothrombin to thrombin in stage II, and for the stabilization of the fibrin clot in stage III. The activity of many laboratory anticoagulants is based on the removal of ionized calcium from the blood by such calcium-binding substances as EDTA, oxalate, and citrate.

Plasma calcium deficiencies resulting from disease seldom cause clinical bleeding tendencies because coagulation can take place with less calcium than is needed for other physiologic functions. Calcium levels low enough to interfere with the clotting mechanism would be incompatible with life and would cause tetany or cardiac arrest before the deficiency could prolong coagulation. Decreased plasma calcium concentrations (hypocalcemia) may occur following massive transfusions or exchange transfusions using citrated rather than heparinized blood.

Factor V (Proaccelerin)

Factor V (proaccelerin), also known as the labile factor, is essential for speeding the conversion of prothrombin to thrombin in stage II of the coagulation sequence. Factor V deteriorates rapidly in specimens at room temperature but is more stable and remains available for replacement therapy in fresh-frozen citrated plasma. A deficiency of factor V may be detected by prolonged clotting time, prothrombin time, and partial thromboplastin time tests.

Decreased factor V levels may occur with:

Acquired deficiencies (severe liver disease, DIC, fibrinolysis, radioactive phosphorus therapy, surgery, circulating factor V inhibitors)

Congenital deficiencies (parahemophilia)

Factor VII (Proconvertin)

Factor VII (proconvertin) is also known as the stable factor. It is essential for the activation of factor X in the presence of extrinsic tissue thromboplastin and helps accelerate the conversion of prothrombin to thrombin during stage II of the coagulation sequence. Factor VII is the first plasma factor to be depressed after the administration of coumarin anticoagulants. The depression of factor VII is followed by the successive reduction of factors IX, X, and II. Conversely, the synthesis and activity of factor VII reappear rapidly, rising to normal levels within 5–6 hours after the cessation of coumarin therapy and administration of adequate vitamin K. A factor VII deficiency may be detected by a prolonged prothrombin time test.

Decreased factor VII levels may occur in:

Acquired deficiencies (hepatic carcinoma, hepatitis, obstructive jaundice, vitamin K deficiency, dicumarol therapy, hemorrhagic disease of the newborn, prolonged administration of broad-spectrum antibiotics, kwashiorkor)

Congenital deficiencies, although these are rare

Increased factor VII levels may occur in late normal pregnancy, thromboembolic conditions, and oral contraceptive therapy.

Factor VIII (Antihemophilic Factor)

Factor VIII (antihemophilic factor, or AHF), also known as hemophilic factor A, is an important precursor required for the generation of intrinsic plasma thromboplastin in stage I of the coagulation sequence. Decreased levels of factor VIII reduce normal thromboplastic activity, which in turn diminishes the conversion of prothrombin to thrombin, causing prolonged bleeding. Congenital factor VIII deficiency can be inherited as a sex-linked, recessive disorder that is transmitted by females but is manifested almost exclusively in males, who experience symptoms in both the heterozygous and homozygous states.

Individuals with little or no factor VIII activity are classified as severe hemophiliacs, those with levels between 1% and 5% of normal as moderate, and those whose levels are 6%–30% of normal as mild. The degree of factor VIII deficiency in classic hemophilia generally parallels the severity of the bleeding symptoms, which range from massive, life-threatening hemorrhage to a slow oozing following trauma or surgery. Surgery is possible in individuals with hemophilia if plasma AHF levels are maintained at more than 10%–25% of normal for minor procedures and 30%–60% of normal for major surgery. The factor VIII level in these individuals may be raised approximately 14% by the rapid transfusion of 1 L of fresh-frozen plasma or as high as desired using human factor VIII concentrate.

Absence of factor VIII produces abnormal coagulation time, prothrombin consumption time, partial thromboplastin time, and thromboplastin generation time test values. However, results of some laboratory procedures may be within the normal range if factor VIII deficiencies are moderate to mild. For example, clotting time and prothrombin consumption time are normal in blood containing 2% and 10%, respectively, of the usual factor VIII activity, whereas partial thromboplastin time is normal only when the patient has more than 30%–40% of the usual factor VIII activity.

Decreased factor VIII levels may occur with:

Acquired deficiencies (DIC, fibrinolysis, and circulating factor VIII inhibitors due to childbirth, lupus erythematosus, multiple myeloma, rheumatoid arthritis, penicillin sensitivity, carcinoma)

Congenital deficiencies (hemophilia A or classic hemophilia, von Willebrand's disease)

Increased factor VIII levels may occur with:

Adrenalin therapy	Macroglobulinemia
Coronary artery disease	Muscular exercise
Coumarin anticoagulants, sudden cessation	Oral contraceptives
Hyperthyroidism	Pregnancy
Hypoglycemia	Surgery

Factor IX (Plasma Thromboplastin Component)

Factor IX (plasma thromboplastin component, or PTC), also known as hemophilic factor B or Christmas factor, is essential for the generation of intrinsic plasma thromboplastin in stage I of the coagulation sequence. Factor IX influences the amount of thromboplastin available to convert prothrombin to thrombin but does not influence the rate at which it is produced. A congenital deficiency of factor IX produces a hemorrhagic disease clinically indistinguishable from classic hemophilia. It is inherited as a sex-linked characteristic similar to factor VIII deficiency. Individuals with Christmas disease require about 1 L of fresh-frozen plasma daily to control bleeding following an acute hemorrhagic episode or minor surgery. Factor IX deficiency may be detected by prolonged coagulation time, partial thromboplastin time, prothrombin consumption time, and thromboplastin generation time tests.

Decreased factor IX levels may occur with:

Circulating factor IX inhibitors

Congenital deficiency, hemophilia B (Christmas disease)

Dicumarol and related anticoagulant therapy

Hemorrhagic disease of the newborn

Liver disease

Nephrotic syndrome

Vitamin K deficiency (insufficient dietary intake, poor intestinal absorption)

Factor X (Stuart-Prower Factor)

Factor X (Stuart-Prower factor) is essential for the prompt conversion of prothrombin to thrombin in stage II coagulation by both the intrinsic and extrinsic thromboplastin systems. Factor X also is required for the generation of intrinsic plasma thromboplastin in stage I coagulation and is activated by extrinsic tissue thromboplastin in the presence of factor VII. A deficiency of factor X may produce abnormal coagulation time, prothrombin time, partial thromboplastin time, and prothrombin consumption time test results.

Decreased factor X levels may occur with:

Congenital deficiencies, although these are rare

Dicumarol and related anticoagulant therapy

Hemorrhagic disease of the newborn

Liver disease, hepatic trauma

Vitamin K deficiency

Increased factor X levels may occur with oral contraceptives and pregnancy.

Factor XI (Plasma Thromboplastin Antecedent)

Factor XI (plasma thromboplastin antecedent, or PTA), also known as hemophilic factor C, is required for the evolution of intrinsic plasma thromboplastin in stage I coagulation. Factor XI is activated by factor XII and in turn activates factor IX to continue the cascade effect of the coagulation sequence. A congenital deficiency of factor XI is not a sex-linked trait because it occurs in both males and females. Individuals with a factor XI deficiency may exhibit a mild bleeding tendency following surgery or a tooth extraction. A deficiency of factor XI may be detected by prolonged clotting time, partial thromboplastin time, prothrombin consumption time, and thromboplastin generation time tests.

Decreased factor XI levels may occur in:

Circulating factor XI inhibitors

Congenital deficiencies, although these are rare

Congenital heart disease

Dicumarol and related anticoagulant therapy

Liver disease

Newborn infants

Paroxysmal nocturnal hemoglobinuria

Vitamin K deficiency (due to intestinal malabsorption)

Factor XII (Hageman Factor)

Factor XII (Hageman factor), also known as the glass contact factor, initiates the entire coagulation mechanism and is essential for the normal generation of intrinsic plasma thromboplastin in stage I. Factor XII is activated following injury by contact with collagen and other subendothelial connective tissues within the body. It also may be activated outside the body following venipuncture when the blood comes in contact with a surface such as glass or micronized silica. Activated factor XII in turn triggers the Fletcher factor, which has a reciprocal effect that causes factor XII activity to stimulate factor XI to speed up the clotting sequence. It also plays an important role in fibrinolysis by converting plasminogen to plasmin. Because the absence of factor XII generally is not associated with any clinically recognizable bleeding disorders, an unsuspected deficiency may be detected during the coagulation workup by prolonged prothrombin consumption time, partial thromboplastin time, coagulation time, and thromboplastin generation time tests.

Decreased factor XII levels may occur in:

Congenital deficiencies (rarely)	Newborn infants
Liver disease (on occasion)	Pregnancy

Increased factor XII levels may occur with increased exercise and physical labor.

Factor XIII (Fibrin Stabilizing Factor)

Factor XIII (fibrin stabilizing factor, or FSF), also known as fibrinase, is an enzyme present in blood, tissues, and platelets that is necessary to stabilize the cross-linkage of fibrin strands to form a firm clot. Factor XIII is activated by thrombin in the presence of calcium. Only 10% of the normal plasma concentration of factor XIII is needed to ensure complete hemostasis and as little as 2% is needed to control hemorrhage. A deficiency of factor XIII results in a weak clot that does not support the growth of fibroblasts, resulting in delayed or poor wound healing, prolonged post-traumatic bleeding, and abnormal scar formation.

Decreased factor XIII levels may occur in:

Agammaglobulinemia	Myeloma
Circulating factor XIII inhibitors	Newborn infants
Congenital deficiencies (rarely)	Pernicious anemia
Lead poisoning	Severe liver disease

Increased factor XIII levels may occur in:

Infants born to mothers who experienced hemorrhagic episodes during pregnancy

Myocardial infarctions (accompanying reduced fibrinolytic activity with reduced heparin tolerance)

Premature infants

Fletcher Factor (Prekallikrein)

Fletcher factor (prekallikrein) is a normal plasma protein that is triggered by factor XII activity during the formation of intrinsic plasma thromboplastin in stage I of the coagulation sequence. Prekallikrein is converted by activated factor XII to its active form, the enzyme kallikrein, which in turn speeds up factor XII activity. In addition, activated Fletcher factor helps stimulate the conversion of plasminogen to plasmin during fibrinolysis and clot dissolution in stage IV coagulation. Fletcher factor deficiency, an inherited (autosomal recessive), clinically asymptomatic defect, is identified by a prolonged activated partial thromboplastin time test.

COAGULATION PROFILE

A **coagulation profile** is a series of selected studies that evaluates all stages of the coagulation process and is performed during presurgical screening or the investigation of hemorrhagic disorders. A sample coagulation screening panel might consist of the following tests:

Bleeding time	Prothrombin time
Whole blood clotting time	Antithrombin III
Clot retraction	Thrombin time
Platelet count	Fibrinogen level
Platelet adhesion and aggregation	Fibrin-fibrinogen degradation products
Activated partial thromboplastin time	

This entire group of tests should be performed during the initial investigation of hemostasis to detect coagulation deficiencies and pinpoint the particular problem involved. Although this screening panel generally indicates bleeding disorders in asymptomatic individuals, it occasionally misses deficiencies responsible for clinically mild symptoms, which may be significant during periods of stress such as surgery. These tests also do not reveal all clotting defects because some procedures are too insensitive and more specific studies are needed with other screening tests for correct interpretation. Thus, in a patient with a significant clinical history of a bleeding tendency, further investigation and more extensive tests are needed, even when screening test results are normal.

A detailed clinical history should be obtained from the patient to identify any personal or family episodes of unusual bleeding before surgery or during routine investigation. The history should include careful patient questioning to determine the type, degree, and duration of bleeding following trauma, dental extraction, or minor surgery; the age at which symptoms of a bleeding tendency were first noticed; and any episodes of spontaneous bleeding. A complete history also should include a list of medications the patient is currently taking, particulary coumarin drugs, aspirin and aspirin-containing compounds, antihistaminics, anti-inflammatory agents, barbiturates, and certain tranquilizers.

SPECIMEN COLLECTION AND HANDLING

Coagulation studies are most reliable when performed on specimens collected without traumatizing surrounding tissues to prevent contamination with tissue fluid containing thromboplastin. When collecting specimens for coagulation studies, the use of two syringes is recommended to ensure an uncontaminated blood flow. The first few milliliters of blood aspirated after entering the vein should be discarded and the second syringe used to collect the specimen.

▶▶ *Nursing Responsibilities and Implications*

1. Withhold aspirin or aspirin-containing products, as well as other platelet-active agents, whenever possible, for up to 1 week before the coagulation profile.

2. Apply a tourniquet, use the sterile technique, and perform an atraumatic venipuncture with a 19- or 20-gauge needle.

3. Withdraw 2–3 mL of blood into a plastic or siliconized glass syringe or vacuum tube to rinse tissue fluid from the needle. Do not collect blood from an indwelling venous catheter because it may contain residual heparin, which could interfere with coagulation test results.

4. Remove the tourniquet as soon as a good blood flow is established to avoid excessive stasis.

5. Detach the first syringe or tube from the needle without removing it from the vein.

6. Attach a second syringe or vacuum tube to the needle and collect the entire sample of blood to be used for coagulation testing.

7. Transfer blood into appropriate containers without delay and mix thoroughly with the proper anticoagulant solutions, taking care to avoid air bubbles. Collect one EDTA tube, two citrate tubes, and at least two plain serum tubes to ensure an adequate specimen for the complete coagulation profile. Remember to fill vacuum tubes completely to provide the exact volume of blood for the amount of anticoagulant solution present.

8. Deliver all tubes to the laboratory promptly. When specimens must be tested by a special reference laboratory, they must be quick-frozen and transported in small aliquots of citrated plasma on dry ice to prevent the precipitation or deterioration of factors I, V, and VIII.

9. Observe the venipuncture site for seeping in patients with suspected coagulation defects.

TESTS OF VASCULAR AND PLATELET FUNCTION

Bleeding Time

Bleeding time is a test of hemostatic efficiency that records the duration of active bleeding from a standardized superficial puncture wound of the skin. A bleeding time test helps evaluate platelet and vascular response to injury by estimating the integrity of the primary hemostatic plug. Interaction of vascular and platelet factors such as the number and functional activity of platelets along with the elasticity of capillary walls determines the duration and degree of bleeding. The bleeding time test is a reliable preoperative screening method for platelet disorders and may be used to investigate suspected hemorrhagic disease in individuals with a history of bleeding or easy bruising.

Clinical Significance
Bleeding time may be prolonged by various vascular disorders, as well as by diseases associated with a low platelet count (thrombocytopenia) or defective platelet function (thromb-

asthenia and thrombocytopathy). The inverse relationship between bleeding time and platelet count provides an index of platelet activity, with counts below $100,000/\mu L$ producing prolonged test results. An abnormal bleeding time accompanied by an adequate platelet count suggests defective platelet function, which must be further investigated with clot retraction, prothrombin consumption, and platelet aggregation studies.

Coagulation disorders such as hemophilia generally are accompanied by a normal bleeding time, although delayed bleeding may recur at the puncture site 24 hours after the test. Ingestion of as little as 10 grains of aspirin 2 hours before testing will prolong bleeding time by 2–3 minutes or longer in most healthy individuals. Individuals with von Willebrand's disease exhibit markedly prolonged bleeding time test results following aspirin intake.

Normal Values

The normal values for the bleeding time test are:

Duke bleeding time	1–5 minutes
Ivy bleeding time	1–7 minutes

Variations

A **prolonged bleeding time** may occur with:

Acute leukemia

Aplastic anemia

Aspirin intake

Congenital heart disease

Disseminated intravascular coagulation

Fibrinolytic activity

Hemorrhagic disease of the newborn

Hypothyroidism

Idiopathic thrombocytopenic purpura

Infectious mononucleosis

Multiple myeloma

Pernicious anemia

Prolonged oral anticoagulant therapy

Purpura hemorrhagica

Schönlein-Henoch purpura

Scurvy

Secondary thrombocytopenia purpura due to allergy; collagen diseases, including lupus erythematosus; drug sensitivity due to sulfonamides or chlorothiazaide compounds; infections such as measles, mumps, streptococcus, or typhus; lymphoproliferative disorders such as Hodgkin's disease

Severe deficiency of factors I, II, V, VII, VIII, IX, or XI

Severe liver disease (cirrhosis, obstructive jaundice)

Thrombasthenia (Glanzmann's disease)

Thrombocytopathia

von Willebrand's disease

Methodology

In the bleeding time test, a small cut or puncture wound is made in the fingertip, earlobe, or forearm with an appropriate instrument and the duration of bleeding is timed. The test continues until the flow of blood ceases but should be discontinued after 20 minutes if the blood flow shows no signs of stopping. Considerable skill and practice are required to produce a uniform incision, and the results may be affected by the technique of the person performing the test. Normal values for the bleeding time test must be determined by each laboratory according to the puncture site and type of lancet used in testing.

The Duke method uses the fingertip or earlobe and is difficult to standardize for reproducibility because of variations in capillary blood supply and skin thickness. The Ivy bleeding time uses an area on the inner surface of the forearm with no visible superficial veins and is the method of choice because the incision is more easily controlled. A blood pressure cuff on the upper arm is inflated to 40 mm Hg and makes the test more sensitive by increasing venous pressure to ensure capillary filling without interfering with venous return. Two puncture wounds approximately 3 mm deep should be made with a sterile lancet or template on an area cleansed with alcohol, carefully avoiding small surface veins. A stopwatch is started at the time of incision, and drops of blood are gently blotted with a filter paper every 30 seconds without exerting pressure on the wound.

Tourniquet Test

The **tourniquet test**, also known as the capillary fragility test, is a nonspecific evaluation of capillary resistance to conditions of increased pressure and anoxia. The procedure is influenced by the capillaries and the ability of platelets to occlude small gaps between endothelial cells of the capillary walls to contribute to normal hemostasis. Although it is one of the least scientific studies, the tourniquet test measures capillary weakness and helps to identify platelet deficiencies or functional defects in individuals with inadequate hemostasis.

Clinical Significance

The tourniquet test uses the positive pressure of an inflated blood pressure cuff to limit venous return and produce a condition of increased pressure or hypoxia within the capillaries. Decreased resistance to the intravascular pressure exerted by 100 mm Hg causes capillary rupture, which leads to bleeding and the formation of petechiae in some individuals. When petechiae appear as a result of routine tourniquet use during specimen collection, it is inadvisable to do the actual tourniquet test. However, a positive tourniquet test reaction in women over 40 years of age may not be pathologic.

Normal Values

Most healthy individuals do not develop petechiae as a result of the tourniquet test; test results may be interpreted as follows:

Normal	0–10 petechiae
Questionable	10–20 petechiae
Abnormal hemostatic function	>20 petechiae

Variations

Increased capillary fragility (positive tourniquet test) is associated with numerous conditions:

Strongly positive results may occur with:

Idiopathic thrombocytopenic purpura

Scurvy

Secondary thrombocytopenic purpura due to aplastic anemia, acute leukemia, scarlet fever, measles, influenza, chronic nephritis

Thrombasthenia

Moderately positive results may occur with Glanzmann's disease, liver disease such as cirrhosis or obstructive jaundice, and vascular purpura.
Weakly positive results may occur with:

Dysproteinemia	Senile purpura
Hereditary hemorrhagic telangiectasia	Severe factor VII, fibrinogen, or prothrombin deficiency
Polycythemia vera	
Premature infants	Vitamin K deficiency
Schönlein-Henoch purpura	von Willebrand's disease

Methodology

In the tourniquet test, a blood pressure cuff is applied in the normal manner and maintained midway between the systolic and diastolic pressures, with a maximum value of 100 mm Hg. The arm is inspected carefully before testing, and any preexisting blemishes, bruises, or petechiae are noted to standardize the procedure and prevent false-positive test results. The blood pressure cuff should be released after 5 minutes and the forearm observed for the presence of petechiae at least 1 inch from the cuff.

Reactions may be reported as negative or from 1+ to 4+, depending on the number of petechiae that appear within a 5 cm circle, as follows:

Grade	Petechiae
1+	0–10
2+	10–20
3+	20–50
4+	>50

Clot Retraction

The **clot retraction test** is a simple procedure that estimates the number of platelets and their function and evaluates fibrinogen quantity and utilization. A normal blood clot, containing sufficient numbers of adequately functioning platelets, rapidly decreases in size, pulls away from the sides of a test tube, and expresses 40%–60% of its serum as it contracts. After 4 hours of incubation at 37 C, there should be a well-defined clot surrounded by a volume of clear serum approximately equal to the volume of the clot. Laboratory observation of clot size and characteristics may be useful in diagnosing platelet deficiency or dysfunction, decreased fibrinogen concentration, and excessive fibrinolytic activity.

Clinical Significance

The degree of clot retraction is related to the number of platelets and their ability to function. Because complete retraction only occurs when the platelet count is within normal limits, a decrease in platelets below 100,000/μL will result in slow or incomplete clot retraction. Abnormal platelet function (thrombasthenia) also reduces clot retraction, and this reduction is accompanied by the formation of a characteristically soft clot. However, a platelet count over 100,000/μL does not improve normal clot retraction or reduce the amount of time required for the retraction. In fact, an excessively high platelet count may actually impede retraction.

Clot retraction depends upon an adequate plasma fibrinogen level and total red blood cell mass, with the degree of retraction apparently decreasing as erythrocyte concentrations increase. On the other hand, a small, firm, completely retracted clot with unclotted red blood cells (red blood cell fallout) may be the result of hypofibrinogenemic states or excessive fibrinolysis within the clot. Rapid red blood cell fallout during retraction, especially in a soft, shaggy clot, frequently can be the first indication of disseminated intravascular coagulation (DIC).

Normal Values
A normal clot retracts as follows:

Partial retraction	1–2 hours
Complete retraction	12–24 hours

Variations
Reduced or impaired clot retraction may occur with:

Acute leukemia

Aplastic anemia

Factor XIII deficiency

Fibrinolytic activity, increased

Hodgkin's disease

Hyperfibrinogenemia

Hypofibrinogenemia (less than 150 mg/dL)

Idiopathic thrombocytopenic purpura

Multiple myeloma

Polycythemia vera

Secondary thrombocytopenia, severe

Thrombasthenia (Glanzmann's disease, or hereditary hemorrhagic thrombasthenia)

Methodology
Clot retraction studies require at least 5 mL of whole blood collected without anticoagulants in a plain or siliconized glass tube (red-stoppered tube). The specimen should be incubated at 37 C or allowed to stand undisturbed at room temperature and examined for retraction at the end of 2, 6, 12, and 24 hours. Observations are recorded as complete retraction, partial retraction, or no retraction. Laboratory reports of clot retraction also may include the time required for retraction to begin, time required for complete retraction, consistency of the clot, amount of serum expressed from the clot, and volume of cells not included in the clot.

Platelet Count

The **platelet count** is an actual enumeration of thrombocytes present in the blood. Platelets are the tiny fragments of cytoplasm that are released into the bloodstream from the large megakaryocytes in the bone marrow. Circulating platelets are reported in thousands per microliter or cubic millimeters of whole blood. However, an evaluation of the findings should take into consideration that direct counting methods are subject to a 10%−20% error. This error is related to the inherent cell characteristics of platelets that cause them to fragment, clump, and adhere to exposed tissue surfaces and collecting implements, making accurate dilution and counting procedures difficult. Platelet determinations are most reliable when accompanied by an estimated count and morphologic observation from a stained peripheral blood smear.

Clinical Significance

Sufficient normal platelets are required to maintain vascular integrity and support hemostasis through such functions as adhesion, aggregation, vasoconstriction, thromboplastic activity, and clot retraction. Any significant variation in the number of circulating platelets, whether due to changes in bone marrow production or accelerated platelet destruction and utilization, interferes with the coagulation mechanism and may result in hemorrhage or thrombosis. The number of functional platelets may be influenced by many diseases; however, the count must be greatly altered for serious bleeding problems to occur. Conditions such as acute thrombocytopenic purpura and the consumption coagulopathy associated with DIC usually are characterized by a hemorrhagic tendency due to an abnormal platelet count.

Normal Values

The clinically significant values for the platelet count are:

Normal range	150,000−400,000/μL
Severe bleeding disorders	<50,000/μL or >1,000,000/μL

Variations

An **increased platelet count** (thrombocytosis) may occur with:

Acute blood loss (peak values occur at 7−10 days)	Iron deficiency anemia
Acute posthemorrhagic anemia	Multiple myeloma
Adrenalin injections	Myelofibrosis
Asphyxia	Polycythemia vera
Bone trauma (fractures)	Postpartum
Carcinoma	Postsplenectomy
Chronic granulocytic leukemia	Reticulocytosis
Exercise, sudden	Sickle cell anemia
Hemolytic anemia	Surgery (peak values occur 5−10 days postoperatively)
Inflammatory conditions or infections	

A **decreased platelet count** (thrombocytopenia) may occur with:

Acute infections (septicemia)	Aplastic anemia
Acute leukemia	Autoimmune diseases

Cirrhosis of the liver

Collagen diseases

Defibrination syndrome, DIC

Drug sensitivity (acetazolamide, amidopyrine, barbiturates, chloramphenicol, chlorothiazide compounds, meprobamate, oxytetracycline, phenylbutazone, quinidine, quinine, salicylate compounds, streptomycin, sulfonamides, thiazides, tolbutamide)

Hemolytic disease of the newborn

Hypersplenism

Idiopathic thrombocytopenic purpura

Incompatible blood transfusion

Lymphoproliferative disorders

Massive blood replacement (10 units or more with stored blood)

Megaloblastic anemia (vitamin B_{12} and folic acid deficiencies)

Menstrual cycle

Metastatic carcinoma

Multiple myeloma

Myelofibrosis

Vaccine injections

X-ray irradiation

Methodology

Platelet counts require 5 mL of blood collected in a tube containing EDTA anticoagulant (lavender-stoppered tube) with a minimum of agitation to prevent cell fragmentation. Capillary blood from a finger puncture should be collected, obtaining a large, freely flowing drop of blood, using swift manipulation to avoid platelet aggregation on exposed tissue fibrils.

Platelet Adhesion and Aggregation

Platelet adhesion and aggregation studies test the ability of platelets to adhere to foreign surfaces and each other during hemostasis. Adequately functioning platelets normally adhere to collagen and microfibrils exposed by vascular injury, causing the release of a substance that stimulates platelet clumping and formation of the hemostatic plug. A number of qualitative platelet defects, together with several unrelated conditions, may interfere with these normal functions and produce bleeding disorders characterized by a prolonged bleeding time. Laboratory tests of platelet adhesion and aggregation are used to detect abnormal platelet function and help diagnose hereditary and acquired platelet deficiencies. However, because of difficulty in standardization and methodology, platelet adhesion studies are offered in progressively fewer laboratories.

Clinical Significance

Platelet adhesion studies, also known as the glass bead retention tests, evaluate platelet function by measuring their adhesiveness to foreign surfaces such as glass beads or glass wool in the laboratory. Adhesiveness is calculated by passing a sample of blood through a column of glass beads and performing a platelet count on the resulting specimen. The difference between this value and a count performed prior to the adhesion test represents the number of platelets retained by the glass due to adhesion. However, test results may be influenced by the clumping of platelets to each other, which can make accurate test interpretation difficult because aggregation may be independently abnormal.

   Platelet aggregation tests evaluate the ability of platelets to adhere to each other by measuring their reaction when mixed with several known aggregating agents in the laboratory. Aggregation is calculated by mixing a suspension of the patient's platelets with

TABLE 10-1 Platelet Aggregation Response in Selected Conditions

Giant Platelet Syndromes	Aggregating Agent			
	Adenosine Diphosphate	Epinephrine	Collagen	Ristocetin
Bernard-Soulier disease	Normal or decreased	Normal or decreased	Normal	Absent
von Willebrand's disease	Normal	Normal	Normal	Absent
Thrombasthenia	Absent	Absent	Absent	Normal
Storage pool disease	Normal or decreased	Absent	Normal or decreased	Normal
Release defect	Normal or decreased	Absent	Normal or decreased	Normal
Intermediate type	Normal	Decreased	Normal or decreased	Normal

agents that induce clumping such as adenosine diphosphate (ADP), collagen, epinephrine, and ristocetin. When aggregation occurs, the number of platelets occurring as separate particles in the suspension appears to decrease and the amount of light transmitted through the solution increases. Test results are recorded for each aggregating agent as the percentage of change in light transmittance through each specimen, with different platelet abnormalities producing a unique pattern of aggregation responses (Table 10-1).

Normal Values
The normal values for platelet adhesion and aggregation* studies are:

Glass bead retention   50%–90%

*Normal values for platelet aggregation studies are not indicated qualitatively on the test result sheet but rather are reported in descriptive terms, which must be established by the individual laboratory.

Variations
Decreased platelet adhesiveness may occur with:

Anemia, severe

Azotemia

Bernard-Soulier syndrome

Chédiak-Higashi syndrome

Macroglobulinemia

Multiple myeloma

Myeloid metaplasia

Plasma cell dyscrasias

Thrombasthenia, acquired and familial

Thrombocytopathy

Uremia

Von Willebrand's disease

Increased platelet adhesiveness may occur with:

Carcinoma	Hyperlipemia	Pregnancy
Hypercoagulability	Oral contraceptives	Thrombosis

Decreased platelet aggregation may occur with:

Afibrinogenemia	Glycogen storage disease (von Gierke's disease)
Bernard-Soulier syndrome	
Chédiak-Higashi syndrome	Hemocystinuria
Cirrhosis	Hemorrhagic thrombocythemia
Drug therapy	Myeloid metaplasia
Antibiotics	Plasma cell dyscrasias
Anticoagulants	Platelet release defects
Antihistamines, some	Polycythemia vera
Anti-inflammatory drugs	Preleukemia
Aspirin-containing drugs	Scurvy
Cardiovascular drugs (vasodilators and antilipemics)	Sideroblastic anemia
	Uremia
Psychotropic drugs	Von Willebrand's disease
Glanzmann's disease (thrombasthenia)	Waldenström's macroglobulinemia

Increased platelet aggregation may occur with:

Athermatosis	Hypercoagulability
Diabetes mellitus	Hyperlipemia

Methodology

Platelet adhesion studies using the glass bead retention method require 10 mL of blood collected with EDTA anticoagulant (lavender-stoppered tube). Platelet aggregation studies require 10 mL of blood collected in a plastic syringe and transferred carefully, with minimal agitation, to a tube containing sodium citrate anticoagulant (blue-stoppered tube). Specimens must be delivered to the laboratory immediately for testing within 3 hours to prevent platelets from losing the ability to aggregate.

▶▶ Nursing Responsibilities and Implications

1. Withhold all medications for 7–10 days prior to testing, if possible, because many drugs interfere with platelet aggregation while they are in the bloodstream (Table 10-2).

2. Note on the laboratory slip any medications the patient has taken in the previous 7–10 days.

3. Instruct the patient to fast overnight prior to testing to avoid lipemia, which affects the test results; water is permitted.

4. Maintain pressure at the puncture site after removing the needle; continue to observe for bleeding.

TABLE 10-2   Drugs That Interfere With Platelet Function

Acetylsalicylic acid	Ibufenac
*Alphaprodine	Ibuprofen
Carbenicillin	*Imipramine
Cephalothin	*Indomethacin
*Chlordiazepoxide	Mefenamic acid
Chloroquine	Methylprednisone
*Chlorpromazine	Naproxen
Clofibrate	Nitrofurantoin
Cyproheptadine	Nortriptyline
Dextropropoxyphene	Oxyphenbutazone
Diazepam	Penicillin G
*Diphenhydramine	*Phenylbutazone
Dipyridamole	*Prochlorperazine
Furosemide	*Promethazine
*Glyceryl guaiacolate	Propranolol
Heparin	Sulfinpyrazone
Hydrocortisone	Vitamin E

*Drugs known to affect platelet function tests in newborns when taken by the mother during gestation.

TESTS OF OVERALL COAGULATION

Whole Blood Clotting Time

Whole blood clotting time, also known as the Lee-White coagulation time, is an insensitive test of the overall ability of blood to clot. Although it is influenced by many external conditions and is difficult to reproduce accurately, this procedure measures the time required for the interaction of all factors involved in the coagulation sequence. The sensitivity of this standard clotting time method can be increased, however, by drawing the blood directly into a contact activator such as a Celite tube, a variation known as the activated coagulation time (ACT) test.

Laboratory determinations of whole blood clotting time generally are used to demonstrate gross abnormalities of hemostasis, monitor and control heparin therapy, and detect the presence of circulating anticoagulants. Test results of the ACT closely parallel the significance of the activated partial thromboplastin time (APTT) in its sensitivity to factor VIII deficiency and the effects of heparin therapy. The clot formed during the whole blood clotting time procedure may be retained and inspected after 2, 12, and 24 hours for clot retraction or signs of fibrinolysis.

Clinical Significance

The whole blood clotting time may be prolonged by deficiencies of any coagulation factor except factor VII, which participates only in the extrinsic clotting system. However, it is not an adequate screening test for mild to moderate hemorrhagic disorders because it does not detect plasma factor deficiencies until their concentrations are less than 2%–3% of normal. Thus, although a prolonged clotting time indicates that a serious problem exists, a normal clotting time does not exclude the presence of a hemorrhagic disorder or ensure adequate hemostasis.

Normal Values

The normal and clinically significant values for the whole blood clotting time are:

Plain glass tube	5–15 minutes
Siliconized tube	24–45 minutes
Activated clotting time	
Normal	<2 minutes and 10 seconds
Borderline	2 minutes and 15 seconds
Prolonged	2 minutes and 20 seconds

Variations

A **prolonged whole blood clotting time** may occur with:

Afibrinogenemia

Anticoagulant therapy

Circulating anticoagulants

Dysproteinemia

Factor V, VII, IX, X, XI, or XII deficiency

Fibrinolysis, excessive

Hemorrhagic disease of the newborn

Hypofibrinogenemia

Hypoprothrombinemia

Leukemia

Liver disorders

Methodology

The whole blood clotting time test requires 5 mL of blood collected using the two-syringe method and transferred immediately into three small test tubes without anticoagulants. Exactly 1 mL of blood should be emptied gently into each tube. The tubes should be kept at room temperature. The last tube filled should be tilted gently at 30-second intervals. Once clotting is observed in this tube, the procedure should be repeated with the second tube and then the first tube. The whole blood clotting time is the total time elapsed between venipuncture and complete clotting of the first tube filled.

The ACT test also requires blood collected by the two-tube method, with at least 1 mL drawn into the first tube and discarded. With the needle still in place, the tourniquet should be removed and the first tube replaced with a vacuum Celite tube. Timing begins after this tube has been filled and mixed. After waiting 1 minute, the tube should be tilted every 5 seconds until a clot appears. Whole blood clotting time tests should not be performed on capillary blood because specimens obtained from a finger puncture contain tissue thromboplastin and yield falsely decreased test results.

Circulating Anticoagulants

Circulating anticoagulants are highly specific IgG immunoglobulins that neutralize certain clotting factors, predisposing the patient to abnormal hemostasis and prolonging a number of coagulation test results. Although some coagulation inhibitors, such as antithrombin III, are naturally occurring proteins (see Antithrombin III later in this chapter), many nontherapeutic anticoagulants in the bloodstream are antibodies acquired during a variety of diseases. The most frequently encountered of these pathologic anticoagulants is directed against factor VIII, although inhibitors of factors I, V, IX, X, XI, XII, and XIII also may be developed. Laboratory detection of circulating coagulation inhibitors and their level of activity is used to potentially guide effective replacement therapy with appropriate factor concentrates.

Clinical Significance
The level of circulating anticoagulant activity is especially important in hemophilic individuals and must be determined before replacement therapy with factor VIII concentrates can begin. Administration of such factor concentrates to patients with inhibitors usually stimulates the formation of more antibodies within 3–4 days, producing a vicious cycle because the in vivo half-life of factor VIII is so short. Thus, for such concentrates to be effective at all, the inhibitor activity of the circulating anticoagulant must be neutralized before an effective level of factor VIII can be achieved. Factor I, V, IX, X, XI, and XII inhibitors also have been described but are rare and produce short-lived symptoms that may vary from mild to severe.

The presence of coagulation factor antibodies is indicated by prolonged clotting time, prothrombin time (PT), or partial thromboplastin time (PTT) results that cannot be corrected by the addition of normal plasma during substitution studies. These two tests are the best screening measures for circulating anticoagulants because most clotting inhibitors affect these tests of overall coagulation but do not necessarily alter the results of other studies. Once a circulating coagulation inhibitor has been detected, other tests may be performed to help determine the coagulation stage and factor affected by anticoagulant activity.

Normal Values
Circulating anticoagulants or inhibitors are not normally found in the blood. Clinically significant amounts are present when circulating anticoagulants reduce the activity of a coagulation factor by 50% or more.

Variations
Factor I inhibitors may occur with:

Afibrinogenemia

Fibrin-fibrinogen degradation products (FDP)

Macroglobulinemia

Multiple myeloma

Factor V inhibitors may occur with streptomycin therapy, major surgery, and blood transfusions.

Factor VIII inhibitors may occur with:

Abortions

Advancing age

Cutaneous penicillin allergy

Disseminated intravascular coagulation (DIC)

Factor VIII transfusions

Immunologic disorders

Macroglobulinemia

Plasma cell dyscrasias

Postpartum period (especially after the firstborn child)

Rheumatoid arthritis

Systemic lupus erythematosus

Factor IX, X, XI, XII, and XIII inhibitors may occur with:

Collagen-vascular disease

Infectious disorders

Malignancies

Systemic lupus erythematosus

Methodology

Detection of circulating coagulation inhibitors requires 5 mL of blood collected in a tube containing sodium citrate anticoagulant (blue-stoppered tube).

Partial Thromboplastin Time

The **partial thromboplastin time** (PTT) is a general test of the entire coagulation mechanism that detects deficiencies of all plasma clotting factors except factors VII and XIII and platelets. Partial thromboplastin time results are most useful in identifying abnormalities of intrinsic thromboplastin formation. Test results are more likely to be prolonged by stage I defects than by deficiencies in the later stages of coagulation. The activated partial thromboplastin time (APTT), in which activators are added to the regular PTT test reagent, is a sensitive variation of the test that shortens the clotting time and gives a narrower range of normal values. Laboratory determination of PTT and APTT may be used to monitor heparin anticoagulant therapy and provide a valuable aid to the diagnosis of coagulation disorders.

Clinical Significance

The partial thromboplastin time test lacks the necessary sensitivity to identify mild deficiencies of single plasma factors because the results are prolonged only when levels of these coagulation factors drop below 25%–35% of normal. The test also cannot detect minor clotting defects because they may produce normal or only slightly prolonged test values that may be masked by increased concentrations of other factors. Occasionally, prolonged PTT or APTT values may be the only abnormal coagulation finding. If this is so, its clinical significance is questionable, and additional testing is required.

Differential APTT methods, also known as substitution tests or factor assays, may be performed to identify precisely which factors are lacking when the routine screening test is prolonged. Deficiencies of individual factors are qualitatively evaluated by substituting known reagents for each factor, one at a time, to determine which combination corrects the clotting defect and produces normal test results. The actual concentration of individual clotting factors is measured by performing an APTT using the patient's plasma and a variety of test plasmas, each known to lack a specific factor. Such factor assays are used to differentiate mild, moderate, and severe hereditary deficiency patterns and to follow the course of acquired factor inhibitors.

Normal Values

The normal and clinically significant values for the partial thromboplastin time are:

Activated partial thromboplastin time

Normal range	30−40 seconds
Borderline	40−46 seconds
Prolonged	>46 seconds

Partial thromboplastin time

Normal range	40−100 seconds
Factor deficiency	>120 seconds

Variations

A **prolonged partial thromboplastin time** may occur with:

Abruptio placentae

Anticoagulant therapy

Circulating anticoagulants

Cirrhosis of the liver and obstructive jaundice

Disseminated intravascular coagulation (DIC)

Factor V, VIII, IX, X, XI, or XII deficiency

Fibrinolysis, excessive

Hemorrhagic disease of the newborn

Hypofibrinogenemia and afibrinogenemia

Prothrombin deficiency

Salicylate therapy

Vitamin K deficiency

von Willebrand's disease

A **decreased partial thromboplastin time** may occur with acute hemorrhage and extensive cancer (unless there is a great deal of liver involvement).

Methodology

Partial thromboplastin time procedures require 5 mL of blood collected in sodium citrate or sodium oxalate anticoagulant (blue- or black-stoppered tube) and delivered to the laboratory immediately for prompt testing. Tubes must be completely filled with blood to prevent falsely prolonged test results due to the effect of excess anticoagulant. Plasma specimens should be refrigerated when testing cannot be performed immediately because some factors deteriorate rapidly at room temperature, causing falsely prolonged test results.

Plasma Recalcification Time

Plasma recalcification time, also known as plasma clotting time, is a test of overall co-agulation activity, the results of which are equal in significance to results obtained from whole blood coagulation time procedures. Because the anticoagulants used to prevent clotting during specimen collection remove only calcium from the blood, plasma contains all the other factors necessary for clot formation. Therefore, normal plasma rapidly forms a fibrin clot when the proper amount of calcium is replaced in the laboratory. However, a number of plasma and platelet deficiencies, as well as certain coagulation inhibitors, prevent normal clotting following recalcification and produce prolonged test results. Laboratory determinations of plasma recalcification time are used to identify the presence of naturally occurring anticoagulants and detect clotting deficiencies.

Clinical Significance

The rate of plasma clotting depends on the concentration of plasma coagulation factors as well as the quantity and quality of platelet function, and reflects the concentration of platelet factor 3. Thus, plasma recalcification proceeds much more rapidly and provides a more accurate assessment of coagulation activity if the test is performed on platelet-rich plasma.

Normal Values

The normal values for the plasma recalcification time are:

Platelet-rich plasma	90–150 seconds
Platelet-poor plasma	110–240 seconds

Variations

An **increased plasma recalcification time** may occur with:

Circulating anticoagulants

Factor V, VIII, IX, X, XI, or XII deficiency

Fibrinogen deficiency

Heparin therapy

Prothrombin deficiency, severe

Thrombocytopenia, severe

Methodology

Plasma recalcification time tests require 5 mL of blood collected with sodium citrate anticoagulant (blue-stoppered tube) and delivered to the laboratory immediately for prompt testing. An unnecessary delay between specimen collection and testing may produce unreliable test results because of changes in temperature and pH.

TESTS TO EVALUATE STAGE I COAGULATION

Prothrombin Consumption Time

Prothrombin consumption time (PCT), also known as the serum prothrombin time, is an indirect measurement of the capacity of stage I coagulation to generate intrinsic plasma thromboplastin. During normal clotting, the thromboplastin converts at least 75%

of the available prothrombin to thrombin and leaves little or no prothrombin remaining in the serum. However, a deficiency in the factors that produce thromboplastin reduces the amount of prothrombin consumed and leaves a high concentration of the substance in the serum.

The PCT test measures the residual prothrombin in serum after clotting has occurred and reflects a deficiency of those factors that form thromboplastin as well as a platelet dysfunction. Laboratory determinations of PCT are helpful in detecting and confirming stage I coagulation defects and also may be used as a screening test.

Clinical Significance

Prothrombin consumption time test results are abnormal when the levels of factors active during stage I (factors VIII, IX, X, XI, and XII) drop to 10% or less of normal or when platelets are reduced in number or efficiency. The speed with which PCT specimens clot reflects the amount of prothrombin remaining in the serum and is inversely proportional to the amount of thromboplastin generated during stage I coagulation. Thus, a prolonged PCT test result indicates that little prothrombin remained in the serum; therefore, ample thromboplastic activity occurred during the original clotting process. On the other hand, a decreased PCT test result indicates that defective prothrombin conversion occurred during the original coagulation process, and further testing is needed to determine which factor deficiency is responsible. The PCT is more sensitive to stage I defects than the whole blood clotting time but is not as sensitive as the partial thromboplastin time (PTT) or the thromboplastin generation time (TGT) tests.

Normal Values

The clinically significant values for the prothrombin consumption time are:

Normal	>25 seconds
Borderline	20–25 seconds
Abnormal	<20 seconds

Variations

An **abnormal prothrombin consumption time** may occur with:

Circulating anticoagulants	Heparin therapy
Cirrhosis of the liver	Obstructive jaundice
Dysproteinemia	Thrombasthenia
Factor V deficiency, severe	Thrombocytopenia (less than 50,000/μL)
Factor VII deficiency, severe	
Factor VIII, IX, X, XI, or XII deficiency	von Willebrand's disease
Hemorrhagic disease of the newborn	

Methodology

Prothrombin consumption time tests require 5 mL of blood collected in a nonsiliconized glass tube using the two-syringe technique with a minimum of trauma. Specimens must be allowed to clot undisturbed because both hemolysis and undue agitation of the test tube accelerate prothrombin consumption. The test also may be performed on the serum specimen remaining after performing the whole blood clotting time.

Thromboplastin Generation Time

The **thromboplastin generation time** (TGT) is a complex two-phase procedure used to detect deficiencies of the factors required for thromboplastin formation in stage I of the coagulation sequence. The powerful coagulant activity of thromboplastin normally is produced when specimens of the patient's serum, adsorbed plasma, and platelet concentrate are combined in a tube. If all the necessary factors are present, this mixture begins to form a fibrin clot shortly after it is added to a thrombin-fibrinogen reagent. The time required to produce this clot is prolonged by a deficiency of any of the factors required for thromboplastin generation, although factor VIII, IX, XI, and XII deficiencies are most common. Laboratory determinations of TGT currently are confined to distinguishing factor VIII deficiency (classic hemophilia) from factor IX deficiency (Christmas disease) in the differential diagnosis of hemophilia.

Clinical Significance

Thromboplastin generation time is useful in detecting severe single-factor deficiencies but cannot be relied on to detect mild defects or disorders. For example, the TGT test probably will yield normal results when factor VIII levels are at least 10% of normal, although significant clinical symptoms may occur with levels in the 10%–30% range. However, the TGT test is not appropriate for extensive diagnostic use or routine screening of stage I coagulation activity and is now rarely performed because simpler procedures are now available to identify specific clotting defects. Such stage I coagulation deficiencies are evaluated more easily by substitution tests or factor assays using the APTT test. However, the TGT test may be used to confirm an abnormal PTT because it is more sensitive to deficiencies of stage I coagulation factors than either the PTT or PCT.

Normal Values

The normal values for the thromboplastin generation time are:

Clot formation	8–14 seconds any time during 6 minutes of the test

---

Variations

A **prolonged thromboplastin generation time** may occur with:

Circulating anticoagulants

Factor V deficiency

Factor VIII deficiency (classic hemophilia)

Factor IX deficiency (Christmas disease)

Factor X, XI, or XII deficiency

Platelet deficiency

Methodology

The standard thromboplastin generation time procedure requires 10 mL of blood collected in sodium citrate or sodium oxalate anticoagulant (blue- or black-stoppered tube) along with 10 mL collected in a plain glass tube (red-stoppered tube). Both specimens should be drawn with a minimum of trauma using the two-syringe method and delivered to the laboratory immediately for prompt analysis.

TESTS TO EVALUATE STAGE II AND III COAGULATION

Prothrombin Time

Prothrombin time (PT) is a popular test for detecting deficiencies in the extrinsic clotting system that provides an overall evaluation of stages II and III of the coagulation sequence. The procedure measures the time required for clot formation when a tissue thromboplastin reagent is added to plasma, thus bypassing the intrinsic plasma thromboplastin formation in stage I. Any prolongation of this clotting time indicates less than normal concentration of one or more factors of the extrinsic thromboplastin system. Laboratory determinations of PT may be used to detect and diagnose hemorrhagic disorders. Prothrombin time tests also are frequently performed to monitor the course of oral coumarin therapy.

Clinical Significance

Although the PT test measures the activity of prothrombin, fibrinogen, and factors V, VII, and X, it is relatively insensitive to changes in the prothrombin level. Test results are affected promptly and significantly by alterations of factors V and VII but are prolonged by only 2 seconds when the prothrombin level is reduced to 10% of normal. Abnormal PT values unrelated to therapeutic anticoagulant administration may be investigated by a series of substitutions with various corrective reagents to determine the deficient factor.

Prothrombin time values may be influenced by the administration of a number of drugs that alter protein-binding patterns, inhibit the formation of intestinal microorganisms, or induce the production of certain enzymes. For example, salicylates, phenylbutazone, and indomethacin can displace protein-bound anticoagulants, which makes more anticoagulants available to inhibit clotting, thus increasing the PT. In addition, broad-spectrum antibiotics and some oral sulfonamides alter the intestinal flora responsible for producing vitamin K, inhibiting the formation of clotting factors and increasing the PT.

On the other hand, drugs such as barbiturates, griseofulvin, and glutethimide increase the rate of anticoagulant metabolism and decrease the PT. If any of these drugs are withdrawn from a patient who has been stabilized on a regimen of an anticoagulant plus the drug, a critical change in the prothrombin level may result. A partial list of the most commonly used drugs that affect the PT is presented in Table 10-3.

Because relatively minor changes in PT values may reflect considerable physiologic alterations, the safest method of reporting test results is to note the PT of both the patient and the control in seconds. Control values indicate the activity of the reagents used at the time of testing and may vary somewhat from day to day. Prothrombin time results also may be reported as a percentage of normal activity, which expresses the relationship of pro-

TABLE 10-3 Drugs That Commonly Affect the Prothrombin Time

Increased Prothrombin Time	Decreased Prothrombin Time
Acetaminophen	Anabolic steroids
Allopurinol	Antacids
Aminosalicylic acid	Antihistamines
Anabolic steroids	Ascorbic acid
Aspirin	Aspirin
Cathartics	Barbiturates
Chloral hydrate	Chloral hydrate
Chloramphenicol	Colchicine
Chlorthalidone	Corticosteroids
Clofibrate	Digitalis
Dicumarol	Diuretics
Diuretics	Ethchlorvynol
Disulfiram	Glutethimide
Ethacrynic acid	Griseofulvin
Glucagon	Oral contraceptives
Guanethidine	Tetracycline
Heparin	Vitamin K
Indomethacin	
Mefenamic acid	
Mercaptopurine	
Methyldopa	
Methylphenidate	
Nalidixic acid	
Neomycin	
Phenylbutazone	
Phenyramidol	
Propylthiouracil	
Quinidine	
Quinine	
Streptomycin	
Sulfinpyrazone	
Sulfonamides	
Thyroid	
Tolbutamide	

thrombin concentration to the clotting time. Percentage values are obtained by comparing the PT in seconds with a reference curve prepared from the results of tests performed on several dilutions of normal plasma.

Normal Values

The range of normal values for the prothrombin time is 11–15 seconds.

Variations
An **increased prothrombin time** may occur with:

Afibrinogenemia

Circulating anticoagulants

Cirrhosis

Disseminated intravascular coagulation (DIC)

Drug therapy (see Table 10-3)

Dysfibrinogenemia

Factor V, VII, or X deficiency

Fibrin degradation products (FDP)

Fibrinolytic activity, increased

Hemolytic jaundice

Hemorrhagic disease of the newborn

Hypofibrinogenemia (<100 mg/dL)

Leukemia, acute

Obstetric complications

Obstructive jaundice

Pancreatitis, chronic

Polycythemia vera

Prothrombin deficiency

Sprue

Vitamin K deficiency

A **decreased prothrombin time** may occur with:

Drug therapy (see Table 10-3)

Multiple myeloma

Myocardial infarction

Pulmonary embolism

Thrombophlebitis, acute

Methodology
Prothrombin time determinations require 5 mL of blood collected in sodium oxalate or sodium citrate anticoagulants (black- or blue-stoppered tubes) and delivered to the laboratory immediately for prompt analysis. Test tubes must be filled to capacity with blood to prevent falsely elevated test results caused by the effect of extra anticoagulant. When testing cannot be performed promptly, plasma specimens should be refrigerated because some factors deteriorate rapidly at room temperature, falsely prolonging the PT.

Stypven Time

The **Stypven time** test, also known as Russell's viper venom assay, is a PT variation used to differentiate a factor VII deficiency from a factor X deficiency. The Stypven reagent requires factors V and X and platelets to produce thromboplastic activity that affects the coagulation mechanism in the same way as tissue thromboplastin but does not require factor VII. Thus, the Stypven time is prolonged if the patient's blood lacks factor X but is unaffected by a factor VII deficiency. Laboratory determinations of the Stypven time are used primarily to verify factor X deficiency when a prolonged PT is corrected during substitution studies by the addition of a serum reagent containing factors VII and X.

Clinical Significance
Routine factor assays cannot differentiate between deficiencies of factor VII and X because most substitution studies used to investigate prolonged PT results employ a serum reagent containing both factors. Thus, the Stypven time test is indicated when a prolonged PT result is corrected only by this aged serum reagent during follow-up studies. If use of the Stypven reagent produces a normal test time, the patient's plasma lacks factor X; if test results remain prolonged with the Stypven reagent, factor VII is probably deficient.

Normal Values

The normal and clinically significant values for the Stypven time test are:

Normal range	8–19 seconds
Borderline	19–22 seconds
Prolonged	>22 seconds

Variations

A **prolonged Stypven time** may occur with a factor V, X, or prothrombin deficiency.

Methodology

Stypven time determinations require 5 mL of blood collected in a silicone syringe and transferred gently to a tube containing sodium citrate anticoagulant (blue-stoppered tube). Specimens should be collected following an overnight fast to avoid obtaining lipemic plasma, which may interfere with the test results.

▶▶ **Nursing Responsibilities and Implications**

1. Instruct the patient to fast overnight; water is permitted.

2. Handle the specimen gently to prevent hemolysis.

Thrombin Time

The **thrombin time** is a screening test used to detect hemostatic levels of fibrinogen and evaluate its conversion to fibrin in stage III of the coagulation sequence. The test measures the time required for clot formation after thrombin is added to plasma; any significant prolongation of this clotting time indicates a fibrinogen deficiency, which should be investigated further. Laboratory determinations of thrombin time frequently are performed as an emergency procedure to detect life-threatening fibrinogen deficiencies and reported as the time required for fibrin clot formation. A variation of this procedure, the **thrombin clotting time**, also may be used to monitor the patient's response to heparin therapy, with test results reported in heparin activity equivalents.

Clinical Significance

Most thrombin time methods are insensitive to mild decreases in fibrinogen concentration or reactivity because they do not detect deficiencies until the level falls below 100 mg/dL. Test results are affected significantly, however, by any defect or alteration in the structure of the fibrinogen molecule (**dysfibrinogenemia**). Thrombin time results also are prolonged by increased plasmin concentrations and the presence of fibrin-fibrinogen degradation products (FDP) resulting from increased fibrinolytic activity.

Prolonged thrombin time values also are due to the presence of therapeutic anticoagulants in the blood resulting from contamination during specimen collection through a catheter previously used for heparin infusion. Another thrombin time variation, the **reptilase time test**, was therefore developed to detect the presence of adequate fibrinogen levels without interference from heparin or increased concentrations of plasmin and

FDP. Thus, normal reptilase time test results with a prolonged thrombin time are evidence that the patient has normal fibrinogen concentrations but has received heparin or that heparin contamination has occurred.

Normal Values

The clinically significant values for the thrombin time test and its variations are:

Thrombin time
  Normal   10–15 seconds

Thrombin clotting time
  Therapeutic range   0.2–0.4 U/mL

Reptilase time
  Normal   <20 seconds

Variations

An **increased thrombin time** may occur with:

Afibrinogenemia

Circulating anticoagulants

Dysfibrinogenemia

Hemorrhagic disease of the newborn

Heparin anticoagulant therapy

Hypofibrinogenemia (less than 100 mg/dL)

  Acute leukemia

  Disseminated intravascular coagulation (DIC)

  Lymphomas

Obstetric complications

Poor nutrition

Surgical procedures

Increased fibrinolytic activity

  Cirrhosis of the liver

  Hemorrhage

  Stress

  Shock

Increased fibrinogen-fibrin degradation products (FDP)

Polycythemia vera

Methodology

Thrombin time determinations require 5 mL of blood collected without hemolysis in sodium oxalate or sodium citrate anticoagulants (black- or blue-stoppered tube). However, sodium citrate is preferable if the test is being used to monitor heparin therapy. Specimens for thrombin time should be delivered to the laboratory immediately for prompt analysis.

Antithrombin III

Antithrombin III (AT III), the primary natural inhibitor of the coagulation sequence, is a plasma protein that limits intravascular clotting by slowly inactivating thrombin and several other coagulation factors. Antithrombin III activity is greatly enhanced by the presence of even small amounts of heparin, which markedly accelerates thrombin inhibition. Antithrombin III is also known as heparin cofactor because concentrations above 60% of normal are essential for efficient heparin therapy, and levels below 40% can decrease the therapeutic response to heparin.

Antithrombin III concentrations vary slightly according to age and sex, with lower levels normally occurring in women between 19 and 60 years of age and in men above 60 years of age. Although excess AT III may increase the potential for hemorrhage, low levels are more clinically significant because they frequently are associated with thrombosis. Laboratory determinations of AT III aid the diagnosis, treatment, and prevention of thrombosis.

Clinical Significance

Antithrombin III levels may be reduced significantly by congenital abnormalities, although most deficiencies result from stress situations such as surgery, pregnancy, infection, or trauma. Antithrombin III levels below 80% of normal are a major factor in the development of deep vein thrombosis following surgery and indicate a predisposition to thrombosis under other conditions. For example, AT III levels between 50% and 70% of normal indicate a moderate risk of pulmonary embolism or thrombophlebitis of the lower extremities, whereas concentrations less than 50% of normal indicate a significant risk of thromboembolic disorders. Thus, AT III determinations should be performed immediately before and after surgery to identify patients who are in a hypercoagulable state and at risk for the development of deep or superficial vein thrombosis.

All women over 30 years of age should have AT III determinations before oral contraceptives are prescribed because estrogen-containing drugs can reduce AT III levels by approximately 15%−20%. Tests also should be performed on any patient with a strong personal or family history of recurrent thromboembolic episodes as well as patients receiving oral anticoagulants or heparin. Although a single heparin injection does not affect AT III levels, continuous intravenous infusion or repeated injections of heparin significantly reduce AT III concentrations; the potential for recurrent thrombotic episodes exists when therapy is discontinued abruptly.

Normal Values

The normal values for antithrombin III vary with individual procedures but generally are:

Percent activity	
Plasma	80%−130%
Serum	15%−35% lower than plasma concentrations
Quantitative values	18−40 mg/dL
	7.8−11.0 μmol/min/mL

Variations

Decreased antithrombin III levels may occur with:

Arteriosclerosis	Cirrhosis
Burns	Congenital AT-III deficiency
Cardiovascular disease	Diabetes mellitus, maturity-onset

Disseminated intravascular coagulation (DIC)

Fibrinolytic agents, therapeutic

Heparin administration

Hepatic abscess

Hepatitis

Hemocystinuria

L-Asparaginase therapy

Liver disease

Malignancies

Nephrotic syndrome

Oral contraceptives, estrogen-containing

Proteinuria

Postoperative period, immediate

Postpartum

Pulmonary embolism

Stroke

Surgery

Increased antithrombin III levels may occur with:

Androgen therapy

Factor V or VII deficiency

Hemophilia A and B

Oral anticoagulants (dicumarol)

Progesterone

Renal transplantation

Methodology

Antithrombin III determinations require 5 mL of blood collected with sodium citrate (blue-stoppered tube) or without anticoagulants (red-stoppered tube). Although plasma is the preferred test specimen, serum may be used but will produce significantly lower test results because AT III consumes coagulation enzymes during the clotting process. For accurate, reproducible AT III test results, specimens should be collected without hemolysis or lipemia.

▶▶ Nursing Responsibilities and Implications

1. Instruct the patient to fast overnight; water is permitted.

2. Handle the specimen gently to prevent hemolysis.

Fibrinogen Assay

Fibrinogen assays measure the amount of fibrinogen available for fibrin formation in stage III of the coagulation sequence. A number of different procedures may be used to determine the amount of fibrinogen. Fibrinogen assay procedures are more sensitive than most thrombin time methods; however, the results may be compromised somewhat by the presence of early fibrinogen-fibrin degradation products, which also clot with the thrombin reagent. Laboratory determinations of fibrinogen concentration are used in the routine diagnosis and treatment of hemorrhagic disorders. They also may be ordered on an emergency basis during surgical or obstetric bleeding.

Clinical Significance

The most common emergency use of fibrinogen determinations is during obstetric delivery, when plasma levels can drop precariously low and result in massive hemorrhage if not promptly corrected. In such instances the detection of a fibrinogen deficiency enables the physician to identify the correct preventive or corrective measure to be taken before a life-threatening hemorrhage occurs. Thus, most emergency requests for fibrinogen analysis are not concerned with exact concentrations but whether sufficient fibrinogen is present to form a clot and control bleeding.

> **Normal Values**
> The range of normal values for fibrinogen assays is 200–400 mg/dL.

Variations
Decreased fibrinogen levels may occur with:

Abortion, septic	Fibrinolytic activity, increased
Acute leukemia	Hemorrhage, severe
Afibrinogenemia, congenital	Liver damage, severe
Anaphylactic shock	Metastatic carcinoma
Burns, severe	Obstetric complications
Congenital hypofibrinogenemia	Scurvy
Disseminated intravascular coagulation (DIC)	Surgery

Increased fibrinogen levels may occur with:

Inflammatory conditions	Pregnancy
Pneumonia	Rheumatic fever

Methodology
Fibrinogen assays require 5 mL of blood collected with a minimum of trauma in tubes containing sodium oxalate or sodium citrate anticoagulants (black- or blue-stoppered tube). Tubes should be filled to capacity to ensure proper proportions of anticoagulant and blood. Specimens should be delivered to the laboratory immediately for prompt analysis.

TESTS TO EVALUATE STAGE IV COAGULATION

Fibrin-Fibrinogen Degradation Products

Fibrin-fibrinogen degradation products (FDP), also known as fibrin(ogen) split products, are the partially digested fragments of fibrin that result from clot degeneration and lysis following hemostasis. The normal rate of clot breakdown by the fibrin-dissolving enzyme plasmin causes low levels of FDP to enter the bloodstream, where they are removed by the liver and reticuloendothelial system. However, because plasmin digests fibrinogen as well as fibrin, increased fibrinolytic activity results in the excessive production of the FDP fragments X, Y, D, E, A, B, and C. Clinical conditions that stimulate intravascular fibrinolysis produce FDP levels high enough to interfere with platelet function in the formation of the hemostatic plug and prevent unconsumed fibrinogen from clotting.

In addition, very high FDP levels resulting from disorders such as disseminated intra-vascular coagulation (DIC) produce symptoms of bleeding similar to those of coagulation factor deficiencies. Thus, although fibrin degradation during normal clot lysis is vital to the prevention of thrombosis, increased fibrinolysis can cause severe hemorrhage, even though intravascular clotting was the initiating factor. Laboratory determinations of FDP concentration are used to detect increased fibrin and fibrinogen breakdown and fre-quently are included in the initial screening tests of hemostatic function to aid diagnosis of local or disseminated intravascular coagulation.

Clinical Significance
Increased fibrinolytic activity and high FDP levels may occur when the coagulation mecha-nism is stimulated by tissue thromboplastin released from the placenta or by damage to the vascular endothelium. Thromboplastin also may be released into the bloodstream by disease, trauma, bacterial endotoxins, intravenous hemolysis, stasis, or antigen-antibody complexes. The presence of thromboplastin in the bloodstream activates the coagulation process, causing clot formation at the site of injury or accumulation of unlocalized fibrin deposits in the veins.

As the inappropriate release of tissue thromboplastin continues, uncontrolled fibrin formation progresses, depleting coagulation factors to the extent that further clotting is severely prolonged or prevented entirely. Thus, disorders such as DIC cause the fibrino-lytic mechanism to remove these clots and fibrin deposits, producing high levels of FDP in the blood. These high FDP levels, combined with complete depletion of coagulation fac-tors, generate so much inhibitory activity that clotting cannot occur and generalized bleeding begins. Measurement of FDP concentrations, usually an emergency procedure ordered for patients with unexplained hemorrhaging, should be performed as soon as a diagnosis of DIC is suspected and before blood transfusion therapy is begun.

Normal Values
The normal values for fibrin-fibrinogen degradation products are:

Blood	2–8 μg/mL
Urine	<0.25 μg/mL

Variations
Increased levels of serum fibrin-fibrinogen degradation products may occur with:

Mild to moderate increases
- Alcoholic cirrhosis
- Aneurysms
- Brain damage
- Blood transfusion, incompatible
- Burns
- Carcinomatosis
- Deep vein thrombosis

- Disseminated intravascular coagulation
- Internal bleeding, newborns
- Myocardial infarction
- Parturition
- Pregnancy, late
- Respiratory distress, newborns
- Sepsis

Shock	Moderate to marked increases
Surgical complications	Abruptio placentae
Tissue damage, massive	Eclampsia
	Pulmonary embolism

Increased levels of urinary fibrin-fibrinogen degradation products may occur with:

Hydronephrosis	Proliferative glomerulonephritis
Lupus nephritis	Renal disease, active
Membranous glomerulonephritis	

Methodology

Measurement of FDP requires 5 mL of blood collected without anticoagulants (red-stoppered tube) before transfusion therapy is initiated. Fibrin-fibrinogen degradation products do not coagulate; therefore, they remain in the serum specimen, where they may be detected after fibrinogen is removed through clotting.

Euglobulin Lysis Time

The **euglobulin lysis time** is a sensitive test of systemic fibrinolysis that measures the rate of deterioration of a clot artificially prepared from thrombin and the euglobulin proteins of plasma. The euglobulin fraction contains clotting factors, as well as all the factors necessary for fibrinolysis, including fibrinogen, plasmin, plasminogen, and plasminogen activator, but has very little antiplasminogen to inhibit fibrinolysis. Therefore, increased fibrinolytic activity shortens the time required for lysis of a euglobulin clot; the shorter the lysis time, the more powerful the fibrinolytic activity. Laboratory determinations of the euglobulin lysis time are used to detect increased amounts of the fibrinolysins and to measure the adequacy of plasmin and plasminogen activator function.

Clinical Significance

An accelerated euglobulin lysis time indicates increased activity of plasminogen activators, which occurs during disorders characterized by excessive fibrinolytic activity, including DIC and primary hyperfibrinolysis. The time required for euglobulin lysis also may be abnormally short in patients who have normal fibrinolytic activity but have little fibrin to be lysed because fibrinogen concentrations are reduced. Test results are unaffected by heparin, and accurate results are obtained in patients receiving this anticoagulant because all heparin is removed in the laboratory during preparation of the euglobulin fraction.

Normal Values

The normal values for the euglobulin lysis time are:

Normal lysis	>2 hours
Increased fibrinolysis	<2 hours

Variations

A **decreased (abnormal) euglobulin lysis time** may occur with:

Disseminated intravascular coagulation (slightly abnormal lysis)

Liver disease

Malignancies, certain

Oral contraceptives

Primary hyperfibrinolysis (very abnormal lysis)

Methodology

Euglobulin lysis time tests require 5 mL of blood collected in sodium citrate anticoagulant (blue-stoppered tube) and delivered promptly to the laboratory. Testing must be performed immediately after the blood is drawn to prevent the loss of fibrinolytic activity that occurs when plasma is stored. If testing cannot be performed immediately, the plasma should be separated from the cells and frozen to reduce the rate at which fibrinolytic activity is lost.

Precautions

To prevent vascular irritation, which will falsely accelerate the euglobulin lysis time, the following precautions should be observed:

1. Do not rub the intended puncture site excessively with the alcohol swab.

2. Instruct the patient not to pump the fist before the venipuncture.

3. Release the tourniquet immediately after entering the vein.

Paracoagulation Tests

The **paracoagulation studies**, including the **ethanol gelation** and **protamine sulfate** tests, are a group of assays used to detect the presence of soluble fibrin monomer complexes during the evaluation of fibrinolysis. The action of thrombin on fibrinogen during normal coagulation produces fibrin strands, which form a stable fibrin clot. However, fibrinolysins present during such disorders as DIC attack fibrinogen to produce soluble fibrin monomer complexes, which prevent clot formation and lead to hemorrhage. Laboratory detection of fibrin monomer paracoagulation aids the diagnosis of DIC during the investigation of intravascular clotting disorders and may be used to differentiate DIC from primary or secondary fibrinolysis.

Clinical Significance

Paracoagulation tests indicate the presence of circulating fibrin monomer complexes caused by secondary fibrinolysis associated with DIC by the formation of a fibrin gel with an ethanol reagent. A protamine sulfate reagent also acts on soluble fibrin monomer complexes and FDP caused by plasmin activity to produce fibrin strands in the presence of secondary fibrinolysis. However, neither ethanol nor protamine sulfate produces any visible reaction during primary fibrinolysis because no soluble fibrin monomer complexes are present on which these reagents may act. False-negative test results may be encountered in patients with severe hypofibrinogenemia; false-positive reactions may be caused by dysproteinemia or hyperfibrinogenemia, and further investigation is needed to support a diagnosis of DIC.

Normal Values
The normal values for paracoagulation tests are:

Ethanol gel

Normal	Normal (granular precipitate)
Abnormal	Positive (gel formation)

Protamine sulfate

Normal	Negative (no fibrin strands)
Abnormal	Positive (visible fibrin strands)

Variations
Positive paracoagulation tests (ethanol gel and protamine sulfate) occur with DIC.

Negative paracoagulation tests occur with primary or secondary fibrinolytic syndromes.

Methodology
The ethanol gelation and protamine sulfate paracoagulation tests require 5 mL of blood collected with sodium citrate anticoagulant (blue-stoppered tube).

Precautions
To prevent false-positive ethanol and protamine sulfate paracoagulation test results the following precautions should be observed:

1. Obtain the specimen without trauma.

2. Do not delay mixing the blood and anticoagulant.

Plasminogen

Plasminogen, the inactive precursor of the fibrin-splitting enzyme plasmin, is a protein incorporated into the clot during coagulation that normally remains dormant until hemostasis is restored. Plasminogen is converted to plasmin by several enzymes, the most important of which is produced by the endothelial cells lining blood vessel walls but which also appear in the urine, plasma, and tissues. This conversion of plasminogen to plasmin activates the physiologic fibrinolytic process responsible for the ultimate dissolution of fibrin clots in blood vessels, soft tissues, and body cavities. Laboratory determinations of plasminogen concentration are used to evaluate fibrinolysis and the cause of increased FDPs and may be used to differentiate congenital and acquired hypofibrinogenemias.

Clinical Significance
Plasminogen concentrations are significant in hypofibrinogenemia because decreased levels occur in the acquired form, indicating a serious secondary disease process, whereas normal levels accompany the congenital form. Decreased plasminogen concentrations also may indicate that the patient is predisposed to recurrent thrombosis because of an abnormality in the plasminogen molecule or a congenital defect in the release of plasminogen activators. Conversely, inhibitors of the plasminogen-plasmin fibrinolytic system, such as α_2-antiplasmin, prevent random fibrinolysis by limiting plasmin activity to sites of fibrin deposition.

> **Normal Values**
> The normal values for plasminogen concentrations are:
>
> 20 mg/dL
> 2.5−5.2 U/mL

Variations
Increased plasminogen levels may be associated with:

Infancy	Pregnancy
Infection, acute bacterial	Stress
Inflammation, acute phase	Surgery
Malignant disease	Thrombophlebitis
Myocardial infarction	Trauma
Oral contraceptives, long-term use	Tuberculosis

Decreased plasminogen levels may be associated with:

Cirrhosis, advanced	Liver disease
Coronary artery bypass surgery	Nephrosis, severe
Disseminated intravascular coagulation	Thrombolytic therapy (streptokinase, urokinase)
Fibrinolysis, primary	

Methodology
Plasminogen determinations require 5 mL of blood collected with sodium citrate anticoagulant (blue-stoppered tube).

ANTICOAGULANT THERAPY AND ASSOCIATED TESTS

Heparin

Heparin is a direct anticoagulant that interferes with the clotting mechanism by retarding the thrombin-fibrinogen reaction immediately after its administration. Heparin prolongs the entire clotting process by preventing the generation of plasma thromboplastin, retarding the conversion of prothrombin to thrombin, and neutralizing the action of thrombin on fibrinogen. However, to achieve its maximum anticoagulant activity, heparin requires the presence of a naturally occurring clot inhibitor, the heparin cofactor antithrombin III. (See Antithrombin III earlier in this chapter.) The anticoagulant effects of heparin disappear within 4−6 hours after each dose because it is rapidly inactivated by liver enzymes and excreted by the kidneys.

Clinical Significance
Heparin is administered routinely intravenously or through subcutaneous or intramuscular injections because it is not absorbed from the gastrointestinal tract and is thus ineffective

when given orally. Heparin activity must be monitored carefully to establish the therapeutic range and maintain a constant anticoagulant effect through intermittent or continuous heparin injection. The patient's response to therapy generally is monitored before every heparin injection to evaluate the residual activity and determine the dose necessary to maintain the desired therapeutic effect. The use of heparin is contraindicated in patients with gastrointestinal bleeding, suspected intracranial hemorrhage, blood dyscrasias involving abnormal hemostasis, thrombocytopenia, severe liver or kidney disease, and brain or spinal cord surgery.

On the other hand, high doses of heparin are employed in a number of clinical situations such as during coronary bypass surgery when the heart-lung machine is used. However, the high heparin dosages used during these procedures to prevent the development of significant clots usually also cause routine monitoring tests to be incoagulable. Thus, alternate laboratory monitoring methods have been developed; the activated whole blood clotting time (ACT), which is performed before, during, and immediately after heparinization, currently is the most useful method. (See Whole Blood Clotting Time earlier in this chapter.)

Therapeutic Monitoring

Many coagulation tests can be used to monitor routine heparin therapy, including the activated partial thromboplastin time (APTT), whole blood clotting time, activated whole blood clotting time (ACT), and thrombin clotting time. Traditionally, the whole blood clotting time was used to monitor the anticoagulant effects of heparin therapy, although this method is time-consuming and difficult to standardize. Recently, however, the APTT has been used to follow response to heparin therapy in most patients because it is more sensitive and much easier to reproduce.

The desired therapeutic range for coagulation test values depends on the particular laboratory procedure used and the time interval between specimen collection and the previous heparin injection. For example, APTT test results obtained approximately 60 minutes after heparin infusion should be prolonged to about twice the normal or preheparinization level. When anticoagulant therapy is changed from heparin to a coumarin derivative, the effect of the coumarin cannot be determined for at least 6 hours following the last heparin injection.

Therapeutic Values
Laboratory values during heparin therapy should be maintained as follows:

Intermittent injection

Whole blood clotting time	Twice the preheparin value (but >20−25 minutes)
Thrombin clotting time	0.2−0.4 U/mL

Continuous infusion

Activated partial thromboplastin time	60−100 seconds

Heart-lung machine

Activated whole blood clotting time	480 seconds

Coumarin Derivatives

Coumarin derivatives are indirect anticoagulants administered orally to prevent clotting and inhibit the growth of existing clots by blocking the synthesis of certain coagulation factors. These compounds delay or prevent the synthesis of vitamin K-dependent factors (II, VII, IX, and X) by the liver, causing them to disappear from the blood according to their individual degradation rates. Thus, coumarin derivatives act slowly to inhibit coagulation, requiring 10 hours after the first dose to exert a minimum anticoagulant effect and 2–5 days to develop maximum activity. In addition, the effects of such coumarin anticoagulants as warfarin and bishydroxycoumarin are cumulative and may persist for 3–14 days after therapy has been discontinued.

Clinical Significance
Coumarin derivatives provide an effective means of treating active thrombotic or thromboembolic episodes in individuals who are predisposed to clot formation. However, therapeutic response to coumarin derivatives may be affected by a variety of physiologic and pathologic conditions, as well as by diet and exercise. For example, responsiveness to coumarin therapy may be decreased by conditions such as excessive vitamin K intake or poor absorption of the coumarin resulting from gastrointestinal disease, hyperlipemia, diabetes mellitus, and thyrotoxicosis. In contrast, vitamin K deficiency, advanced age, cachexia, hepatic insufficiency, preexisting hemorrhagic tendency, and hypermetabolic states can enhance the effect of coumarin and increase the bleeding tendency.

Patient response to therapy also may be influenced by the interaction of coumarin with a number of other drugs taken simultaneously. Such drugs either enhance the action of coumarin and accentuate its therapeutic effects or suppress coumarin metabolism and decrease the anticoagulant effect by shortening its duration of activity. Thus, careful monitoring is required when drugs are added to or deleted from the total therapeutic regimen to detect any change in patient response. A partial list of the drugs that increase or decrease patient sensitivity to coumarin is presented in Table 10-4.

Therapeutic Monitoring
Prothrombin time determinations currently are used to monitor coumarin therapy. Prothrombin time methods are more sensitive than the whole blood clotting time for following the course of coumarin therapy because the whole blood clotting time will not be affected until the prothrombin results fall to 10% of normal activity. Prothrombin time test results during coumarin therapy should be prolonged to one and one-half to two and one-half times the patient's pretreatment level.

Therapeutic Values
Prothrombin time test results during coumarin therapy should be maintained as follows:

18–29 seconds

20%–30% of normal activity

TABLE 10-4   Drugs That Interfere With Coumarin Anticoagulation

Drugs That Increase Coumarin Sensitivity	Drugs That Decrease Coumarin Sensitivity
Acetaminophen	Antacids
Alcohol	Ascorbic acid
Allopurinol	Barbiturates
Anabolic steroids	Carbamazepine
Chloral hydrate	Chloral hydrate
Chloramphenicol	Cholestyramine
Chlorthalidone	Chlortetracycline
Clofibrate	Colchicine
Disulfiram	Cortisone-prednisone
Ethacrynic acid	Diuretics
Glucagon	Ethchlorvynol
Indomethacin	Glutethimide
Methylphenidate	Haloperidol
Metronidazole	Oral contraceptives
Neomycin	Rifampin
Nortriptyline	Xanthines
Phenylbutazone	
Phenytoin	
Quinine	
Quinidine	
Sulfonamides	
Thyroid preparations	

REFERENCES

Barber, J. 1978. Basic coagulation. *Lab. Med.* 9(4):40.

Bauer, J. D. 1982. *Clinical laboratory methods.* 9th ed. St. Louis: The C. V. Mosby Co.

Collins, R. D. 1975. *Illustrated manual of laboratory diagnosis.* 2nd ed. Philadelphia: J. B. Lippincott Co.

Doucet, L. R. 1981. *Medical technology review.* Philadelphia: J. B. Lippincott Co.

Dougherty, W. M. 1976. *Introduction to hematology.* 2nd ed. St. Louis: The C. V. Mosby Co.

Eastham, R. D. 1970. *Clinical haematology.* 3rd ed. Baltimore: Williams & Wilkins Co.

French, R. M. 1980. *Guide to diagnostic procedures.* 5th ed. New York: McGraw-Hill Book Co.

Gambino, S. R., and Altman, P. 1979. Fibrin degradation products (FDP); the FDP test. *Lab 79.*

Garb, S. 1976. *Laboratory tests in common use.* 6th ed. New York: Springer Publishing Co.

Henry, J. B. 1984. *Clinical diagnosis and management by laboratory methods.* 17th ed. Philadelphia: W. B. Saunders Co.

Larson, F. C. 1982. *Clinical significance of tests on the DuPont Clinical Analyzer.* Wilmington, Del.: DuPont Industries.

Lenahan, J. G., and Smith, K. 1978. *Hemostasis*. 13th ed. Morris Plains, N.J.: General Diagnostics, Division of Warner-Lambert Co.

Maslow, W. C., et al. 1980. *Hematologic disease*. Boston: Houghton Mifflin Co.

McGann, M. A., and Triplett, D. A. 1982. Interpretation of antithrombin III activity. *Lab. Med.* 13(12):742.

————. 1983. Laboratory evaluation of the fibrinolytic system. *Lab. Med.* 14(1):18.

Miale, J. B. 1982. *Laboratory medicine—hematology*. 6th ed. St. Louis: The C. V. Mosby Co.

Ortho Diagnostics, Inc. 1975. *A closer look at hemostasis*. Raritan, N.J.: Ortho Diagnostics, Inc.

————. 1982. *Ortho diagnostic systems: Seminar manual*. Raritan, N.J.: Ortho Diagnostics, Inc.

Rader, M. 1981. Coagulation factor disorders. *Diagn. Med.* 4(5):57.

Raphael, S. S., et al. 1983. *Laboratory technology*. 4th ed. Philadelphia: W. B. Saunders Co.

Seiverd, C. 1983. *Hematology for medical technologists*. 5th ed. Philadelphia: Lea & Febiger.

Sirridge, M. 1983. *Laboratory evaluation of hemostasis*. 3rd ed. Philadelphia: Lea & Febiger.

Soloway, H. B. 1978. Monitoring heparin therapy: How and why. *Diagn. Med.* 1(1):33.

Starr, A., Schmidt, P., and Dede, D. 1977. Proper handling of specimens for coagulation studies. *Lab. Med.* 8(11):26.

Strand, M. M., and Elmer, L. A. 1983. *Clinical laboratory tests*. 3rd ed. St. Louis: The C. V. Mosby Co.

Swanson, J. O. 1978. Preoperative coagulation testing. *Lab. Med.* 9(5):28.

Tilkian, S. M., Conover, M. B., and Tilkian, A. G. 1983. *Clinical implications of laboratory tests*. 3rd ed. St. Louis: The C. V. Mosby Co.

Vega Diagnostics. 1980. *Antithrombin III by RIA*. Pasadena, Calif.: Vega Diagnostics.

Vollmer, K. 1975. *The coagulation factors*. Miami, Fla.: Dade Division of American Hospital Supply Corp.

Widmann, F. K. 1983. *Clinical interpretation of laboratory tests*. 9th ed. Philadelphia: F. A. Davis Co.

11

Serology/Immunology

ANTIGEN-ANTIBODY REACTIONS 579
T- and B-Lymphocytes · Immunoglobulins · Complement
SPECIMEN COLLECTION FOR SEROLOGIC STUDIES 585
SEROLOGIC TESTS FOR AUTOIMMUNITY 586
Test for Antinuclear Antibodies · Tests for Deoxyribonucleic
Acid Antibodies · Tests for Antimitochondrial and Anti-Smooth Muscle
Antibodies · Test for the Rheumatoid Factor · Test for Thyroid
Antibodies
SEROLOGIC TESTS FOR FEBRILE AGGLUTININS 593
Widal Test for Typhoid and Paratyphoid Fevers · Weil-Felix Test for
Rickettsial Diseases · Agglutination Test for Brucellosis · Agglutination
Test for Tularemia
SEROLOGIC TESTS FOR FUNGAL INFECTIONS 598
SEROLOGIC TESTS FOR MYCOPLASMAL INFECTIONS 602
Test for Cold Agglutinins · Test for Mycoplasmal Antibodies · Test for
Streptococcus MG Agglutinins
SEROLOGIC TESTS FOR PARASITIC INFECTIONS 605
Test for Toxoplasmosis · Tests for Other Parasitic Infections
SEROLOGIC TESTS FOR STREPTOCOCCAL INFECTIONS 609
Test for Antistreptolysin O Titer · Tests for Antideoxyribonuclease B and
Antihyaluronidase · Test for C-Reactive Protein
SEROLOGIC TESTS FOR SYPHILIS 614
Tests for Nontreponemal Antibodies · Tests for Treponemal Antibodies
SEROLOGIC TESTS FOR TORCH DISEASES 619
SEROLOGIC TESTS FOR VIRAL INFECTIONS 620
Tests for Cytomegalovirus · Tests for Viral Hepatitis · Test for Herpes
Simplex Virus · Tests for Infectious Mononucleosis · Test for Rubella

Clinical immunology is a rapidly evolving field in which the ability of the immune system to respond to invasion by foreign elements is evaluated. The immune system also serves as a defense against the body's own aberrant cells that have developed through mutation. Thus, the field of clinical immunology includes the study of autoimmune antibodies that are produced to rid the body of potentially harmful tumor cells.

Serology is the portion of clinical immunology concerned with detecting, identifying, and measuring specific antibodies that develop in the blood in response to exposure to disease-producing antigens. The field of serology includes a number of tests that are used to diagnose autoimmune diseases resulting from antithyroid, antinuclear, and antismooth antibodies, as well as infectious and noninfectious diseases produced by microorganisms.

Although infectious diseases generally are diagnosed by isolating microorganisms through routine culture, serologic procedures to identify disease-specific antibodies frequently are used when morphologic identification is impossible or impractical. Serologic antibody procedures also allow retroactive diagnosis of infectious diseases because certain antibodies remain in the blood even after the acute phase of the disease has subsided. However, because antibodies cannot be demonstrated by simple physical or chemical means, detection and identification depend on observing visible reactions with specific antigens in various test reagents. Visible antigen-antibody reactions may be produced by a number of techniques, including precipitation, agglutination, immunodiffusion, hemagglutination, complement fixation, immunoelectrophoresis, fluorescent antibody, and enzyme-labeled immunoassay procedures.

ANTIGEN-ANTIBODY REACTIONS

The concepts of antigen and antibody formation are totally interrelated.

An **antigen** is any protein, carbohydrate, lipoprotein, lipopolysaccharide, or nucleoprotein whose presence provokes an immunologic response and induces antibody formation. Although most antigens are substances such as microorganisms that are actually foreign to the body, they also may be physiologically normal constituents mistakenly perceived as foreign by the body. Therefore, substances such as bacteria, viruses, protozoa, worms, bacterial and plant toxins, pollen, venoms, mismatched blood, certain foods and drugs, nuclear proteins, and DNA may act as antigens.

An **antibody** is a substance produced by the body following contact with an antigen that attempts to neutralize or incapacitate the antigen. Antibodies are immunoglobulins secreted by plasma cells and some lymphocytes contained in the spleen, lymph nodes, thymus, tonsils, and adenoids in response to stimulation of the immune system. Antibodies provide immunity or resistance to a substance by reacting solely and specifically with the particular antigen that has stimulated their production.

T- and B-Lymphocytes

Two separate but interrelated categories of lymphocytes, T-lymphocytes and B-lymphocytes, with different functions play a dominant role in governing the reactivity and response of the immune system to invasion.

T-lymphocytes, governed by the thymus gland, are primarily associated with cell-mediated immune responses such as delayed hypersensitivity, transplant or graft rejection, bacterial and viral killing, and tumor immunity. T-lymphocyte levels (normally 45%–

85%, 500–2400 T cells/μL) generally correlate with the functional status of the cell-mediated immunologic system. T-lymphocytes assist B-lymphocytes in responding to antigenic stimulation. Under abnormal circumstances, T-lymphocytes may attack the host's own tissue cells if surface properties are altered sufficiently to be perceived by the T cells as foreign. This property is important in surveillance against tumor development and is at least partly responsible for the development of autoimmune disease.

   B-lymphocytes, derived from the fetal liver and bone marrow, are antibody-producing cells that synthesize immunoglobulins to specific antigens and give rise to plasma cells. They have demonstrable surface immunoglobulins. Each B-lymphocyte produces only one type of antibody or immunoglobulin molecule throughout its life, although subsequent contact with its specific antigen stimulates these reactive B cells to further immune activity. Such immune activity causes the transformation of B-lymphocytes, first into larger cells and eventually into several plasma cells which manufacture antibodies that interact specifically with the same antigen that stimulated their synthesis. B-lymphocyte levels (normally 4%–23%, 50–200 B cells/μL) correlate with the status of the humoral immunologic system.

   Because complex interaction and cooperation between T- and B-lymphocytes are required for immune competence, any change in either or both cell types suggests the possibility of immunodeficiency disease. Therefore, quantitation of the actual number of circulating T- and B-lymphocytes can confirm the clinical diagnosis and aid in classifying lymphocytic leukemia, lymphomas, primary and secondary immunodeficiency diseases, and autoimmune diseases. For example, an increase in B-lymphocytes is associated with lymphoproliferative malignancies, including acute and chronic lymphocytic leukemia, Waldenström's macroglobulinemia, and multiple myeloma, whereas B-lymphocyte decreases accompany infantile sex-linked agammaglobulinemia and common variable immunodeficiency. On the other hand, an increase in T-lymphocytes occurs with autoimmune disorders such as Graves' disease, whereas a decrease in T-lymphocytes occurs in systemic lupus erythematosus, Wiskott-Aldrich syndrome, Hodgkin's disease, thymic hypoplasia (DiGeorge's syndrome), lymphomas, and immunosuppressive therapy. Once the diagnosis of immunodeficiency disease is made, the therapeutic response also may be evaluated by monitoring changes in the percentages of T and B cells.

Immunoglobulins

Immunoglobulins are proteins secreted by B-lymphocytes and released into the bloodstream, lymph, and gastrointestinal, respiratory, and urinary tracts, where they destroy potential pathogens. Immunoglobulins occur in the blood as the γ-globulin fraction of serum protein, which is divided by immunoelectrophoresis into five classes. (See Serum Protein Electrophoresis and Immunoelectrophoresis in Chapter 4.)

   Immunoglobulin G (IgG) antibodies produce antibacterial and antiviral activity by neutralizing the toxins of gram-positive bacteria and viruses in the bloodstream and tissue spaces. IgG antibody production develops rather late in the immune response to new antigens but continues at high levels well after the antigen has been eliminated. Once specific IgG antibodies are produced, subsequent exposure to the same antigen causes them to reappear rapidly. IgG antibodies are not directly cytotoxic but kill cells by activating complement or phagocytic cells. Maternal IgG antibodies are the only immunoglobulins that are transported across the placenta of immunized mothers and are the fetus's and neonate's sole source of defense against infection.

   Immunoglobulin A (IgA) antibodies are responsible for gastrointestinal and respiratory tract immunity and constitute the first line of defense against invasion by a variety of pathogenic organisms. The bulk of IgA is contained in surface secretions such as tears, saliva, sweat, mucus, colostrum, and breast milk, and the remainder appears in the serum. Although the complete function of IgA antibodies against bacteria is unclear, the major role seems to be repelling viruses that invade the host through the respiratory and gastrointestinal tracts.

Immunoglobulin M (IgM) antibodies are the first antibodies formed in response to primary contact with any new antigen and are the most efficient immunoglobulins in stimulating the activity of the complement system. IgM antibodies are particularly effective against microorganisms and are responsible for the initial response to endotoxins of gram-negative bacteria and antigens of the ABO group. IgM production usually continues as long as the antigen remains, ceases when the antigen has been eliminated, and falls rapidly after the onset of IgG antibody synthesis. Thus, persistent IgM antibody production suggests that the antigen is still present.

Immunoglobulin D (IgD) antibodies are present in trace amounts in plasma. IgD is the predominant immunoglobulin on the surface of B-lymphocytes. The functions of IgD are unknown, and their biologic activity or significance has not yet been identified.

Immunoglobulin E (IgE) antibodies are responsible for many allergic conditions governed by atopic and anaphylactic hypersensitivity reactions, as well as for fixed tissue responses and skin sensitivity. The most common causes of increased IgE levels are parasitic infestations, hay fever, asthma, certain types of eczema, and systemic reactions to insect venoms, penicillin, and other drugs or chemicals. The clinical significance of variations in plasma levels are not well understood, and no apparent correlation exists between the severity of symptoms and IgE levels. Thus, IgE antibody tests are not widely used in clinical practice because their usefulness in the differential diagnosis of allergic and nonallergic conditions has not yet been established. However, a recently developed procedure, the **radioallergosorbent test** (RAST), aids the diagnosis of allergic diseases by estimating circulating IgE antibody levels, identifying the offending allergens, and evaluating the effects of treatment. The RAST test screens patients for hypersensitivities to most common allergens by testing serum with different allergen complexes and measuring the amount of IgE directed toward each allergen (Table 11-1). Because effective treatment of allergies decreases IgE antibody levels, the RAST test also helps evaluate the success of treatment of allergic diseases by monitoring variations in antibody concentration to specific allergens produced by changes in therapy and lifestyle.

Complement

The **complement system** is comprised of a group of nine distinct globulins, designated C1 to C9, that interact in a specific cascading sequence to control immunologic responses following antigen-antibody interactions. These serum proteins normally remain inactive in the bloodstream until their enzymelike activity is stimulated by alteration of IgG, IgM, or IgA antibodies following union with their respective antigens. Complement activity therefore gains specificity from the role of antibodies in seeking, identifying, and binding antigens to help the immune system destroy foreign substances and defend the host's integrity. Complement activity enhances phagocytosis, aids the lysis of bacteria by antibodies, and is associated with inflammatory responses in defense against infection with pathogenic organisms.

Clinical Significance

Complement is consumed by increased utilization during the hyperimmune activity that occurs in many systemic diseases and causes serum complement levels to fall during the

TABLE 11-1 Allergens Detected by the RAST* Test

Foods	Grasses	Weeds	Trees
Almond	Bahia	Common ragweed	Beech
Barley	Bermuda	Dandelion	Birch
Blue mussel	Brome	English plantain	Cedar
Brazil nut	Common reed	False ragweed	Cottonwood
Buckwheat	Cultivated oat pollen	Firebrush	Elm
Carrot	Cultivated rye	Giant ragweed	Hazelnut
Casein	Cultivated wheat pollen	Goldenrod	Maple
Celery	Johnson grass	Lamb's quarter	Oak
Cheese	Kentucky blue	Mugwort	Olive
Chicken	Meadow fescue	Nettle	Sycamore
Coconut	Meadow foxtail	Ox-eye daisy	Walnut
Codfish	Orchard	Rough marsh elder	White ash
Corn	Perennial rye	Rough pigweed	White pine
Crab	Red top	Russian thistle	Willow
Egg white	Sweet vernal	Scale	
Egg yolk	Timothy	Sheep sorrel	
Gluten	Velvet	Western ragweed	
Hazelnut		Wormwood	
Lobster			
Milk			
Oat			
Orange			
Parsley			
Pea			
Peanut			
Pork			
Rice			
Rye			
Potato			
Salmon			
Sesame seed			
Shrimp			
Soybean			
Strawberry			
Tomato			
Tuna			
Wheat			
White bean			

*RAST = radioallergosorbent test.

Epidermals	Molds	Insects	Miscellaneous
Cat epithelium	*Alternaria tenuis*	Bee venom	Castor bean
Chicken feathers	*Aspergillus fumigatus*	Cockroach	Coffee bean
Cow dander	*Candida albicans*	Imported fire ant	House dust
Dog dander	*Cladosporium herbarum*	Paper wasp	Insulin
Dog epithelium	*Mucor racemosus*	White-faced hornet	Ispaghula
Duck feathers	*Penicillium notatum*	Yellow hornet	Silk
Goat epithelium		Yellow jacket	Wild silk
Goose feathers			
Guinea pig dander			
Hampster epithelium			
Horse dander			
Mouse epithelium			
Mouse urine			
Pigeon droppings			
Rabbit epithelium			
Rat epithelium			
Sheep epithelium			
Swine epithelium			

active phase. Complement levels are decreased significantly in patients with systemic lupus erythematosus (SLE), acute and chronic glomerulonephritis, chronic active hepatitis, subacute bacterial endocarditis, exacerbations of rheumatic fever, malaria, autoimmune hemolytic anemia, and severe rheumatoid arthritis. Complement components are also acute-phase reactants and become increased in acute inflammatory diseases and necrotizing disorders. Thus, profiling of complement activity recently has been shown to have diagnostic value in identifying complement-depleted individuals and evaluating patients with clinically significant congenital or acquired complement disorders.

Serologic evaluation of total hemolytic complement activity helps determine the functional adequacy of the entire complement sequence and is used to diagnose and monitor immune-mediated diseases. The test for total hemolytic activity measures the ability of complement in serum to hemolyze 50% or 100% of a sheep cell reagent coated with antisheep antibody. Results are expressed in terms of CH_{50} and CH_{100} units respectively, which are derived and interpreted from levels in normal serum known to cause 50% or 100% hemolysis.

However, because individual complement components, particularly C3 and C4, correlate very well with total complement activity, these levels frequently are substituted for total hemolytic complement assays to evaluate acquired disease states. For example, C3 activity, which is diminished significantly in active SLE and certain types of glomerulonephritis, is useful in assessing the clinical course of renal involvement. Decreased C3 levels usually are associated with kidney involvement and herald the exacerbation of renal impairment 1 or 2 months before it occurs and help evaluate the response to treatment. On the other hand, elevated C3 levels may occur with acute-phase plasma protein responses, infections, inflammatory and necrotizing disorders, and rheumatoid arthritis.

Likewise, because the C4 component also is significantly diminished in active SLE and lupus nephritis, simultaneous determinations of C3 and C4 levels help distinguish acute glomerulonephritis from SLE nephritis. Deficiencies of the C5 to C9 components accompany, and may be responsible for, connective tissue or collagen-like states.

Normal Values

The normal and clinically significant values for total complement and complement components are:

Total complement

50–200 CH_{100} U/mL	Normal
40–85 CH_{50} U/mL	Normal
>85% of normal value	Normal
50%–80% of normal value	Suggests decrease in complement activity
<50% of normal value	Significant decrease in complement activity

Complement (C3)

65–220 mg/dL	Normal

Complement (C4)

15–40 mg/mL	Normal

Methodology

Measurement of total hemolytic complement levels (CH_{50} and CH_{100}) requires 5 mL (for each test) of blood collected in a tube without anticoagulants (red-stoppered tube). Determination of complement C2 to C4 components requires 3 mL of blood (for each component) collected without anticoagulants; measurement of C1, C5, and C6 requires 3 mL of blood (for each component) collected in EDTA (lavender-stoppered tube).

SPECIMEN COLLECTION FOR SEROLOGIC STUDIES

Serologic evaluation of disease ideally should include tests performed on two blood specimens, an acute-phase specimen and a convalescent-phase sample, drawn at least 2–3 weeks apart. Because it takes time for the body to react to invading microorganisms, serologic studies are more effective when specimens are collected later in the course of the disease and during the convalescent period. The nurse must recognize that although positive serologic test results frequently are conclusive evidence of disease, there is a time lag between the clinical presence of disease and increased antibody titers.

Demonstration of increasing antibody concentrations between acute- and convalescent-phase specimens often forms the basis for diagnosis and provides a retrospective confirmation of an admission diagnosis. Therefore, patients admitted with a history of exposure to an infectious agent should be placed in isolation until the positive antibody reaction has had time to develop. However, a single elevated antibody titer, although indicative of increased immune reactivity, is inconclusive by itself.

The patient's history of vaccination or exposure to infectious agents, along with test titers in individuals from the same geographic area, must be considered when interpreting serologic test results, particularly single titers.

▶▶ *Nursing Responsibilities and Implications*

1. Note on the laboratory slip any pertinent clinical data such as probable diagnosis, presenting symptoms, concurrent disorders, drug therapy, and type and date of previous vaccinations or infections.

2. Instruct the patient to refrain from fluids or food for 8 hours prior to the test to limit lipemic activity, which may interfere with the test results; water is permitted.

3. If applicable, draw the specimen before any skin test antigen is administered because skin testing may stimulate immunoglobulin production and cause a falsely elevated antibody titer.

4. Draw the specimen before administering antimicrobial agents or other drugs such as γ-globulin that may cause a falsely decreased antibody titer.

5. Perform a nontraumatic venipuncture to limit hemolysis, which will cause unreliable test results.

6. Prevent self-contamination with the specimen, syringe, or needle.

7. Send the specimen to the laboratory immediately after it is obtained to ensure accurate results; if prompt testing is not possible, separate serum from clotted cells and refrigerate; if testing must be delayed more than 72 hours or if the specimen is to be sent to another laboratory for further studies, freeze the serum as quickly as possible.

8. If the test is positive for infectious disease, teach the patient the importance of adhering to the prescribed medical regimen, including follow-up supervision.

9. If the test is positive for infectious disease, notify the infection control nurse or public health agency to determine what special precautions are necessary; make certain that those infectious diseases that are reportable under state or local health regulations are reported to the proper authorities; inform the patient that certain diseases, such as sexually transmitted diseases, will result in mandatory inquiries from the authorities.

SEROLOGIC TESTS FOR AUTOIMMUNITY

Autoimmunity is the process by which the body fails to recognize particular substances, such as hormones or tissue components, as belonging to itself and develops antibodies to destroy them. There are two groups of autoimmune reactions: those directed against specific organ products or cells such as thyroglobulin and red blood cells and those that interact with antigenic structures shared by many different tissues, organs, or body processes such as DNA, nuclear protein, and mitochondria. Autoantibodies are detrimental to the host and can result in a variety of autoimmune diseases that eventually may be fatal.

Test for Antinuclear Antibodies

Antinuclear antibodies (ANA) are autoimmune immunoglobulins produced by the body against one or more nuclear antigens present in its own tissues. These autoantibodies may react with the whole nucleus or any of its components, including nuclear proteins, single- or double-stranded DNA, nucleoli, and histones. Antinuclear antibodies generally develop in patients with untreated active SLE, although they may appear in other collagen diseases such as scleroderma, dermatomyositis, rheumatoid arthritis, and hypersensitivity states. Positive ANA reactions also occur in patients with myasthenia gravis, leprosy, infectious mononucleosis, malignancy, Hashimoto's disease, drug-induced lupus syndromes, and diseases associated with liver damage due to autoimmunity or viral infection.

Patients with ANA experience antigen-antibody reactions that are accompanied by complement fixation and a subsequent drop in circulating complement levels. The combination of autoantibody, antigen, and circulating complement forms an immune complex. This immune complex precipitates within the blood vessels of many organs and causes vasculitis and glomerulonephritis.

The most sensitive screening test for ANA activity in patients with SLE and clinically similar connective tissue or collagen-vascular disorders is the indirect fluorescent antibody (IFA) procedure. When ANA are present in the serum, the nuclei of test cells stain in a variety of patterns that reflect the distribution of the various antigens within the nucleus. Thus, fluorescent nuclear staining patterns produced by a patient's ANA, which may be diffused, peripheral, speckled, or nucleolar, are governed by the predominant antibody associated with the specific disease.

A **diffused or homogeneous pattern** results from staining of the entire nucleus due to antibodies that react with DNA-nucleoprotein-histone complexes. This pattern characteristically appears in high titers in SLE but also may be seen in low titers in rheumatoid arthritis and other diseases.

A **peripheral or marginal pattern** results from staining of the nuclear membrane due to antibodies directed against DNA. This pattern is seen primarily in Sjögren's syndrome, scleroderma, and dermatomyositis, although it also may occur in SLE.

A **speckled pattern** reflects specks of staining dispersed throughout the nucleus due to antibodies directed against saline-extractable nuclear antigens. This pattern usually occurs in scleroderma, Raynaud's syndrome, Sjögren's syndrome, polymyositis, and mixed connective tissue disease.

A **nucleolar pattern** reflects staining of the nucleolar membranes due to antibodies that react with RNA-nucleoprotein complexes. This pattern usually occurs in patients with scleroderma as well as those with Sjögren's syndrome, SLE, and rheumatoid arthritis.

Clinical Significance

The greatest diagnostic value of ANA testing is in the differential diagnosis of connective tissue diseases in patients with a complicated clinical picture that includes symptoms that resemble those of rheumatoid arthritis. Antinuclear antibody tests also have some value in monitoring the therapeutic efficacy of various medications because effective treatment of SLE causes ANA titers to decrease. Negative ANA results virtually rule out the diagnosis of connective tissue disease, particularly SLE, unless the patient is under treatment.

Antinuclear antibody determinations are not diagnostic by themselves, and additional tests are needed to interpret the significance of positive results for any given autoimmune disorder. Positive results for total ANA should be confirmed by anti-DNA antibody tests because DNA antibodies seldom appear in any condition other than SLE. Although ANA titers may not correlate with the clinical course of a particular autoimmune state, some correlation does appear to exist between ANA titers and the severity of the disease. Thus, it is imperative that test results be correlated with the patient's age, sex, clinical condition, medical history, and additional laboratory findings before a definite diagnosis is made.

Normal Values

The normal and clinically significant values for antinuclear antibodies are:

$<1:20$	Negative; normal
$1:20-1:80$	Little diagnostic significance; may be seen in rheumatoid arthritis or scleroderma
$1:80-1:200$	Suggests connective tissue disease
$>1:200$	Strong evidence for connective tissue disease

Variations

False-positive antinuclear antibody tests may occur in apparently healthy individuals, especially those over 50 years of age, and in patients receiving many commonly prescribed drugs, including:

Aminosalicylic acid	Ethosuximide	Hydroxytryptophan
Carbidopa	Griseofulvin	Isoniazid
Diphenylhydantoin	Hydralazine	Mephenytoin

Methyldopa	Procainamide	Streptomycin sulfate
Methylthiouracil	hydrochloride	Sulfadimethoxine
Penicillin	Propylthiouracil	Tetracycline
Phenylbutazone	Quinidine	Trimethadione

False-negative antinuclear antibody tests may occur in patients with SLE who are undergoing steroid therapy.

Methodology
Antinuclear antibody determinations require 5 mL of blood collected without trauma and without anticoagulants (red-stoppered tube).

▶▶ Nursing Responsibilities and Implications
See Specimen Collection for Serologic Studies—Nursing Responsibilities and Implications.

Tests for Deoxyribonucleic Acid Antibodies

Deoxyribonucleic acid antibodies (anti-DNA) are autoimmune immunoglobulins that react with both the single-stranded denatured form of DNA (sDNA) and the double-stranded native form (nDNA). Tests for anti-sDNA concentrations are not clinically significant because this autoantibody appears in several inflammatory conditions and produces positive results in several collagen-vascular diseases. Tests for anti-nDNA concentrations, however, are diagnostic for active spontaneous SLE because this antibody develops only in patients with this disease.

Anti-nDNA antibody titers correlate well with the clinical course of SLE because levels fall during the chronic phase or remission but rise during the acute phase or relapse. In addition, increased anti-nDNA levels also correlate with the onset of lupus nephritis and some drug-induced syndromes. Conversely, reduced anti-nDNA levels signify an improvement in clinical status in response to therapy, and, although negative test results do not eliminate the diagnosis of SLE, they do suggest the absence of active nephritis. Therefore, laboratory tests for anti-nDNA activity provide valuable diagnostic and prognostic information for the differential diagnosis of SLE but must be interpreted in light of the patient's total clinical condition.

Clinical Significance
The presence of anti-nDNA antibodies following the diagnosis of SLE is considered an indication of recurrent active disease or a poor response to therapy. Therefore, periodic monitoring of anti-nDNA antibody titers helps evaluate the clinical course of SLE, and persistently low titers signify a successful response to long-term therapy. On the other hand, rising anti-nDNA titers, associated with a fall in the complement level, indicate renal involvement because anti-nDNA–DNA–complement complexes are involved in the development of lupus nephritis. (See Complement earlier in this chapter.)

Periodic determination of anti-nDNA and complement levels may be helpful in patient management because SLE with renal involvement usually is associated with high anti-nDNA levels and depressed serum complement levels. Although a syndrome closely resembling SLE with increased anti-nDNA titers may follow the prolonged use of procainamide or similar drugs, there is no renal involvement, and complement levels remain normal. Thus, the combined determination of anti-nDNA titers and complement levels aids the differential diagnosis of lupuslike syndromes.

Normal Values

The normal and clinically significant anti-DNA antibody values are:

Radioimmunoassay tests

<1.0 μg of DNA/mL	Nonspecific
1.0−2.5 μg of DNA/mL	SLE in remission; other autoimmune disturbances
>10 μg of DNA/mL	Active SLE

Indirect fluorescent antibody tests

<1:10	Negative; normal
>1:10 with high ANA titer	Highly suggestive of SLE
1:10−1:20 with low ANA titer	Suggestive of disease other than SLE

Variations

False-positive anti-DNA antibody tests may occur in patients receiving certain drugs, particularly hydralazine.

False-negative anti-DNA antibody tests may occur in patients undergoing steroid therapy.

Methodology

Native DNA antibody determinations require 5 mL of serum collected without hemolysis and without anticoagulants (red-stoppered tube).

▶▶ *Nursing Responsibilities and Implications*

See Specimen Collection for Serologic Studies—Nursing Responsibilities and Implications.

Tests for Antimitochondrial and Anti-Smooth Muscle Antibodies

Antimitochondrial and anti-smooth muscle antibodies are autoimmune immunoglobulins that frequently develop against certain liver antigens in patients with primary biliary cirrhosis, chronic active hepatitis, and cryptogenic cirrhosis. **Antimitochondrial antibodies** appear predominantly in patients with primary biliary cirrhosis, less frequently in patients with chronic active hepatitis or cryptogenic cirrhosis, and only rarely in patients with other disorders. Primary biliary cirrhosis occurs most often in women 30−60 years of age and is characterized by a chronic inflammatory breakdown of the small intrahepatic biliary ducts and tubules. However, there is no correlation between antimitochondrial antibody titers and disease activity or duration of symptoms, suggesting that the antibody appears during the course of the disease and persists.

Conversely, **anti-smooth muscle antibodies** appear most often in patients with chronic active hepatitis, less frequently in patients with primary biliary cirrhosis, and only rarely in patients with cryptogenic cirrhosis. Chronic active hepatitis, also called lupoid hepatitis, is a chronic liver disease that usually affects young females and causes progressive necrosis of hepatic parenchymal cells and deteriorating liver function. However, because anti-smooth muscle antibodies may accompany infectious mononucleosis, acute viral hepatitis, and infiltrative tumors, their presence suggests that they also occur in response to damaged liver cells.

Tests for these antimitochondrial and anti-smooth muscle antibodies are not diagnostic by themselves but help differentiate primary biliary cirrhosis, chronic active hepatitis, and cryptogenic cirrhosis from other liver diseases. Although these autoantibodies do not appear to cause liver disease, they persist for many years during certain autoimmune disorders and make certain diagnoses more probable than others. It is therefore imperative that test results be interpreted in light of the patient's entire clinical condition.

Clinical Significance
Tests for antimitochondrial antibodies have been recommended as a substitute for surgical exploration to confirm the diagnosis of primary biliary cirrhosis suggested by clinical, laboratory, or histologic manifestations. The presence of high antimitochondrial antibody titers in obstructive jaundice favors a diagnosis of primary biliary cirrhosis over surgically treatable extrahepatic biliary obstruction, drug-induced cholestatic jaundice, or viral hepatitis. However, these autoantibodies are of little help in differentiating primary biliary cirrhosis from certain types of viral hepatitis because they also appear in some patients with non-B chronic active hepatitis.

Normal Values
The normal and clinically significant values for antimitochondrial and anti-smooth muscle antibodies are:

Antimitochondrial antibodies

<1:10	Normal
>1:20	Positive for antimitochondrial antibodies; suggests primary biliary cirrhosis
>1:80	Strong evidence of primary biliary cirrhosis

Anti-smooth muscle antibodies

<1:20	Normal
<1:40	Diagnostically insignificant
>1:80	Strong evidence of chronic active hepatitis

Variations
False-positive antimitochondrial antibody tests may occur in low titers in healthy patients and those with autoimmune diseases associated with primary biliary cirrhosis and drug-induced jaundice.

   False-positive anti-smooth muscle antibody tests may occur in low titers in healthy patients between 50 and 70 years of age and those with:

Asthma, intrinsic	Infiltrative tumors	Viral hepatitis, acute
Infectious mononucleosis with liver damage	Malignant diseases	Yellow fever

Methodology

Antimitochondrial and anti-smooth muscle antibody determinations require 5 mL of blood collected without hemolysis in a tube without anticoagulants or preservatives (red-stopped tube).

▶▶ ## Nursing Responsibilities and Implications

See Specimen Collection for Serologic Studies—Nursing Responsibilities and Implications.

Test for the Rheumatoid Factor

The **rheumatoid factor** (RF) is an autoantibody produced in the synovium as a result of chronic infection, autoimmunity, or connective tissue defects in patients with rheumatoid arthritis. Rheumatoid factor appears in the serum and synovial fluid several months after the onset of rheumatoid arthritis and is detectable for months or years despite therapy. In general, the presence of RF is not affected by analgesic and anti-inflammatory drugs, although gold salt therapy decreases the RF titer.

Test results on synovial fluid generally correlate strongly with those performed on serum, although patients who are seronegative occasionally will have positive synovial fluid test results. In addition, because the RF is at least partially responsible for inflammatory responses and patient morbidity, there is a correlation between high titers and severe rheumatoid disease. Thus, demonstration of the RF is useful in diagnosis when rheumatoid arthritis is suspected but not for assessing the severity of illness or following therapy.

Clinical Significance

Rheumatoid factor tests are useful in differentiating rheumatoid arthritis from rheumatic fever because patients with rheumatic fever or the juvenile form of rheumatoid arthritis often have negative test results. Tests are positive in approximately 90% of patients who exhibit the classic symptoms of advanced rheumatoid arthritis but also may be positive in patients with many chronic inflammatory illnesses. However, RF tests detect only 50% of patients with atypical signs of rheumatoid arthritis and frequently are negative early in the disease, when an accurate diagnosis is needed most.

Normal Values

The normal and clinically significant values for rheumatoid factor are:

Qualitative	Negative
Quantitative	
$<1:20$	Normal
$<1:40$	Chronic inflammatory diseases
$1:40-1:60$	Diagnostic for rheumatoid arthritis
$>1:60$	Advanced rheumatoid arthritis

Variations
False-positive tests for the rheumatoid factor may occur in healthy individuals over 60 years of age and those with a variety of other chronic inflammatory conditions, including:

Cirrhosis	Osteoarthritis
Dermatomyositis	Paraproteinemia
Diabetes mellitus	Polyarteritis nodosa
Hepatic neoplasms	Pulmonary interstitial fibrosis
Hepatitis	Sarcoidosis
Hypertension	Schistosomiasis
Juvenile rheumatoid arthritis	Scleroderma
Kala-azar	Subacute bacterial endocarditis
Leprosy	Syphilis
Liver disease, chronic	Systemic lupus erythematosus
Lymphomas	Tuberculosis
Macroglobulinemia	Viral infections
Mixed connective tissue disease	Yaws

Methodology
Rheumatoid factor determinations require 5 mL of blood collected in a tube without anticoagulants (red-stoppered tube).

▶▶ Nursing Responsibilities and Implications
There are no specific nursing responsibilities for rheumatoid factor determinations. Food and fluid restrictions usually are not necessary.

Test for Thyroid Antibodies

Thyroid antibodies are autoimmune immunoglobulins that occur during various thyroid diseases against the patient's own thyroid tissues and eventually destroy the thyroid gland. Clinically significant thyroid antibodies include **antithyroglobulin**, directed against the thyroglobulin present in thyroid tissue follicles, and **antimicrosomal antibodies**, found in the cytoplasm of thyroid epithelial cells. These antibodies generally appear about 4 weeks after the onset of symptoms in patients with Hashimoto's disease, Graves' disease, primary myxedema, nontoxic goiter, and thyroid carcinoma. They also may be found in the sera of patients with fibrous thyroiditis and de Quervain's disease, as well as in most children with lymphocytic thyroiditis.

Antithyroglobulin and antimicrosomal antibody tests are valuable in the differential diagnosis of thyroid enlargement because varying titers of these antibodies occur in thyroid conditions. However, the presence of thyroid antibodies is not diagnostic of any particular condition because they also occur in 15% of apparently healthy people and in up to 20% of older individuals. It is therefore imperative that thyroid antibody tests be correlated with the patient's clinical condition and additional histopathologic or laboratory data.

Clinical Significance

High thyroid antibody titers usually indicate Hashimoto's disease or Graves' disease, whereas negative results virtually exclude these conditions. Thus, thyroid antibody testing is most useful in distinguishing Hashimoto's disease from simple nontoxic goiter, thyroid carcinomas, de Quervain's disease, and fibrous thyroiditis. Immunofluorescent thyroid antibody techniques appear to be particularly valuable in detecting antibodies in juvenile lymphocytic thyroiditis when other tests are negative, whereas low antithyroglobulin antibody titers may be significant in pediatric Hashimoto's disease.

Normal Values

The normal and clinically significant values for antithyroglobulin and anti-microsomal thyroid antibodies are:

<1:100	Normal
>1:1000	Hashimoto's disease, Graves' disease, autoimmune diseases

---

Variations

False-positive thyroid antibody tests may occur in patients with such nonthyroid disorders as:

Addison's disease	Hypoparathyroidism
Allergic disorders	Liver disease
Atrophic gastritis	Myasthenia gravis
Connective tissue disorders	Pernicious anemia
Diabetes mellitus	Sjögrens syndrome

Methodology

Antithyroglobulin and antimicrosomal thyroid antibody determinations require 5 mL of blood collected in a tube without anticoagulants (red-stoppered tube).

▶▶ Nursing Responsibilities and Implications

There are no specific nursing responsibilities for antithyroglobulin and antimicrosomal antibody determinations. Food and fluid restrictions usually are not necessary.

SEROLOGIC TESTS FOR FEBRILE AGGLUTININS

Serologic tests for febrile agglutinins diagnose infectious diseases by detecting antibacterial antibodies directed against certain microorganisms. Diseases most commonly detected by febrile agglutination tests are the enteric fevers, typhoid and paratyphoid; the rickettsial diseases, Rocky Mountain spotted fever and typhus; and brucellosis and tularemia. Bacterial cultures are the best means of isolating and identifying the organisms responsible for a febrile condition; tests for febrile agglutinins should never be considered a substitute for this process.

Febrile agglutination tests help identify the causative agent of a fever of unknown origin when the patient is tested late in the disease or previous antibiotic therapy suppresses the organism involved. Although febrile disease must not be diagnosed solely on serologic reports, this indirect method of diagnosis provides a retrospective opportunity to pinpoint a particular disease. Test results are reported as the highest serum dilution (titer) in which there is a positive reaction with the test antigen, although a single agglutination test is of little value.

Because many individuals have agglutinins due to immunization, tests should be performed every 3–5 days after the onset of the disease to demonstrate a change in antibody titer. A significant rise in titer between paired serum specimens usually occurs in the first 8–15 days of the illness, and a progressive increase in titer is the primary evidence of infection. When the tests are performed late in the disease, titers gradually decline over a period of time. Improved serologic techniques and a significant decrease in the incidence of enteric fevers, rickettsial diseases, brucellosis and tularemia, however, have discouraged the widespread use of tests for febrile agglutinins in the investigation of fever.

Widal Test for Typhoid and Paratyphoid Fevers

The **Widal test** is an agglutination procedure formerly used to detect *Salmonella typhi* and *S. paratyphi* antibodies in the indirect diagnosis of typhoid and paratyphoid fevers. Because all *Salmonella* organisms have flagella, both the body of the bacteria (somatic or O portion) and its flagella (flagellar or H portion) can act as antigens in stimulating antibody production. In addition, *S. typhi* has an extra surface antigen (Vi) that also stimulates antibody formation in the infected host.

Detectable *Salmonella* antibodies begin developing by the end of the first week following infection, produce elevated O agglutinin titers within 4 weeks, and rise to peak titers in the third to sixth week. Antibodies to O antigens increase markedly during the active stage of *Salmonella* infection, persist for only a few months, and usually return to insignificant levels 6 months after recovery. Although titers may remain negative early in the disease, they will not decrease in the presence of continued infection or when the individual is a carrier.

Antibodies to H antigens, on the other hand, do not indicate recent typhoid infections as reliably as O agglutinins because they are not always demonstrable in *Salmonella* infections. Titers of H agglutinins rise more slowly and peak later than O agglutinin titers following exposure to typhoid and may remain elevated for years after the organism has disappeared. Antibodies to Vi antigens also increase during typhoid infection and often remain elevated even after O or H agglutinins have returned to normal. Persisting Vi antibodies were once believed to indicate a chronic carrier state, but this correlation has now been discredited. Thus, a documented increase in O agglutinin titers is far more reliable and diagnostically significant than either H or Vi antibodies for diagnosing recent *Salmonella* infections.

Clinical Significance

The Widal test must be interpreted in light of the patient's total clinical picture and immunization history because positive results are not significant and may occur following recent typhus vaccination. Test results also may be misleading in patients with febrile illnesses from other causes such as liver disease or hypergammaglobulinemia that characteristically produce chronically high *Salmonella* antibody levels. Users of illicit drugs also have higher than normal levels of *Salmonella* agglutinins, which probably reflects poor hygienic practice and increased contact with enteric organisms of all sorts.

Negative Widal test results do not necessarily rule out infection but are best used as baseline data for subsequent comparative testing. Although a single test result is not diagnostic unless the titer is unusually high, a positive test result occurring several days after a negative test result is usually significant. However, improved culture techniques and effective antimicrobial therapy have made agglutinin tests obsolete.

Normal Values

The clinically significant values for the *Salmonella* antigens are:

O antigen

1 : 40−1 : 80	Normal; natural agglutinin in endemic area; recent typhoid immunization
Fourfold increase in paired serum samples within 10−14 days	Clinically significant; diagnostic in unvaccinated patients
>1 : 160 and rising	Current *Salmonella* infection

H antigen

1 : 40−1 : 80	Normal; natural agglutinin in endemic area; recent typhoid immunization
1 : 80−1 : 160	Recent vaccination; past typhoid infection; anamnestic reaction

Vi antigen

>1 : 10	Clinically significant

Variations

False-positive Widal test reactions may occur in patients with hypergammaglobulinemia due to liver disease or narcotic addiction, those with recent typhoid vaccination, typhoid carriers, and individuals with an anamnestic response. False elevations of the typhoid agglutinin titer also may occur when O antigens produced by infection with other enteric bacilli cross-react with *Salmonella* test antigens.

False-negative Widal test results may occur early in the infectious stage of typhoid fever before agglutinins have developed and in overwhelming infections when the body's defenses are too depleted to produce agglutinins. Patients with agammaglobulinemia, leukemia, advanced carcinoma, immunosuppressive disorders, certain congenital deficiencies, or general debilitation also may be unable to produce detectable febrile agglutinins despite the presence of documented typhoid infection. Antibiotic therapy, particularly when given early in the course of typhoid fever, may prevent or depress a rise in the agglutinin titer or inhibit the development of detectable antibodies.

Methodology

The Widal test for *Salmonella* agglutinins requires 5 mL of blood collected in a tube without anticoagulants (red-stoppered tube) and without hemolysis. Specimens should be collected before instituting specific antibiotic therapy, which could depress or diminish the agglutinin titer.

▶▶ *Nursing Responsibilities and Implications*

See Specimen Collection for Serologic Studies—Nursing Responsibilities and Implications. Food or fluid restrictions usually are not necessary.

Weil-Felix Test for Rickettsial Diseases

The **Weil-Felix test** is an agglutination procedure used for the indirect diagnosis of rickettsial diseases such as Rocky Mountain spotted fever and typhus. The test uses three strains of *Proteus* X bacilli (*Proteus* OX19, *Proteus* OX2, and *Proteus* OXK) that cross-react with antigens similar to those carried by certain rickettsiae. *Proteus* agglutinins may appear as early as the fifth or sixth day of infection but are always present by the tenth or twelfth day. Peak titers occur early in the convalescent period after several weeks of illness, begin to decrease in 6–8 weeks, and return to undetectable levels within 3–5 months of clinical recovery.

Clinical Significance

Patients with epidemic typhus, murine (endemic) typhus, and Rocky Mountain spotted fever (tickborne typhus) characteristically develop strong agglutinins to *Proteus* OX19. Test reactions with *Proteus* OX2 antigens are positive in patients with spotted fevers such as boutonneuse tick fever, Siberian tick fever, and Queensland tick fever. *Proteus* OXK reaction is positive with scrub typhus (tsutsugamushi disease) but also may indicate relapsing fever, a nonrickettsial disease caused by a spirochete.

Although *Proteus* OX19 test antigen is widely used in diagnosing typhus infections, results are nonspecific and do not identify the precise rickettsial organisms responsible for the disease. The differential diagnosis of rickettsial infections is possible with complement fixation tests, which permit both immediate and retrospective identification of specific antibodies. However, specific microimmunofluorescence tests using rickettsial antigens produce more reliable results for the diagnosis of Rocky Mountain spotted fever than the Weil-Felix test.

Normal Values

The clinically significant values for *Proteus* antigens in the diagnosis of rickettsial disease are:

Agglutination tests

>1:80	Clinically significant in unvaccinated individuals
>1:160 or fourfold increase in paired serum samples within 7 days	Diagnostic for rickettsial infection
<1:200	Nonspecific after recent vaccination or in endemic areas

Complement fixation tests

>1:8	Diagnostic

Variations

False-positive Weil-Felix reactions may be encountered in patients with recent or concurrent *Proteus* infection (as in the urinary tract) due to the formation of specific anti-*Proteus* agglutinins. False-positive test results also occur in recently vaccinated individuals, those living in areas where typhus is endemic, and patients with leptospirosis, *Borrelia* infections, or severe liver disease.

False-negative Weil-Felix reactions may result from aborted or delayed antibody production in patients receiving early antibiotic therapy before the first test specimen is drawn. Patients with confirmed rickettsial infections also may fail to develop *Proteus* agglutinins, which suppress test response and cause an incorrect laboratory diagnosis. However, although certain patients with typhus, rickettsialpox, spotted fever, trench fever, or Q fever do not react to the Weil-Felix test, this does not rule out these diseases.

Methodology

The Weil-Felix test requires 5 mL of blood collected without hemolysis in a tube without anticoagulants (red-stoppered tube). Specimens must be obtained before instituting specific antibiotic therapy, which could interfere with the test results by depressing or diminishing agglutinin titers.

▶▶ ## Nursing Responsibilities and Implications

See Specimen Collection for Serologic Studies—Nursing Responsibilities and Implications. Food or fluid restrictions usually are not necessary.

Agglutination Test for Brucellosis

The **agglutination test for brucellosis** detects antibodies generated by any of three closely related *Brucella* species and is used in the indirect diagnosis of human brucellosis or undulant fever. These organisms are transmitted to humans from infected animals (*B. abortus* from cattle, *B. suis* from hogs, and *B. melitensis* from goats) and mimic many diseases, the severity and clinical symptoms of which vary considerably. Because diagnosis based on clinical symptoms alone usually is quite difficult and often impossible, serologic identification of these organisms is important when culture techniques are not possible. Although response to *Brucella* infection varies in different individuals, higher agglutinin titers generally are more suggestive of active infection.

In patients with acute brucellosis, detectable agglutinin titers develop in the second week of illness, reach diagnostically significant levels during the third or fourth weeks, and peak between the fourth and eighth weeks. Agglutinin titers normally decrease gradually or disappear completely during clinical improvement, although in most patients slightly elevated titers remain for 5 or more years following apparent recovery from active brucellosis. Patients who have recovered from brucellosis may exhibit a temporary rise in *Brucella* antibody titers that confuses test interpretations and is stimulated by any subsequent unrelated febrile illness. These titers rise rapidly to significant levels within a few days, only to drop precipitously to negative titers 7–10 days later.

Chronic brucellosis is more difficult to diagnose because test titers may fluctuate over many months, and there is no definite criterion for judging their significance. Thus, *Brucella* infection cannot be ruled out on the basis of low test titers alone because high agglutinin levels do not develop in some patients, even though they may have brucellosis. When chronic brucellosis is strongly suspected but cannot be confirmed through routine agglutination tests, an extra test reagent may be added to the *Brucella* antigen for addi-

tional sensitivity. This technique is known as the **antihuman globulin** (AHG) or **Coombs'**
test. (Coombs' test is discussed in Chapter 12.)

Clinical Significance

Agglutination tests for *Brucella* organisms must be interpreted in light of additional patient
data such as the current clinical findings, medical history, recent vaccinations, and geographic location. For example, patients immunized with *Brucella* vaccines develop high
antibody titers, although they remain uninfected. Early antibiotic therapy reduces the
chances of isolating the *Brucella* organism by culture methods but does not hinder the
development of specific antibodies or interfere with the diagnostic value of this test.

Normal Values

The clinically significant titers for *Brucella* antigens are:

1 : 20 – 1 : 80	Normal in farmers or endemic areas without clinical infection; chronic brucellosis; recovery stage of acute infection
>1 : 160	Past or present infection
1 : 320	Diagnostically significant
Fourfold increase within 2 weeks	Active infection

Variations

False-positive test results occasionally may occur in cross-reactions with *Brucella* test
antigens and agglutinins produced by patients with tularemia, cholera, and *Proteus* OX19
infections. However, such cross-reactions do not appear in all patients with tularemia, and
any reaction with *Brucella* antigens generally is much weaker than in specific tests for
tularemia agglutinins. False-positive *Brucella* test reactions also may occur in individuals
who recently were vaccinated against cholera because antibodies common to both organisms persist for 2½ years following vaccination. Although the patient's history in these
situations should suggest the possibility of such a cross-reaction, more specific tests are
available to distinguish these conditions when clinical evidence is inconclusive.

Methodology

Agglutination tests for *Brucella* infections require 5 mL of blood collected without trauma
in a tube without anticoagulants (red-stoppered tube). Specimens should be delivered to
the laboratory as soon as possible for prompt testing.

▶▶ Nursing Responsibilities and Implications

See Specimen Collection for Serologic Studies—Nursing Responsibilities and Implications. Food or fluid restrictions usually are not necessary.

Agglutination Test for Tularemia

The **agglutination test for tularemia** is widely used for the indirect diagnosis of febrile
infections produced by *Francisella tularensis*. Because *F. tularensis* is difficult to isolate by

culture methods, this test has become the most reliable diagnostic aid for rabbit fever and deer fly fever. Patients with such tularemia infections begin to develop specific *F. tularensis* antibodies within 1–3 weeks after the onset of illness, although detectable titers generally appear during the second week. Agglutinin titers reach maximum levels in 2–3 months and begin to decline slowly 1 year after clinical recovery but may remain detectable for many years after the infection or throughout the individual's life.

Clinical Significance

Clinical findings and patient history must be considered carefully when establishing a diagnosis of tularemia because cross-agglutination reactions occasionally produce false-positive test results. A negative test does not rule out tularemia but only indicates that the specimen was taken before detectable antibody formation occurred. A fourfold rise in titer in specimens drawn every 3–5 days indicates active infection, whereas a single elevated titer is very suggestive of infection at some time, although not necessarily indicative of current or recent infection. Because elevated titers persist for such long periods of time, however, the rise between acute and convalescent sera is almost mandatory for a positive diagnosis.

Normal Values

The clinically significant titers for *Francisella* antigens are:

$<1:40$	Normal, uninfected individuals
$>1:80-1:160$	Infection, current or past
$>1:640$	Peak agglutinin titer

Variations

False-positive results occasionally occur from cross-agglutination reactions between the *F. tularensis* organism and *Brucella abortus* or *Proteus vulgaris* (OX19). These errors can be eliminated by conducting parallel serum testing with all three antigens to identify the responsible organism; a higher titer usually is obtained with the specific test antigen.

Methodology

Agglutination tests for tularemia require 5 mL of blood collected without hemolysis in a tube without anticoagulants (red-stoppered tube). Specimens should be collected before starting specific antibiotic therapy, which could depress or diminish the agglutinin titer, and delivered to the laboratory for prompt testing.

▶▶ ### Nursing Responsibilities and Implications

See Specimen Collection for Serologic Studies—Nursing Responsibilities and Implications. Food or fluid restrictions usually are not necessary.

SEROLOGIC TESTS FOR FUNGAL INFECTIONS

Serologic tests for fungal antibodies play an important role in the diagnosis of mycotic infections and supplement cultural or histopathologic evidence of a disorder. Both ordinarily harmless and pathogenic fungi may become virulent in debilitated hosts and produce systemic infections that can mimic bacterial disease and may go undetected without special diagnostic efforts. Although recovery and identification of the etiologic agent from clinical specimens are required for definitive identification of mycotic infections, cultural proof occasionally cannot be obtained and other laboratory procedures must be utilized. (See Fungus Cultures in Chapter 9.)

Serologic fungal antibody tests provide the clinician with valuable diagnostic information in a much shorter time than is required for fungal cultures to become positive. Thus, when interpreted properly and combined with the patient's clinical history, serologic tests generally provide enough information to allow a tentative or presumptive diagnosis of mycotic infection. Test antigens for some fungal infections contain common components and cross-react with other fungi to give false-positive reactions, although titers are greater against test antigens from the causative organism. False-negative test results may occur in patients in whom antibody production is diminished by immunosuppression from cancer, underlying disease, chemotherapy, or prior treatment with broad-spectrum antibiotics.

Clinical Significance

Systemic infections can be divided into the so-called primary diseases and secondary or opportunistic invasions. Primary infections, including blastomycosis, coccidioidomycosis, and histoplasmosis, are produced by pathogenic organisms, afflict previously healthy persons, and must be recognized and treated individually. Opportunistic or secondary fungal infections, including aspergillosis and cryptococcosis, occur when certain fungi normally present in the environment attack patients with other diseases who cannot mount an effective defense.

Aspergillus is a common opportunistic fungus that causes lung or gastrointestinal tract infections, which often are difficult to diagnose and produce severe but nonspecific symptoms.

Blastomyces organisms frequently produce pulmonary symptoms, although the respiratory tract is not always the site of primary infection. Although serologic cross-reactions may occur in patients with coccidioidomycosis or histoplasmosis, these titers are usually lower than those produced by blastomycosis. Decreasing serologic test titers indicate disease regression.

Coccidioides antibodies develop during the first 3 weeks of infection and are diagnostic of fungal infection but are not useful for predicting the course or prognosis of the disease. False-positive serologic cross-reactions may occur in patients with histoplasmosis, whereas false-negative results often occur in patients with solitary pulmonary lesions. Low titers of *Coccidioides* antibodies therefore should be followed by repeat testing at 2- to 3-week intervals.

Cryptococcus organisms produce a brief inflammatory lung infection and rapidly disseminate throughout the body, including the central nervous system, where they may cause prolonged illness. *Cryptococcus* organisms frequently coexist with tuberculosis, diabetes, and hematologic malignant diseases, causing symptoms of cryptococcosis to be masked by those of the primary affliction. Cryptococcal antigens circulate within the host during cryptococcosis and may be demonstrated in serum or cerebrospinal fluid by immunologic procedures even in patients in whom no organism can be detected. The presence of the rheumatoid factor in the patient's serum may interfere with the test results.

Histoplasma organisms are yeastlike fungi that cause a variety of clinical manifestations. Antibody titers are increased within 6 weeks after infection. These titers generally persist for weeks or months and then fall rapidly. However, they may remain elevated for up to 1 year and continue to stimulate dermal sensitivity reactions even after clinical recovery. Serologic procedures are valuable in diagnosing and establishing the prognosis of histoplasmosis and in distinguishing hypersensitivity reactions or chronic infections from active cases. Although rising antibody titers suggest continuing or progressive infection and decreasing titers indicate regression, several follow-up specimens should be drawn at 2- to 3-week intervals to detect fluctuating antibody levels. False-positive cross-reactions occur in patients with aspergillosis, blastomycosis, or coccidioidomycosis, although antibody titers in these conditions are usually lower than those produced by histoplasmosis.

Normal Values

The normal and clinically significant values for selected fungal infections are:

Aspergillosis

<1:8	Negative; normal
Fourfold rise in paired serum specimens	Highly suspicious of infection

Blastomycosis

<1:8	Negative; may indicate regression of infection
1:8−1:16	Highly suggestive of active infection
>1:32	Indicates active infection

Coccidioidomycosis

<1:2	Negative; normal
1:2−1:4	May indicate active or prior infection
>1:16	Indicates active infection; parallels the severity of infection

Cryptococcosis

<1:8	Negative; normal
Fourfold rise in paired serum specimens	Highly suspicious of infection

Histoplasmosis

1:8−1:16	Highly suspicious of infection
>1:32	Diagnostic of active infection

Methodology

Serologic detection of fungal antibodies requires 10 mL of blood collected aseptically in a tube without anticoagulants (red-stoppered tube). Specimens for serologic testing should be collected at 2- to 3-week intervals to detect increasing antibody titers against the responsible organism.

▶▶ Nursing Responsibilities and Implications

See Specimen Collection for Serologic Studies—Nursing Responsibilities and Implications. Food or fluid restrictions usually are not necessary.

SEROLOGIC TESTS FOR MYCOPLASMAL INFECTIONS

Mycoplasma pneumoniae is a nonbacterial organism responsible for the respiratory disease formerly known as "primary atypical pneumonia" and "viral" pneumonia, which is characterized by fever and a nonpurulent cough. Although culture methods for *Mycoplasma* are available, serologic tests, including those for cold agglutinin titers and mycoplasmal antibodies, are preferable for the diagnosis of mycoplasmal pneumonia.

Test for Cold Agglutinins

Cold agglutinins are autoimmune antibodies produced by *Mycoplasma pneumoniae* infections that agglutinate human red blood cells incubated at temperatures between 0 and 10 C but is reversible at 37 C. Production of cold agglutinins increases markedly during the first week of *M. pneumoniae* infection, before the appearance of antimycoplasmal antibodies, and peaks during the third or fourth week. However, unlike specific antimycoplasmal antibodies that persist for many months, cold agglutinin titers disappear rapidly following the sixth week of infection. Cold agglutinin titers often are related to the severity and duration of illness, although significant titers may be seen in mild cases.

Clinical Significance
Pneumonitis (a form of primary atypical pneumonia) is the only common respiratory disease in which significantly increased cold agglutinin titers consistently occur. High cold agglutinin titers accompanied by a fourfold or greater rise in concentration suggest a recent *M. pneumoniae* infection but also may occur in the absence of such infections. For example, these antibodies exist in very low concentrations in many healthy persons but are not of pathologic importance unless the body temperature is lowered artificially.

Cold agglutinins and *Streptococcus* MG agglutinins are not related to each other, but both are associated with primary atypical pneumonia. However, tests for either one or both of these substances may be negative in this condition. Consequently, when *M. pneumoniae* is suspected to be the causative agent of nonbacterial pneumonia, tests for both agglutinins should be performed on each serum sample. (See Test for *Streptococcus* MG Agglutinins later in this chapter.)

Normal Values
The normal values for cold agglutinins are:

<1:32	Normal; conditions unrelated to *M. pneumoniae*
>1:40	Acute *M. pneumoniae* infection

Variations
False-positive test results for cold agglutinins may appear in the blood of patients with malaria, peripheral vascular disease, congenital syphilis, severe anemia, hepatic cirrhosis, and common respiratory diseases. Thus, test results should be interpreted together with

the entire clinical picture and other diagnostic studies to prevent an inaccurate diagnosis of nonbacterial pneumonia.

Because **false-negative test results** may occur when specimens are refrigerated for prolonged periods of time, blood for cold agglutinin determinations should be stored at room temperature before serum is separated from red blood cells for testing. Refrigeration causes absorption of all or most of the cold agglutinins by the red blood cells, removing these antibodies from the serum and interfering with the test values.

Methodology

Cold agglutinin determinations require 5 mL of blood drawn into a warm tube or syringe and taken immediately to the laboratory in a 37 C water bath. If a water bath is not available or the specimen cannot be delivered to the laboratory promptly, blood for cold agglutinin testing should be stored at room temperature. These same procedures also should be followed when a patient who is known to have these antibodies has blood drawn for type and crossmatch or for hematologic procedures.

▶▶ ### Nursing Responsibilities and Implications

In addition to the guidelines listed under Specimen Collection for Serologic Studies— Nursing Responsibilities and Implications, the nurse should proceed as follows:

1.   Inform the patient that there are no food or fluid restrictions.

2.   Store the specimen at room temperature.

Test for Mycoplasmal Antibodies

Diagnostically significant elevations of mycoplasmal antibodies may be detected in the serum of most patients with *Mycoplasma pneumoniae* infection about 7–10 days after the onset of illness. However, because these antibodies often persist after the condition has cleared, a single specimen is not too helpful for the diagnosis of recent mycoplasmal infections. In addition, mycoplasmal antibodies also develop in the serum of some patients with pancreatitis caused by lipid alterations induced by the liberation of pancreatic enzymes. Therefore, a fourfold rise in titer between specimens collected at the onset of disease and those 2–3 weeks later provides the best specific diagnostic evidence of current or recent mycoplasmal infection.

Normal Values

The normal and clinically significant values for mycoplasmal antibodies are:

<1:2	Normal
<Fourfold rise in specimens 10–21 days apart	Inconclusive for mycoplasmal infections
>Fourfold rise in titer in paired serum specimens	Suggests recent mycoplasmal infection
<1:256, single specimen	Inconclusive
>1:256, single specimen	Strongly suggests recent mycoplasmal infection

Variations
False-positive mycoplasmal antibody tests may occur in patients receiving antibiotics.

Methodology
Mycoplasmal antibody determinations require 5 mL of blood collected from a fasting patient in a tube without anticoagulants (red-stoppered tube).

▶▶ **Nursing Responsibilities and Implications**
See Specimen Collection for Serologic Studies—Nursing Responsibilities and Implications. Food or fluid restrictions usually are not necessary.

Test for *Streptococcus* MG Agglutinins

Patients with pneumonitis (a form of primary atypical viral pneumonia produced by *Mycoplasma pneumoniae*) frequently develop an additional but unrelated antibody to *Streptococcus* MG bacteria. *Streptococcus* MG antibodies increase during the second or third week of infection and reach maximum levels in the fifth or sixth week. Agglutinin titers begin to decrease shortly after peak concentrations are reached and gradually return to preinfection levels.

Clinical Significance
Although *Streptococcus* MG is not the causative agent of primary atypical pneumonia, many patients with this syndrome develop increased *Streptococcus* MG agglutinins late in the disease or during convalescence. Slightly elevated titers also may develop in individuals without atypical pneumonia because *M. pneumoniae* often is present in the normal flora of the upper respiratory tract of many persons. Thus, detection of elevated *Streptococcus* MG agglutinin titers has become an additional aid in the diagnosis of mycoplasmal pneumonia. In addition, *Streptococcus* MG agglutinin titers frequently correlate closely with cold agglutinin titers in the presence of mycoplasmal pneumonia. However, the absence of *Streptococcus* MG agglutinins does not necessarily exclude the diagnosis of primary atypical pneumonia because early antibiotic therapy may inhibit their development.

Normal Values
The normal values for *Streptococcus* MG are:

<1:10	Normal
>1:20 with a fourfold rise in titer	*M. pneumoniae* infection

---

Methodology
Streptococcus MG agglutinin determinations require 5 mL of blood collected in a tube without anticoagulants (red-stoppered tube).

▶▶ **Nursing Responsibilities and Implications**
See Specimen Collection for Serologic Studies—Nursing Responsibilities and Implications. Food or fluid restrictions usually are not necessary.

SEROLOGIC TESTS FOR PARASITIC INFECTIONS

Serologic tests are particularly useful in the diagnosis of parasitic infections when it is difficult to identify organisms by examination of blood or feces. Serologic tests for parasitic infections generally are used to detect and assess toxoplasmosis, amebiasis, trichinosis, and hydatid disease caused by *Echinococcus*. Although antibody titers against parasitic organisms are often quite high, acute infections are best diagnosed by a fourfold titer rise, and chronic infections are characterized by a persistent, stable titer.

Although a great deal of meaningful information often can be gained from a single test specimen, especially in high-risk populations, diagnosis cannot be based on a single serologic result. Maximum information is gathered from sequential or paired serum specimens (acute and convalescent) taken 2–3 weeks apart and accompanied whenever possible by appropriate laboratory tests. (See also Specimens for Microbiologic Examination—Stool in Chapter 9.) A significant titer is the test result most closely associated with clinical disease or exposure; a diagnostic titer is one that unequivocally indicates infection.

Test for Toxoplasmosis

Toxoplasma gondii, the organism that causes toxoplasmosis, is a ubiquitous parasite that infects many species of birds, reptiles, and mammals and is one of the most common latent infectious agents of humans. The greatest risk of transmission to humans occurs from eating infected raw or undercooked meat, particularly mutton and pork; travel or residence in rural areas where the disease is common; or the ingestion of contaminated soil. Primary *T. gondii* infection stimulates the production of IgM antibodies, which usually appear within the first week following infection, peak in 3–4 weeks, and generally become undetectable within 3–4 months. Subsequent toxoplasmal antibodies of the IgG class usually become detectable 3 weeks after primary infection, peak at 2–6 months, decrease slowly, and persist at detectable levels throughout life.

Toxoplasmosis is usually asymptomatic or characterized by a lymph node infection resembling infectious mononucleosis in immunocompetent adults. As one of the four TORCH diseases, it may produce a congenital infection with a wide range of manifestations in newborns. (See Serologic Tests for TORCH Diseases later in this chapter.) Toxoplasmosis can result in serious complications in immunocompromised adults, particularly those undergoing immunosuppressive therapy, who are at increased risk of toxoplasmosis. Toxoplasmosis therefore must be considered in the differential diagnosis of illnesses of unknown etiology with central nervous system symptoms in infants or immunocompromised patients. Thus, toxoplasmal antibody tests are a valuable aid in the diagnosis of toxoplasmosis or evaluation of an individual's immune status but must be correlated with the clinical findings.

Clinical Significance

Transplacental infection of the fetus may occur if the mother acquires an acute toxoplasmal infection during pregnancy. Infection may result in stillbirth, spontaneous abortion, premature birth, or congenital toxoplasmosis. Although women who have serologic evidence of toxoplasmal infection prior to becoming pregnant rarely give birth to infected neonates, those who develop toxoplasmal antibodies during pregnancy may transmit congenital toxoplasmosis. Thus, toxoplasmal antibodies in infants under 4 months of age are probably of maternal origin, whereas those found after 4–6 months result either from early postnatal or congenital infection. A negative initial titer followed by a positive titer suggests self-acquired infection. The incidence of congenital infection varies according to the trimester during which the mother becomes infected, with the highest incidence of transmission to the fetus occurring in the third trimester. However, the greatest risk to the developing fetus occurs when maternal infection is acquired in the first trimester.

The major sequelae of congenital toxoplasmosis in fetuses infected during the first two trimesters include hydrocephaly or microcephaly, psychomotor retardation, bilateral retinochoroiditis, and cerebral calcification. Congenital toxoplasmosis is also manifested by other clinical signs, including abnormal cerebrospinal fluid, convulsions, jaundice, fever, splenomegaly, hepatomegaly, lymphadenopathy, vomiting, diarrhea, pneumonitis, and rash. However, these initial symptoms of congenital toxoplasmosis are occasionally nonspecific and may lead to misdiagnosis on clinical grounds, even in infected infants who have the generalized form of the disease. Infected infants who demonstrate no clinical symptoms at birth also may develop blindness, mental retardation, deafness, epilepsy, spasticity, and palsy.

Normal Values
The normal and clinically significant values for toxoplasmal antibodies are:

Total indirect hemagglutination
(IHA) antibody

<1:16	Negative; susceptibility to acute toxoplasmal infection
1:16−1:64	Reflects past exposure to *Toxoplasma*; rising titer may signify early stages of disease
>1:64	Clinically significant
>1:256	Indicates relatively recent exposure to *Toxoplasma* or acute infection
>1:1024	Very significant of toxoplasmosis

Indirect immunofluorescence
(IIF)-IgM antibody

>1:2	Significant of congenital toxoplasmal infection in neonates
>1:32	Significant of recent or early toxoplasmal infection in adults

---

Variations
False-positive toxoplasmal antibody tests may occur in serum containing high levels of rheumatoid factor or in specimens from patients with antinuclear antibodies.

Methodology
Determination of toxoplasmal antibodies requires 5 mL of blood collected without hemolysis in a tube without anticoagulants (red-stoppered tube). Collection of acute and convalescent specimens is recommended for pregnant women with known or suspected *T. gondii* exposure.

▶▶ *Nursing Responsibilities and Implications*

See Specimen Collection for Serologic Studies—Nursing Responsibilities and Implications. Food or fluid restrictions usually are not necessary.

Tests for Other Parasitic Infections

Serologic tests to detect and identify a variety of parasitic infections are most helpful when diagnostic forms cannot be demonstrated readily in blood or stool specimens. However, the sensitivity and specificity of certain procedures are problematic, and interpretation of test results can be difficult.

Amebiasis.   A number of sensitive serologic tests for antibodies to invasive *Entamoeba histolytica* are available, which become more sensitive as the parasite's invasiveness increases. Although they do not detect amebic cyst carriers, these tests produce positive results in the majority of patients with liver abscesses and acute amebic dysentery. Thus, a negative serologic test for amebic antibodies suggests strongly that amebic abscess is not the cause of the patient's clinical symptoms. However, although amebic antibody titers gradually decrease over time, serologic test results may remain positive for up to 2 years after successful therapy.

Echinococcosis.   Echinococcosis, a disease caused by *Echinococcus granulosus*, usually is diagnosed by serologic procedures, although low antibody titers do not necessarily indicate current infection because test antigens may cross-react with antibodies produced by other conditions. Thus, increased antibodies may be observed in patients with liver cirrhosis, collagen diseases, and other parasitic infections. Because antibody titers usually decrease rapidly within 3 months after surgical removal of a hydatid cyst and continue to drop for 1 year, failure to observe such a decline usually indicates incomplete cyst removal.

Malaria.   In recent years several sensitive serologic antibody procedures have been developed for the diagnosis of malaria, a disease caused by *Plasmodium vivax, P. falciparum, P. malariae,* and *P. ovale.* Increased antibody titers generally indicate that the patient has acquired malaria at some time and also may identify the infecting species in many early primary infections. However, these tests generally are not used to diagnose clinical infections but are particularly useful in epidemiologic surveys and the detection of infected blood donors.

Schistosomiasis.   Several sensitive and specific serologic procedures are available to detect schistosomiasis, a disease caused by *Schistosoma japonicum, ˙S. mansoni,* and *S. haematobium.* Test results are sometimes difficult to interpret because reagents to detect schistosomal infections often cross-react with antibodies produced by other parasitic diseases. In addition, patients in endemic areas frequently have been exposed to *Schistosoma* organisms and exhibit variable immunologic responses that prevent serologic procedures from differentiating between present clinical involvement and chronic multiple exposure. Thus, detailed travel and exposure histories are invaluable in patients who present diagnostic difficulties.

Trichinosis.   Serologic tests to detect antibodies to *Trichinella spiralis*, the causative agent of trichinosis, become positive 3 weeks after the onset of primary infection. Titers rise slowly for several weeks, gradually reach peak levels in about 2 months, and eventually decline over a 2-year period. Although low antibody titers during infection are significant for trichinosis, active clinical cases usually are accompanied by much higher titers, and a fourfold titer increase is required for definite diagnosis. However, low titers should be interpreted with caution because they may represent old or residual antibodies rather than the formation of new antibodies.

Trypanosomiasis. Serologic procedures for *Trypanosoma brucei* antibodies are usually positive in patients with Gambian and Rhodesian trypanosomiasis and positive for *T. cruzi* antibodies in patients with South American trypanosomiasis. South American trypanosomiasis, also known as Chagas' disease, may be spread by blood transfusions or by the bite of the *Triatoma* bug. The African form is spread by the bite of the tsetse fly. In their dormant state, these diseases may be exacerbated by immunosuppressive therapy. However, because of the chronic nature of these diseases, stable titers in the low to moderate range are difficult to interpret.

Normal Values

The normal and clinically significant values for selected parasitic infections are:

Amebiasis

<1:10	Negative; normal
>1:128	Clinically significant for amebic infections
Fourfold titer rise	Diagnostic for amebic infections

Echinococcosis

<1:80	Negative; normal
>1:128	Significant for *Echinococcus* exposure
>1:256	Diagnostic of *Echinococcus* infections

Malaria

<1:10	Negative; normal
>1:64	Indicates past or present malaria infections

Schistosomiasis

Negative	Normal; no past *Schistosoma* exposure
Positive	Indicates past or present clinical involvement

Trichinosis

Negative	Normal
>1:5	Significant for *Trichinella spiralis* infections
Fourfold titer rise	Diagnostic of *Trichinella spiralis* infections

Trypanosomiasis

<1:10	Negative; normal
>1:32 by complement fixation	Significant for acute Chagas' disease
>1:128 by indirect hemagglutination	Significant for Chagas' disease

Methodology

Serologic detection of antibodies for the diagnosis of many parasitic infections requires 5 mL of blood collected in a tube without anticoagulants (red-stoppered tube).

▶▶ ### Nursing Responsibilities and Implications

See Specimen Collection for Serologic Studies—Nursing Responsibilities and Implications. Food or fluid restrictions usually are not necessary.

SEROLOGIC TESTS FOR STREPTOCOCCAL INFECTIONS

Many patients infected with Lancefield group A β-hemolytic streptococci develop antibodies against several of the toxic extracellular enzymes produced by this organism, including streptolysin, deoxyribonuclease, and hyaluronidase. Thus, although not specific for any particular disease, the presence of these antibodies provides reliable evidence of acute streptococcal infections such as scarlet fever, tonsillitis, otitis media, or puerperal sepsis. These diseases frequently follow similar courses, and they can be followed by serial titers or serum levels of streptococcal antibodies, which are more valuable than single titers.

Serologic identification of streptococcal antibodies also is helpful in following the course of poststreptococcal sequelae such as rheumatic fever and acute hemorrhagic glomerulonephritis, which develop 2–3 weeks after the original acute infection. Poststreptococcal diseases are believed to represent allergic reactions to all β-hemolytic streptococci, including the group A strain in which symptoms develop after the organisms have disappeared. Thus, although active streptococcal infections are diagnosed easily by culture, retrospective demonstration of streptococcal antibodies aids diagnosis after the acute stage of illness has passed. The best single test for previous streptococcal infections is the antistreptolysin O (ASO) titer, but greater documentation results when this test is combined with antihyaluronidase (AH) and antideoxyribonuclease B (anti-DNase B) determinations.

Test for Antistreptolysin O Titer

Antistreptolysin O (ASO) antibodies are immunoglobulins to the streptococcal enzyme streptolysin O that develop in the serum of many individuals recently infected with Lancefield group A streptococci. Antistreptolysin O levels in patients with acute streptococcal diseases usually rise significantly 2–5 weeks after infection, reach peak levels 2–4 weeks later, and remain elevated for variable periods. Titers begin falling approximately 4–6 weeks after peaking and gradually return to preinfection levels within 6–12 months.

Normal ASO values vary widely because most patients have experienced streptococcal infections at one time or another, although elevated titers probably are caused by recent infections. However, ASO titers remain elevated in patients with poststreptococcal rheumatic fever and glomerulonephritis even after the initial infection has subsided. Thus, although elevated or rising titers do not indicate whether the acute phase of the infection has passed, high titers persisting for several months strongly suggest a continuing infection.

Clinical Significance

Antistreptolysin O titers of newborns are usually similar to maternal titers but drop sharply before 6 months of age as immunoglobulins received from the maternal bloodstream are eliminated. Children under 2 years of age seldom have ASO titers because streptococcal infections before this age are uncommon. Children 5–12 years of age exhibit high normal titers without apparent infection. Thus, individuals, especially school-aged children who are exposed repeatedly to streptococci, can have ASO antibody levels as high as 200 units without clinical evidence of recent streptococcal infection.

A twofold rise in titer in paired serum specimens collected at 10- to 14-day intervals normally is considered to be reliable evidence of recent streptococcal infection. However, such twofold increases in titer may occur but not exceed the upper limits of normal, making it impossible to confirm or eliminate streptococci as a possible cause of illness. On the other hand, single titers frequently have relative significance when compared with the accepted normal limits of test results and when they are considered with other laboratory findings in light of the patient's clinical symptoms. Thus, although information provided by a single titer is limited, such interpretation becomes necessary when ASO titers are not measured until the patient is well into the convalescent stage and peak titers already have been reached.

Patients with recent group A streptococcal infections may exhibit elevated titers of 200–2500 units, whereas those with rheumatic fever may have titers as high as 7500 units. Generally, the greater the antibody response (higher number of units), the more severe the infection. However, early antibiotic or corticosteroid therapy may inhibit streptolysin O production, in which case patients with rheumatic fever fail to show the anticipated ASO increase. Thus, persistently elevated ASO titers, especially following antibiotic therapy, are considered strong evidence of rheumatic fever.

Normal Values

The normal and clinically significant values for antistreptolysin O titers are:

Normal	0–200 Todd units
Adults	<120 Todd units
Children	
<2 years	<50 Todd units
2–5 years	<100 Todd units
5–19 years	<200 Todd units
Streptococcal infections	
Adults	>125 Todd units
School-aged children	>250 Todd units
Acute glomerulonephritis	>350 Todd units
Acute rheumatic fever	>500 Todd units

Variations
False-positive antistreptolysin O titers may occur in the absence of streptococcal infections as a result of:

Contaminated serum (*Bacillus cereus, Pseudomonas* species)	Hyperglobulinemia
	Inhibition of test antigen, nonspecific
Hyperbetalipoproteinemia	Lipemic sera, markedly
Hypercholesterolemia	Liver disorders, certain

Falsely decreased antistreptolysin O titers may occur in patients with streptococcal infections accompanied by antibiotic or corticosteroid therapy, antibody deficiency syndromes, and nephrotic syndromes.

Methodology
Identification of antistreptolysin O antibodies requires 5 mL of blood collected aseptically in a tube without anticoagulants (red-stoppered tube).

▶▶ Nursing Responsibilities and Implications
See Specimen Collection for Serologic Studies—Nursing Responsibilities and Implications. Food or fluid restrictions usually are not necessary.

Tests for Antideoxyribonuclease B and Antihyaluronidase

Antideoxyribonuclease B (anti-DNase B) and **antihyaluronidase** (AH) are antibodies against specific toxic extracellular enzymes that develop in many individuals who recently have recovered from group A streptococcal infections. These antibodies inhibit the activity of the deoxyribonuclease B and hyaluronidase exozymes in the serum of patients with acute rheumatic fever, pyodermic skin infections, or poststreptococcal sequelae such as glomerulonephritis. Thus, serologic detection of increasing anti-DNase B or AH titers is a good indication of present or past group A streptococcal infections.

An additional test, the **streptozyme (STZ) procedure**, is used as a simple screening method for all antibodies to extracellular antigens produced during streptococcal pharyngitis, rheumatic fever, pyoderma, glomerulonephritis, or other related conditions. Streptozyme tests detect more positive specimens than any other single test for streptococcal antibodies, although single determinations are not as significant as serial titrations performed at weekly or biweekly intervals. Sequential determinations performed for up to 6 weeks following streptococcal infections help evaluate the patient's antibody response and guide clinical conclusions regarding the course of the disease and its treatment. In addition, factors that produce false-positive ASO tests, such as lipemia and liver disease, do not influence the AH, anti-DNase B, or STZ tests.

Clinical Significance
The anti-DNase B test is probably the best single procedure for the serologic detection of recent hemolytic streptococcal infection and frequently is preferred over ASO titers when acute rheumatic fever or poststreptococcal glomerulonephritis is suspected. Antideoxyribonuclease B levels increase more reliably than ASO antibodies following streptococcal skin infections, whereas the incidence of elevated titers equals that of ASO titers in acute rheumatic fever but decreases in poststreptococcal glomerulonephritis. Determination

of anti-DNase B levels commonly is used to evaluate complications of streptococcal pyoderma such as acute poststreptococcal glomerulonephritis because titers generally develop later, rise higher, and persist longer than ASO titers. Tests for anti-DNase B also are particularly useful in evaluating possible Sydenham's chorea, which has a long latent period, because the peak rise in titer occurs later than the peak elevation in ASO titers.

Conversely, AH antibody titers are elevated in most patients with streptococcal respiratory infections but less often in skin infections and have less significance than ASO titers when used alone. Therefore, because titers peak and decline before ASO antibodies reach peak levels, tests for AH antibodies are most useful as a secondary test accompanying the ASO titer to confirm a diagnosis of streptococcal infection.

Normal Values
The normal and clinically significant values for antideoxyribonuclease B, antihyaluronidase, and streptozyme tests are:

Streptozyme	Negative
Antideoxyribonuclease B	
Adults	<85 units
Children	
Preschool	<60 units
School-aged	<170 units
Antihyaluronidase	
Normal	<250 units
Rheumatic fever	>1024 units

Variations
False-negative antideoxyribonuclease B determinations may occur in individuals with hemorrhagic pancreatitis whose serum contains endogenous deoxyribonuclease B enzymes.

Methodology
Antideoxyribonuclease B and antihyaluronidase determinations require 5 mL of blood collected aseptically in a tube without anticoagulants (red-stoppered tube). The streptozyme test requires 5 mL of blood collected in a tube without anticoagulants or with heparin (green-stoppered tube).

▶▶ ### Nursing Responsibilities and Implications
See Specimen Collection for Serologic Studies—Nursing Responsibilities and Implications. Food or fluid restrictions usually are not necessary.

Test for C-Reactive Protein

C-reactive protein (CRP) is an abnormal plasma protein that appears in the bloodstream during the acute stage of various infectious and noninfectious inflammatory disorders but is undetectable in healthy persons. C-reactive protein appears in the serum

12–14 hours after the onset of an inflammatory process, reaches peak levels within 48–72 hours, and rapidly falls as the condition abates. Persistently elevated test results indicate a continuation of the inflammatory process, whereas the reappearance of CRP following successful treatment indicates an exacerbation of the condition. Because CRP values usually decrease following adequate treatment of the inflammatory process, levels normally increase again only if the disease is reactivated.

Elevated CRP values may occur in many diseases, including rheumatic fever, rheumatoid arthritis, and acute bacterial or viral infections such as active pulmonary tuberculosis, pneumococcal pneumonia, and active streptococcal pharyngitis. Likewise, CRP has been demonstrated in patients with disseminated lupus erythematosus, myocardial infarction, malignant tumors, gout, pregnancy after the first trimester, and various oral contraceptive preparations or intrauterine devices. C-reactive protein concentrations also rise after surgical trauma, reach peak levels 2 days after surgery, and gradually subside in the absence of surgical complications but remain high if inflammation develops.

Thus, the presence of CRP in the serum, peritoneal or synovial fluid, and serous exudates reflects to some degree the extent and severity of the inflammatory condition or tissue necrosis. However, although CRP is a clinically significant acute-phase reactant, its lack of specificity eliminates it as a diagnostic tool. C-reactive protein generally is used to assess the clinical course of disease and evaluate the progress of therapy in patients with acute rheumatic fever or rheumatoid arthritis.

Clinical Significance

Because healthy individuals do not have demonstrable CRP in their serum or tissue fluids, the presence of any amount of this protein indicates an active inflammatory process. C-reactive protein values increase more quickly during infection or tissue destruction than the erythrocyte sedimentation rate (ESR) and are a more significant indicator of an acute inflammatory process than an elevated ESR. In addition, CRP determinations give fewer false-positive reactions than other indicators of inflammation such as temperature, white blood cell count, and the ESR.

Because CRP usually is found during the acute phases of rheumatic fever and rheumatoid arthritis, test values are used to monitor the response to therapy in patients with these diseases. However, despite adequate therapy, elevated CRP levels frequently reappear and remain elevated in patients with rheumatic fever when treatment is discontinued, indicating a continuation of rheumatic activity. Elevated CRP levels, particularly in cerebrospinal fluid, aid the differential diagnosis of meningitis and are more sensitive in differentiating bacterial from nonbacterial meningitis than any other single test. C-reactive protein tests also may be used to distinguish upper urinary tract infections with renal involvement from lower urinary tract infections.

Normal Values

The normal and clinically significant values for C-reactive protein are:

Qualitative	Negative
Quantitative	<12 mg/L

Variations

False-positive C-reactive protein tests may occur in older individuals as a result of various degenerative, subclinical, or occult diseases. Normal or negative sera also may produce false-positive test results when specimens are refrigerated or frozen for several days before testing.

Methodology

C-reactive protein determinations require 5 mL of blood collected without anticoagulants (red-stoppered tube) and delivered to the laboratory as soon as possible for prompt testing.

▶▶ **Nursing Responsibilities and Implications**

See Specimen Collection for Serologic Studies—Nursing Responsibilities and Implications.

SEROLOGIC TESTS FOR SYPHILIS

Syphilis, a disease caused by the pathogenic spirochete *Treponema pallidum*, usually is contracted through sexual contact, although congenital infection also may result from primary or chronic infection of the mother during pregnancy. The first symptom of syphilis is a solitary lesion or primary chancre that develops at the invasion site (usually the anogenital region) about 3 weeks after initial contact with the organism. These firm, inflamed, ulcerated lesions release an exudate containing live spirochetes, which are visible by dark-field microscopic examination.

Primary lesions heal spontaneously within 2–4 weeks, and the spirochetes invade neighboring tissues, where, if untreated, they produce secondary lesions, including sore throat, fever, and skin rash, within 2 weeks to 6 months. Infectious spirochetes from these secondary lesions may be demonstrated by dark-field examination and may recur during the next 2–4 years, after which symptoms subside and the disease becomes latent. After years of dormancy, the infection may move into the tertiary stage, in which a variety of characteristic disorders can occur. Syphilis that remains untreated over a period of many years can cause severe bone, visceral, cardiovascular, mental, and central nervous system damage and can result in death.

The presence of spirochetes, whether obtained from active primary or secondary lesions or from affected lymph nodes, confirms the diagnosis of syphilis. However, because primary lesions produce only mild discomfort and frequently pass unnoticed, the patient often fails to seek medical attention until spirochetes are no longer present in the lesion. In addition, dark-field procedures are not always reliable because even small doses of penicillin taken before the chancre appears can greatly impair identification of the causative agent.

Therefore, because specimens from lesions are seldom available for dark-field identification of treponemal spirochetes, serologic tests to detect antibodies produced by *T. pallidum* infection generally are used to diagnose syphilis. Serologic tests for syphilis are divided into two general groups: nontreponemal antibody tests, including VDRL (Venereal Disease Research Laboratories) and RPR (Rapid Plasma Reagin) to detect reagin, and treponemal antibody tests, including FTA-ABS (fluorescent treponemal antibody absorption) (Table 11-2). Syphilis should be diagnosed only after complete evaluation of clinical findings and laboratory tests to identify the antibodies that develop following *T. pallidum* invasion.

In many states serologic tests for syphilis are mandatory for marriage applicants and maternity patients before or after delivery to reduce the incidence of congenital syphilis.

TABLE 11-2   Expected Serologic Findings in Syphilis

Stage	Latent Period	VDRL*	FTA-ABS†
Primary	2–6 weeks	Early: >50% reactive Late: >75% reactive	85% reactive
Secondary	9–12 weeks	>98% reactive (unusually high titer >1:32)	100% reactive
Latent	6 months to 2 years	>60% reactive (unusually low titer)	97% reactive
Tertiary	10–40 years	70% reactive (unusually low titer)	95% reactive
After treatment	—	Variable	Reactive for years or life despite therapy

*Venereal Disease Research Laboratories.
†Fluorescent treponemal antibody absorption test.

The greatest risk of congenital infection results from transplacental transmission of treponemal spirochetes to the fetus during the first 4 months of gestation if the mother remains untreated. Although treatment late in pregnancy cures both the mother and fetus, it will not prevent congenital anomalies. Therefore, proper prenatal care and early treatment are vital in the prevention of fetal infection and anomalies.

Although it is easy to diagnose syphilis in infants who are born with a variety of overt clinical symptoms, diagnosis is problematic in apparently normal infants whose mothers are known syphilitics. For example, passive transfer of antibodies from the mother to fetus may cause the reagin and FTA-ABS tests to be reactive in infants who lack evidence of infection. Any treponemal antibodies detected in the infant's blood as a result of passive transmission from the mother will not exceed the maternal titer and will rapidly decrease in 2–4 months. Thus, an apparently normal infant with a reactive VDRL creates a diagnostic problem of whether the reaction is caused by the passive transfer of maternal antibodies or active infection in the infant. In addition, serologic tests also should be performed on all infants with congenital syphilis because a reactive VDRL test on cerebrospinal fluid provides reliable evidence of neurosyphilis.

Tests for Nontreponemal Antibodies

Nontreponemal antibody tests are designed to detect the presence of a nonspecific antibody-like substance, called **reagin**, that is stimulated by the invasion of *T. pallidum* into the body. However, as the amount of time following the appearance of primary syphilis chancres increases, the possibility of isolating treponemal organisms decreases. Therefore, serologic tests for syphilis depend on demonstrating antibodies stimulated by the treponemal organisms and usually respond to reagin or treponemal antibodies 1–3 weeks after appearance of the primary lesion.

The most common and reliable nontreponemal tests currently used to detect reagin are the **VDRL (Venereal Disease Research Laboratories)** and **ART (automated reagin test)** procedures. Although nontreponemal screening procedures are useful for detecting primary and secondary syphilis, reagin tests are generally negative during the early, contagious phase of the disease. When clinically suspicious symptoms are accompanied by negative test results, serologic studies should be continued weekly for 8 weeks to detect any developing reagin or antibodies. These antibodies produce reactive test results that remain at significant levels until sufficient therapy is administered. However, because late syphilis produces variable titers, VDRL screening tests may decline or even become nonreactive in some patients as untreated syphilis progresses to the late latent or tertiary phase.

These serologic screening tests may be used both qualitatively and quantitatively to detect the presence of syphilis reagin in serum or cerebrospinal fluid. All qualitatively reactive specimens are tested with serial dilutions and reported as the highest titer producing a reaction to confirm the diagnosis of syphilis and follow the course of treatment.

Clinical Significance

VDRL titers usually respond to therapy by reverting to nonreactive levels during primary and secondary syphilis, although this reversion rarely occurs in latent or tertiary syphilis. In general, the longer the syphilis has been established before treatment begins, the longer some degree of test reactivity persists before the test reverts to nonreactive. Occasionally, however, even massive and prolonged treatment fails to reduce nontreponemal antibody titers to nonreactive levels, and screening tests remain reactive.

Test results are reported with the terms "reactive" (definite flocculation with test antigen), "weakly reactive" (slight flocculation), and "nonreactive" (no flocculation) replacing the older terms "positive," "doubtful," and "negative." The terminology has been changed to prevent false presumptions concerning the presence or absence of syphilis in a patient. However, when tests do not confirm the diagnosis of syphilis in a patient with clinical evidence of the disease, more specific treponemal antibody tests, such as the FTA-ABS, are warranted.

Normal Values

The normal and clinically significant values for nontreponemal antibody tests are:

Qualitative	Nonreactive
Quantitative	
<1:8	Biologic false-positives
>1:32	Advance of disease from primary to secondary stage

Variations

Reactive or weakly reactive test findings indicate the presence of reagin, which almost invariably results from a treponemal infection. However, reagin also may be found in a number of patients who are not infected with treponemes due to conditions other than syphilis. These results are known as biologic false-positives and may be either acute or chronic.

Acute biologic false-positives, in which the VDRL reverts to nonreactive within 6 months, generally are associated with:

Atypical pneumonia

Bejel

Chickenpox

DPT immunization in children

Infectious hepatitis

Infectious mononucleosis

Malaria

Measles

Pneumococcal pneumonia

Scarlet fever

Smallpox vaccination

Subacute bacterial endocarditis

Tuberculosis

Chronic biologic false-positives, in which the reaction persists for more than 6 months, have been associated with:

Hyperglobulinemia

Leprosy

Leptospirosis

Periarteritis nodosa

Pinta

Rheumatic fever

Rheumatoid arthritis

Systemic lupus erythematosus

Thyroiditis

Vaccinia

Yaws

Other factors that contribute less frequently to the problem of biologic false-positives include:

Advanced age (eighth decade)

Collagen vascular diseases

Common cold

Heroin addiction

Hypertensive drugs

Pregnancy

Tissue regeneration

When false-positive reactions are suspected, serologic studies should be repeated at 3- to 6-month intervals because positive reactions due to acute disease usually disappear spontaneously within this period. If positive reactions persist in the absence of recognizable disease, treponemal antibody tests are needed to differentiate between true and false-positive reactions.

False-negative VDRL reactions occasionally occur with:

Early syphilis, when the reagin concentration is too low to detect

Errors in test interpretation

Late latent or tertiary syphilis

Presence of alcohol in the blood

Methodology

VDRL screening tests for reagin require 5 mL of blood collected in a tube without anti-coagulants (red-stoppered tube). Blood specimens should be drawn without trauma to prevent hemolysis and before meals to avoid the formation of excessive bile or chyle in the serum. Although mild lipemia does not interfere with VDRL reactions, excessive amounts can obscure the test antigen particles and interfere with the test results.

▶▶ ### Nursing Responsibilities and Implications

See Specimen Collection for Serologic Studies—Nursing Responsibilities and Implications. Food or fluid restrictions may or may not be imposed, depending on the laboratory, but alcohol intake must be avoided for 24 hours prior to testing.

Tests for Treponemal Antibodies

Several treponemal antibody tests are available to diagnose syphilis by detecting specific antibodies produced during infection with the *T. pallidum* spirochete. The **fluorescent treponemal antibody absorption test (FTA-ABS)** is the most sensitive and reliable of the treponemal antibody tests currently available for detecting all stages of syphilis when the diagnosis is in doubt. This confirmatory procedure generally is used to differentiate patients with syphilis from patients with biologic false-positive reactions to VDRL tests.

A variation of this test, the **FTA-ABS IgM**, is highly reliable for diagnosing congenital syphilis because IgM antibodies in fetal or infant blood correlate well with active *T. pallidum* infection. Therefore, detection of antitreponemal IgM antibodies in the blood of newborns is interpreted as evidence of congenital syphilis because these specific antibodies do not cross the placenta. However, a negative FTA-ABS IgM test does not exclude the possibility of *T. pallidum* infection because the neonate may have been infected too late in the pregnancy for the IgM antibody to develop.

The **Treponema pallidum immobilization (TPI) test** is the original treponemal antibody test and the reference procedure for all other tests for syphilis. Although the TPI is difficult to perform, it is still the method of choice for detecting neurosyphilis when the cerebrospinal fluid VDRL gives nonreactive or equivocal results. Additional serologic studies may be necessary to detect treponemal antibodies if early infection is suspected and test results are nonreactive.

Clinical Significance

The FTA-ABS is the most dependable procedure for detecting syphilis in the very early or late stages. For example, it is useful in patients who present diagnostic problems such as those with a reactive VDRL but no clinical evidence of syphilis or clinical symptoms of late syphilis and a nonreactive VDRL. In either case reactive FTA-ABS provides good evidence of past or present syphilis, although it cannot differentiate syphilis from other treponemal diseases such as pinta, yaws, and bejel.

On the other hand, a borderline FTA-ABS cannot be interpreted properly, and follow-up or repeat testing is needed to clarify the results. The FTA-ABS also cannot measure the effectiveness of treatment because therapy usually does not remove specific treponemal antibodies following infection, and tests may remain reactive for life. Thus, it is important to recognize that persistent serologic reactivity may be due either to syphilis that has been cured or to reinfection.

Normal Values

The normal and clinically significant FTA-ABS values are:

Reactive	Confirms the presence of treponemal antibodies
Borderline	Inconclusive; low antibody concentration or technical errors
Nonreactive	No treponemal antibodies detected

Variations

False-positive FTA-ABS reactions occasionally may occur in patients with:

Antinuclear antibodies

Autoimmune disorders

   Rheumatoid arthritis

   Systemic lupus erythematosus

Chronic infection

Cirrhosis of the liver

Diabetes mellitus

Hypergammaglobulinemia

Lymphoma

Pregnancy

Scleroderma

Senescence

Smallpox vaccination

Treponematosus

   Bejel

   Pinta

   Yaws

Methodology

Treponemal antibody tests require 5 mL of blood collected without anticoagulants (red-stoppered tube).

▶▶ **Nursing Responsibilities and Implications**

See Specimen Collection for Serologic Studies—Nursing Reponsibilities and Implications. Food or fluid restrictions usually are not necessary.

SEROLOGIC TESTS FOR TORCH DISEASES

The acronym TORCH has come into general use to represent a group of specific diseases that cause particular problems during pregnancy because of the potential for serious effects on the developing fetus. The letters T, R, C, and H represent toxoplasmosis, rubella, cytomegalovirus, and herpes simplex; the letter O encompasses a variety of disorders, including listeriosis and syphilis.

Testing for toxoplasmosis is discussed under Serologic Tests for Parasitic Infections, testing for syphilis is discussed under Serologic Tests for Syphilis, and testing for rubella, cytomegalovirus, and herpes simplex is discussed under Serologic Tests for Viral Infections.

SEROLOGIC TESTS FOR VIRAL INFECTIONS

Tests for Cytomegalovirus

Cytomegalovirus (CMV) is a common herpesvirus that frequently resides as a latent, localized, asymptomatic infection in many adults but, under certain circumstances, also may cause an active, symptomatic infection. Latent CMV may be reactivated and produce a clinical illness that resembles infectious mononucleosis in patients with immunologic deficiencies or those receiving multiple transfusions or immunosuppressive therapy following organ transplants. The highest risk of primary CMV infection occurs, however, when tissues from a seropositive donor are transplanted into a seronegative recipient. Pregnant women with primary infection also may transmit congenital CMV to the fetus through the placenta, by contact with an infected cervix during birth, or in maternal milk or colostrum. Pregnant women who demonstrate mononucleosis-like symptoms should be tested for CMV.

In the majority of fetal CMV infections, no immediate clinical evidence of abnormalities is found, but about half of the neonates born to infected mothers eventually manifest intensely damaging congenital defects. If the fetus survives, the newborn may be mentally retarded due to microcephaly or other cerebral problems. Frequently, sensorimotor abnormalities are present. Congenitally infected infants frequently appear normal at birth but later manifest bone abnormalities, growth retardation, deafness, visual defects, and chronic gastroenteritis. Other significant fetal problems such as hepatosplenomegaly, increased IgM, conjugated hyperbilirubinemia, cerebral calcifications, jaundice, thrombocytopenia purpura, petechiae, rash, and interstitial pneumonia, which may be present at birth, also have been associated with congenital CMV infection.

Clinical Significance

Viral cultures for the definitive diagnosis of primary or congenital CMV infection should be accompanied by serologic studies on paired acute and convalescent serum samples to confirm the diagnosis. The first serum sample (acute phase) should be taken as soon as clinical signs of infection are recognized, and the second sample (convalescent phase) should be taken 1–2 weeks later. A fourfold increase in antibody titer is the classic requirement for diagnosis of recent or current primary CMV infection, although this finding may not substantiate a latent CMV infection.

Paired serum samples also help confirm suspected exposure to CMV infection when the first serum specimen is collected as soon after exposure as possible. The absence of detectable antibody in the serum at the time of exposure indicates susceptibility; a second sample tested 3–4 weeks later will determine if infection has resulted. Because titers may fluctuate in the apparent absence of active infection, it is more important to show that antibodies were absent in the first specimen but present in the second specimen.

Serologic studies also provide a valuable aid in determining immune status, although testing during pregnancy to evaluate fetal risk is difficult because no specific antibody titer indicates active CMV infection. Antibodies detected in infants under 4 months of age may be of maternal origin, whereas those present in infants over 4–6 months of age are usually due to early postnatal or congenital infection. IgM antibodies often are produced in infants congenitally infected with CMV, are detectable at birth or shortly thereafter, and persist for 200 days or more following primary infection. Thus, the presence of IgM antibodies in children under 2 years of age may be helpful in documenting primary infection but not necessarily a current or very recent infection. Test interpretation has several pitfalls, however, because IgM antibodies appear not only during primary infection but also during reinfection and frequently produce false-positive and false-negative results.

Normal Values

The clinically significant cytomegalovirus values are:

Indirect fluorescent antibody tests

IgG antibodies

<1:16	Susceptibility to CMV infection
>1:16 on a single serum sample	Positive for CMV antibodies; not diagnostic of recent infection
<Twofold increase in paired serum samples	Positive for CMV antibodies; not diagnostic of recent infection
>Fourfold increase in paired serum samples	Diagnostic of recent or current CMV infection

IgM antibodies

<1:8	No detectable CMV IgM antibodies
>1:8	Positive for current infection

Variations

False-positive cytomegalovirus IgM test reactions may result from cross-reactivity with the rheumatoid factor and human herpesviruses, including Epstein-Barr virus, varicella, and herpes simplex virus.

Methodology

Serologic studies for CMV require 5 mL of blood collected aseptically in a tube without anticoagulants (red-stoppered tube). Because clear serum is essential for most serologic studies, specimens should be collected without hemolysis, lipemia, or bacterial contamination, which may interfere with indirect fluorescent antibody tests.

▶▶ **Nursing Responsibilities and Implications**

See Specimen Collection for Serologic Studies—Nursing Responsibilities and Implications. Food or fluid restrictions usually are not necessary.

Tests for Viral Hepatitis

The term **viral hepatitis** includes at least three different diseases, each produced by a separate organism: hepatitis A virus (HAV), hepatitis B virus (HBV), and the uncharacterized group of non-A, non-B (NANB) hepatitis viruses. Recovery from type A hepatitis produces a long-lasting immunity against the HAV organism, whereas recovery from type B hepatitis provides long-lasting immunity against that virus. However, these viruses do not provide cross immunity, and individuals who are immune to HBV can still contract HAV and vice versa.

Hepatitis A, formerly called infectious hepatitis, is an acute disease with a characteristically short incubation period of 2–6 weeks. In this form of hepatitis, chronic or carrier states usually do not develop. Patients with HAV complain of sudden fever, gastrointestinal tract disorders, lethargy, headaches, and anorexia within 1 month of exposure to HAV, followed by right upper quadrant pain and jaundice. Because HAV usually is transmitted by infected milk, water, or food, infections often occur following the ingestion of raw or undercooked seafood, usually shellfish, caught in waters contaminated with human waste. Although fecal-oral contamination is the more common mode of HAV infection, personal contact with infected individuals also may contribute to the spread of the disease via the respiratory tract.

Excretion of HAV in blood and feces usually occurs 2–3 weeks before the onset of clinical symptoms and lasts for a short time. Thus, although HAV usually is undetectable by the time the patient consults a physician, its specific antibodies appear early in the acute phase of the disease and persist for years after recovery. Therefore, measurement of HAV antibodies is more useful in diagnosis than detecting HAV antigens.

Hepatitis B, previously known as serum hepatitis, has a 6- to 26-week incubation period. Chronic carriers frequently occur, a state that is related closely to age and socioeconomic and geographic factors. Type B hepatitis usually is associated with parenteral drug abuse or post-transfusion sequelae because the infection is spread primarily by contact with blood and other body fluids. Therefore, individuals who have received multiple blood transfusions, patients on hemodialysis, individuals with hemophilia, newborns, homosexual men, parenteral drug abusers, and health care professionals are particularly at risk of infection.

The onset of hepatitis B is insidious and characterized by jaundice, which develops slowly and persists for many months, and the gradual development of fatigue, arthralgia, and arthritis. Clinical manifestations of hepatitis B may range from subclinical infections, to liver damage with jaundice, to fulminant hepatitis that may lead to early death in severe cases. Individuals in close contact with an infected person may contract the infection, especially the sexual partners of patients with hepatitis B.

The appearance of HBV surface antigens indicates an infection of unknown duration because the causative agent of this disease is present in the viral coat of the hepatitis B organism. As the disease progresses, hepatitis B core and "e" antigens appear and may be used to follow the disease through convalescence, development of chronic active hepatitis, or the chronic carrier state. Occasionally, the antibody to hepatitis core antigen may be the only indicator of HBV activity if testing occurs after clearance of the surface antigen but before the appearance of its antibody. The presence of hepatitis B surface and "e" antigens for 8–10 weeks or longer following initial testing generally indicates the development of a chronic carrier state and the possibility of cirrhosis.

The high incidence of chronic infections and chronic carriers without specific HAV or HBV markers makes non-A, non-B (NANB) hepatitis a tremendous source of public health concern, particularly in blood donor screening. Non-A, non-B hepatitis may include systemic liver diseases accompanied by cytomegalovirus, Epstein-Barr virus, rubella, herpes simplex virus, or enteroviruses. Such disorders currently are diagnosed by excluding the possibility of HAV and HBV because at present there are no serologic markers specific for the NANB virus. Non-A, non-B hepatitis mainly is transmitted through contaminated blood to individuals who have received multiple blood transfusions, although patients with hemophilia, individuals receiving hemodialysis, and parenteral drug abusers are also at increased risk of infection.

Clinical Significance

The clinical symptoms associated with hepatitis A, hepatitis B, and NANB hepatitis often are so similar that it is impossible to make a definitive diagnosis without the use of serologic markers. Hepatitis A and hepatitis B viruses produce a variety of antigens and antibodies in human blood that follow distinctive serologic patterns during the course of infection. Therefore, it is possible not only to diagnose the type of hepatitis by identifying these serologic patterns but also to monitor the stages of the infection and determine the probable prognosis. Tests for serologic markers also are used to evaluate asymptomatic patients for infectivity or carrier status, determine the immune status of individuals at risk of exposure, and identify candidates for HBV vaccination.

There are at least seven distinct serologic markers associated with HAV and HBV, the identification of which may be used to evaluate susceptibility, infection, or immunity to the disease. These markers, which may be identified singly or in panels, include the hepatitis A antibody (anti-HAV), hepatitis B surface antigen (HBsAg) and antibody (anti-HBs), hepatitis B core antibody (anti-HBc), and the hepatitis B "e" antigen (HBeAg) and antibody (anti-HBe). A screening panel for viral hepatitis measures anti-HAV, HBsAg and anti-HBs, and anti-HBc; no routine tests are available at present for the clinical diagnosis of hepatitis A viral antigen. The panel of tests to evaluate the significance of hepatitis B markers includes HBsAg, anti-HBs, and anti-HBc; the hepatitis B "e" panel includes HBeAg and anti-HBe markers.

The presence of **hepatitis A antibody (anti-HAV)** indicates that the patient has been exposed to HAV but does not differentiate between a recent acute infection and one that is past or preexisting. Two specific antibody markers, anti-HAV IgM and anti-HAV IgG, provide a valuable guide to previous exposure and immunity. Anti-HAV IgM antibodies appear 2–4 weeks after exposure to HAV and are detectable for only 4–8 weeks during the acute phase of the infection. Detection of the anti-HAV IgM antibody usually coincides with the appearance of clinical symptoms and is the best serologic marker for confirming a recent acute HAV infection. Anti-HAV IgG antibody replaces anti-HAV IgM as a serologic marker during the convalescent phase of hepatitis A. Anti-HAV IgG antibodies persist for life, granting immunity from reinfection by HAV.

Hepatitis B surface antigen (HBsAg), the earliest indicator of hepatitis B infection, develops 2–4 weeks before demonstrable liver disease or the appearance of clinical symptoms. The HBsAg marker normally reaches peak concentrations at the onset of clinical disease and declines to undetectable levels within 4–6 weeks. However, because HBsAg may persist after the clinical signs of acute infection and liver damage have disappeared, its presence in the patient's serum also may be an indicator of chronic infection. Therefore, all blood, stool, sputum, and other specimens that are reactive for HBsAg should be considered capable of transmitting HBV. Hepatitis B surface antigen previously was known as Australia antigen or hepatitis-associated antigen, but these terms are outdated and confusing because several hepatitis-associated antigens have been identified.

Antibody to hepatitis B surface antigen (anti-HBs) appears during the latter phase of hepatitis B infection, normally 2–16 weeks after HBsAg is no longer detectable, and may persist for years. However, although this marker generally is not detected until the infection has been eradicated, it also can coexist with circulating antigens. Thus, the presence of anti-HBs usually indicates clinical recovery and subsequent immunity to HBV but cannot be taken as evidence that the infection has been overcome. Anti-HBs also may appear in the blood following passive transmission in blood products.

Antibody to hepatitis B core antigen (anti-HBc) is an early indicator of recent acute hepatitis B infection that usually persists for many years. Anti-HBc develops shortly after the appearance of HBsAg and remains as a lifelong marker, indicating past infection as well as active infection in the acute/chronic period. This core antibody marker is the best and most reliable indicator of recent acute HBV infection in the absence of HBsAg and anti-HBs. Thus, the presence of anti-HBc in a patient currently or recently ill or in one who recently has received blood strongly suggests hepatitis B infection.

Hepatitis B "e" antigen (HBeAg) is an early indicator of acute active infection that becomes detectable before the onset of symptoms and usually persists for only 3–6 weeks. The appearance of HBeAg represents the most infectious period of the disease and identifies patients who pose the greatest threat of transmitting hepatitis B infection. Because this marker disappears after infection ceases and the patient recovers completely, its presence indicates ongoing or very recent hepatocellular infection or progression to a chronic, infectious carrier state. Persistence of HBeAg for longer than 3 months after the onset of acute illness suggests an unfavorable clinical prognosis and a risk to the patient of chronic liver disease.

The presence of **antibody to hepatitis B "e" antigen (anti-HBe)** indicates termination of active hepatitis B, diminished viral reactivity, and a good prognosis for resolution of acute infection. The anti-HBe marker develops after anti-HBc but before anti-HBs and persists for many years, indicating both recovery and immunity to HBV. The combined presence of anti-HBe and anti-HBc in the absence of HBsAg and anti-HBs also confirms the recent acute stage of hepatitis B infection. The presence of anti-HBe in patients who are chronic carriers of HBsAg indicates an asymptomatic, "healthy" carrier state. Measurement of both HBeAg and anti-HBe provide more useful information than separate determinations of either marker and should be ordered only in patients with recent hepatitis B infection documented by the presence of HBsAg, anti-HBs, or anti-HBc.

Normal Values

The normal and clinically significant values pertaining to viral hepatitis are:

Hepatitis A Antibodies

Anti-HAV IgM	Anti-HAV IgG	Significance
Negative	Negative	Susceptible to HAV infection
Positive	Negative	Onset of acute hepatitis A infection
Negative	Positive	Convalescent phase; immunity to HAV reinfection

Hepatitis B Profile

HBsAg	Anti-HBs	HBeAg	Anti-HBe	Anti-HBc	Significance
Negative	Negative	Negative	Negative	Negative	Susceptible to HBV infection; early incubation after HBV exposure
Positive	Negative	Negative	Negative	Negative	Very early stage of acute hepatitis B infection; patient infectious
Positive	Negative	Positive	Negative	Negative	Early stage of acute hepatitis B; very infectious, greatest risk of transmitting infection

(continued)

Normal Values *(Continued)*

Positive	Negative	Positive	Negative	Positive	Acute phase of HBV infection; chronic carrier, remains infectious
Positive	Negative	Positive	Positive	Positive	Late in acute phase; improvement of chronic carrier
Positive	Negative	Negative	Positive	Positive	Late in acute phase; improvement of chronic carrier
Negative	Negative	Negative	Positive	Positive	Convalescent phase
Negative	Negative	Negative	Negative	Positive	Convalescent phase; may remain many years after acute viremic state
Negative	Positive	Negative	Positive	Positive	Recovery phase; no longer infectious
Negative	Positive	Negative	Negative	Positive	Recovery phase; remains for years
Negative	Positive	Negative	Negative	Negative	Past infection; passive immunization with surface antibody

Methodology

Complete evaluation of viral hepatitis requires 15 mL of blood collected in a tube without anticoagulants (red-stoppered tube). Individual HAV and HBV antigen or antibody tests require 5 mL of blood collected without anticoagulants.

▶▶ Nursing Responsibilities and Implications

See Specimen Collection for Serologic Studies—Nursing Responsibilities and Implications. Food and fluid restrictions usually are not necessary.

Test for Herpes Simplex Virus

Herpes simplex virus (HSV) is a common infectious agent with two structural variants containing similar antigens that produce a variety of clinical disorders. However, HSV-1 and HSV-2 recently have been commonly isolated from sites classically infected by the other type. Herpes simplex virus type 1 (HSV-1) invades the eyes, mouth, or upper respiratory tract, where it is a common cause of cold sores and severe sporadic encephalitis in adults. Herpes simplex virus type 2 (HSV-2) infects the urogenital tract, where it is transmitted by sexual contact. Herpes simplex virus also can be transmitted to the neonate during vaginal delivery. Herpes simplex virus has been implicated in cervical cancer and aseptic meningitis. Herpes simplex virus generally remains latent following primary infection but may be reactivated by fever, emotional stress, or hormonal imbalance and is accompanied by recurrent clinical symptoms.

Nurses, dental workers, and hospital personnel may contract HSV infections if minor abrasions on their fingers or hands come in contact with saliva, lesions, or mucous membranes contaminated with the virus. Primary or recurrent HSV infections acquired early in pregnancy increase the risk of abortion or congenital herpes as the virus ascends to the fetus from lesions in the genital tract. Many cases of neonatal herpes develop after birth and are associated with transfer of the organism from lesions in the mother, father, or hospital personnel or HSV in breast milk.

However, the greatest risk of neonatal herpes occurs at delivery as the infant comes in contact with infected genital secretions during passage through the birth canal of a mother with active genital herpes. The effects of neonatal herpes may be nonexistent or range from mild eye infection and skin rash to a fatal systemic infection of the liver, heart, or adrenals. Newborns severely affected with congenital herpes may develop central nervous system disorders resulting in permanent brain damage with microcephaly and intracranial calcification.

Clinical Significance

Herpes antibodies usually appear during the first week of primary infection and persist for 6 months but may be detectable throughout the patient's life. Herpes antibodies found in infants under 4 months of age are normally of maternal origin, whereas those found in infants over 6 months of age generally result from early postnatal or congenital infection. Although viral cultures are most useful in the accurate diagnosis of herpes infections, serologic tests are an important guide to the immune status of pregnant women and successful management of genital herpes.

However, because HSV-1 and HSV-2 share common antigens, detection of one type of antibody may not be diagnostic for that infective agent unless the serum shows no antibody titer for the other type. Thus, serologic tests for herpes simplex infections usually are performed with HSV-1 antigen, and if the initial test is negative, a second test is performed with HSV-2 antigen before the serum is reported as negative. If a sample is negative on HSV-1 substrate and positive on HSV-2 substrate, it is considered to indicate HSV-2 infection. In addition, a fourfold or greater rise in antibody titer between acute and convalescent serum specimens is required to indicate infection because no single serologic test should be considered diagnostic.

Normal Values

The normal and clinically significant values for herpes simplex virus are:

$<1:10$	Negative for herpes simplex antibodies
$1:10-1:100$	Early (7 days) primary herpes simplex infection
$1:100-1:500$	Current late primary herpes simplex infection
$>1:500$	Established latent herpes simplex infection

Methodology

Herpes simplex virus antibody determinations require 5 mL of blood collected aseptically in a tube without anticoagulants (red-stoppered tube). Because clear serum is essential for serologic testing, specimens must be free from hemolysis, bacterial contamination, and lipemia.

▶▶ ## Nursing Responsibilities and Implications

See Specimen Collection for Serologic Studies—Nursing Responsibilities and Implications.

Tests for Infectious Mononucleosis

Infectious mononucleosis (IM) is an acute infectious disease that primarily affects children or young adults and is characterized by abnormal lymphocytes, numerous monocytes, and the production of heterophil antibodies. Laboratory identification of high heterophil antibody titers or specific Epstein-Barr virus (EBV) antibodies, combined with the clinical and hematologic profiles characteristic of IM, are considered diagnostic for this disease.

The term **heterophil** refers to a group of antibodies that react with antigens other than the specific antigen responsible for its production. Heterophil antibody tests are nonspecific screening procedures for the presence of agglutinins reacting to the red blood cells of sheep or horses that are associated with IM. Sheep and horse red blood cells apparently share a common antigen with the EBV and are used as a reagent to detect infection because heterophil antibodies agglutinate them.

Heterophil antibody tests become positive 3–10 days after infection, reach peak concentrations within 3 weeks, and remain elevated for 6 weeks or more. However, because tests may remain negative for up to 4 weeks after infection, repeat testing is often necessary when clinical symptoms persist. Heterophil antibody titers normally subside gradually during the 8–12 weeks following complete recovery and eventually disappear but may remain elevated for up to 1 year after onset of the disease.

Heterophil antibody procedures include the Paul-Bunnell test, which detects the presence of these antibodies, and the Davidsohn differential test, which identifies various heterophil antibodies from their characteristic agglutination patterns. Most elevated Paul-Bunnell tests require further investigation with the Davidsohn differential test to verify the diagnosis of IM. The degree of titer elevation in the Davidsohn differential test is unimportant because any positive result is diagnostic for the disease.

The **Epstein-Barr virus** (EBV) is a herpesvirus that infects human lymphoid cells and has been identified as the causative agent of IM. Infection with the EBV stimulates the production of antibodies to several viral antigens, the most well defined being against the protein coat known as the viral capsid antigen (EB-VCA). Antibodies to EB-VCA develop 1–2 weeks after the onset of IM, reach peak titers within 3–4 weeks, and decline to lower titers, which persist indefinitely.

IgG antibodies to EB-VCA appear in all individuals with past EBV infection who remain carriers, whereas IgM antibodies to EB-VCA are found only in individuals with primary infection. Thus, the absence of EBV antibodies excludes the diagnosis of acute IM and identifies individuals who have never been infected and are susceptible to primary infection. The persistence of EBV titers provides a dependable indicator of immunity, although in rare instances the disease may recur. The elevation of EBV titers does not correlate with the severity of IM.

Clinical Significance

The presumptive heterophil antibody test (Paul-Bunnell test) is currently the most popular procedure for diagnosing acute IM, although it is not absolutely specific for the disease. Heterophil antibodies occur in low titers in most healthy people and in higher titers in patients with other diseases; negative results do not exclude a diagnosis of IM. Measurement of EBV antibody titers, on the other hand, is indicated in patients with negative heterophil antibody tests who exhibit symptoms of a disease resembling IM that cannot be differentiated clinically from IM due to EBV. Serologic studies specific for EBV antibodies are seldom indicated, however, in patients with acute IM because the Davidsohn differential test is diagnostic for the disease.

Two serum specimens are needed to confirm active EBV infection. The first blood specimen (acute serum) should be obtained as soon as possible after the onset of clinical signs of infection, and the second specimen (convalescent serum) should be obtained 1–2 weeks later. Conversion of a single EBV antibody titer from negative to positive or a fourfold increase in antibody titers between acute and convalescent serum specimens is considered diagnostic for a current infection.

Normal Values

The normal and clinically significant test values for infectious mononucleosis are:

Antibodies to Epstein-Barr virus
(EB-VCA)

<1:20	Normal; susceptibility to IM
1:20–1:320 on single specimen	Immunity to IM; not diagnostic for current or recent infection
>1:320 on single specimen	Current or recent infection
<Twofold increase in paired serum samples	Not diagnostic for current or recent infection
>Fourfold increase in paired serum samples	Diagnostic for current infection

Heterophil antibodies

<1:56	Normal; found in healthy patients
1:64–1:224 on single specimen	Inconclusive; requires Davidsohn differential
>1:224	Diagnostic for IM

Davidsohn differential

Any positive result is diagnostic for IM

Variations

False-positive heterophil antibody tests may occur in patients with a variety of upper respiratory tract infections and serum sickness following vaccine injection of horse or rabbit serum. Misleading heterophil antibody titers also may appear following blood transfusions to which blood-group specific substances have been added to neutralize the isoagglutinins.

Methodology
Detection of heterophil or EBV antibodies requires 5 mL of blood collected in a tube without anticoagulants (red-stoppered tube). Because clear serum is essential in most serologic procedures, specimens must be free from hemolysis, bacterial contamination, and lipemia. Acute serum samples should be obtained as soon as possible after the onset of illness, and a second, or convalescent, specimen should be obtained 14–21 days later.

▶▶ ### Nursing Responsibilities and Implications
See Specimen Collection for Serologic Studies—Nursing Responsibilities and Implications.

Test for Rubella

Rubella, also known as German measles or 3-day measles, is a mild, exanthematous viral disease of children and young adults that rarely produces complications. Although the disease itself has little clinical significance, maternal exposure to the rubella virus during the first trimester of pregnancy has the potential to cause congenital malformations or spontaneous fetal abortion. The most common effect of maternal infection is retardation of normal fetal growth, resulting in mental retardation, microcephaly, nerve deafness, cataracts, retinopathy, congenital heart defects, and pulmonary stenosis. The extent of these birth defects depends on the stage of fetal development when the mother becomes infected with rubella. The earlier in the pregnancy the exposure occurs, the larger the risk; the greatest threat of birth defects occurs during the first 2 months of gestation.

Antibody levels rise extremely rapidly during infection with rubella virus, peak within 5–7 days after the onset of the rash, and remain high for many years. Because any amount of antibody produced by prior infection or vaccination will protect the fetus, it is important to know the immune status of pregnant women who are exposed to rubella. Therefore, rubella antibody tests help identify women who are susceptible to the disease and determine whether a rash or illness that develops during the first trimester of pregnancy is due to rubella. In addition, serologic tests to detect antibodies to rubella virus are valuable in determining the immune status of women of childbearing age, preschool children, and hospital personnel.

Clinical Significance
Serologic tests for rubella antibodies are primarily useful when a pregnant woman is exposed to rubella or contracts an illness that resembles rubella. The absence of antibodies at the time of exposure indicates susceptibility to rubella virus. However, because rubella antibodies persist at static levels for many years, a single determination can give little diagnostic information. Therefore, a fourfold or greater rise in antibody titer in two consecutive samples collected 1–2 weeks apart indicates recent rubella infection, whereas a stable or declining titer indicates past infection.

The presence of rubella antibodies shortly after exposure to the disease indicates prior infection and immunity that protects the fetus; negative results in the second sample indicate that infection has not occurred. A rising titer in subsequent specimens, however, confirms the diagnosis of rubella infection and probable damage to the fetus. On the other hand, when the initial specimen contains rubella antibodies and subsequent specimens have significantly higher titers, there is no way to determine the significance. For example, the increase may result from primary rubella infection and threaten the fetus or be due to secondary infection and renewed antibody production with no risk to the fetus.

Early postnatal or congenital rubella infection is confirmed by detecting antibodies in the infant's serum above and beyond those transferred passively from the mother (i.e., those that remain 4–6 months after birth). Antibodies in infants under 4 months of age frequently are acquired from the mother and normally fall at the rate of one twofold titer dilution per month. Diagnosis of congenital rubella is aided by serologic tests of acute and convalescent sera, with evidence of infection suggested by a rise in the antibody level.

Normal Values
The clinically significant values for rubella antibodies are:

Hemagglutination inhibition test

<1 : 8	Susceptibility to rubella infection
1 : 8	Immunity uncertain
>1 : 8	Immunity from prior infection or vaccination
>1 : 64	Resistance to rubella infection

Fluorescent antibody test

<1+ fluorescence	Susceptibility to rubella infection
>1+ fluorescence	Positive for rubella antibodies

Methodology
Determination of rubella antibody titers requires 5 mL of blood collected in a tube without anticoagulants (red-stoppered tube). The first sample should be collected no later than 3 days after the onset of illness.

▶▶ Nursing Responsibilities and Implications
See Specimen Collection for Serologic Studies—Nursing Responsibilities and Implications. Food or fluid restrictions usually are not necessary.

REFERENCES

Abbott Laboratories, Diagnostics Division. 1981. *Differential diagnosis and immunologic assessment of viral hepatitis.* North Chicago, Ill.: Abbott Laboratories.

Aloisi, R. M. 1979. *Principles of immunology.* St. Louis: The C. V. Mosby Co.

Bailey, W., and Scott, G. 1982. *Diagnostic microbiology.* 6th. ed. St. Louis: The C. V. Mosby Co.

Bauer, J. D. 1982. *Clinical laboratory methods.* 9th ed. St. Louis: The C. V. Mosby Co.

BBL Division of Becton-Dickinson, and Co. 1974. *Antistreptolysin O titration.* Cockeysville, Md.: BBL Division of Becton-Dickinson, and Co.

Beckmann Instruments, Inc. 1974. *Diagluto I.M. test.* Fullerton, Calif.: Beckmann Instruments, Inc.

Behring Diagnostics, American Hoechst Corp. 1976. *Rapilatex-RF test.* Somersville, N.J.: Behring Diagnostics, American Hoechst Corp.

Bio-Science Laboratories. 1981. *T and B lymphocyte quantitation.* Van Nuys, Calif.: Bio-Science Laboratories.

———. 1982. *The Bio-Science handbook.* 13th ed. Van Nuys, Calif.: Bio-Science Laboratories.

Bologna, C. V. 1971. *Understanding laboratory medicine.* St. Louis: The C. V. Mosby Co.

Calbiochem-Behring Corp. 1980. *Rubella antibody test.* LaJolla, Calif.: Calbiochem-Behring Corp.

———. 1981. *Antistreptolysin O test.* LaJolla, Calif.: Calbiochem-Behring Corp.

Chang, Y. 1983. A guideline to serologic tests for syphilis. *Diagn. Med.* 6(3):51.

———. 1983. Serologic markers of viral hepatitis. *Diagn. Med.* 6(4):28.

Collins, R. D. 1975. *Illustrated manual of laboratory diagnosis.* 2nd ed. Philadelphia: J. B. Lippincott Co.

Commonwealth of Pennsylvania, Department of Public Health. *Teacher's guide to venereal disease education.* Harrisburg, Pa.: Commonwealth of Pennsylvania, Department of Public Health.

Delaat, A. 1984. *Microbiology for the allied health professions.* 3rd ed. Philadelphia: Lea & Febiger.

Diagnostic Products, Organon Inc. 1968. *Rheumanosticon test.* West Orange, N.J.: Diagnostic Products, Organon Inc.

Difco Laboratories. 1976. *Bacto-febrile antigen.* Detroit, Mich.: Difco Laboratories.

Doucet, L. D. 1981. *Medical technology review.* Philadelphia: J. B. Lippincott Co.

Drew, W. L. 1981. Cytomegalovirus. *Clin. Microbiol. Newsletter* 3(16):105.

Electro-Nucleonics Laboratories. 1978. *Antimitochondrial antibody.* Bethesda, Md.: Electro-Nucleonics Laboratories.

———. 1978. *Anti-nDNA test.* Bethesda, Md.: Electro-Nucleonics Laboratories.

———. 1979. *Antibody to herpesvirus hominis.* Bethesda, Md.: Electro-Nucleonics Laboratories.

———. 1979. *Toxoplasma antibody.* Bethesda, Md.: Electro-Nucleonics Laboratories.

———. 1980. *Antibody to rubella virus.* Bethesda, Md.: Electro-Nucleonics Laboratories.

———. 1981. *Antibody to cytomegalovirus.* Bethesda, Md.: Electro-Nucleonics Laboratories.

———. 1981. *Antibody to Epstein-Barr virus.* Bethesda, Md.: Electro-Nucleonics Laboratories.

Fife, K. H., and Corey, L. 1980. Recent advances in the diagnosis of hepatitis. *Lab. Med.* 11(10):649.

French, R. M. 1980. *Guide to diagnostic procedures.* 5th ed. New York: McGraw-Hill Book Co.

Guttmann, R. D., et al. 1981. *Immunology.* Kalamazoo, Mich.: The Upjohn Co.

Henry, J. B. 1984. *Clinical diagnosis and management by laboratory procedures.* 17th ed. Philadelphia: W. B. Saunders Co.

Hyland Division, Travenol Laboratories, Inc. 1974. *CR-test.* Costa Mesa, Calif.: Hyland Division, Travenol Laboratories, Inc.

Kallestad Laboratories, Inc. 1981. *Total IgE Test.* Austin, Tex.: Kallestad Laboratories, Inc.

Lancanster, R. C. 1975. *Listen, look, and learn—serology.* Bethesda, Md.: American Society of Clinical Pathologists.

Larsen, F. C. 1983. *Clinical significance of tests available on the DuPont Automatic Clinical Analyzer.* Wilmington, Del.: DuPont Industries.

Lederle Diagnostics. 1973. *Febrile antigen test.* Pearl River, N.Y.: Lederle Diagnostics.

Lennette, E. H., Spaulding, E. H., and Truant, J. P., editors. 1980. *Manual of microbiology.* 3rd ed. Washington, D.C.: American Society for Microbiology.

Litton Bionetics Laboratory Products. 1980. *Epstein-Barr viral capsid antigen test.* Kensington, Md.: Litton Bionetics Laboratory Products.

———. 1980. *TORCH (Toxoplasma gondii, rubella, CMV, herpes simplex virus) screening test.* Kensington, Md.: Litton Bionetics Laboratory Products.

Marymont, J. H., and Herrmann, K. L. 1982. Rubella testing—an overview. *Lab. Med.* 13(2):83.

MetPath. 1983. *Reference manual.* Teterboro, N.J.: MetPath.

Microbiological Associates. 1980. *ANA and anti-ds DNA test.* Walkersville, Md.: Microbiological Associates.

Microbiological Research Corp. 1979. *Herpes simplex virus test.* Bountiful, Utah: Microbiological Research Corp.

———. 1980. *Test for toxoplasmosis.* Bountiful, Utah: Microbiological Research Corp.

Morse, C. D. 1981. Usefulness of febrile agglutinins. *Clin. Microbiol. Newsletter* 3(16):107.

Nuclear-Medical Laboratories. 1979. *Detection of hepatitis surface antigens.* Dallas, Tex.: Nuclear-Medical Laboratories.

Ophoven, J. 1979. Infectious mononucleosis: serologic aspects. *Lab. Med.* 10(4):203.

Parker, J. 1981. Malignant lymphomas. *Diagn. Med.* 4(3a):77.

Peter, J. B., and Dawkins, R. L. 1979. Evaluating autoimmune diseases. *Diagn. Med.* 2(5):2.

Peter, J. B., Cherry, J. D., and Bryson, Y. J. 1982. Improving diagnostics of congenital infections. *Diagn. Med.* 5(4):61.

Peter, J. B., Bryson, Y. J., and Lovett, M. A. 1983. Genital herpes: urgent questions, elusive answers. *Diagn. Med.* 6(2):7.

Raphael, S. S., editor. 1983. *Medical laboratory technology.* 4th ed. Philadelphia: W. B. Saunders Co.

Rippey, J. H. 1979. Tests for rheumatoid factor. *Lab. Med.* 10(2):97.

Smith, A. L. 1981. *Principles of microbiology.* 9th ed. St. Louis: The C. V. Mosby Co.

Strand, M. M., and Elmer, L. A. 1983. *Clinical laboratory tests.* 3rd ed. St. Louis: The C. V. Mosby Co.

Taborn, J. D., and Walker, S. E. 1979. Rheumatoid factor: a review. *Lab. Med.* 10(7):392.

Tilkian, S. M., Conover, M. B., and Tilkian, A. G. 1983. *Clinical implications of laboratory tests.* 3rd ed. St. Louis: The C. V. Mosby Co.

Van Lente, F. 1982. Rediscovering C-reactive protein. *Diagn. Med.* 5(3):95.

Walls, K. W., and Smith, J. W. 1979. Serology of parasitic infections. *Lab. Med.* 10(6):329.

Widmann, F. K. 1983. *Clinical interpretation of laboratory tests.* 9th ed. Philadelphia: F. A. Davis Co.

Zeus Scientific, Inc. 1979. *Thyroid antibody test system.* Raritan, N.J.: Zeus Scientific, Inc.

12

Immunohematology and Transfusion Therapy

BLOOD TYPES 634
ABO System · Rh System · Other Blood Group Systems

ANTIBODY DETECTION 642
Direct Antiglobulin Test (Direct Coombs' Test) · Antibody Screen
(Indirect Coombs' Test) · Antibody Identification

COMPATIBILITY TESTING 646
Specimen Collection and Handling · Routine Crossmatch · Emergency
Crossmatch · Crossmatching Blood for Newborns and Infants

TRANSFUSION THERAPY 649
Selection of Blood and Alternate Donor Groups · Administration of
Blood · Massive Transfusions

COMPONENT THERAPY 652
Whole Blood · Red Blood Cells · Granulocytes · Platelets
· Cryoprecipitated Antihemophilic Factor · Plasma

TRANSFUSION REACTIONS 661
Investigation of Transfusion Reactions · Acute Hemolytic Transfusion
Reactions · Bacterial Reactions · Circulatory Overload · Febrile
Reactions · Hypersensitivity Reactions · Transmission of Disease via
Transfusion

SELECTION AND SCREENING OF BLOOD DONORS 669
Criteria for Selecting Blood Donors · Criteria for Excluding Blood Donors

Immunohematology is the study of the highly reactive antigens present on red blood cells and their respective serum antibodies. An antigen is any protein substance that can induce an immune response within the body by stimulating the production of a specific antibody capable of reacting against it. Erythrocyte antigens (agglutinogens) are chemical structures that give specific characteristics to the surface of red blood cells and cause them to agglutinate in response to corresponding antibodies (agglutinins).

At least 50 distinct red blood cell characteristics have been identified, and every individual's red blood cells demonstrate a unique combination of antigens. This individuality is not limited to red blood cells, however, because all nucleated body cells, including leukocytes and platelets, also demonstrate a similar, but completely unrelated, degree of differentiation. Individuals usually do not produce antibodies against the numerous antigens on their own cells but will develop antibodies against any foreign antigen present. This is the basis for such problems as hemolytic disease of newborns and incompatible blood transfusions.

Routine immunohematologic studies include blood typing, antibody detection and identification (Coombs' antiglobulin tests), and compatibility testing (crossmatch), which are required for thorough evaluation of both patient and donor blood before transfusion. These immunohematologic studies generally are performed on the cells and serum of clotted blood specimens, which must be collected carefully to prevent hemolysis. Specimens for immunohematologic studies must be labeled clearly with the patient's name and hospital identification number to help avoid the potentially disastrous results of incorrect identification.

BLOOD TYPES

Blood types are inherited characteristics determined by various antigens present on the red blood cells or certain cellular chromosomes and governed by the laws of genetics. At least 13 independent and well-defined blood group systems have been determined by the presence or absence of these numerous properties. The ABO and Rh blood group systems are the most clinically important in crossmatching because the A, B, and Rh substances are strongly antigenic if transfused into individuals who lack them. The HLA antigens of nucleated body cells, as well as a number of additional red blood cell systems, also have been discovered to exist in conjunction with the ABO and Rh groups.

ABO System

The **ABO system** contains four main blood groups: A, B, AB, and O, along with subgroups of group A, designated A_1 and A_2. Blood group letters refer to the antigen or agglutinogen present on the red blood cell surface. Thus, type A blood cells have A agglutinogen, type B cells have B agglutinogen, type AB cells have both A and B agglutinogens, and type O cells have no agglutinogens. Depending on which antigen is present on the red blood cells, the person's serum will contain the reciprocal antibody or agglutinin that reacts with all agglutinogens absent from the blood. Therefore, type A blood serum contains anti-B agglutinin, type B blood serum contains anti-A agglutinin, type AB blood serum contains no agglutinins, and type O blood serum contains both anti-A and anti-B agglutinins (Table 12-1).

TABLE 12-1 Summary of Relationship Between Agglutinogens and Agglutinins in Complete ABO System*

Blood Group	Genotype	Agglutinogen (Antigens on Erythrocytes)	Agglutinin (Antibodies in Serum)	Serum Agglutinates Cells of Groups						Approximate Frequency (%) in United States
				O	A_1	A_2	B	A_1B	A_2B	
O	OO	O	Anti-A_1 Anti-A_2 Anti-B	−	+	+	+	+	+	45
A_1	A^1A^1 A^1A^2 A^1O	A_1	Anti-B	−	−	−	+	+	+	31
A_2	A^2A^2 A^2O	A_2	Anti-B	−	−	−	+	+	+	10
B	BB BO	B	Anti-A_1 Anti-A_2	−	+	+	−	+	+	10
A_1B	A^1B	A_1; B	None	−	−	−	−	−	−	3
A_2B	A^2B	A_2; B	None	−	−	−	−	−	−	1

* + equals agglutination; − equals no agglutination.

Inheritance of ABO Blood Groups

ABO blood groups are determined by a pair of genes composed of various combinations of genes designated O, A, and B. Every individual inherits one gene from each parent to produce a genetic formula, or genotype, which is either homozygous (same gene from each parent) or heterozygous (different genes from each parent). The recognizable blood groups, or phenotypes, resulting from various genetic combinations are governed by the dominant or recessive characteristics of each gene. Thus, the four main ABO blood groups may have the following possible genotypes: type O, genotype OO; type A, genotype AA or AO; type B, genotype BB or BO; and type AB, genotype AB. It can be seen from this that the genes for both A and B are dominant over the recessive O but are codominant and have equal expression when they appear together.

Specific genotypes cannot be identified by laboratory testing and may be determined only through detailed family studies and the evaluation of parental phenotypes. However, the possible phenotypes of children can be predicted from the phenotypes of both mother and father when genetic inheritance patterns are understood (Table 12-2). The principles of ABO blood group inheritance have important legal applications in cases of disputed paternity because careful interpretation of phenotypes can exclude persons with certain ABO groups from parentage.

TABLE 12-2   Blood Types of Parents and Possible Blood Types of Offspring

Parental Phenotypes	Corresponding Parental Genotypes	Possible Phenotypes of Offspring	Impossible Phenotypes of Offspring
O + O	OO + OO	O	A, B, AB
A + A	AA + AA	A	O, B, AB
	AA + AO	A	O, B, AB
	AO + AO	A, O	B, AB
A + O	AA + OO	A	O, B, AB
	AO + OO	A, O	B, AB
A + B	AA + BB	AB	O, A, B
	AO + BB	B, AB	O, A
	AA + BO	A, AB	O, B
	AO + BO	O, A, B, AB	None
A + AB	AA + AB	A, AB	O, B
	AO + AB	A, B, AB	O
B + B	BB + BB	B	O, A, AB
	BO + BB	B	O, A, AB
	BO + BO	B, O	A, AB
B + O	BB + OO	B	O, A, AB
	BO + OO	O, B	A, AB
B + AB	BB + AB	B, AB	O, A
	BO + AB	A, B, AB	O
AB + O	AB + OO	A, B	O, AB
AB + AB	AB + AB	A, B, AB	O

Rules governing the inheritance of the basic ABO system may be summarized as follows:

1. Agglutinogens A or B cannot appear in a child unless they are present in one or both parents.

2. A parent of group AB must transmit agglutinogens for either A or B and therefore cannot have a child of group O.

3. A parent of group O cannot have a child of group AB.

4. Agglutinogens A_1 or A_2 cannot appear in a child unless they are present in at least one of the parents. Thus, a parent of group A_1B cannot have a child of group A_2. On the other hand, a parent of group A_1 with the genotype A^1A^2 can have an A_2 child. Evaluation of genotypes is particularly important in the interpretation of this rule because phenotype A_1 may be the result of genotypes A^1A^1, A^1A^2, or A^1O.

ABO Typing

The ABO blood type is determined in the laboratory by mixing a saline suspension of the patient's red blood cells with anti-A and anti-B antisera. When these anti-A and anti-B agglutinins come in contact with the corresponding agglutinogen, the red blood cells agglutinate. Type A blood cells, containing group A agglutinogens, will agglutinate with the anti-A serum mixture; the anti-B serum will not agglutinate with the type A blood cells. Reverse typing, which mixes patient's serum with type A and B red blood cells, also is performed to confirm these findings.

Similar reactions between red blood cells and serum also take place in the body during a transfusion with an incompatible blood type. Thus, if a patient with type A blood inadvertently receives a transfusion of either type B or O whole blood, the anti-A agglutinins in the donor blood will hemolyze the recipient's A cells.

Rh System

The **Rh system** identifies blood as positive or negative according to the presence or absence of a particular Rh antigen, designated as Rh_0 or D, on the red blood cell surface. This $Rh_0(D)$ factor may be inherited in conjunction with any of the ABO blood types and, next to A and B agglutinogens, is the most clinically important antigen in blood banking. However, the $Rh_0(D)$ factor is only part of a large and complicated system, which also includes the related red blood cell characteristics or antigens designated as rh', rh", hr', and hr" or as C, E, c, and e, respectively.

Unlike the ABO blood group agglutinins, antibodies to Rh antigens do not occur naturally or spontaneously in the serum. Thus, anti-Rh_0(anti-D) antibodies almost always result from exposure of an Rh-negative individual to Rh-positive cells either through transfusion or pregnancy. An Rh-negative individual who receives a transfusion of Rh-positive blood will slowly develop anti-Rh_0(anti-D) agglutinins against the $Rh_0(D)$ factor on the red blood cells. Although this has no immediate ill effect, the individual is sensitized and will agglutinate the red blood cells of any subsequent Rh-positive transfusion, causing a serious reaction.

Sensitization to the $Rh_0(D)$ factor also can occur during pregnancy when antigen from the red blood cells of an Rh-positive fetus seeps into the maternal bloodstream through the placenta. The fetus has inherited the $Rh_0(D)$ positive factor from the father. The anti-Rh_0(anti-D) antibodies produced in an Rh-negative mother may then return to

TABLE 12-3 Most Common Rh Phenotypes and Genotypes*

Reactions With Serum Containing							
Anti-Rh₀ (D)	Anti-rh' (C)	Anti-rh" (E)	Anti-rh' (c)	Anti-rh' (e)	Phenotypes	Possible Genotypes	Approximate Percentage in United States
Rh-positive (approx. 85%)							
+	+	+	+	+	Rh_1Rh_2 (CcDEe)	R^1R^2 (CDe/cDE)	13
+	+	−	+	+	Rh_1rh (CcDe)	R^1r (CDe/cde)	33
+	+	−	−	+	Rh_1Rh_1 (CCDe)	R^1R^1 (CDe/CDe)	17
+	−	+	+	+	Rh_2rh (cDEe)	R^2r (cDE/cde)	13
+	−	+	+	−	Rh_2Rh_2 (cDEE)	R^2R^2 (cDE/cDE)	3
+	−	−	+	+	Rh_0(cDe)	R^0r (cDe/cde)	2
Rh-negative (approx. 15%)							
−	−	−	+	+	rh (cde)	rr (cde/cde)	14
−	−	+	+	+	rh"rh (cdEe)	r"r (cdE/cde)	1
−	+	−	+	+	rh'rh (Ccde)	r'r (Cde/cde)	1

*A number of additional Rh phenotypes and genotypes are possible, although most are rare. + equals present; − equals absent.

the fetus through the placental barrier, causing agglutination and hemolysis of fetal red blood cells, a condition known as erythroblastosis fetalis. A firstborn child usually shows no ill effects from this maternal sensitization, although with subsequent pregnancies the maternal anti-Rh_0(anti-D) concentration increases to clinically significant levels and can produce serious reactions in the fetus. However, because administration of specific Rh immune globulin (RhoGAM) to nonsensitized women is now routine, few Rh-negative women produce anti-Rh_0(anti-D) as a result of an Rh-positive pregnancy.

Inheritance of Rh Blood Types

The presence or absence of Rh_0(D), as well as the particular combination of rh'(C) or hr'(c) and rh" (E) or hr"(e) on the red blood cell surface, is determined by a single pair of genes or gene complexes. Every individual inherits one gene or complex from each parent, producing a genetic formula or genotype that is homozygous (same set of Rh factors) or heterozygous (different sets of Rh factors). The specific assortment of antigens or factors detectable on the red blood cells of an individual is the phenotype. Because all Rh factors are codominant, the phenotype of a homozygous individual can have only three main Rh factors, whereas that of a heterozygous individual may demonstrate either four or all five factors (Table 12-3).

Laboratory identification of the specific gene combinations responsible for a particular phenotype is difficult because any of the demonstrable Rh antigens may be part of either or both genetic packages. Thus, an individual with the phenotype Rh_1Rh_2(CcDEe) may be the result of any one of six possible genotypes, although some of these are quite rare. However, useful assumptions can be made about possible genotypes by carefully interpreting parental phenotypes according to the principles of genetic inheritance. These complex studies of possible Rh antigen combinations are important in population surveys, tests for the exclusion of parentage, and evaluating hemolytic disease of the newborn resulting from anti-Rh_0(anti-D).

Rules governing Rh inheritance permit the following conclusions:

1. The Rh factors Rh_0(D), rh'(C), rh"(E), hr'(c), and hr"(e) cannot appear in a child unless the corresponding factor is present in one or both parents.

2. A parent lacking the rh'(C) factor must have a child with the hr'(c) factor, and a parent lacking the hr'(c) factor must have a child with the rh'(C) factor.

3. A parent lacking the rh"(E) factor must have a child with the hr"(e) factor, and a parent lacking the hr"(e) factor must have a child with the rh"(E) factor.

Rh Typing

The Rh blood type is determined in the laboratory by testing the patient's red blood cells with specific antibodies to detect the presence or absence of the corresponding Rh antigen. Thus, testing with anti-Rh_0(anti-D) typing serum agglutinates all cells containing the Rh_0(D) factor and leads to the designation Rh-positive. On the other hand, nonagglutination of cells with anti-Rh_0(anti-D) typing serum indicates the absence of Rh_0(D) antigen and leads to the designation Rh-negative.

An additional testing technique, performed only on Rh-negative blood, rules out weakly Rh-positive blood, which may not react with the typing serum on immediate reading. This procedure demonstrates an important Rh factor variant known as D^u in a few individuals who are classified as Rh-negative, D^u-positive. These individuals generally are considered to be weakly Rh-positive and may correctly receive either Rh-positive or Rh-negative blood during transfusion therapy.

Because to date no antibody has been discovered that reacts specifically with the reciprocal antigen to $Rh_o(D)$, designated as $Hr_o(d)$, no anti-Hr_o(anti-d) typing serum is available for clinical use. Although in routine clinical procedures, including pretransfusion compatibility studies, Rh typing consists of testing with anti-Rh_o(anti-D) serum only, tests may be performed for any of the five common Rh factors. Testing with the additional typing serums anti-rh'(anti-C), anti-rh"(anti-E), anti-hr'(anti-c), and anti-hr"(anti-e) usually is performed in special cases such as family studies to estimate the probability of certain Rh genotypes. Detection of all Rh factors, including $Rh_o(D)$, is important to the prognosis of future pregnancies in Rh-immunized women to predict possible fetal phenotypes from the phenotypes of both parents.

Other Blood Group Systems

Aside from the antigens described in the ABO and Rh blood group systems, the red blood cell surface contains at least 300 other antigens that can be detected by specific antibodies. The most clinically significant of these additional antigens include the Fy antigens of the Duffy system; the K, k, Kp, Ku, and Js antigens of the Kell system; and the Jk antigens of the Kidd system. Antigens associated with the MNS, Lewis, Lutheran, Ii, or P systems produce relatively few clinical problems but occur frequently enough that their presence must be identified. These additional blood group antigens have practical significance only when antibodies to one or more of them cause a transfusion reaction or hemolytic disease of the newborn. Other red blood cell antigens rarely have clinical importance but contribute to the understanding of human genetics and frequently are used as genetic markers for population surveys or family inheritance patterns.

On the other hand, nucleated cells, including circulating leukocytes, platelets, and most tissue cells, contain antigens of the **HLA system** (human leukocyte antigen or histocompatibility locus A) on their surface membranes. These antigens are located on certain autosomal chromosomes and are classified into five different series, designated A, B, C, D, and DR (D-related), that combine to determine an individual's HLA type. An almost infinite number of antigen combinations and HLA phenotypes are possible because there are at least 20 distinct group A antigens, 40 B antigens, 8 C antigens, 12 D antigens, and 10 DR antigens.

Testing for HLA antigens, which is far more complicated than red blood cell typing, is most clinically useful in the areas of organ transplantation, platelet and granulocyte transfusions, disease associations, and paternity testing. Although first valued for its role in tissue rejection and organ transplant survival, increasing knowledge of the HLA system may provide better insight into diagnosis, treatment, prognosis, and prevention of disease. For example, HLA typing may be used to select compatible platelet or granulocyte donors and to investigate febrile reactions following granulocyte transfusion or therapeutic unresponsiveness to platelet infusion resulting from HLA incompatibility. (See Transfusion Reactions later in this chapter.) Likewise, the presence of certain HLA antigens has been associated with increased susceptibility to a number of diseases and may predispose an individual to the development of these conditions (Table 12-4). This does not imply, however, that these diseases occur only in individuals with specific HLA types, that certain individuals necessarily will develop these disorders, or that the antigens occur only in individuals with these diseases.

TABLE 12-4   HLA Antigens and Disease Associations

HLA Antigen	Disease
A1	Psoriasis vulgaris
A3	Idiopathic hemochromatosis
A10	Pemphigus vulgaris
B8	Addison's disease, idiopathic Celiac disease Chronic active hepatitis Dermatitis herpetiformis Graves' disease Juvenile dermatomyositis Myasthenia gravis Pernicious anemia Sarcoidosis Sjögren's syndrome Systemic lupus erythematosus
B13	Psoriasis vulgaris Psoriatic arthritis
B14	Idiopathic hemochromatosis
Bw15	Insulin-dependent diabetes Pernicious anemia
B17	Psoriasis vulgaris Psoriatic arthritis
B27	Ankylosing spondylitis Psoriatic arthritis Reiter's syndrome Rheumatoid arthritis, juvenile Sacroiliitis *Salmonella* arthritis Uveitis, acute or chronic juvenile
B35	de Quervain's disease Graves' disease
Bw35	Subacute thyroiditis
B37	Psoriasis vulgaris
B38	Psoriatic arthritis
B40	Multiple sclerosis Rheumatoid arthritis, juvenile
Bw47	Adrenal hyperplasia, congenital
B52	Takayasu's disease
B54	Insulin-dependent diabetes, juvenile

(continued)

TABLE 12-4 HLA Antigens and Disease Associations (*continued*)

HLA Antigen	Disease
Cw1	Sacroiliitis
Cw4	Schizophrenia
Cw6	Psoriasis vulgaris
DR2, Dw2	Goodpasture's syndrome Multiple sclerosis
Dw3	Addison's disease, idiopathic Celiac disease Chronic active hepatitis Dermatitis herpetiformis Graves' disease Hashimoto's disease Insulin-dependent diabetes, juvenile Myasthenia gravis Sjögren's syndrome Systemic lupus erythematosus
DR4, Dw4	Buerger's disease Insulin-dependent diabetes mellitus Rheumatoid arthritis, adult
DR7	Celiac disease

ANTIBODY DETECTION

Antibody detection tests, such as the antiglobulin or Coombs' tests, are nonspecific procedures to detect the presence of antibodies (immunoglobulins) on the red blood cell surface or in serum. Although most antibodies agglutinate cells containing specific antigens immediately, other antibody molecules (incomplete antibodies) merely coat the surface of cells with the corresponding antigen without completing the agglutination reaction. This incomplete antigen-antibody reaction merely sensitizes the cells and remains invisible; it can be demonstrated only by the addition of Coombs' antiglobulin serum, which causes sensitized red blood cells to agglutinate.

The two main applications of the antiglobulin reaction are the direct test, which demonstrates red blood cell sensitization, and the indirect test, which detects immune antibodies in the bloodstream. The **direct antiglobulin test** is performed on the patient's red blood cells to determine if an incomplete antibody already has become attached to them. The test is positive if the red blood cells agglutinate, making the original undetected antigen-antibody reaction visible and indicating that the antiglobulin serum has combined all the antibody molecules simultaneously. The indirect test, known as the **antibody screen**, is performed on the patient's serum that is incubated with a red blood cell reagent to detect antibodies in the serum that correspond to known antigens on the test cells.

Direct Antiglobulin Test (Direct Coombs' Test)

The **direct antiglobulin test** (DAT) is used in hematology and transfusion services to detect the presence of complement or immune γ-globulin antibodies adsorbed on the red blood cell surface. The test reaction is called direct because it requires only the addition of Coombs' serum directly to the patient's cells, which have been washed to remove excess serum, which could give false antiglobulin test reactions. Red blood cells that have been sensitized in vivo will agglutinate and produce visible clumping when they are combined with the anti–γ-globulin antibodies of the Coombs' serum.

The appearance of agglutination indicates a positive test and may be reported as $1+$ to $4+$ according to the degree of clumping, which depends on the relative concentration of antibodies coating the cells. The major clinical value of the DAT is the early diagnosis of hemolytic disease of the newborn or autoimmune hemolytic anemia and the investigation of red blood cells sensitized by drugs or hemolytic transfusion reactions. However, although the direct antiglobulin test indicates that some antibody has become attached to the red blood cell surface, it cannot identify the exact nature of that antibody. (See Antibody Identification later in this chapter.)

Clinical Significance

Positive DAT reactions resulting from hemolytic disease of the newborn usually are due to anti-ABO, anti-Rh, anti-Kell, and other warm antibodies adsorbed on the red blood cell surface. In these instances red blood cell sensitization occurs in utero, and testing of umbilical cord blood at birth can indicate whether an infant will be affected. Many hospitals therefore routinely perform direct antiglobulin tests on the umbilical cord blood of all infants as a precaution. Such routine testing can detect any red blood cell sensitization that is not apparent but might develop and cause a hemolytic reaction within several days after delivery.

Direct antiglobulin test reactions also may be used to differentiate autoimmune hemolytic anemia, in which antibodies react with the patient's own red blood cells, from hemolytic anemias resulting from other causes. Thus, IgG or IgM autoantibodies associated with autoimmune hemolytic anemia are demonstrated by a positive DAT, whereas red blood cells associated with hemolytic anemias such as hereditary spherocytosis produce a negative DAT. Likewise, drug-induced antibodies often cause positive DAT results because the drug or an immune complex of the drug and antibody may coat the red blood cell surface and initiate complement activity.

Normal Values

The direct antiglobulin test is normally negative.

Variations

Positive direct antiglobulin test results may occur with:

Autoimmune hemolytic anemia	Cephaloridine
Drug therapy (may persist for months)	Cephalosporin
α-Methyldopa	Cephalothin
Aminopyrine	Chlorpromazine

Isoniazid	Hemolytic anemia, drug-induced
Para-aminosalicylic acid	Hemolytic disease of the newborn
Penicillin	Infection
Phenacetin	Malignancy
Quinidine	Normal health
Quinine	Renal disease
Streptomycin	Rheumatoid arthritis
Sulfonamides	Systemic lupus erythematosus
Elderly individuals	Transfusion reaction

False-negative direct antiglobulin test results may accompany heparin administration in individuals with acquired hemolytic anemia.

Methodology

Direct antiglobulin tests require at least 10 mL of venous blood collected without anticoagulants (red-stoppered tube). In neonates the specimen should be collected from the umbilical cord after it has been clamped and cut.

▶▶ Nursing Responsibilities and Implications

1. Indicate on the laboratory request slip the patient's age, history of transfusion or pregnancy, and any drug therapy.

2. Handle the specimen gently to prevent hemolysis.

3. Send the specimen to the laboratory immediately for testing within 24 hours.

Antibody Screen (Indirect Coombs' Test)

The **antibody screen** (indirect Coombs' test) is used to detect serum antibodies other than those of the ABO system that may cause red blood cell sensitization and to determine certain blood group antigens. The test reaction is considered indirect because two steps are required before the antigen-antibody interaction can be demonstrated. Thus, when serum with unknown antibodies is exposed to red blood cells containing a number of known specific antigens, the antibodies will react to the corresponding antigens and coat the test cells with immunoglobulins. Subsequent addition of antiglobulin (Coombs') serum will agglutinate these sensitized red blood cells if the individual's serum contains antibodies to one or more of the test cell antigens.

The absence of agglutination following the addition of antiglobulin serum indicates that the serum being tested lacks antibodies to the particular antigens present on the test cells. Visible agglutination of the red blood cells, on the other hand, indicates a positive test reaction, which may be reported from ± to 4+ according to the amount of clumping. However, although a positive antibody screen indicates the presence of an unexpected antibody in the serum, it cannot identify the exact nature of that antibody. A variation of the antibody screen uses serum containing a known specific antibody to detect a particular antigen on an individual's red blood cells. (See Antibody Identification later in this chapter.)

Clinical Significance

The antibody screen is an important procedure that is used routinely to detect the following:

Antigens such as Rh variant Du, Kell, or Duffy, which are not demonstrated by other techniques

Antiglobulin consumption (special studies)

Donor-recipient incompatibility during pretransfusion crossmatching

γ-Globulin neutralization (special studies)

Leukocyte antibodies (special studies)

Mixed agglutination reactions (special studies)

Platelet antibodies (special studies)

Unexpected or irregular antibodies

The antibody screen generally is used in compatibility testing for blood transfusions to detect antibodies in the serum of the recipient resulting from a previous transfusion. Incubation of a mixture of the donor's red blood cells and the recipient's serum with anti-globulin serum can determine if the proposed transfusion will cause a hazardous antigen-antibody response. A positive agglutination reaction indicates incompatibility, whereas a negative test result is considered a compatible crossmatch.

The antibody screen also may be used to demonstrate the presence of red blood cell antibodies such as anti-Rh or anti-Kell from a previous blood transfusion or pregnancy. One important application of the antibody screen is the testing of maternal serum before delivery in a woman with suspected or potential Rh and other red blood cell factor problems. A positive antibody screen in the mother can alert the physician to the possibility of severe hemolytic problems in the neonate.

Normal Values
Results of the antibody screen are normally negative.

Methodology
See Direct Antiglobulin Test—Methodology.

▶▶ Nursing Responsibilities and Implications
See Direct Antiglobulin Test—Nursing Responsibilities and Implications.

Antibody Identification

The detection of unexpected red blood cell antibodies during antibody screening procedures usually occurs in individuals who have been exposed to foreign red blood cell antigens through pregnancy, previous transfusion, or injection. Occasionally, the serum of individuals with no known exposure to foreign red blood cell antigens may demonstrate red blood cell antibodies other than anti-A and anti-B. The precise identification of these irregular antibodies is always important but is of particular concern to the obstetric patient before delivery so that preparations can be made for a possible exchange transfusion in the neonate.

The exact identity of unexpected antibodies in the patient's serum can be determined by testing the serum against a series of red blood cells representing all common blood group antigens. A panel of 10 or 15 red blood cell samples generally is used, with various antigen combinations contained in each sample. Thus, proper application and interpretation of the distinct patterns of antigen-antibody reactions facilitate the identification of one or more antibodies.

Clinical Significance

Exact identification of unexpected or irregular antibodies is most important during the investigation of the following:

Discrepancy between ABO and serum grouping

Hemolytic disease of the newborn

Incompatible crossmatch

Multiparous women with a history of jaundiced infants

Positive antibody screening

Positive direct antiglobulin test

Serum of blood donors

Serum of blood transfusion recipients

Transfusion reaction

Methodology

Antibody identification requires two specimens of venous blood: 7 mL of whole blood in a tube with EDTA (lavender-stoppered tube) and 20 mL of clotted blood (red-stoppered tube).

▶▶ **Nursing Responsibilities and Implications**

See Direct Antiglobulin Test—Nursing Responsibilities and Implications.

COMPATIBILITY TESTING

Compatibility testing is the inclusive term given to the series of procedures performed before transfusion to ensure the suitability of blood from a particular donor for a specific recipient. Laboratory procedures required before transfusion include ABO grouping and Rh typing of the recipient, detection and identification of unexpected antibodies on both recipient and donor blood, and crossmatching of recipient and donor blood. The most complex of these procedures is the crossmatch, which combines a sample of the recipient's serum with the donor's red blood cells to detect antibodies that might damage transfused cells and cause hemolytic transfusion reactions.

The crossmatching procedure includes several incubation temperatures and cell suspension media to aid the detection of antigen-antibody interactions capable of producing the agglutination and hemolysis responsible for transfusion reactions. Compatibility is indicated by the absence of agglutination or hemolysis when serum and red blood cell samples are combined under test conditions that are optimal for antibody activity. A compatible crossmatch, however, does not rule out the presence of unexpected donor or recipient antibodies and cannot guarantee normal donor cell survival or prevent recipient immunization.

Specimen Collection and Handling

Compatibility testing and crossmatching procedures require 5 mL of blood collected without anticoagulants (red-stoppered tube) from a fresh venipuncture site. Specimens for crossmatching procedures must be less than 48 hours old and should be free of hemolysis, which could mask the detection of a hemolyzing reaction during testing. When a number of transfusions for the same recipient are requested within several days, a fresh blood specimen should be collected within 24 hours of the next scheduled transfusion to perform the later crossmatches. This precaution is essential to detect any newly formed antibodies in the recipient's bloodstream as a result of the previous transfusions. Each staff member involved in the transfusion process must be constantly aware of the many possibilities for error, including nontechnical mistakes such as inadequate or incorrect identification, which can result in the patient's death.

Precautions
To ensure reliable crossmatching and compatibility testing, the following precautions should be observed:

1. Do not collect blood specimens from the tubing used for intravenous fluid infusion or from the vein receiving it. If use of the infusion line is unavoidable, however, the tubing should be flushed with saline and the first 5 mL of blood discarded before the specimen is collected.

2. Clearly label all specimen tubes for crossmatch with the patient's full name, identification number, and date.

3. Do not submit blood specimens to the laboratory if there is any doubt about the identity of the sample. A new blood specimen must be collected if there is any discrepancy or question about the source of the original sample.

▶▶ Nursing Responsibilities and Implications

1. Include on the laboratory request form the patient's full name, hospital identification number, age, sex, clinical diagnosis, medications, history of pregnancies or previous transfusions, the number of units ordered, and the type of blood component requested.

2. Verify the patient's identity using the wristband before collecting the blood specimen for crossmatch.

3. Perform a venipuncture and collect a fresh blood specimen according to the procedure described in Chapter 4 under Performing a Venipuncture.

4. Label the blood specimen at the patient's bedside immediately after collection to prevent any confusion regarding its source.

Routine Crossmatch

The **routine crossmatch**, the safest test to ensure complete compatibility, requires 45–60 minutes and is divided into three distinct phases—protein, thermo, and antiglobulin—each with different incubation times and temperatures. The **protein phase** is performed at room temperature and can detect any incompatibility of the ABO system or agglutination reactions resulting from anti-Rh or other antibodies such as anti-M and anti-P_1. The

thermo phase requires incubation at 37 C for 15−30 minutes and can detect incompatibility due to weak anti-Rh antibodies and certain other Rh antibodies such as anti-C, anti-E, or anti-c. The **antiglobulin phase** requires the addition of Coombs' serum to demonstrate incompatibility resulting from clinically significant antibodies such as anti-Kell, anti-Kidd, anti-Lewis, and anti-Duffy, which are seldom detected in the other phases.

Emergency Crossmatch

Emergency crossmatching procedures or the release of blood before completion of routine compatibility studies is warranted only when the need to replace blood volume is greater than the risk of a transfusion reaction. The decision to administer a blood transfusion before completion of complete pretransfusion studies may be justified, however, only when the physician considers the possible incompatibility to be the lesser danger. Thus, although the recipient may possess antibodies or develop delayed immunity to certain factors in the transfused blood, the patient's welfare is best served by the calculated but definite risk of emergency transfusion procedures. Many blood banks require that the responsible physician sign a legal release or acknowledgement of increased risk whenever compatibility testing cannot be performed and blood is administered that has not been crossmatched.

Three degrees of emergency crossmatch may be utilized, depending on the severity of the patient's condition and the urgency of the need for blood. When a delay of 30−45 minutes is acceptable, the routine crossmatch is performed and completed, although the procedure in one set of tubes is shortened by reducing the incubation periods. A recently developed technique using low ionic strength solutions (LISS) to perform a complete emergency crossmatch in 10−15 minutes is of particular value in these circumstances. This practice is relatively safe during emergencies if the unexpected antibody screen is negative.

When 15−30 minutes are safely available, the patient's ABO group and Rh type should be determined and uncrossmatched, type-specific blood administered. A complete crossmatch is then performed while the patient is receiving the blood. When the emergency is most extreme and no time is available for testing, uncrossmatched, type-specific or group O Rh-negative blood with low isoagglutinin titers and no irregular antibodies may be administered. The risks of emergency transfusion are reduced if the patient's blood group and Rh type and the results of unexpected antibody screening are already known. (See Selection of Blood and Alternate Donor Groups later in this chapter.)

Crossmatching Blood for Newborns and Infants

Crossmatching procedures to determine the compatibility of blood for transfusion to newborns and infants are not reliable when performed with the infant's serum. Because natural antibodies are not produced until a few months after birth, any antibodies in the serum of very young infants are the result of transplacental transmission from the maternal bloodstream. Thus, pretransfusion testing to select blood for an infant less than 1 month old must be performed with serum from the mother. However, when the infant is between 1 and 3 months old, the crossmatch should include serum from both mother and infant because some actively formed antibodies may already be present at this age.

TRANSFUSION THERAPY

For safe and effective transfusion therapy, the pathophysiology of the disorder under treatment and the composition and physiologic functions of the transfused component should be understood completely. (See Component Therapy later in this chapter.) Thus, transfusion therapy must be guided by a careful evaluation of the patient's clinical condition as well as the etiology and course of the disease. Basic medical indications for transfusion therapy include the restoration and maintenance of oxygen-carrying capacity, blood volume, coagulation properties, and leukocyte functions. The therapeutic benefits anticipated from transfusion of whole blood or its derivatives must outweigh the possibility of serious hemolytic, pyrogenic, allergic, and hypersensitivity reactions or circulatory overload. (See Transfusion Reactions later in this chapter.)

Selection of Blood and Alternate Donor Groups

Any substance containing red blood cells must be tested to ascertain that the cells belong to the same ABO and Rh groups as the recipient and must be crossmatched with the recipient's blood to ensure compatibility before transfusion. Whenever possible, the recipient must receive crossmatched, compatible, group-specific blood. (See Compatibility Testing earlier in this chapter.) At times, however, it is impossible for the recipient to receive group-specific blood, and the physician may request transfusion of group O Rh-negative blood to any other ABO group without compatibility testing. The hazards associated with transfusion of type O blood as an alternate donor group may be minimized by removal of the plasma and administration of packed cells whenever circumstances permit. Group O packed cells or low-titer whole blood may be given in the following circumstances:

- During an extreme emergency (see Emergency Crossmatch earlier in this chapter).
- When no other blood is available.
- When the recipient's blood group cannot be determined.
- When no other blood is available that lacks a specific factor to which the patient is sensitized.

Only group O blood that has been screened to ensure the absence of immune anti-A and anti-B antibodies may be used for transfusion in recipients with type A, B, or AB blood. Because the red blood cells of group O blood contain neither A nor B antigens, they will not be harmed by whatever antibodies are present in the recipient's serum. Likewise, the low anti-A and anti-B antibody titers of group O blood usually cause little harm to the cells of type A or B recipients. Group O blood, on the other hand, is seldom administered to type AB recipients because their cells contain both A and B antigens and can be hemolyzed by the anti-A and anti-B antibodies of group O blood.

Group AB recipients, however, may receive type A or type B blood with no ill effects because their serum contains neither anti-A nor anti-B antibodies and will not destroy cells from any ABO group. Likewise, the anti-B and anti-A antibodies contained in the serum of type A and type B donors, respectively, are rapidly diluted and neutralized before the recipient's group AB cells can be damaged. Although type AB recipients can receive either type A or B donor blood, only one of the two (usually group A because it is more common) should be administered to any recipient.

Likewise, transfusions with whole blood or red blood cells of an alternate ABO group should be continued even if the recipient's own blood type becomes available. A decision to change back to group-specific blood may be hazardous to the recipient, particularly following massive transfusions of an alternate blood group. For example, if a type B recipient receives group O blood followed by group B cells, a severe reaction may result from the anti-B antibodies in the group O whole blood. The following is a summary of alternate donor group selection:

Recipient's Group	First Choice	Second Choice
O	O	None
A	O	None
B	O	None
AB	A or B	O

Administration of Blood

For safe and effective transfusion therapy, careful attention to detail must accompany each step of the preparation and administration of blood. Hospital personnel must be aware of the possible complications associated with the infusion of blood and must be alert for any changes in the recipient that could be attributed to the transfusion process.

Precautions

To help ensure the success of transfusion therapy, the following precautions should be observed:

1. Do not rely only on a label attached to the blood container or the name written on the patient's bed to ensure correct identification before transfusion; use several cross-checks, including the patient's wristband.

2. Observe strict aseptic technique while performing the venipuncture and starting the transfusion.

3. Agitate the blood container gently from time to time during the transfusion to help maintain a uniform, trouble-free blood flow.

4. Complete transfusions within 4 hours to avoid the dangers of bacterial proliferation and red blood cell hemolysis.

5. Do not administer any solution other than physiologic saline through the same tubing as blood because it may cause hemolysis or clotting. This prohibits filling or flushing blood administration sets with a solution of dextrose in water. Likewise, intravenous solutions containing calcium, such as lactated Ringer's solution and many of the other balanced electrolyte solutions, are also unsuitable for use in the transfusion of blood because they may cause citrated blood to clot.

6. Return blood to the blood bank for storage when the transfusion cannot be started within 15 minutes after the blood arrives.

▶▶ Nursing Responsibilities and Implications

1. Check with extra caution the identity of the patient and the unit of blood to be transfused; strict identification is even more essential when the patient is unconscious. Specific hospital nursing procedure should be followed.

2. Determine the temperature, pulse, respiratory rate, and blood pressure of the recipient before the transfusion is started.

3. Mix the blood container gently but thoroughly before starting the transfusion because red blood cells settle to the bottom of the unit and plasma rises to the top.

4. Perform a venipuncture using an 18- or 19-gauge needle for the transfusion of whole blood and packed red blood cells; smaller needles may be used to administer other blood products such as fresh-frozen plasma, platelets, granulocytes, albumin, and antihemophilic factor. (The procedure for performing a venipuncture is discussed in Chapter 4.)

5. Administer 25–50 mL of blood slowly for the first 30 minutes to minimize the volume of blood infused in case the patient experiences an immediate reaction.

6. Observe the recipient closely during the first 15 minutes of transfusion and at 15-minute intervals thereafter to detect any adverse transfusion reactions as soon as possible. The transfusion must be discontinued immediately at the first indication of symptoms such as fever, lower back pain, difficulty in breathing, or nausea. (See Transfusion Reactions later in this chapter.)

7. Establish a uniform rate of blood flow that is neither too rapid nor too slow. Administer whole blood at a rate of 500 mL/2 hours and packed red blood cells at a slower rate; transfuse chronically anemic patients even more slowly, at a rate of 2mL/kg/hr.

8. Check the rate of blood flow frequently because any change in the height of the bed or intravenous pole during transfusion may alter the established rate. Blood flow also may be altered by changes in the position of the needle within the vein or tonicity of the vein, as well as by repositioning the extremity receiving the infusion.

9. Remove the needle when the transfusion is completed and apply pressure to the infusion site for a few minutes to avoid hematoma formation.

10. Rinse the infusion set with normal saline solution before starting the infusion of other solutions or drugs. If a subsequent transfusion is necessary, a new infusion set must be used.

11. Return any unused units of blood to the blood bank immediately. Only those units in which the container closure has not been pierced and that have been kept refrigerated will be accepted for reissue.

Massive Transfusions

Massive transfusion is defined as the replacement of more than half of a patient's normal blood volume during a 12-hour period. The immediate and long-term complications of massive transfusion of stored blood usually are overlooked but may include the following:

Acid-base changes

Adenine nephrotoxicity

Alloantibody development

Circulatory overload

Citrate toxicity

Decreased antithrombin III

Decreased coagulation factors V and VIII and platelets

Decreased ionized calcium

Dilution of coagulation factors

Disease transmission

Hyperkalemia

Hypoglycemia

Hypothermia

Increased circulating anticoagulants

Increased plasma ammonia

Increased plasma hemoglobin

Intravascular consumption of coagulation factors

Thrombasthenia

Thrombocytopenia

COMPONENT THERAPY

Once the need for transfusion has been determined, the deficient blood component should be identified and, whenever possible, replaced with only that specific substance rather than whole blood. The use of blood components prevents the unnecessary transfusion of red blood cells, thus avoiding possible red blood cell antibody production and minimizing the hazards of immunization. This practice provides the maximum benefits of transfusion therapy but reduces the risk to the patient and minimizes the number of complications that may result from the transfusion of unnecessary components. The individual derivatives that can be obtained from whole blood include red blood cells, plasma, cryoprecipitated antihemophilic factor, certain coagulation factors, platelet concentrate, and leukocyte concentrate. Choice of the appropriate blood fraction, dosage, and rate of administration must be guided by the patient's clinical status.

Whole Blood

Whole blood collected from selected human donors contains all the cellular and plasma components needed to replace red blood cell mass and restore blood volume. Thus, the administration of whole blood increases the recipient's total blood volume and oxygen-carrying capacity. It is most useful in treating acute massive blood loss. Fresh whole blood (less than 24 hours old) also may be used to replace coagulation factors I, V, and VIII and platelets in the treatment of hemophilia A, thrombocytopenia, and disseminated intravascular coagulation.

However, whole blood should not be used if more efficient specific components are available because patients with adequate blood volume but deficient oxygen-carrying capacity derive little benefit from whole blood plasma. (See Red Blood Cells later in this chapter.) Likewise, in the absence of hypovolemia, coagulation disorders should be treated with specific blood components because the labile coagulation factors deteriorate unpredictably and refrigeration decreases platelet survival. (See Platelets, Cryoprecipitated Antihemophilic Factor, and Plasma later in this chapter.) In addition, infusion of large amounts of whole blood may increase bleeding due to coagulation factor deficiency and cause circulatory overload and congestive heart failure in patients with precarious cardiac function.

Decisions regarding the need for whole blood transfusion and the amount of whole blood to be administered must be based on the patient's clinical condition rather than laboratory values for hemoglobin concentration. The rate of whole blood infusion also depends on the patient's clinical status but should not take longer than 4 hours per unit. Blood may be warmed to avoid hypothermia during massive transfusion whenever it is clinically advisable, but the temperature should not exceed 37 C. Whole blood must be administered through a filter designed to remove such microaggregates as fibrin clots, white blood cells, platelets, and other debris that may develop during the storage of blood.

Indications

The administration of whole blood is indicated for:

Acute blood loss	Hypovolemic shock
Exchange transfusions (blood < 6 days old)	Replacement of nonlabile coagulation factors (in association with mass transfusions)
Extracorporeal circulation	Replacement of surgical blood loss

Contraindications

To help ensure the success and safety of whole blood administration, the following contraindications should be observed:

1. Do not administer whole blood to correct anemia that can be treated with red blood cell components or specific medications such as iron, B_{12}, or folic acid.

2. Do not use whole blood to correct a deficiency of labile clotting factors such as platelets and factor VIII.

3. Do not administer whole blood to correct conditions that respond to specific blood components.

4. Do not administer ABO or Rh incompatible blood unless withholding blood might result in loss of life. (See Selection of Blood and Alternate Donor Groups earlier in this chapter.)

5. Do not use whole blood for fluid replacement when volume expansion can safely and adequately be achieved with saline, lactated Ringer's solution, albumin, or plasma protein fractions.

Side Effects and Hazards

The expected benefits of whole blood transfusion must be carefully weighed against the hazards and potential side effects (see Transfusion Reactions later in this chapter) such as:

Allergic reactions	Metabolic complications (massive transfusions)
Alloimmunization of the recipient	
Bacterial contamination	Acidosis
Circulatory overload	Citrate toxicity
Febrile reactions	Depletion of coagulation factors and platelets
Hemolytic transfusion reaction	
Hypersensitivity reactions	Hypokalemia
Iron overload	Hypothermia
	Transmission of infectious disease

Red Blood Cells

Red blood cells are the concentrated component remaining when plasma is separated and removed from whole blood by a natural sedimentation process or by centrifugation. Administration of red blood cells is the treatment of choice for symptoms associated with deficient oxygen-carrying capacity in patients whose blood volume does not need to be increased. Thus, transfusion of red blood cells replaces red blood cell mass in patients with cardiac disease, severe or chronic anemia, and restricted sodium, potassium, or citrate intake whose blood volume is adequate. Red blood cell infusion also minimizes the risks of circulatory overload or cardiovascular failure in patients who react poorly to rapid shifts of blood volume and is preferred during surgery unless massive hemorrhage is anticipated.

The four red blood cell preparations primarily intended to increase the recipient's oxygen-carrying capacity include packed red blood cells, washed red blood cells, frozen red blood cells, and leukocyte-poor red blood cells.

Approximately 300 mL of **packed red blood cells**, with a hematocrit of 65%–85%, remains after most of the plasma is removed from a unit of whole blood; each unit of packed cells raises an adult's hematocrit by 3%.

Washed red blood cells contain almost no plasma and few leukocytes, which markedly reduces the antibodies introduced during transfusion to previously sensitized individuals and decreases the possibility of sensitization in patients who require frequent transfusions.

Frozen red blood cells are preserved by the addition of glycerol and may be stored for up to 3 years. Techniques used in the freeze-thaw-wash procedure to prepare cells for transfusion remove almost all plasma proteins, platelets, and leukocytes, which reduces the risk of sensitization to leukocyte and platelet antigens. Thus, frozen red blood cells are recommended as a source of red blood cell mass in patients receiving immunosuppressive therapy or multiple transfusions over a prolonged period. The prolonged shelf-life of frozen red blood cells also makes them ideal for the storage of blood drawn in anticipation of later autotransfusion during elective surgery in individuals with rare antibodies.

Leukocyte-poor red blood cells are derived from whole blood or red blood cells that are specially treated with a combination of filtration, washing, and sedimentation procedures to remove leukocytes and platelets. These red blood cell modification techniques remove 70%–90% of the 3–4 billion leukocytes usually present in each unit of blood, making it acceptable for transfusion to individuals with leukocyte antibodies. The highest concentration of these leukocyte antibodies are most likely to be found in multiparous women and patients who have received multiple transfusions or tissue transplants.

When individuals with leukocyte antibodies are infused with blood containing incompatible white blood cells, immune damage to donor leukocytes may result in febrile transfusion reactions, with potentially fatal results. The frequency and severity of these febrile leukocyte reactions are related directly to the number of incompatible leukocytes transfused. Administration of leukocyte-poor red blood cells helps to prevent HLA immunization in patients who are expected to require platelet or granulocyte transfusions or patients who are potential bone marrow transplant recipients.

The volume and rate of red blood cell infusion should be based on the patient's clinical condition and the degree of hematocrit replacement required but must not exceed 4 hours per unit. Because the high hematocrit of packed red blood cells produces greater viscosity and slows the infusion rate, 50–100 mL of physiologic saline may be added to the cells immediately before administration to resuspend the cells. Red blood cells must be administered through a filter designed to remove fibrin clots and other particles, which can cause pulmonary microemboli in patients receiving large quantities of stored blood. Red blood cells may be warmed to avoid hypothermia during transfusion of large amounts of blood, but the temperature should not exceed 37 C.

Indications

Administration of **packed red blood cells** is indicated for:

Administration of group O blood to nongroup O recipients

Exchange transfusions in hemolytic disease of the newborn

Multiple transfusions over a prolonged period of time

Priming renal dialysis and extra-corporeal heart-lung units

Replacement of red blood cell mass without increasing plasma volume

Anemia, chronic

Burns

Debilitated patients

Elderly patients

Heart failure, active or incipient

Transfusion therapy in patients requiring restricted sodium or citrate intake

Kidney disease

Liver disease

Administration of **washed red blood cells** is indicated for recipients with IgA or IgE hypersensitivity; recipients with paroxysmal nocturnal hemoglobinuria; and transfusion of group O red blood cells to nongroup O recipients.

Administration of **frozen red blood cells** is indicated for:

Autotransfusion of individuals with rare antibodies

Long-term transfusion therapy

Organ transplant candidates

Rare blood-type inventories

Transfusion following repeated (more

than three) febrile reactions to leukocyte or platelet antibodies

Transfusion of patients requiring leukocyte-poor red blood cells

Transfusion of patients with paroxysmal nocturnal hemoglobinuria

Administration of **leukocyte-poor red blood cells** is indicated for:

Bone marrow or organ transplant recipients

Multiple or frequent transfusions

Newborns

Prevention of graft versus host disease in immunodeficient patients

Transfusion following repeated (more than three) febrile transfusion reactions to leukocyte antibodies

Transfusion of patients with hyperkalemia

Contraindications

To help ensure safe and effective red blood cell administration, the following contraindications should be observed:

1. Do not administer red blood cells to treat anemia that can be corrected with specific products such as iron, B_{12}, or folic acid.

2. Do not use red blood cells to correct coagulation deficiencies.

3. Do not administer red blood cells that are not ABO-compatible with the recipient's plasma.

4. Do not treat shock with red blood cell infusions.

5. Do not administer leukocyte-poor red blood cells to patients who have demonstrated a single febrile transfusion reaction (see Transfusion Reactions later in this chapter).

Side Effects and Hazards

The hazards and potential side effects of red blood cell administration are similar to those associated with transfusion of whole blood (see Transfusion Reactions), including:

Allergic reactions

Febrile reactions

Hemolytic transfusion reactions

Hypersensitivity reactions

Intravascular hemolysis (if frozen red blood cells are not washed adequately after thawing to remove glycerol)

Transmission of infectious diseases

Granulocytes

Granulocyte concentrate is the transfusion product composed of the buffy coat collected from the whole blood of a single donor and suspended in 200–500 mL of anticoagulated plasma. Depending on the specific method used to prepare this blood component for infusion, a unit of granulocyte concentrate may contain more than 20 billion granulocytes along with varying amounts of platelets and erythrocytes. Transfused granulocytes provide a source of bactericidal activity in patients with neutropenia and migrate to the sites of infection during septicemia that is unresponsive to appropriate antibiotic therapy or other treatment. Granulocyte transfusions generally are indicated by an absolute neutrophil count of 500/μL or less, although the overall status of the patient and the likelihood of marrow recovery also must be considered.

The amount of granulocyte concentrate required for the treatment of neutropenia varies according to the cause of the disorder and the patient's clinical condition. The course of therapy currently recommended for the treatment of neutropenia is 1 unit of granulocyte concentrate daily until bone marrow function resumes or the infection disappears. The apparent cure of an infection is indicated by healing of the infected area, negative blood cultures, or a sustained reduction in fever. Because the circulating granulocyte pool repopulates last, however, patients frequently begin to recover from neutropenia-related infection before the granulocyte count rises in the peripheral blood.

Repeated granulocyte infusions are always necessary but carry the risk of transfusion-related reactions because of the presence of varying amounts of erythrocytes in each unit. Thus, granulocyte concentrate must be crossmatched with the prospective recipient to ensure compatibility and help reduce the severity of such transfusion reactions as pulmonary distress and febrile or allergic reactions. If pulmonary distress occurs during granulocyte transfusion, the transfusion must be discontinued and intravenous hydrocortisone administered; future granulocyte transfusions in such patients should be administered slowly and preceded by intravenous steroid administration. The severity of febrile or allergic reactions does not require that the transfusion be terminated, but these reactions can be reduced or avoided by slowing the infusion rate and administering meperidine and diphenhydramine.

Indications

Administration of granulocyte concentrate is indicated for the treatment of infection or septicemia that is unresponsive to antibiotic therapy, in the presence of severe neutropenia.

Contraindications

To ensure safe and effective administration of granulocyte concentrate, the following contraindications should be observed:

1. Do not use granulocyte concentrate to treat infections that respond to antibiotic therapy.

2. Do not use granulocyte concentrate to treat neutropenia in which bone marrow function is not expected to resume.

3. Do not use granulocyte concentrate unless donor and recipient ABO types are compatible.

Side Effects and Hazards

The hazards and potential side effects of granulocyte administration are similar to many of the risks associated with whole blood and red blood cell transfusion (see Transfusion Reactions later in this chapter), including:

Allergic reactions

Febrile reactions

Graft versus donor disease in immuno-deficient or immunosuppressed patients

Hemolytic transfusion reactions

Hypersensitivity reactions

Pulmonary distress (wheezing, cough, pulmonary edema)

Sensitization to HLA and red blood cell antigens

Transmission of disease

Platelets

At present, two types of **platelet preparations** are available, which consist of megakaryocyte cytoplasmic fragments separated from fresh whole blood and suspended in 30–80 mL of the original plasma. Single-unit concentrates usually contain 70%–80% of the platelets in 1 unit of blood and increase the platelet count of an average adult by 5000–10,000/μL. Plateletpheresis concentrates, on the other hand, contain platelets from the equivalent of 6 units of blood, all from a single donor, and raise the adult platelet count by 30,000–50,000/μL. Platelet preparations are used to correct hemostatic disorders and prevent or control bleeding episodes resulting from quantitative platelet deficiencies (thrombocytopenia) or functional platelet abnormalities (thrombasthenia).

Transfusion of platelet preparations is indicated in patients with rapidly falling or low platelet counts, usually less than 25,000/μL, hemorrhaging patients with platelet counts under 50,000/μL, or surgical candidates with platelet counts below 100,000/μL. The decision to administer platelet transfusions must be based on the condition of the patient's own circulating platelets and the cause of the thrombocytopenia. Although the amount of platelet concentrate required to improve hemostasis is determined by the severity of the thrombocytopenia, the usual dose is 6–8 units.

However, the anticipated increase in the platelet count will not occur if the transfused platelets are rapidly destroyed. Disorders such as disseminated intravascular coagulation (DIC), splenomegaly, fever and sepsis, and acute hemorrhage can shorten the survival of transfused platelets, often to as little as 1 hour. Survival of transfused platelets also may be reduced by the formation of platelet antibodies, as occurs in idiopathic thrombocytopenic purpura, or sensitization to HLA antigens. These HLA antigens are present on the surface of all nucleated body cells, including platelets, and may be responsible for the ineffective response to frequent platelet transfusions. (See other blood group systems earlier in this chapter.)

Formation of HLA and platelet antibodies in patients following organ transplantation or repeated transfusions or pregnancies is not unusual. However, routine platelet counts performed 1 hour after transfusion can detect impaired platelet survival and identify patients who have developed HLA antibodies during past transfusions. Because antibodies generally develop after the infusion of about 20 units of platelet concentrate, evaluation of HLA composition of prospective donor-recipient pairs is desirable in candidates for long-term platelet therapy. Selection of donors based on HLA typing may ensure longer post-transfusion platelet survival in patients who do not respond to platelet concentrates from random donors.

The blood bank must be notified in advance of the need for platelet concentrate so that personnel have enough time to perform the special preparation techniques. Platelet products normally remain viable for 72 hours at room temperature, but the infusion must be completed within 4 hours after the preparation leaves the blood bank to prevent bacterial proliferation. Platelet concentrate must be administered through special infusion sets, which include a nonwettable mesh clot filter and needle to prevent platelet aggregration. The use of normal infusion sets for the administration of platelet products can unintentionally remove platelets during transfusion because platelets tend to adhere to foreign surfaces.

Indications

Platelet administration is indicated for the treatment of:

Hemorrhage, postoperative	Chemotherapy
Thrombasthenia (in association with clinically significant hemorrhage)	Drug idiosyncrasies
	Hypersplenism
Thrombocytopenia and bleeding due to:	Leukemia
	Lupus erythematosus
Aplastic anemia	Radiation
Cancer	Uremia

Contraindications

To ensure safe and effective infusion of platelet concentrate, the following contraindications should be observed:

1. Do not use platelet concentrate to treat bleeding episodes due to rapid platelet destruction associated with idiopathic thrombocytopenic purpura, platelet antigens, fever, sepsis, or disseminated intravascular coagulation (DIC).

2. Do not administer platelet concentrate to treat plasma coagulation deficiencies such as hemophilia A (factor VIII deficiency).

3. Do not use platelet concentrate to treat conditions that are unrelated to thrombocytopenia or thrombasthenia.

Side Effects and Hazards

The hazards and potential side effects of platelet administration are similar to several of the risks associated with whole blood transfusion (see Transfusion Reactions earlier in this chapter), including:

Allergic reactions	Hypersensitivity reactions	Immunization to HLA antigens
Circulatory overload	Immunization to certain red blood cell and platelet antigens	
Citrate toxicity		Transmission of disease
Febrile reactions		

Cryoprecipitated Antihemophilic Factor

Cryoprecipitated antihemophilic factor (AHF) is a preparation that contains the antihemophilic factor (factor VIII) obtained from a single unit of whole blood by slowly thawing fresh-frozen plasma. Cryoprecipitated AHF provides a source of factors VIII and XIII and fibrinogen to help prevent and control hemorrhage or bleeding in certain coagulation deficiencies. The average container of cryoprecipitated AHF supplies 80–100 units of factor VIII and 200–250 mg of fibrinogen in approximately 15 mL of plasma. Each unit of cryoprecipitated AHF is equal to the factor VIII activity found in 1 mL of fresh plasma with normal coagulation function. (The significance and function of coagulation factors are discussed in Chapter 10.)

The amount of cryoprecipitated AHF that must be administered is not completely predictable because the activity of factor VIII after transfusion can vary from patient to patient. Therefore, the duration of therapy must be determined by the type and location of the hemorrhage and the patient's clinical condition. The number of containers of cryoprecipitated AHF required to achieve and maintain a hemostatic level can be calculated according to the following formula:

$$\frac{\text{Desired factor VIII level (\%)} \times \text{Patient's plasma volume (mL)}}{100 \times \text{Average number of factor VIII units per container (80)}}$$

Cryoprecipitated AHF therapy may be required for 10 days or longer after surgery to maintain hemostasis and prevent hemorrhage in patients with certain coagulation defects. Treatment of hemophilia A usually requires rapid infusion (10 mL/min) of the loading dosage that is expected to produce the desired level of factor VIII, followed by smaller maintenance doses every 12 hours. Repeated infusions two to three times per day usually are necessary to maintain hemostatic levels because the half-life of factor VIII is 8–12 hours; smaller amounts given less frequently generally are sufficient to correct deficiencies in von Willebrand's disease. Larger doses of cryoprecipitated AHF or concentrates with higher activity may be required to maintain hemostasis when circulating antibodies to factor VIII are present in the patient's blood.

Cryoprecipitated AHF should be thawed in a water bath at 37 C within 15 minutes and should not be refrigerated or refrozen after thawing. The thawed product may be maintained at room temperature for up to 6 hours before use if the container remains unopened but must be infused within 4 hours once the container has been opened. Cryoprecipitated AHF must be administered intravenously through an appropriate infusion filter. Patient response to treatment with cryoprecipitated AHF should be monitored with periodic laboratory studies such as fibrinogen assays or the activated partial thromboplastin time (APTT) to assess factor VIII levels.

Indications

Administration of cryoprecipitated AHF is indicated for the treatment of:

Bleeding associated with factor VIII deficiency

Factor XIII deficiency

Fibrinogen deficiency

Hemophilia A

von Willebrand's disease

Contraindications

Administration of cryoprecipitated AHF is contraindicated for the treatment of undefined coagulation defects.

Side Effects and Hazards

The hazards and potential side effects of cryoprecipitated AHF administration are similar to several of the risks associated with whole blood transfusion (see Transfusion Reactions later in this chapter), including:

Allergic reactions

Febrile reactions

Hemolysis (following the infusion of a large volume of an ABO-incompatible product)

Positive direct antiglobulin test (following the infusion of a large volume of an ABO-incompatible product)

Transmission of disease

Plasma

Plasma for infusion is prepared from the clear liquid portion of anticoagulated whole blood obtained from a single donor that has been separated from the red blood cells and frozen for storage. Plasma that is removed and frozen within 6 hours of collection is known as **fresh-frozen plasma** and is a source of coagulation factors, including fibrinogen, factor IX, and the labile factors V and VIII. An average container (250 mL) of fresh-frozen plasma contains 200 units of both factor VIII and factor IX and 400 mg of fibrinogen along with other coagulation factors. Plasma that is frozen between 6 hours and 26 days after collection provides plasma proteins and fluid for volume expansion, but only limited quantities of the coagulation factors are intact.

The amount of the plasma to be administered and the rate of infusion depend on the patient's clinical condition and ability to tolerate the volume being infused. Ideally, plasma should be ABO-compatible with the recipient's blood group but may be administered without regard to Rh type. Because serious reactions may develop during the administration of plasma products, the nurse should observe the patient's condition and vital signs as a reference before initiating the transfusion. The patient's condition should be reevaluated approximately 15 minutes later and at the end of the infusion to ensure that the transfusion is proceeding uneventfully and that no adverse reactions have occurred.

Frozen plasma should be thawed, with gentle agitation, in a 37 C water bath immediately before use. Plasma must be infused through an appropriate filter within 6 hours after thawing, and the infusion must not contain any additional medications or solutions.

Indications

Administration of **fresh-frozen plasma** is indicated for the control of bleeding in conditions in which factors V, VIII, and IX and fibrinogen must be replaced; control of bleeding in patients in whom the synthesis of plasma coagulation factors is limited because of severe liver disease; and correction of dilutional hypocoagulability in patients who receive massive transfusions.

Administration of **single-donor plasma** is indicated for the replacement of blood volume in patients with hypovolemic shock; replacement of plasma proteins in selected patients with severe hypoproteinemia; and replacement of plasma factor IX.

Administration of **albumin** is indicated for the treatment of:

Burns, extensive

Hyperbilirubinemia

Liver failure, acute

Nephrosis, acute

Preparation for cardiopulmonary bypass (preoperative)	panied by pulmonary interstitial edema (adults)
Protein loss, severe	Toxic conditions
Respiratory distress syndrome accom-	Traumatic shock, acute

Contraindications
To ensure safe and effective infusion of plasma components, the following contraindications should be observed:

1. Do not administer fresh-frozen plasma to correct coagulation defects that can be treated with specific therapy such as vitamin K, cryoprecipitated AHF, or factor VIII concentrates.

2. Do not administer plasma to replace labile coagulation factors such as factors V and VIII.

Side Effects and Hazards
The hazards and potential side effects of plasma infusion are similar to the risks associated with the infusion of whole blood (see the following section on Transfusion Reactions), including:

Allergic reactions	Hypothermia (when large volumes are required)
Circulatory overload	
Citrate toxicity (when large volumes are required)	Positive direct antiglobulin test (resulting from ABO-incompatibility of plasma antibodies with the recipient's red blood cells)
Febrile reactions	
Hemolysis (rare)	Transmission of disease
Hypersensitivity reactions	

TRANSFUSION REACTIONS

A **transfusion reaction** is any unfavorable event that occurs in a patient during or shortly after the infusion of whole blood or blood components as a result of that transfusion. Although current compatibility testing techniques generally prevent the administration of blood or blood components containing antibodies to red blood cell antigens, adverse transfusion reactions may be caused by incompatible leukocytes, platelets, or plasma proteins. Regardless of the cause, prompt recognition and treatment of serious transfusion reactions can save lives and decrease morbidity. Because there are no effective means of predicting or preventing most of these reactions, every transfusion must be considered a potentially hazardous procedure.

Several types of immediate and delayed transfusion reactions can occur in varying degrees of severity during the administration of blood or blood components.

Immediate transfusion reactions include:

Bacterial reactions, which result from the infusion of infected blood or the use of transfusion apparatus contaminated with pyrogens.

Circulatory overload, which results from the massive infusion of stored blood.

Febrile reactions, which result from the infusion of blood contaminated with pyrogens or the presence of antileukocyte or antiplatelet antibodies.

Hemolytic transfusion reactions, which result from the infusion of incompatible whole blood or red blood cells.

Hypersensitivity reactions, which result from immunization to food and drug immunoglobulins, the presence of antileukocyte or antiplatelet antibodies, or the infusion of blood containing antigens in recipients with corresponding antibodies.

Delayed transfusion reactions may occur several days or weeks after the infusion of blood or certain blood components and include:

Development of hemosiderosis and post-transfusion hemochromatosis

Formation of antileukocyte or antiplatelet antibodies

Formation of immune antibodies to coagulation factors

Hemolysis of donor red blood cells by recipient antibodies

Immunization to red blood cell antigens

Suppression of erythropoiesis, temporary

Thrombophlebitis

Transmission of disease (cytomegalovirus infection, malaria, syphilis, viral hepatitis)

Investigation of Transfusion Reactions

The appearance of untoward clinical symptoms such as chills, fever, urticaria, changes in blood pressure, and oliguria either during or following blood transfusions may result from several conditions, including a hemolytic transfusion reaction. The presence or absence of certain clinical symptoms, however, does not conclusively eliminate a specific cause of the reaction because some reactions are almost completely asymptomatic and escape diagnosis unless the patient is monitored carefully. Symptoms such as urticaria, on the other hand, may occur in more than one type of reaction and therefore are not sufficient evidence alone for a definitive diagnosis.

Thus, a thorough and orderly investigation must be initiated whenever any transfusion reaction involving more than urticaria occurs to confirm or rule out hemolysis and determine the cause of the reaction. A report detailing any transfusion reaction should include the patient's history of previous transfusions, transfusion reactions, or sensitization caused by pregnancy, as well as the amount of blood administered and the rate of infusion. The report also should include information regarding any other intravenous therapy administered.

▶▶ *Nursing Responsibilities and Implications*
In the event of a suspected hemolytic transfusion reaction, the nurse should proceed as follows:

1. Discontinue the transfusion immediately if all blood has not already been given; keep the intravenous line open with a slow infusion of physiologic saline so that medication can be administered immediately if necessary.

2. Return the remaining blood or blood component, with the administration set intact,

to the blood bank at once, even if only a few drops remain in the bottle or plastic container.

3. Obtain both a clotted and a heparin- or EDTA-anticoagulated post-transfusion blood specimen (red-stoppered tube and green- or lavender-stoppered tube) from the recipient as soon as a reaction is suspected. Collect blood specimens carefully to avoid hemolysis because hemoglobinemia is evidence of a hemolytic transfusion reaction.

4. Collect a urine sample from the recipient as soon as a transfusion reaction is suspected.

5. Submit a transfusion reaction report promptly, stating the reason for returning the remaining blood and describing the clinical symptoms of the transfusion reaction.

6. Monitor the patient's vital signs frequently, including urinary output.

7. Collect all urine voided by the patient.

8. Obtain repeat post-transfusion blood and urine samples from the patient 5–24 hours after the transfusion reaction and 3–5 days later.

9. Do not administer further transfusions of blood or blood components until the cause of the reaction has been established.

Acute Hemolytic Transfusion Reactions

Acute hemolytic reactions result from the infusion of incompatible blood and are potentially the most serious side effect of transfusions, although they are less common than other transfusion reactions. Red blood cell destruction during hemolytic reactions is caused by incompatibility between donor red blood cells and ABO or Rh antibodies in the recipient's plasma. Administration of incompatible blood due to errors in crossmatching is rare, however, because compatibility testing techniques have become more sensitive, although adequate laboratory procedures are no guarantee against subsequent hemolytic reactions. Most hemolytic reactions therefore result from carelessness in checking the patient's identity, clerical errors in identifying or labeling specimens, crossmatching blood for the wrong patient, or giving blood intended for one patient to another.

Hemolytic transfusion reactions usually occur immediately after the administration of as little as 50–100 mL of incompatible blood or shortly following the transfusion. Hemolytic reactions also may be delayed and appear as long as 2–10 days after an incompatible transfusion, usually in patients with a history of previous transfusions or pregnancies. Delayed hemolytic reactions generally are caused by undetected recipient antibodies, which rapidly increase in strength as donor red blood cells containing the corresponding antigen remain in the bloodstream. The time interval between the infusion of blood and the onset of any symptoms may divert suspicion from the transfusion as the cause of hemolysis.

Occasionally, the only indication of hemolysis or an incompatible transfusion is a rapid and unexpected decrease in the recipient's hemoglobin level, hematocrit, and red blood cell count, which leads to anemia. The initial symptoms of hemolytic reactions also may be minimal and almost impossible to detect in patients under deep anesthesia who are unable to complain of discomfort. Except for signs of shock, the first indication of a reaction in most anesthetized patients is an unexplained oozing from the operative wound due to a rapidly developing coagulation defect. Because the other symptoms of hemolytic reaction are masked by anesthesia, prompt recognition of the cause and significance of this blood seepage is critical. Likewise, symptoms such as chills and fever may be mild or absent during hemolytic reactions in infants, although infants appear pale and feel cold to the touch in the phase corresponding to chills in the adult.

Signs and Symptoms

Clinical symptoms of an immediate, severe hemolytic reaction are not the same in all patients but vary in severity according to the amount of blood infused, the nature of the antibodies, and the patient's condition. The clinical events that occur during severe transfusion reactions generally are reversible with adequate medical support and may include:

Anuria	Hemoglobinuria (within 2−4 hours)
Anxiety	Hyperbilirubinemia (within 6−12
Azotemia (after 24 hours)	hours)
Back and chest pain	Hypotension
Bilirubinuria	Increased pulse rate
Chills	Jaundice (within 1−2 days)
Cyanosis	Nausea and vomiting
Diaphoresis	Oliguria
Disseminated intravascular coagulation	Pallor
Dyspnea	Pain at the infusion site
Fever	Renal failure, acute
Flushing	Rigor
Hemoglobinemia (within 2−4 hours)	Shock

Bacterial Reactions

Bacterial reactions are caused by the transfusion of blood, plasma, or intravenous fluids contaminated with pathogenic organisms or their pyrogenic toxins. Pyrogens are the products of bacterial metabolism present in any medium in which bacteria have grown, regardless of whether viable organisms remain. Bacterial reactions usually are due to coagulase-positive staphylococci or gram-negative bacilli, including *Pseudomonas*, which are able to multiply rapidly even at 4 C. Bacterial contamination of blood or blood components is rare, however, because of the increased use of disposable equipment and strict adherence to aseptic techniques and blood bank regulations.

Blood must remain refrigerated until it is given to the patient to prevent bacterial contamination because few organisms can grow rapidly enough at 4 C to constitute a real danger. Thus, blood should be exposed to room temperatures only during transfusion, and the seal on blood containers should not be opened until it is to be administered. Each container of blood should be examined carefully before the transfusion for evidence of bacterial contamination such as hemolysis or an unusual color.

Signs and Symptoms

A transfusion of blood containing bacteria or pyrogens results in a severe, life-threatening, influenza-like reaction characterized by:

Anuria	Fever, high (onset within 1 hour)
Bleeding, profuse	Hypotension, marked
Chills (onset within 1 hour)	Renal necrosis, acute
Diarrhea	Shock
Disseminated intravascular coagulation	Vomiting

Circulatory Overload

Circulatory overload results from the sudden expansion of the recipient's blood volume following a transfusion of blood or fluid in unusually large amounts or at an excessively rapid rate. Although blood volume is readjusted to normal levels within 24 hours after a transfusion in most individuals, this adjustment may be delayed in infants, elderly patients, and individuals with compromised cardiac or pulmonary status, chronic anemia, impaired renal function, or hypoproteinemia. Circulatory overload in these individuals may precipitate serious complications of transfusion therapy such as left heart failure, pulmonary congestion, and pulmonary edema and requires immediate treatment.

Circulatory overload may be prevented by adjusting both the rate and volume of blood or fluid administration according to the patient's age and initial blood volume. Individuals who are susceptible to circulatory overload should be transfused with packed red blood cells at a rate no faster than 1 mL per kilogram of body weight per hour; intravenous fluids should never be administered faster than 5 mL/min. Intravenous fluids must be administered much slower in children, elderly patients, and individuals with heart disease, as well as when impending cardiac decompensation is suspected. Infusion of blood or volume expanders as rapidly as possible is acceptable and frequently necessary, however, when the patient's blood volume is substantially reduced (shock).

Signs and Symptoms
The symptoms of circulatory overload are the same as those associated with congestive heart failure, including:

Cardiac arrest (in severely anemic patients)	Cyanosis	Edema, peripheral
Coughing	Dyspnea	Headache, severe

Febrile Reactions

Febrile reactions, the most common adverse effect of transfusions, are the result of cytotoxic antibodies in donor or recipient plasma directed against leukocyte or platelet antigens. Febrile transfusion reactions are caused by leukocyte incompatibility in patients who receive repeated platelet infusions because of leukocyte contamination of platelet preparations. Patients who receive multiple blood transfusions and previously pregnant women are particularly prone to febrile transfusion reactions, as are patients with Hodgkin's disease, lymphomas, and liver disease.

Febrile reactions are not easy to identify, however, because they cannot be differentiated from the early stages of hemolytic reactions. Transfusion recipients who display repeated febrile reactions probably should receive only leukocyte-poor packed red blood cells or HLA-compatible or identical platelets. Premedication with antipyretics may modify reactions in some patients receiving continued or repeated transfusions, whereas other patients may benefit from antihistamines or steroid therapy.

Signs and Symptoms

Febrile reactions to antileukocyte or antiplatelet antibodies generally occur immediately but may be delayed several hours and are characterized by:

Anxiety	Leukopenia (rare)
Chest pain (within 5 minutes)	Malaise (up to 8 hours)
Chills (up to 8 hours)	Myalgia
Coughing (within 5 minutes)	Nausea (within 5 minutes)
Fever (up to 8 hours)	Palpitations (within 5 minutes)
Flushing (within 5 minutes)	Shock (rare)
Headache (up to 8 hours)	Vomiting (up to 8 hours)
Increased diastolic pressure (up to 8 hours)	

Hypersensitivity Reactions

Hypersensitivity reactions following the transfusion of whole blood or blood components are the secondary result of immunization to substances such as food and drug antigens or foreign immunoglobulins in the donor material. Hypersensitivity reactions range in severity from the relatively mild allergic dermal response to the more severe and potentially fatal anaphylactoid reaction. Most dermal reactions are produced by the infusion of food or drug antigens to which the recipient is sensitive or the passive transfer of allergic antibodies. Anaphylactoid reactions may be caused by food and drug allergens or by the formation of anti-immunoglobulin antibodies in the recipient's blood during the administration of products containing IgA to patients who are deficient in that immunoglobulin.

Patients who are prone to hypersensitivity reactions or who complain of pruritus during a transfusion should be treated with antihistamines such as diphenhydramine to prevent or minimize allergic reactions. Anaphylactoid reactions, however, are extremely dangerous and must be treated immediately with epinephrine, steroids such as cortisone, and oxygen. Patients who receive multiple blood transfusions, previously pregnant women, and individuals who are deficient in IgA are at risk of anaphylactoid reactions and in some cases should be pretreated with steroids before transfusion therapy is instituted. Antihistamines and steroids should be administered only when indicated and must be injected into the patient and not into the container of blood.

Signs and Symptoms

The **most common manifestations** of allergic hypersensitivity reactions develop during transfusion, are of little consequence, and consist of:

Edema, facial and periorbital	Pruritus
Erythema, localized	Urticaria (hives, nettle rash, wheals)

More serious manifestations of hypersensitivity reactions resemble anaphylaxis, require the immediate cessation of the transfusion, and include:

Abdominal pain	Diarrhea	Fever
Asthmatic attacks	Dizziness	Headache
Bronchial spasm	Edema (facial,	Nausea
Chills	laryngeal, glottis)	Vomiting

Immediate anaphylactoid reactions are rare and are characterized by:

Drop in blood pressure	Shock	Wheezing
Flushing	Shortness of breath	

Delayed anaphylactoid reactions with symptoms resembling those of serum sickness may occur 1–5 days after the infusion of blood, plasma, or plasma fractions and include:

Arthritis	Malaise	Pericarditis
Fever	Myalgia	

Transmission of Disease via Transfusion

Transmission of disease from donor to recipient, a serious complication associated with the transfusion of blood or blood components, may occur in spite of careful donor selection and testing prior to infusion. Disease may be caused by many infectious agents present in the blood of normal donors that are inconsequential when transfused to immunocompetent hosts but produce devastating results in immunocompromised recipients. Diseases that may be transmitted by transfusion therapy involving whole blood and its derivatives include viral infections such as acquired immune deficiency syndrome (AIDS), cytomegalovirus (CMV), hepatitis, and syphilis, as well as malaria, a protozoal disease.

Acquired Immune Deficiency Syndrome (AIDS)
Acquired immune deficiency syndrome (AIDS) is an incurable, terminal disease that destroys the body's natural defense system, allowing a variety of fatal cancers and virulent infections to develop. Acquired immune deficiency syndrome usually affects homosexual and bisexual men, intravenous drug users, and hemophiliacs. The disease may be transmitted by transfusion of blood from donors suspected of carrying the causative virus. A number of children, individuals with hemophilia, and patients recovering from cardiovascular bypass surgery have contracted AIDS following massive transfusion of platelets or plasma preparations derived from blood obtained from asymptomatic donors. A screening test to detect the virus during its long incubation period in potential blood donors has been developed and is in widespread use.

Cytomegalovirus
Cytomegalovirus (CMV) infection, a condition resembling infectious mononucleosis, is caused by a herpesvirus and may develop 3–6 weeks after massive transfusion of fresh blood. Although post-transfusion CMV infection seldom results in clinical disease, trans-

mission of the virus may produce arthralgia, fever, hepatic dysfunction, hepatomegaly, leukopenia, lymphocytosis, pneumonia, skin rashes, and splenomegaly. This post-transfusion syndrome is especially threatening, however, during pregnancy, immunosuppressive therapy, or homograft transplantation, as well as to infants and immunocompromised patients, who may develop life-threatening interstitial pneumonitis, encephalitis, or chorioretinitis.

The risk of transmitting CMV infection is particularly high in granulocyte transfusions because the virus is concentrated in the viable leukocytes, although it also may be found in erythrocytes, plasma, and serum. Thus, it may be necessary to use leukocyte-poor blood as an alternative to finding seronegative donors to avoid transfusion-induced CMV infection in susceptible patients. This precaution is particularly appropriate during exchange transfusions in infants of seronegative mothers because the fresh blood used to transfuse pediatric patients is more likely to contain higher concentrations of live virus. (Serologic tests for cytomegalovirus are discussed in Chapter 11.)

Hepatitis

Post-transfusion hepatitis remains the most common serious consequence of transfusion of blood or blood products such as plasma, antihemophilic factor, factor VIII and IX concentrates, and fibrinogen. Viral hepatitis traditionally has been subclassified into two types: hepatitis A, formerly called infectious hepatitis, and hepatitis B, also known as serum hepatitis. Hepatitis A is clinically mild, has a short incubation period of 2–6 weeks, and is spread by fecal-oral transmission or blood transfusion, although transmission by transfusion occurs rarely. Hepatitis B is clinically severe, has an incubation period of 6–26 weeks, and is transmitted by the infusion of blood or plasma that is infected or administered through contaminated needles or syringes.

Although individuals who have had clinical hepatitis are immediately rejected as donors, others with no evident disease may donate blood while in the incubation stage and present an extreme hazard to transfusion therapy. However, because individuals with hepatitis B demonstrate a specific antigen early in the disease, often before chemical abnormalities or clinical symptoms occur, a screening test for its presence is performed on all donor blood. This mandatory testing to detect carriers of the hepatitis B virus has excluded most high-risk donors and dramatically reduced the incidence of post-transfusion hepatitis.

The elimination of blood containing hepatitis B virus from transfusion services, however, has uncovered the existence of a previously unsuspected virus as an important cause of transfusion-associated hepatitis. This clinically mild disorder, termed non-A, non-B (NANB) hepatitis, has an incubation period of 2–15 weeks and may produce serious long-term effects such as chronic liver disease and a potentially fatal cirrhosis. Unfortunately, because there is no reliable test as yet to detect NANB hepatitis, prevention depends on careful screening of donors for clinical symptoms and follow-up of recipients to detect post-transfusion hepatitis. (Serologic tests for hepatitis virus are discussed in Chapter 11.)

Malaria

Individuals who have had **malaria** generally are rejected as blood donors because transfusion of their blood or red blood cells carries the risk of transmission. Likewise, prospective donors who have visited or lived in endemic areas may not give blood until at least 36 months after discontinuing treatment with malarial suppressive medication. Antimalarial drugs may prevent symptoms such as chills and fever without eradicating parasites, which may remain in the body for years after the initial attack. *Plasmodium vivax* cannot survive for more than 96 hours in blood stored at 4 C, although *P. malariae* and *P. falciparum* can survive indefinitely under the usual blood storage conditions.

Syphilis

The transmission of **syphilis** following an infusion of stored blood or blood components is theoretically possible but not very probable. For the transmission of syphilis, spirochetes must be present in the donor's blood and remain viable at the time of transfusion. However, because spirochetes cannot survive at refrigerator temperatures, only blood products stored at room temperature or transfused very soon after donation have any risk of syphilis transmission.

The use of rapid plasma reagin (RPR) and other screening tests on donor blood can decrease but not eliminate the risk of syphilis transmission because results may be negative while potentially infectious organisms are in the bloodstream. It is still impossible to identify the donor who has been exposed to syphilis and is infected but has not yet developed a chancre, secondary syphilis, or a positive serologic reaction. Thus, a negative serologic test is no guarantee that syphilis will not be transmitted because the donor may be in the latent or incubation phase of the disease.

Potential donors with a history of syphilis generally are rejected immediately regardless of whether their serologic test for syphilis is negative, although adequate treatment may make blood safe for transfusion. Freshly drawn blood products, such as platelet concentrates that must be administered immediately and therefore are not stored before use, present the greatest risk of syphilis transmission. Therefore, blood should be stored for 3 days before transfusion whenever possible to avoid the risk of transmitting treponemal spirochetes, which do not survive refrigeration for 72 hours. (Serologic tests for syphilis are discussed in Chapter 11.)

SELECTION AND SCREENING OF BLOOD DONORS

Blood banks and transfusion services depend on the continued participation of volunteer donors to provide the blood and blood components necessary to meet the needs of the patients they serve. Therefore, conditions surrounding blood donations must be as safe, attractive, well lighted, comfortably ventilated, clean, and convenient as possible. The actual process of donating blood requires approximately 20 minutes and involves little physical pain, although the donor may experience some physiologic reactions to the blood loss such as lightheadedness or fainting.

Careful selection and screening of donors are important in obtaining blood and blood components that are therapeutically effective and free of transmittable diseases. A detailed medical history and limited physical examination immediately before each donation are absolutely necessary to protect the recipient and determine whether giving blood will be harmful to the donor.

Criteria for Selecting Blood Donors

Prospective blood donors must meet the following qualifications:

> *Age*—donors must be between 17 and 65 years of age. Prospective donors between 17 and 21 years of age must have a written letter of consent from a parent or

guardian, unless local law defines the legal age as less than 21. Donors over 65 years of age may be accepted if they have specific written consent from a physician obtained within 2 weeks of donation.

Weight—minimum weight is 49.5 kg.

Temperature—oral temperature should not exceed 37.5 C.

Pulse—pulse must exhibit no pathologic abnormalities and be between 50 and 100 beats/min. A lower pulse rate may be acceptable if the prospective donor is an athlete with a high exercise tolerance.

Blood pressure—systolic blood pressure should be between 90 and 180 mm Hg and the diastolic blood pressure between 50 and 100 mm Hg.

Skin—the skin surrounding the venipuncture site should be free of infection and lesions. Mild skin disorders such as acne, psoriasis, or poison ivy rash are not cause for rejection unless unusually extensive. Donors with boils, purulent wounds, or severe skin infections anywhere on the body should not be accepted.

Hemoglobin—the hemoglobin level should be no less than 12.5 g/dL for female donors and 13.5 g/dL for male donors.

Hematocrit—the hematocrit should be no less than 38% for female donors and 42% for male donors.

Food—all food and liquids other than clear beverages should be withheld for approximately 3 hours before donation.

Interval between donations—a minimum of 8 weeks must elapse between donations. Blood may not be donated more than five times in a 1-year period.

Chronic diseases—donors must be in good general health with no chronic disorders such as cancer or heart, lung, stomach, liver, or kidney disease. Donors with specific diseases such as chronic bronchitis, emphysema, and hypertension may donate only with the written recommendation of their personal physician.

Criteria for Excluding Blood Donors

Prospective blood donors must be excluded for the following reasons:

Pregnancy—women must be excluded from blood donation during pregnancy and for 6 weeks after termination of pregnancy.

Dental surgery—the donor must not have undergone dental surgery or tooth extraction during the previous 72 hours.

Surgical procedures—donors who have had major surgery should be deferred for at least 6 months. Minor surgical procedures such as hemorrhoidectomy, appendectomy, tonsillectomy, minor gynecologic procedures, hernia repair, and varicose vein surgery disqualify a donor only until healing is complete.

Blood or component therapy—donors must be rejected if they have received blood or blood components within the previous 6 months.

Infectious disease—donors with any disease transmittable by blood transfusion such as AIDS, CMV infection, hepatitis, malaria, syphilis, and active pulmonary tuberculosis must be rejected.

Illness—donors must not have a long-term illness, history of convulsions, or abnormal bleeding tendencies and must not be ill at the time of donation. Donors suffering from fever, doubtful rash, acute upper respiratory tract infection, or lymphadenopathy must be rejected.

General appearance—donors who appear ill, excessively nervous, or under the influence of alcohol or drugs should be rejected.

Immunization and vaccination—symptom-free donors who recently have been immunized need not be rejected, with the exception of the following time limits: toxoid, killed viral, bacterial, or rickettsial vaccines—24 hours; smallpox, measles (rubeola), mumps, yellow fever, oral polio vaccine, rabies, and animal serum products—2 weeks; German measles (rubella)—2 months; live virus vaccines—3 months.

Medications—donors should not be taking medications, although oral contraceptives, mild analgesics, minor tranquilizers, vitamins, replacement hormones, or weight-reduction pills generally are not cause for rejection. Donors taking antibiotics, corticosteroids, digitalis, insulin, quinidine, phenytoin, diuretics, nitroglycerine, anticoagulants, or other potent drugs must be evaluated by a physician before being permitted to donate blood.

Drug addiction—any individual with a history of drug addiction is permanently excluded from donation.

Recent tattoo—donors who have received a tattoo within the previous 6 months must be rejected.

Allergies—donors should not have any serious allergies to foods, drugs, or other substances. Individuals who have had bronchial asthma or a hypersensitization injection within the preceding 3 days must be rejected.

▶▶ *Nursing Responsibilities and Implications*

1. Explain the blood donation procedure to each prospective donor and describe what can be expected.

2. Assist the prospective donor in completing the questionnaire concerning the medical history to determine if all qualifications for blood donation are fulfilled.

3. Obtain a signed consent form from the prospective donor at the time of registration.

4. Inform all prospective donors about the potential risk of transmitting AIDS to recipients and encourage donors in high-risk groups, including homosexual and bisexual men, intravenous drug users, and hemophiliacs, to excuse themselves.

5. Assist the Medical Director of the blood bank in performing the limited physical examination of the prospective donor.

6. Give the donor some light refreshment after the blood is drawn and encourage rest for a short time to promote the necessary physiologic readjustment.

7. Instruct operators of heavy machinery, taxicabs, buses and trains, scuba or sky divers, and workers required to climb ladders or scaffolding to wait at least 12 hours after blood donation before returning to work.

8. Instruct donors involved in high-altitude activities requiring accurate judgment and keen reflexes, such as flight crews or ski patrols, to wait 72 hours before resuming these activities.

REFERENCES

American Association of Blood Banks. 1984. *Technical manual.* 11th ed. Washington, D.C.: American Association of Blood Banks.

American Association of Blood Banks and The American Red Cross. 1981. *Circular of information for the use of human blood and blood components.* Washington, D.C.: American Association of Blood Banks and The American Red Cross.

Bauer, J. D. 1982. *Clinical laboratory methods.* 9th ed. St. Louis: The C. V. Mosby Co.

Bio-Science Laboratories. 1982. *The Bio-Science handbook.* 13th ed. Van Nuys, Calif.: Bio-Science Laboratories.

Domen, R. E. 1984. Transfusion therapy of the oncology patient. *Lab. Med.* 15(4):251.

Doucet, L. D. 1981. *Medical technology review.* Philadelphia: J. B. Lippincott Co.

French, R. M. 1980. *Guide to diagnostic procedures.* 5th ed. New York: McGraw-Hill Book Co.

Garb, S. 1976. *Laboratory tests in common use.* 6th ed. New York: Springer Publishing Co.

Henry, J. B. 1984. *Clinical diagnosis and management by laboratory methods.* 17th ed. Philadelphia: W. B. Saunders Co.

Insalaco, J. C. 1984. Massive transfusion. *Lab. Med.* 15(5):325.

Jay, M. 1980. Laboratory investigation of hemolytic disease of the newborn. *Lab. Med.* 11(4):232.

Kalmin, N. D. 1981. Transfusion of cytomegalovirus—a review. *Lab. Med.* 12(8):489.

Kevy, S. V. 1979. Pediatric transfusion therapy. *Lab. Med.* 10(8):459.

Leparc, G. F., and Schmidt, P. J. 1984. Stop! Transfusion reaction. *Diagn. Med.* 7(9):49.

Maehara, K. T. 1983. HLA and disease: an association. *Lab. Med.* 14(10):648.

Miale, J. B. 1982. *Laboratory medicine—hematology.* 6th ed. St. Louis: The C. V. Mosby Co.

Myhre, B. A., and Van Antwerp, R. 1983. Diagnosis of unexpected reactions to transfusion. *Lab. Med.* 14(3):153.

Noto, T. A. 1982. How to interpret a positive DAT. *Diagn. Med.* 6(7):59.

Pagana, K. D., and Pagana, T. J. 1982. *Diagnostic testing and nursing implications.* St. Louis: The C. V. Mosby Co.

Peter, J. B., and Hawkins, B. R. 1981. HLA antigens and disease. *Diagn. Med.* 4(1):2.

Peter, J. B., and Wolde-Miriam, W. 1984. AIDS: putting the puzzle together. *Diagn. Med.* 7(2):56.

Polesky, H. F. 1983. Infections from transfused blood. *Diagn. Med.* 6(6):25.

Raphael, S. S., et al., editors. 1983. *Medical laboratory technology.* 4th ed. Philadelphia: W. B. Saunders Co.

Slonaker, C. E., and Milam, J. D. 1983. Hemotherapy in a large cardiovascular surgical center. *Lab. Med.* 14(12):772.

Strand, M. M., and Elmer, L. A. 1983. *Clinical laboratory tests.* 3rd ed. St. Louis: The C. V. Mosby Co.

Tilkian, S. M., Conover, M. B., and Tilkian, A. G. 1983. *Clinical implications of laboratory tests.* 3rd ed. St. Louis: The C. V. Mosby Co.

Unger, J. L. 1984. Platelet crossmatch techniques: how good are they? *Diagn. Med.* 7(3):59.

Widmann, F. K. 1983. *Clinical implications of laboratory tests.* 9th ed. Philadelphia: F. A. Davis Co.

Wooten, M. J. 1984. Leukocyte-poor, washed red blood cells in transfusion therapy. *Lab. Med.* 15(1):42.

Yesus, Y. W. 1981. Granulocyte transfusion—a review. *Lab. Med.* 12(9):551.

———. 1981. Post-transfusion hepatitis—update. *Lab. Med.* 12(11):703.

APPENDIX A
Organ Panels and Disease Profiles

Laboratory tests of vital blood and urine components can help in making or confirming diagnoses, assessing clinical progress, and guiding and monitoring the effects of therapy. However, because few laboratory tests are diagnostic for any one disease to the exclusion of all other diseases, organ panels or sets of tests frequently are ordered to screen several body systems simultaneously. The characteristic patterns of normal and abnormal test results are used to assess the severity of the condition and focus attention on a particular organ or system that requires more specific testing. Organ panels and disease profiles may include the following tests:

Admission panel (performed on all patients regardless of diagnosis):

Complete blood count (CBC)

Routine urinalysis

Broad-spectrum chemical screening, including:

Albumin

Albumin/globulin (A/G) ratio

Alanine aminotransferase (ALT, formerly SGPT)

Alkaline phosphatase

Aspartate aminotransferase (AST, formerly SGOT)

Bilirubin, direct and total

Blood urea nitrogen (BUN)

Calcium

Chloride

Cholesterol

Creatine phosphokinase (CPK)

Creatinine

Gamma glutamyl transferase (GGT)

Globulin

Glucose

Iron

Lactate dehydrogenase (LDH)

Phosphorus

Potassium

Sodium

Total protein

Triglycerides

Uric acid

Venereal Disease Research Laboratories (VDRL) or other test for syphilis

Anticonvulsant group panel:

Phenobarbital

Phenytoin

Primidone

Mephobarbital

Autoimmune disease profile:

Antimitochondrial antibodies

Antinuclear antibodies (ANA)

Anti-smooth muscle antibodies

Calcium metabolism profile:

Calcitonin

Calcium, total and ionized

Magnesium

Parathyroid hormone (PTH)

Phosphorus

Vitamin D

Cardiac panel:

Aspartate aminotransferase (AST)

Creatine phosphokinase (CPK)

Creatine phosphokinase isoenzymes

Hydroxybutyric dehydrogenase (HBDH)

Lactic dehydrogenase (LH)

Lactic dehydrogenase isoenzymes

Potassium

Coagulation profile:

Activated partial thromboplastin time (APTT)

Antithrombin III (AT III)

Bleeding time

Clot retraction

Fibrin-fibrinogen degradation products (FDP)

Fibrinogen

Platelet adhesion and aggregation

Platelet count

Prothrombin time (PT)

Thrombin time

Whole blood clotting time

Comatose patient profile:

Drug abuse/overdose panel, plus:

Acetaminophen

Alcohol

Blood gases (pH, P_{CO_2}, CO_2)

Blood urea nitrogen (BUN)

Creatinine

Electrolytes

Glucose

Salicylates

Quinine

Coronary risk panel:

Cholesterol, total

Glucose

High-density lipoproteins (HDL)

Lipids, total

Lipoprotein phenotyping

Low-density lipoproteins (LDL)

Phospholipids

Triglycerides

Very low-density lipoproteins (VLDL)

Diabetes mellitus profile:

Glucose, serum (2-hour postprandial) and urine

Glucose tolerance (when not contraindicated by high glucose level)

Ketones, serum and urine

Triglycerides

Dialysis management panel:

Calcium, ionized

Ferritin

Parathyroid hormone (PTH)

Vitamin D

Drug abuse/overdose screen:

Amphetamines	Meperidine	Phencyclidine (PCP)
Barbiturates	Methadone	Phenothiazines
Benzodiazepines	Methamphetamines	Propoxyphene
Codeine	Methaqualone	Tricyclic antidepressants
Heroin	Narcotics	

Electrolyte panel:

Carbon dioxide

Chloride

Potassium

Sodium

Endocrine screening panel:

Dehydroepiandrosterone sulfate
(DHEA)

Follicle-stimulating hormone (FSH)

17-Ketosteroids (17-KS)

Prolactin

Thyroid-stimulating hormone (TSH)

Thyroxine (T_4)

Febrile panel:

Antistreptolysin O titer (ASO)

C-reactive protein (CRP)

Febrile agglutinins

Heterophil

Rheumatoid factor (RF)

Heavy metals screen (urine):

Arsenic

Lead

Mercury

Hepatitis profile:

Hepatitis A antibodies

Hepatitis B core antibodies

Hepatitis B surface antigens and
antibodies

Hepatitis B "e" antigens and antibodies

Hyperal chemistry panel:

Albumin

Alkaline phosphatase

Aspartate aminotransferase (AST)

Bilirubin, total

Blood urea nitrogen (BUN)

Calcium

Creatinine

Electrolytes

Glucose

Iron and iron-binding capacity

Lactate dehydrogenase (LDH)

Magnesium

Nitrogen, 12-hour urine

Phosphorus

Hypertension profile:

Renal panel, plus:

    Blood gases (pH, P_{CO_2}, CO_2)

    Cholesterol

Glucose (2-hour postprandial)

Lactate dehydrogenase (LDH)

Triglycerides

Immunologic evaluation—B-lymphocyte complex:

Antinuclear antibodies (ANA)

Antimitochondrial antibodies

Anti-smooth muscle antibodies

Immunoelectrophoresis

Immunoglobulins (quantitative)

Protein electrophoresis

Rheumatoid factor (RF)

Iron deficiency profile:

Ferritin

Iron

Total iron-binding capacity (TIBC)

Lipid profile:

Cholesterol, total and esters

Glucose

HDL cholesterol

LDL cholesterol

Lipids, total

Lipoprotein electrophoresis

Phospholipids

Triglycerides

Liver panel:

Alanine aminotransferase (ALT)

Alkaline phosphatase

Aspartate aminotransferase (AST)

Bilirubin, direct and total

Cholesterol

Gamma glutamyl transferase (GGT)

Lactate dehydrogenase (LDH) and isoenzymes

Total protein and protein electrophoresis

Urine for bile pigments

Lung maturity profile (amniotic fluid):

Creatinine

Lecithin/sphingomyelin (L/S)

Phosphatidylglycerol

Uric acid

Megaloblastic anemia profile:

Red blood cell folate

Serum folate

Vitamin B_{12}

Neonatal intensive care panel:

Albumin

Calcium

Bilirubin, total

Blood urea nitrogen (BUN)

Electrolytes

Glucose

Pancreatic panel (acute):

Amylase, serum and urine (24-hour or timed collection)

Lipase

Parathyroid/bone panel:

Alkaline phosphatase

Calcium

Phosphorus

Prenatal panel:

ABO and Rh typing

Atypical antibody screen

Complete blood count (CBC)

Rubella

Syphilis serology (VDRL)

Urinalysis

Renal panel:

Blood urea nitrogen (BUN)

Creatinine

Creatinine clearance

Electrolytes

Uric acid

Rheumatoid/arthritic panel:

Antinuclear antibodies (ANA)

Antistreptolysin O titer (ASO)

C-reactive protein (CRP)

Rheumatoid factor (RF)

Serum protein electrophoresis

Uric acid

Stimulants panel:

Amphetamines

Cocaine

Ephedrine

Methamphetamine

Phencyclidine (PCP)

Phenmetrazine

Phenylpropanolamine

Surgical panel:

Coagulation panel, plus:

Aspartate aminotransferase (AST)

Bilirubin, total

Blood urea nitrogen (BUN)

Creatine phosphokinase (CPK)

Glucose

Pseudocholinesterase (PCHE)

Thyroid panel:

Triiodothyronine (T_3) uptake and radioimmunoassay (RIA)

Thyroxine (T_4)

Free thyroxine index (FTI; T_7)

Thyroid-stimulating hormone (TSH)

TORCH panel:

Cytomegalovirus (CMV) antibodies

Herpes virus antibodies

Rubella antibodies

Toxoplasmal antibodies

Tumor marker profile:

α-Fetoprotein (AFP)

β-Human chorionic gonadotropin
(β-HCG)

Carcinoembryonic antigen (CEA)

Prostatic acid phosphatase

APPENDIX B
Blood Specimen Tube Requirements

The following is a general listing of specimen requirements for many laboratory procedures. The stopper colors listed below refer to evacuated collection tube systems.

Color	Tube Contents
Red	No additives
Lavender	EDTA
Green	Heparin
Blue	Sodium citrate
Black	Sodium oxalate
Gray	Glycolytic inhibitor
Yellow	No additive, sterile contents
Brown	Minimal lead content

Red stopper   Studies requiring serum specimens collected without anticoagulants. *Chemistry tests*—two to three tests can be done per 7 mL tube

Acetaminophen

Acetone

Albumin

Alanine aminotransferase (ALT)

Alcohol (do not use alcohol swab)

Aldolase

α_1-Fetoprotein

Amylase

Aspartate aminotransferase (AST)

Barbiturate screen

Bilirubin

Blood urea nitrogen (BUN)

Bromide

Calcium (total)

Carotene

Cholesterol

Cholinesterase

Copper

Cortisol

Creatinine

Creatine phosphokinase (CPK) and isoenzymes

Digitoxin

Digoxin

Electrolytes

Electrophoresis—immunoglobulin, lipoprotein, protein

Ethosuximide

Folate

Follicle-stimulating hormone (FSH)

Free thyroxine (free T_4)

Glucose

Growth hormone (GH)

Iron and total iron-binding capacity (TIBC)

Lactate dehydrogenase (LDH) and isoenzymes

Lead (10 mL tube, chemically clean)

Lipase

Lithium

Luteinizing hormone (LH)

Magnesium

Osmolality

Parathyroid hormone (PTH)

Phenobarbital

Phenytoin

Phospholipids

Phosphorus

Phosphatase, acid

Phosphatase, alkaline

Primidone

Procainamide

Prolactin

Propranolol

Pseudocholinesterase (PCHE)

Salicylate

SMA 12-60, SMAC

Testosterone

Theophylline

Thyroid-binding globulin (TBG)

Thyroid-stimulating hormone (TSH)

Total protein

Total thyroxine (T_4)

Triglycerides

Triiodothyronine (T_3)

Uric acid

Vitamin B_{12}

Hematology tests

Clot retraction

Haptoglobin

Lupus erythematosus (LE) cell preparations

Prothrombin consumption time (PCT)

Immunology/serology tests

α_1-Antitrypsin

Antihyaluronidase

Antinuclear antibodies (ANA)

Antistreptolysin O (ASO)

Antithyroid antibodies

Aspergillus antibodies

Brucella antibodies

Candida antibodies

Ceruloplasmin

CH_{50} (total hemolytic complement)

Cold agglutinins

Complement

C-reactive protein

Cryoglobulin

Deoxyribonuclease B antibodies (anti-DNase B)

Deoxyribonucleic acid antibodies (anti-DNA)

Fluorescent treponemal antibody absorption (FTA-ABS)

Francisella agglutinins

Hepatitis virus antigens

Heterophil antibodies

IgE

Monospot

Rheumatoid factor (RF)

Rubella antibodies

Salmonella agglutinins

Streptococcus MG

Thyroid antibodies

TORCH test

Toxoplasmal antibodies

VDRL

Weil-Felix agglutination

Widal test

Immunohematology tests

Antibody identification (two tubes)

Antibody screen (two tubes)

Antiglobulin test, direct (DAT)

Compatibility (crossmatch [one tube for 3 units])

Erythrocyte typing (ABO, Rh, and extended)

Open-heart evaluation (ABO, Rh genotype, direct antiglobulin test, antibody screen [three tubes])

Prenatal evaluation (ABO, Rh genotype, and antibody screen [two tubes])

Lavender stopper   Studies requiring plasma specimens collected with EDTA anticoagulant.

Chemistry tests

Carcinoembryonic antigen (CEA) (two tubes)

Renin (two tubes, on ice)

Hematology tests

Complete blood count (white blood cell count, red blood cell count, hemoglobin, hematocrit, mean corpuscular volume, mean corpuscular hemoglobin, mean corpuscular hemoglobin concentration)

Differential count

Erythrocyte sedimentation rate (ESR) and zeta sedimentation rate (ZSR)

Glucose-6-phosphate dehydrogenase screen (G-6-PD)

Hemoglobin electrophoresis

Osmotic fragility

Platelet count

Reticulocyte count

Sickle cell preparation

Total eosinophil count

Green stopper   Studies requiring plasma specimens collected with heparin anticoagulant.

Chemistry tests

Ammonia (on ice)

Carboxyhemoglobin

Methemoglobin

Oxygen saturation

pH

Plasma hemoglobin

Immunohematology tests

HLA (human leukocyte A) antibody detection

HLA lymphocyte typing

Immunology/serology tests

T- and B-lymphocyte studies (three heparin tubes and one EDTA tube)

Blue stopper   Studies requiring plasma specimens collected with sodium citrate.
Hematology tests

Coagulation factor assays	Partial thromboplastin time (PTT)
Fibrinogen level	Prothrombin time (PT)
G-6-PD assay (plus one EDTA tube)	Thrombin time (TT)

Gray stopper   Studies requiring plasma specimens collected with a sodium fluoride oxalate glycolytic inhibitor.
Chemistry tests

Glucose	Lactate (on ice)
Glucose tolerance	Lactose tolerance

APPENDIX C
Normal Values

WHOLE BLOOD, SERUM, AND PLASMA (CHEMISTRY)

Test	Specimen	Normal Values*
Acetaminophen	Serum or plasma	Therapeutic range: 4.5−26.0 μg/mL
Acetoacetic acid	Serum	Negative: 0.2−1.0 mg/dL
Acetone	Serum or plasma	Negative: 0.3−2.0 mg/dL Toxic level: >20 mg/dL
ACTH	Plasma	8 AM−10 AM: <80 pg/mL
Albumin	Serum	3.5−5.5 g/dL
Alcohol, ethyl	Serum, plasma, or whole blood	Subclinical: <10 mg/dL <0.005%
Ethyl Isopropyl Methyl		Toxic level: >0.45% Toxic level: >0.15% Toxic level: >0.02%
Aldolase	Serum	Adults: 10−40 IU 3−8 Sibley-Lehninger units/dL Children: approx. two times adult level Newborn: approx. four times adult level
Aldosterone	Serum	Female: 4−31 ng/dL Male: 6−22 ng/dL
α_1-Antitrypsin	Serum	210−500 mg/mL

*Normal values may vary significantly with different laboratory methods.

Source: from Saxton, D. F., et al. 1983. *The Addison-Wesley Manual of Nursing Practice.*
Menlo Park, Calif.: Addison-Wesley Publishing Co.

WHOLE BLOOD, SERUM, AND PLASMA (CHEMISTRY) *continued*

Test	Specimen	Normal Values*	
α_1-Fetoprotein (AFP)	Serum	Gestational Age (weeks)	ng/mL AFP

Gestational Age (weeks)	ng/mL AFP
8	70
12	120
16	200
20	290
24	370
28	430
32	450
36	430
40	360

Males and nonpregnant females: <25 ng/mL

Test	Specimen	Normal Values*
Amikacin	Serum	Therapeutic range: 10–25 µg/mL at peak Toxic level: 135 µg/mL at peak or >10 µg/mL at trough levels
Aminotransferases	Serum	
Aspartate amino-transferase		8–40 U/mL* 3–21 IU/L 5–25 Reitman-Frankel units
Alanine amino-transferase		5–35 U/mL* 5–24 IU/L 5–35 Reitman-Frankel units
Amitriptyline	Serum or plasma	Therapeutic range: 75–200 ng/mL Toxic level: >1000 ng/mL
Ammonia	Whole blood	70–200 µg/dL*
	Plasma	56–150 µg/dL
Amylase	Serum	60–180 Somogyi units/dL
Antidiuretic hormone (ADH)	Plasma	0–2 pg/mL: serum osmolality <285 mOsm/kg 2–12 pg/mL: serum osmolality >290 mOsm/kg
Arsenic	Gastric Hair Nails Whole blood	Negative <65 µg/100 g 90–180 µg/100 g <3 µg/dL
Ascorbic acid tolerance	Plasma	1.6 mg/dL or more

WHOLE BLOOD, SERUM, AND PLASMA (CHEMISTRY) *continued*

Test	Specimen	Normal Values*
Barbiturates	Serum or plasma	
Amobarbital		Therapeutic range: 5–8 μg/mL
		Toxic level: >130 μg/mL
Butabarbital		Therapeutic range: 10–14 μg/mL
		Toxic level: >30 μg/mL
Pentobarbital		Therapeutic range: 1–4 μg/mL
		Toxic level: >5 μg/mL
Phenobarbital		Therapeutic range: 15–35μg/mL
		Toxic level: >40 μg/mL
Secobarbital		Therapeutic range: 3–5 μg/mL
		Toxic level: >5 μg/mL
Base excess	Whole blood	Male: −3.3 to +1.2
		Female: −2.4 to +2.3
Base, total	Serum	145–160 mEq/L
Bicarbonate	Plasma	21–28 mEq/L
Bilirubin	Serum	Direct: 0.1–0.4 mg/dL
		Indirect: 0.2–1.0 mg/dL
		Total: 0.3–1.4 mg/dL
		Children: 0.2–0.8 mg/dL
		Newborn: 1.0–12.0 mg/dL
Blood gases	Whole blood	
pH		Arterial: 7.35–7.45
		Venous: 7.36–7.41
P_{CO_2}		Arterial: 35–45 mm Hg
		Venous: 35–50 mm Hg
P_{O_2}		Arterial: 80–100 mm Hg
Bromide	Serum or plasma	Normal: <20 mg/dL
		Therapeutic range: 20–120 mg/dL
		Toxic level: >120 mg/dL
Bromsulphthalein (BSP) 5 mg/kg	Serum	<0.4 mg/dL or 5% retention after 45 minutes
Calcitonin	Serum or plasma	<425 pg/mL
Calcium	Serum	Adults:
		8.5–10.5 mg/dL
		4.3–5.3 mEq/L
		Children:
		11–13 mg/dL
		6 mEq/L
Carbamazepine	Serum or plasma	Therapeutic range: 5–12 μg/mL
		Toxic level: >9 μg/mL

WHOLE BLOOD, SERUM, AND PLASMA (CHEMISTRY) *continued*

Test	Specimen	Normal Values*
Carbon dioxide (CO₂ content)	Whole blood	Arterial: 19–24 mEq/L Venous: 22–26 mEq/L
	Plasma	Arterial: 21–30 mEq/L Venous: 24–34 mEq/L
Carbon dioxide pressure (Pco₂)	Whole blood	Arterial: 35–45 mm Hg Venous: 35–50 mm Hg
Carbon monoxide (carboxy-hemoglobin)	Whole blood	Nonsmokers: 0%–1.5% saturation Smokers: 1.5%–5.0% saturation Heavy smokers: 5.0%–9.0% saturation
Carcinoembryonic antigen (CEA)	Plasma	0–2.5 ng/mL
Carotene	Serum	50–300 μg/dL (varies with diet)
Cephalin-cholesterol flocculation	Serum	0–1+ after 24 hours 0–2+ after 48 hours
Ceruloplasmin	Serum	18–45 mg/dL
Chlordiazepoxide	Serum or plasma	Therapeutic range: 0.1–3 μg/mL Toxic level: >3 μg/mL
Chloride	Serum	95–108 mEq/L
Cholesterol, total	Serum	Newborn: 50–100 mg/dL 1 year: 70–175 mg/dL Adolescence: 135–240 mg/dL 20–29 years: 144–275 mg/dL 30–39 years: 165–295 mg/dL 40–49 years: 170–315 mg/dL 50–69 years: 175–340 mg/dL Over 70 years: 130–245 mg/dL
Cholesterol, esters	Serum	65%–75% of total cholesterol <210 mg/dL
Cholesterol, fractionated HDL cholesterol LDL cholesterol VLDL cholesterol	Plasma	 29–77 mg/dL 62–185 mg/dL 0–40 mg/dL
Cholinesterase, pseudo-cholinesterase (PCHE)	Serum	Male: 274–532 IU/dL* Female: 204–500 IU/dL*
Citric acid	Serum or plasma	1.7–3.0 mg/dL
Copper	Serum or plasma	Male: 70–140 μg/dL Female: 85–155 μg/dL

WHOLE BLOOD, SERUM, AND PLASMA (CHEMISTRY) *continued*

Test	Specimen	Normal Values*
Cortisol	Plasma	8 AM–10 AM: 5–25 μg/dL 4 PM–midnight: 2–18 μg/dL
Creatine	Serum or plasma	Male: 0.2–0.6 mg/dL Female: 0.6–1.0 mg/dL
Creatine phospho- kinase (CPK)	Serum	Male: 55–170 U/L* 5–35 U/mL Female: 30–135 U/L* 5–25 U/mL
Creatinine	Serum	0.6–1.5 mg/dL
Creatinine clearance	Serum or plasma and urine	Male: 107–141 mL/min Female: 87–132 mL/min
Cryoglobulin	Serum	Negative
11-Deoxycortisol	Plasma	0.05–0.25 μg/dL
Desipramine	Serum or plasma	Therapeutic range: 20–160 ng/mL Toxic level: >1000 ng/mL
Diazepam	Serum or plasma	Therapeutic range: 105–1540 ng/mL Toxic level: 3000–14,000 ng/mL
Dicumarol	Serum or plasma	Therapeutic range: 8–30 μg/mL Toxic level: 42–95 μg/mL
Digitoxin	Serum	Negative Therapeutic range: 17–20 ng/mL
Digoxin	Serum	Negative Therapeutic range: 0.8–2.1 ng/mL
Disopyramide	Serum	Therapeutic range: 2–5 μg/mL Toxic level: not established
Doxepin	Serum or plasma	Therapeutic range: 90–250 ng/mL Toxic level: >1000 ng/mL
Dopamine–β- hydroxylase	Serum or plasma	2–90 IU/L
Electrophoresis, lipoprotein	Plasma	α: 12%–28% 80–310 mg/dL β: 50%–70% 160–400 mg/dL Pre-β: 11%–29% 50–180 mg/dL Chylo- microns: 0%–1% 0–50 mg/dL
Electrophoresis, protein	Serum	Albumin: 3%–68% 3.5–5.5 g/dL α_1: 2%–5% 0.1–0.4 g/dL α_2: 7%–14% 0.4–1.0 g/dL β: 9%–15% 0.5–1.1 g/dL γ: 11%–21% 0.5–1.7 g/dL

WHOLE BLOOD, SERUM, AND PLASMA (CHEMISTRY) *continued*

Test	Specimen	Normal Values*
Erythropoietin	Serum	7–36 mIU/mL
Estradiol	Serum or plasma	Male: 8–50 pg/mL Female: (menstrual cycle) 1–10 days: 20–170 pg/mL 11–20 days: 70–500 pg/mL 21–30 days: 45–340 pg/mL

Estriol	Serum	Gestational Age (weeks)	ng/mL
		25–28	13–23
		29–32	16–26
		33–36	14–32
		37–38	16–44
		39–40	23–42
		Over 40	22–41

Test	Specimen	Normal Values*
Estrogens, total	Serum or plasma	Male: 35–130 pg/mL Female: (menstrual cycle) Follicular: 60–250 pg/mL Midcycle: 120–570 pg/mL Luteal: 75–450 pg/mL

Estrogens, fractionated	Serum	Adult	Estrone	Estradiol	Total
		Male:	102–175	8–50	110–225
		Female: (menstrual cycle)			
		Days			
		1–10	79–250	23–100	102–350
		11–20	131–376	50–290	181–666
		21–30	101–399	40–165	141–564

Units = pg/mL

Test	Specimen	Normal Values*
Ethchlorvynol	Serum or plasma	Therapeutic range: 0.5–6.5 μg/mL Toxic level: >20 mL
Ethosuximide	Serum or plasma	Therapeutic range: 40–100 μg/mL Toxic level: >150 μg/mL
Fats, neutral	Serum or plasma	0–200 mg/dL
Fatty acids, free	Serum	<25 mg/dL; 0.3–1.0 mEq/L
Ferritin	Serum or plasma	Male: 10–273 ng/mL Female: 5–99 ng/mL Children: (6 months–15 years) 7–142 ng/mL
Fibrinogen	Plasma	200–400 mg/dL

WHOLE BLOOD, SERUM, AND PLASMA (CHEMISTRY) *continued*

Test	Specimen	Normal Values*
Flurazepam	Serum or plasma	Therapeutic range: none detected Toxic level: 2000 ng/mL
Folate	Serum Erythrocytes	5−25 ng/mL 166−640 ng/mL
Follicle-stimulating hormone (FSH)	Serum	Male: 4−25 mIU/mL Female: Premenopausal: 4−30 mIU/mL Midcycle peak: 2 × baseline Postmenopausal: 40−250 mIU/mL
Gastrin	Serum or plasma	<100 pg/mL
Gentamicin	Serum or plasma	Therapeutic range: 4−8 μg/mL at peak Toxic level: >10μg/mL at peak or >2 μg/mL at trough
Globulins, total	Serum	1.5−3.5 g/dL
Glucose, fasting	Serum	"True glucose": 65−110 mg/dL All sugars: 80−120 mg/dL
Glucose, 2-hour postprandial	Serum	<145 mg/dL
Glucose tolerance, intravenous	Serum or plasma	Fasting: 65−110 mg/dL 5 minutes: maximum of 250 mg/dL 60 minutes: significant decrease 120 minutes: below 120 mg/dL 180 minutes: fasting level
Glucose tolerance, oral	Serum or plasma	Fasting: 65−110 mg/dL 30 minutes: <155 mg/dL 60 minutes: <165 mg/dL 120 minutes: <120 mg/dL 180 minutes: fasting level or less
Glucose-6-phosphate dehydrogenase (G-6-PD)	Whole blood	4.3−10.8 IU/g of hemoglobin
Gamma-glutamyl transferase (GGT)	Serum	Male: 12−38 mU/mL*; 4−23 IU/L Female: 9−31 mU/mL*; 3.5−13 IU/L
Glutethimide	Serum or plasma	Therapeutic range: 4−12 μg/mL Toxic level: >10 μg/mL
Glycohemoglobin	Whole blood	6.0−8.8% of total hemoglobin
Growth hormone (GH)	Serum	Male: <10 ng/mL Female: <15 ng/mL Children: <10 ng/mL
Haptoglobin	Serum	60−185 mg/dL as hemoglobin binding capacity

WHOLE BLOOD, SERUM, AND PLASMA (CHEMISTRY) *continued*

Test	Specimen	Normal Values*
Hemoglobin	Serum or plasma	Negative; 0.5–5.0 mg/dL
Hemoglobin A₁C quantitative	Whole blood	3.9%–6.4% of total hemoglobin
Hemoglobin A₂ quantitative	Whole blood	2.2%–3.7% of total hemoglobin
Hemoglobin F	Whole blood	<2% of total hemoglobin
Human chorionic gonadotropin (HCG)	Serum	<3 mIU/mL Pregnancy: >10 mIU/L by 10 days after implantation

Human placental lactogen (HPL)	Serum or plasma	Weeks of Pregnancy	μ/mL
		5–27	Less than 4.6
		28–31	2.4–6.1
		32–35	3.7–7.7
		36–40	5.0–8.6

Test	Specimen	Normal Values*
α-Hydroxybutyric dehydrogenase (HBDH)	Serum	150–350 U/mL;* 170–300 IU/L; 56–125 IU/L
17-Hydroxy-corticosteroids (17-OCHS)	Plasma	Male: 7–19 μg/dL Female: 9–21 μg/dL After administration of 25 units of ACTH intramuscularly: 35–55 μg/dL
17-Hydroxy-progesterone	Serum or plasma	Male: 0.4–4.0 ng/mL Female: 0.1–3.3 ng/mL Pregnant: 2.3–7.6 ng/mL Postmenopausal: 0.3–0.9 ng/mL Children: <0.5 ng/mL
Imipramine	Serum or plasma	Therapeutic range: 150–300 ng/mL Toxic level: >1000 ng/mL

Immunoglobulin, fraction	Serum		IgA	IgG	IgM
		Newborn	0	602–1630	0–29
		1–3 months	0–23	146–648	11–116
		4–6 months	3–42	80–512	29–107
		7–12 months	8–54	269–913	32–155
		13–24 months	14–85	123–1005	29–221
		25–36 months	16–75	470–1224	60–225
		3–5 years	23–137	518–1447	42–212
		6–8 years	57–204	688–1533	44–242
		9–11 years	52–256	774–1641	36–240
		12–16 years	52–192	697–1593	39–330

Units = mg/dL

WHOLE BLOOD, SERUM, AND PLASMA (CHEMISTRY) *continued*

Test	Specimen	Normal Values*
Immunoglobulins	Serum	
IgG		Adults: 80%; 800−1600 mg/dL
IgA		Adults: 15%; 50−250 mg/dL
IgM		Adults: 0.5%; 40−120 mg/dL
IgD		0.2%; 0.5−3.0 mg/dL
IgE		0.0002%; 0.01−0.04 mg/dL
Insulin	Plasma	11−240 μIU/mL*
		4−24 μU/mL
Iodine	Serum	
Butanol extracted (BEI)		3.5−6.5 μg/dL
Protein bound (PBI)		4.0−8.0 μg/dL
Iron, total	Serum	60−200 μg/dL
		Male average: 125 μg/dL
		Female average: 100 μg/dL
		Children: 55−185 μg/dL
		Elderly: 60−80 μg/dL
Iron-binding capacity	Serum	Adult: 250−420 μg/dL
		Newborn average: 225 μg/dL
Iron saturation	Serum	Male: 35%−40%
		Female: 30%−35%
Ketone bodies	Serum	2−4 μg/dL
17-Ketosteroids (17-KS)	Plasma	25−125 μg/dL
Lactic acid	Whole blood	Arterial: 3−7 mg/dL
		Venous: 5−20 mg/dL
Lactate dehydro-genase (LDH)	Serum	80−120 Wacker units*
		150−450 Wroblewski units
		71−207 IU/L
LDH (heat stable)	Serum	30%−60% of total LDH
LDH isoenzymes	Serum	LDH_1: 18%−33%
		LDH_2: 28%−40%
		LDH_3: 16%−30%
		LDH_4: 6%−16%
		LDH_5: 2%−13%
Lead	Whole blood	0.01−0.08 mg/dL
Lipase	Serum	Less than 1.5 U/mL*
		14−280 mIU/mL

WHOLE BLOOD, SERUM, AND PLASMA (CHEMISTRY) *continued*

Test	Specimen	Normal Values*
Lipids	Serum	
Total		400–800 mg/dL
Cholesterol		120–260 mg/dL (varies with age)
Triglycerides		0–190 mg/dL
Phospholipids		150–380 mg/dL
Phospholipid phosphorus		8–11 mg/dL
Fatty acids, free		Less than 25 mg/dL
Neutral fat		0–200 mg/dL
Lipoproteins (see Electrophoresis)		
Lithium	Serum	Optimal patient response levels: 0.5–1.5 mEq/L
		Desirable maintenance levels: 0.5–1.0 mEq/L
		Toxicity rarely appears at levels below 1.5 mEq/L
		Moderate toxicity may appear at levels of 1.5–2.5 mEq/L
		Medium to severe reactions appear at levels of 2.0–3.0 mEq/L
Luteinizing hormone (LH)	Plasma	Male: <11 mIU/mL
		Female:
		Midcycle peak <3 × baseline value
		Premenopausal: <25 mIU/mL
		Postmenopausal: >25 mIU/mL
Magnesium	Serum	1.8–3.0 mg/dL
		1.5–2.5 mEq/L
Meprobamate	Serum or plasma	Therapeutic range: 16–27 μg/mL
		Toxic level: >35 μg/mL
Methemoglobin	Whole blood	0.4%–1.5% of total hemoglobin: 0–0.24 g/dL
Methotrexate	Serum or plasma	Toxic level: >41 μg/dL
Myoglobin	Serum	<55 ng/mL
Nitrogen (NPN)	Whole blood	25–40 mg/dL
Osmolality	Serum	275–300 mOsm/kg
Oxygen	Whole blood	
Pressure (Po_2)		Arterial: 95–100 mm Hg
Content		15–23 mL/dL
Saturation		Arterial: 95%–98%
		Venous: 60%–85%
Parathyroid hormone	Serum	<2000 pg/mL

WHOLE BLOOD, SERUM, AND PLASMA (CHEMISTRY) *continued*

Test	Specimen	Normal Values*
pH	Whole blood	Arterial: 7.35−7.45 Venous: 7.36−7.41
Phenobarbital	Serum or plasma	Therapeutic range: 15−35 μg/mL Toxic level: >40 μg/mL
Phenytoin	Serum or plasma	Therapeutic range: 10−20 μg/mL Toxic level: >20 μg/mL
Phosphatase, acid	Serum	0−1.1 U/mL (Bodansky)* 1−4 U/mL (King-Armstrong) 0.13−0.63 U/mL (Bessey-Lowery)
Phosphatase, alkaline	Serum	Adults: 1.5−4.5 U/dL (Bodansky)* 4−13 U/dL (King-Armstrong) 0.8−2.3 U/mL (Bessey-Lowery) Children: 5−14 U/dL (Bodansky)* 15−30 U/dL (King-Armstrong) 3.4−9.0 U/mL (Bessey-Lowery)
Phosphorus	Serum	Adults: 3.0−4.5 mg/dL 1.8−2.6 mEq/L Children: 4.0−7.0 mg/dL 2.3−4.1 mEq/L
Placidyl	Serum or plasma	Therapeutic range: 0.5−6.5 μg/mL Toxic level: >20 μg/mL
Potassium	Serum	3.6−5.0 mEq/L
Primidone	Serum or plasma	Therapeutic range: 5−12 μg/mL Toxic level: >12 μg/mL
Procainamide	Serum or plasma	Therapeutic range: 4−8 μg/mL Toxic level: >12 μg/mL
N-acetyl-procainamide (metabolite)	Serum or plasma	Therapeutic range: 2−8 μg/mL Toxic level: >30 μg/mL
Progesterone	Serum or plasma	Male: <100 ng/mL Female: Follicular phase: 0.3−0.8 ng/mL Luteal phase: 1.2−25.8 ng/mL Normal pregnancy >28 weeks: 45−286 ng/mL Hypertensive pregnancy: 22−210 ng/mL

WHOLE BLOOD, SERUM, AND PLASMA (CHEMISTRY) *continued*

Test	Specimen	Normal Values*
Prolactin	Serum	Male: 0–28 ng/mL Female: Follicular phase: 4–28 ng/dL Luteal phase: 5–40 ng/dL
Propoxyphene	Serum or plasma	Therapeutic range: 0.2–0.8 μg/mL Toxic level: 0.4–14 μg/mL
Prostatic acid Phosphatase	Serum	<0.3 IU/L* <4.0 ng/mL
Protein Total Albumin Globulin A/G ratio	Serum	 Adults: 6.0–8.0 g/dL Infants: 4.7–7.4 g/dL 3.5–5.5 g/dL 1.5–3.5 g/dL 1.5–2.5/L
Protriptyline	Serum or plasma	Therapeutic range: 70–170 ng/mL Toxic level: not established
Pyruvate	Whole blood	0.3–0.9 mg/dL
Quinidine	Serum or plasma	Therapeutic range: 2.3–5.0 μg/mL Toxic level: >6 μg/mL
Renin	Plasma	Normal salt intake (100–180 mEq of sodium): Supine (4–6 hours): 0.5–1.6 ng/mL/hr Upright (4 hours): 1.8–3.6 ng/mL/hr Low salt intake (10 mEq of sodium for 4 days): Supine (4–6 hours): 2.2–4.4 ng/mL/hr Upright (4 hours): 4.0–8.1 ng/mL/hr With diuretic: 6.8–15.1 ng/mL/hr
Salicylates	Serum or plasma	Negative: <2 mg/dL Therapeutic range: <20 mg/dL; arthritic patients: 15–35 mg/dL Toxic level: >40 mg/dL
Serotonin	Whole blood	50–200 ng/mL
Sodium	Serum	135–148 mEq/L
Sulfate	Serum	0.9–6.0 mg/dL 0.2–1.3 mEq/L
Sulfhemoglobin	Serum	Negative
Sulfonamides	Whole blood or serum	Negative; therapeutic range: 5–15 mg/dL

WHOLE BLOOD, SERUM, AND PLASMA (CHEMISTRY) *continued*

Test	Specimen	Normal Values*
Testosterone	Serum or plasma	Male: 400–1200 ng/dL Female: 30–120 ng/dL
Theophylline	Serum	Therapeutic range: 10–20 μg/mL Toxic level: >20 μg/mL
Thymol flocculation	Serum	0–5 units
Thyroglobulin	Serum	<50 ng/mL

Thyroid-stimulating
hormone (TSH)
	Serum	Adult: <4.6 μU/mL
		Cord serum: <20 μU/mL
		Pediatric:
		  1 day: <20 μU/mL
		  Over 2 weeks: <4.6 μU/mL

Thyroid tests
  Protein-bound
  iodine
	Serum	
		4.0–8.0 μg/dL

T_4 (radio-
immunoassay)
		Adult: 4.5–12.0 μg/dL
		  Cord serum: 4.6–18.2 μg/dL
		Pediatric:
		  1 week: 11.0–23.0 μg/dL
		  1 week–1 month: 9.0–18.0 μg/dL
		  1 month–6 months: 7.5–16.5 μg/dL
		  6 months–6 years: 5.5–12.5 μg/dL
		  6 years to 10 years: 5.0–12.5 μg/dL

T_4 (neonatal screen)	Blood spot on filter paper	1–5 days: >4.9 μg/dL 6–8 days: >4.0 μg/dL 9–11 days: >3.0 μg/dL 12–120 days: >3.0 μg/dL
T_4 free T_4 (by column)	Serum	0.9–2.3 ng/dL 4.5–11.0 μg/dL of thyroxine 3.2–7.2 μg/dL of thyroxine iodine
T_4 (Murphy- Pattee) T_3 (radio- immunoassay)		6.0–11.8 μg/dL of thyroxine 3.9–7.7 μg/dL of thyroxine iodine 1.10–2.30 ng/dL
T_3 uptake T_3 free T_7 (free thyroxine index)		25%–35% 250–390 pg/dL 1.3–4.4
Thyroid-binding globulin (TBG)		10–26 μg/dL

Tobramycin	Serum or plasma	Therapeutic range: 4–8 μg/mL at peak
		Toxic level:
		  >10 μg/mL at peak or
		  >2 μg/mL at trough levels

WHOLE BLOOD, SERUM, AND PLASMA (CHEMISTRY) *continued*

Test	Specimen	Normal Values*
Transferrin	Serum	200–400 mg/dL
Triglycerides	Serum	0–29 years: 10–140 mg/dL 30–39 years: 10–150 mg/dL 40–49 years: 10–160 mg/dL 50–59 years: 10–190 mg/dL
Urea clearance	Serum and 24-hour urine	64–99 mL/min (maximum clearance) 41–65 mL/min (standard clearance) or more than 75% of normal clearance
Urea nitrogen (BUN)	Serum	6–20 mg/dL
Uric acid	Serum	Male: 2.1–7.5 mg/dL Female: 2.0–6.6 mg/dL
Valproic acid	Serum or plasma	Therapeutic range: 50–125 μg/mL Toxic level: >150 μg/mL
Vitamin A	Serum	15–60 μg/dL
Vitamin A tolerance	Serum	Fasting: 15–60 μg/dL 3 or 6 hours after administration of 5000 units of vitamin A/kg: 200–600 μg/dL 24 hours after: same as fasting level or slightly above
Vitamin B_1	Whole blood	1.6–4.0 μg/dL
Vitamin B_6	Plasma	3.6–18.0 ng/mL
Vitamin B_{12}	Serum	Male: 200–800 pg/mL Female: 100–650 pg/mL
Vitamin C (ascorbic acid)	Whole blood Plasma	0.7–2.0 mg/dL 0.6–1.6 mg/dL
Vitamin D 25-hydroxy-cholecalciferol	Serum	10–60 ng/mL (lack of exposure to sunlight may reduce range)
Vitamin E	Serum	5–20 μg/mL
Zinc	Serum	50–150 μg/dL

*Normal values may vary significantly with different laboratory methods.

URINE

Test	Specimen	Normal Values*
Acetoacetic acid	Random	Negative
Acetone	Random	Negative
Addis count	12-hour collection	Adult: 0–800,000 RBC/12 hr 0–1,000,000 WBC/12 hr 0–5000 hyaline casts/12 hr Children: 0–600,000 RBC/12 hr 0–2,000,000 WBC/12 hr 0–10,000 hyaline casts/12 hr
ALA (delta-aminolevulinic acid)	24-hour	1.3–7.0 mg/24 hr
Albumin	Random 24-hour	Negative 10–100 mg/24 hr
Aldosterone	24-hour	2–26 µg/24 hr
Alkaline phosphatase	8-hour collection (overnight)	<3.5 U/8 hr
Amitriptyline	Random	Negative
Ammonia	24-hour	0.14–1.5 g/24 hr Infants: 0.56–2.9 g/24 hr
Ammonia nitrogen	24-hour	500–1200 mg/24 hr 20–70 mEq/24 hr
Amylase	2-hour 24-hour	35–260 Somogyi units/hr 80–5000 U/24 hr
Andosterone	24-hour	Male: <5 mg/24 hr Female: <2.5 mg/24 hr
Arsenic	Random 24-hour	<100 µg/L Acceptable industrial exposure: <200 µg/L <0.1 mg/L
Ascorbic acid	Random 24-hour	1–7 mg/dL Less than 50 mg/24 hr
Ascorbic acid tolerance	5- or 6-hour sample	Oral: 10% of administered amount IV: 30%–40% of administered amount
Barbiturates	Random	Negative
Bence-Jones protein	Random	Negative
Bilirubin	Random	Negative; 0.02 mg/dL
Blood, occult	Random	Negative

URINE *continued*

Test	Specimen	Normal Values*	
Bromide	Random	<0.25 mg/dL	
Calcium	Random	1+ turbidity 10 mg/dL	
	24-hour	50−300 mg/24 hr (depends on diet) 25−200 mEq/24 hr	
Catecholamines	Random	0−18 µg/dL	
	24-hour	Less than 100 µg/24 hr (varies with activity)	
Chloride	24-hour	110−254 mEq/24 hr	
Concentration test	Random, after fluid restriction	1.025−1.035	
Copper	24-hour	0−30 µg/dL	
Coproporphyrin	Random	3−20 µg/dL	
	24-hour	Adults: 50−160 µg/24 hr Children: 0−80 µg/24 hr	
Cortisol, free	24-hour	Men: 20−69 µg/24 hr Women: 8−63 µg/24 hr	
Creatine	24-hour	Male: 0−40 mg/24 hr Female: 0−100 mg/24 hr Higher during pregnancy Children: Under 1 year, equal to creatinine level Over 1 year, up to 30% of creatinine level	
Creatinine	24-hour	Male: 20−26 mg/kg/24 hr 1.0−2.0 g/24 hr Female: 14−22 mg/kg/24 hr 0.6−1.8 g/24 hr	
Creatinine clearance	Serum of plasma and urine	Male: 107−141 mL/min Female: 87−132 mL/min	
Epinephrine	24-hour	0−20 µg/24 hr	
Estriol	24-hour	Weeks of Pregnancy	mg/24 hr
		30−32	9−32
		34−36	12−45
		38−40	18−62

URINE *continued*

Test	Specimen	Normal Values*
Estrogens, fractionated Estrone (E$_1$) Estradiol (E$_2$) Estriol (E$_3$)	24-hour, midcycle, nonpregnant	2–25 μg/24 hr 0–10 μg/24 hr 2–30 μg/24 hr

Estrogens, total	24-hour	Male: 4–25 μg/24 hr
		Female:
		    28–100 μg/24 hr (ovulation)
		    22–105 μg/24 hr (luteal peak)
		    4–24 μg/24 hr (at menses)
		    14–20 μg/24 hr (postmenopausal)
		Pregnancy:
		    3–7 mg/24 hr (20 weeks)
		    15–42 mg/24 hr (term)

Follicle-stimulating hormone (FSH)	24-hour	Men: 2–12 IU/day
		Women:
		    Menstrual cycle: 8–60 IU/day
		    During ovulation: 30–60 IU/day
		    Menopause: >50 IU/day

Glucose	Random 24-hour	Negative; 15 mg/dL 130 mg/24 hr
Hemoglobin	Random	Negative
Hemogentisic acid	Random	Negative
Homovanillic acid (HVA)	24-hour	More than 15 mg/24 hr
17-Hydroxy-corticosteroids (17-OHCS)	24-hour	Male: 5–15 mg/24 hr Female: 2–13 mg/24 hr Children: lower values After 25 units of ACTH IM: a twofold to fourfold increase
5-Hydroxyindole-acetic acid (5-HIAA)	Random 24-hour	Negative 1–10 mg/24 hr

17-Ketogenic steroid (17-KGS)	24-hour	Male: 5–23 mg/24 hr
		Female: 3–15 mg/24 hr
		Children:
		    Under 5 years, less than 2 mg/24 hr
		    5–10 years, 3–6 mg/24 hr

Ketone	Random	Negative: 0.3–2.0 mg/dL

URINE *continued*

Test	Specimen	Normal Values*
17-Ketosteroids (17-KS)	24-hour	Male: 8−25 mg/24 hr Female: 5−15 mg/24 hr Children: Under 1 year, less than 1 mg/24 hr 1−4 years, less than 3 mg/24 hr 5−8 years, less than 3 mg/24 hr 9−12 years, approx. 3 mg/24 hr 13−16 years, approach adult levels Over 65: 4−8 mg/24 hr After 25 units of ACTH IM: 50%−100% increase
Androsterone	24-hour	Male: 2.0−5.0 mg/24 hr Female: 0.8−3.0 mg/24 hr
Lactose	24-hour	12−40 mg/24 hr
Lead	24-hour	Less than 100 μg/24 hr; 0.01−0.08 mg/24 hr
Magnesium	24-hour	6.0−9.0 mEq/24 hr
Microscopic examination	Random	RBC: 2−3/high-power field WBC: 4−5/high-power field Hyaline casts: occasional Bacteria: fewer than 1000/mL
Nortriptyline	Random	Therapeutic range: 75−150 ng/mL Toxic level: >1000 ng/mL
Osmolality	Random	Male: 390−1090 mOsm/kg Female: 300−1090 mOsm/kg
	24-hour	Male: 770−1630 mOsm/24 hr Female: 430−1150 mOsm/24 hr
pH	Random	4.6−8.0
Phenolsulfon-phthalein (PSP)	Timed collection after 6 mg of PSP dye IV	15 minutes: 25%−35% of dye excreted 30 minutes: 15%−25% of dye excreted 60 minutes: 10%−15% of dye excreted 120 minutes: 3%−10% of dye excreted
Phenylpyruvic acid	Random	Negative
Phosphorus	24-hour	0.9−1.3 g/24 hr 0.2−0.6 mEq/24 hr
Porphobilinogen	Random 24-hour	Negative 0−2.0 mg/24 hr
Potassium	24-hour	25−100 mEq/24 hr
Pregnanediol	24-hour	Male: 0.5−1.5 mg/24 hr Female: 0.5−7.0 mg/24 hr (nonpregnant)

URINE *continued*

Test	Specimen	Normal Values*
		Pregnant: 10−12 weeks: 5−15 mg/24 hr 18−24 weeks: 13−22 mg/24 hr 28−32 weeks: 27−60 mg/24 hr Children: 0.4−1.0 mg/24 hr
Pregnanetriol	24-hour	Male: 1.0−2.0 mg/24 hr Female: 0.5−2.0 mg/24 hr Children: less than 0.5 mg/24 hr
Protein	Random 24-hour	Negative; 2−8 mg/dL 40−150 mg/24 hr
Reducing substances, total	24-hour	0.5−1.5 mg/24 hr
Sodium	24-hour	40−180 mEq/24 hr
Solids, total	24-hour	55−70 g/24 hr Decreases with age to 30 g/24 hr
Specific gravity	Random	1.016−1.022 (normal fluid intake) 1.001−1.040 (range)
Sugar	Random	Negative
Urea clearance	Serum and 24-hour urine	64−99 mL/min (maximum clearance) 41−65 mL/min (standard clearance) or more than 75% of normal clearance
Urea nitrogen	24-hour	6−17 g/24 hr
Uric acid	24-hour	0.3−0.8 g/24 hr
Urobilinogen	2-hour 24-hour	0.3−1.0 Ehrlich units 0.5−4.0 Ehrlich units/24 hr 0.05−2.5 mg/24 hr
Uroporphyrins	Random 24-hour	Negative 10−30 μg/24 hr
Vanillylmandelic acid (VMA)	24-hour	0.5−14 mg/24 hr
Vitamin B$_1$	24-hour	270−780 μg/24 hr
Vitamin C	24-hour	15−30 mg/24 hr after normal dietary intake
Volume, total	24-hour	Adults: 800−200 mL/24 hr Children: 300−1500 mL/24 hr
Zinc	24-hour	0.15−1.20 mg/24 hr

*Normal values may vary significantly with different laboratory methods.

HEMATOLOGY

Complete Blood Count (CBC)	Normal Values*			
	Adults	Newborn	1 Year	10 Years
Hemoglobin	Male: 14–18 g/dL Female: 12–16 g/dL	14–20 g/dL	11.2–14.0 g/dL	12.5–13.0 g/dL
Hematocrit	Male: 40%–54% Female: 37%–47%	42%–62%	29%–41%	36%–40%
Red blood cell count	Male: 4.5–6.0 million/μL Female: 4.0–5.5 million/μL	4.0–6.3 million/μL	3.6–5.0 million/μL	3.9–5.2 million/μL
White blood cell count	4500–11,000/μL	9000–30,000/μL	6000–18,000/μL	4500–13,500/μL
Neutrophils	54%–75% (3000–7500/μL)	32%–62% (8400/μL)	23% (2700/μL)	31%–61% (3700/μL)
Band neutrophils	3%–8% (150–700/μL)	10%–18% (2500/μL)	8% (1000/μL)	5%–11% (650/μL)
Lymphocytes	25%–40% (1500–4500/μL)	26%–36% (5500/μL)	61% (7000/μL)	28%–48% (3100/μL)
Monocytes	2%–8% (100–500/μL)	5%–6% (1050/μL)	5% (550/μL)	4.0%–4.5% (350/μL)
Eosinophils	1%–4% (50–400/μL)	2.0%–2.5% (400/μL)	2.6% (300/μL)	2.0%–2.5% (200/μL)
Basophils	0%–1% (25–100/μL)	0.5%–1.0% (100/μL)	0.4% (50/μL)	0.5% (40/μL)
Erythrocyte indices				
Mean corpuscular volume (MCV)	76–100 fL	92–115 fL	87–100 fL	80–96 fL
Mean corpuscular hemoglobin (MCH)	25–35 pg	24–38 pg	22–32 pg	27–33 pg
Mean corpuscular hemoglobin concentration (MCHC)	30%–38%	27%–34%	27%–33%	27%–31%
Platelet count	150,000–400,000/μL	150,000–250,000/μL		

HEMATOLOGY *continued*

Other Hematologic Studies	Specimen	Normal Values*
Coagulation studies		
Bleeding time	Capillary blood	Duke method: 1–3 minutes
		Ivy method: 1–7 minutes
Clot retraction	Clotted blood	Partial retraction: 1–2 hours with 40%–60% serum expressed; half the original mass in 2 hours
		Complete retraction: 12–24 hours
Fibrinogen assay	Plasma	200–400 mg/dL
Partial thrombo- plastin time (PTT)	Plasma	Activated: 30–40 seconds
		Nonactivated: 40–100 seconds
Platelet count	Whole blood	150,000–400,000/μL
Prothrombin con- sumption time (PCT)	Serum	Greater than 20 seconds
Prothrombin time	Plasma	11–15 seconds
Thrombin time	Plasma	10–15 seconds
Thromboplastin generation time (TGT)	Serum and plasma	14 seconds or less within 3–5 minutes of thromboplastin generation
Tourniquet test	Patient	1–10 petechiae
Whole blood clot- ting time	Whole blood	Plain tubes: 5–15 minutes
		Siliconized tubes: 24–45 minutes
Eosinophil count	Whole blood	50–400/μL
Erythrocyte sedi- mentation rate (ESR)	Whole blood	
Wintrobe method		Male: 0–9 mm/hr
		Female: 0–20 mm/hr
		Children: 0–15 mm/hr
Westergren method		Male:
		Under 50 years, 0–15 mm/hr
		Over 50 years, 0–20 mm/hr
		Female:
		Under 50 years, 0–20 mm/hr
		Over 50 years, 0–30 mm/hr
		Children: 0–20 mm/hr
Hemoglobin electrophoresis	Whole blood	
A_1		95%–98%
A_2		2%–3%
F		Less than 2%
Lupus erythema- tosus (LE)	Clotted blood	Negative

HEMATOLOGY *continued*

Other Hematologic Studies	Specimen	Normal Values*		
Osmotic fragility	Whole blood	% Saline	% Hemolysis (fresh)	% Hemolysis (incubated)
		0.20	100	95–100
		0.30	97–100	85–100
		0.35	90–99	75–100
		0.40	50–95	65–100
		0.45	5–45	55–95
		0.50	0–5	40–85
		0.55	0	15–70
		0.60		0–40
		0.65		0–10
		0.70		0–5
		0.75		0
Reticulocyte count	Whole blood	Adults: 0.5%–2.0% 25,000–75,000/μL Newborn: 2.5–6.0%		
Cutler		Male: 0–8 mm/hr Female: 0–10 mm/hr Children: 4–13 mm/hr		
Volume, blood	Whole blood	Male: 69 mL/kg Female: 65 mL/kg		
Volume, plasma	Whole blood	Male: 39 mL/kg Female: 40 mL/kg		

Bone Marrow Studies	Specimen	Normal Values*
Differential cell counts	Bone marrow	
Hemocytoblast		0.1%–1.0%
Myeloblasts		0.1%–5.0%
Promyelocytes		0.5%–8.0%
Myelocytes		Neutrophilic: 5%–20% Eosinophilic: 0.1%–3.0% Basophilic: 0%–0.5%
Metamyelocytes		Neutrophilic: 10%–32% Eosinophilic: 0.3%–3.7% Basophilic: 0%–0.3%
Band cells		Neutrophilic: 10%–35% Eosinophilic: 0.2%–2.0% Basophilic: 0%–0.3%

HEMATOLOGY *continued*

Bone Marrow Studies	Specimen	Normal Values*
Segmented cells		Neutrophilic: 7%–30% Eosinophilic: 0.2%–4.0% Basophilic: 0%–0.7%
Lymphocytes		2.7%–24%
Monocytes		0%–2.7%
Plasmacytes		0.1%–1.5%
Megakaryocytes		0.1%–0.5%
Pronormoblasts		0.2%–4.0%
Normoblasts, basophilic		1.5%–5.8%
Normoblasts, polychromatophilic		5.0%–26.4%
Normoblasts, orthochromic		1.6%–21.0%
Reticulum cells		0.1%–2.0%
Myeloid:erythroid (M:E) ratio		Adult: 4:1 (range of 6:1 to 2:1) Newborn: 1.85:1 2 weeks: 11:1 1–2 months: 5.5:1 1–20 years: 2.95:1

*Normal values may vary significantly with different laboratory methods.

SEROLOGY

Test	Normal Values*

Anti-DNA antibodies	Children:
	  0–6: <1:60
	  7–17: <1:70
	Adults: <1:85

Antimitochondrial antibodies	<1:10
Antinuclear antibodies (ANA)	<1:10
Antiparietal cell antibodies	<1:10
Anti-smooth muscle antibodies	<1:10

Antistreptolysin O titer (ASO)	Adults: <120 Todd units
	Children:
	  Under 5 years, <85 Todd units
	  5–19 years, <170 Todd units

Antithyroglobulin antibodies	<1:100

SEROLOGY *continued*

Test	Normal Values*
Antithyroid microsomal antibodies	<1:100
Aspergillus antibodies	<1:8
Australia antigen, hepatitis-associated antigen (HAA)	Negative
Blastomyces antibodies	<1:8
B-lymphocytes	4%−23% B cells 50−500 B cells/mm³
Brucella antigens	<1:80
Cold agglutinins	<1:40
Complement, C3	<1:32
C-reactive protein (CRP)	Negative
Cytomegalovirus (CMV) antibodies	<1:16
Fluorescent treponemal antibody absorption (FTA-ABS)	Nonreactive
Hepatitis A antibodies	Negative
Hepatitis B core antibodies	Negative
Hepatitis B surface antigens	Negative
Herpes simplex virus antibodies	<1:10
Heterophil antibodies	<1:112
Latex fixation	Negative
Legionella antibodies	<1:256
Rheumatoid factor	<1:40
Streptococcus MG agglutinins	<1:20
Thyroid antibodies	<1:32
T-lymphocytes	45%−84% T cells 500−2400 T cells/mm³
Tularemia agglutinins	Less than 1:40
Typhoid agglutinins O H	 Less than 1:80 Less than 1:80
Venereal disease research laboratories (VDRL)	Nonreactive
Weil-Felix (*Proteus* OX2, OXK, and OX19 agglutinins)	Less than 1:32

*Normal values may vary significantly with different laboratory methods.

CEREBROSPINAL FLUID

Test	Normal Values*
Albumin	10−30 mg/dL
Albumin/globulin (A/G) ratio	1.6−2.2/1
Appearance	Clear and colorless
Calcium	2.1−2.7 mEq/L
Carbon dioxide content	25−30 mmol
Cell count	0−10 WBC/μL (60%−100% lymphocytes)
Chloride	Adult: 113−133 mEq/L Children: 120−128 mEq/L
Cholesterol	0.2−0.6 mg/dL
Creatinine	0.5−1.2 mg/dL
Globulin	6−16 mg/dL
Glucose	Adults: 40−80 mg/dL 50%−80% of blood glucose Children: 35−75 mg/dL
5-Hydroxyindoleacetic acid (5-HIAA)	1.5−4.5 mg/dL
Immunoglobulin IgA IgG IgM	 0−0.6 mg/dL 0−5.5 mg/dL 0−1.3 mg/dL
Iron	1−2 mg/dL
Lactate	10−18 mg/dL
Lactic dehydrogenase (LDH)	6−30 IU/L
Magnesium	2.4−3.1 mEq/L
Osmolality	280−290 mOsm/kg
P_{CO_2}	42−52 mm Hg
pH	7.30−7.40
P_{O_2}	40−44 mm Hg
Potassium	2.0−3.5 mEq/L

CEREBROSPINAL FLUID *continued*

Test	Normal Values*
Protein	Adult: 15–50 mg/dL Children: Premature infants, up to 400 mg/dL Newborns, 30–200 mg/dL 1 week–1 month, 30–150 mg/dL 1–6 months, 30–100 mg/dL
Protein electrophoresis	Prealbumin: 3%–6% Albumin: 45%–68% α_1-globulin: 3%–9% α_2-globulin: 4%–10% β-globulin: 10%–18% γ-globulin: 3%–11%
Serology	Negative
Sodium	144–154 mEq/L
Solids, total	0.85–1.70 g/dL
Specific gravity	1.006–1.008
Urea	6–16 mg/dL
Uric acid	0.5–4.5 mg/dL
Volume	90–150 mL
Zinc	2–6 μg/dL

*Normal values may vary significantly with different laboratory methods.

GASTRIC FLUID

Test	Normal Values*
Appearance	Pale gray, translucent, slightly viscous
Fasting residual volume	20–100 mL
pH	1.6–1.8
Basal acid output	1.4–4.0 mEq/hr
Maximal acid output (after histamine stimulation)	5–35 mEq/hr

*Normal values may vary significantly with different laboratory methods.

MISCELLANEOUS VALUES

Test	Specimen	Normal Values*
Chloride	Sweat	4–60 mEq/L
Coombs' test, direct	Serum	Negative
Coombs' test, indirect	Serum	Negative
Diagnex blue (tubeless gastric analysis)	Urine	Free acid present
Sodium	Sweat	10–80 mEq/L

*Normal values may vary significantly with different laboratory methods.

STOOL

Test	Specimen	Normal Values*
Bile	Random	Adults: negative Children: positive
Color	Random	Brown
Coproporphyrin	24-hour	400–1200 μg/24 hr
Fat	72-hour	Total fat: 1–7 g/24 hr (1%–9% of fat intake) 15%–25% of dry weight Neutral fat: 1%–5% of dry weight Free fatty acids: 5%–13% of dry weight Combined fatty acids: 5%–15% of dry weight Microscopic examination: many small fatty acid globules 1–4 μm in diameter
Occult blood	Random	Negative
Ova and parasites	Random	Negative
Protoporphyrin	24-hour	<1800 μg/24 hr
Trypsin	Random	Positive 2+ to 4+ digestion
Urobilinogen	Random	Positive 75–350 mg/100 g
	24-hour	40–250 mg/24 hr
Uroporphyrin	24-hour	10–40 μg/24 hr
Volume	24-hour	100–300 g/24 hr

*Normal values may vary significantly with different laboratory methods.

AMNIOTIC FLUID

Test	Early Gestation	Term
Appearance	Clear	Clear or slightly opalescent
Albumin	0.04 g/dL	0.05 g/dL

	Gestation (weeks)	AFP (μg/mL)
α-Fetoprotein (AFP)	12	43.0
	14	36.0
	16	30.0
	18	24.0
	20	19.0
	22	15.0
	30	3.0
	35	2.0
	40	0.8

Test	Early Gestation	Term
Bilirubin	Greater than 0.075 mg/dL	Greater than 0.025 mg/dL
Chloride	Approx. equal to serum chloride	1–3 mEq/L lower than serum chloride
Cytologic staining		
Oil red O	Greater than 10%	Less than 50%
Nile blue sulfate	0	Less than 20%
Creatinine	Before 28 weeks: 0.8–1.1 mg/dL 30–34 weeks: 1.3–1.7 mg/dL	1.8–4.0 mg/dL (usually greater than 2.0 mg/dL)
Estriol	Below 10 μg/dL	Less than 60 μg/dL
Lipids		
Lecithin	Before 34 weeks: 6–9 mg/dL	After 35 weeks: 15–20 mg/dL
Sphingomyelin	4–6 mg/dL	4–6 mg/dL
L/S ratio		Greater than 2.0
Osmolality	Approx. equal to serum osmolality	Greater than 250 mOsm/kg
P_{CO_2}	33–35 mm Hg	42–55 mm Hg (increases toward term)
pH	7.12–7.38	6.91–7.43 (decreases toward term)
Protein, total	0.36–0.84 g/dL	0.07–0.45 g/dL
Sodium	Approx. equal to serum sodium	7–10 mEq/L lower than serum sodium
Urea	12–24 mg/dL	19–41 mg/dL

AMNIOTIC FLUID *continued*

Test	Early Gestation	Term
Uric acid	2.8–4.7 mg/dL	7.7–12.0 mg/dL
Volume	450–1200 mL	500–1400 mL (increases toward term)

SYMPTOMS OF ELECTROLYTE AND ACID-BASE IMBALANCE

Condition	Symptoms
Sodium (Na^+)	
Hyponatremia	Mild to moderate: weakness, confusion, stupor, apprehension, abdominal cramps
	Severe: hypovolemic shock, death
Hypernatremia	Mild to moderate: dry, sticky mucous membranes, intense thirst, flushed skin, agitation, restlessness, decreased reflexes
	Severe: hypermania and convulsions
Potassium (K^+)	
Hypokalemia	Mild: malaise, thirst, polyuria
	Moderate: muscle weakness, decreased reflexes, loss of muscle tone causing cardiac arrhythmias, weak pulse and falling blood pressure, nausea, vomiting, decreased intestinal motility, decreased respiratory functioning
	Severe: respiratory or cardiac arrest, death
Hyperkalemia	Mild: irritability, nausea, diarrhea, abdominal cramps
	Moderate: weakness, flaccid paralysis, difficulty in breathing and speaking, oliguria leading to anuria
	Severe: ventricular fibrillation, death
Bicarbonate (HCO_3^-)	See blood gases and acid-base balance (below)
Chloride (Cl^-)	
Hypochloremia	Overshadowed by symptoms of accompanying hyponatremia
Hyperchloremia	Overshadowed by symptoms of accompanying hypernatremia
Calcium (Ca^{++})	
Hypocalcemia	Mild to moderate: tingling sensation around mouth and in fingertips; abdominal and skeletal muscle cramps
	Severe: carpopedal spasms and tetany leading to convulsions
Hypercalcemia	Mild to moderate: bone pain, pathologic fractures, flank pain from renal stones
	Severe: intractable nausea and vomiting, dehydration, stupor, coma, cardiac arrest

SYMPTOMS OF ELECTROLYTE AND ACID-BASE IMBALANCE *continued*

Condition	Symptoms
Magnesium (Mg^{++})	
Hypomagnesemia	Mild to moderate: tremors, painful paresthesia, nerve and muscle irritability, increased blood pressure and heart rate
	Severe: disorientation, convulsions
Hypermagnesemia	Mild to moderate: reduced nerve and muscle activity, impaired respiration, lethargy
	Severe: coma, cardiac arrest
Acid-base imbalance and blood gases	
Respiratory acidosis	Impaired respirations, generalized weakness, disorientation, coma
pH: low	
CO$_2$: high	
Pco$_2$: high	
Respiratory alkalosis	Deep, rapid breathing, lightheadedness, tetany, convulsions, unconsciousness
pH: high	
CO$_2$: low	
Pco$_2$: low	
Metabolic acidosis	Deep, rapid (Kussmaul) breathing, weakness, shortness of breath, disorientation, coma
pH: low	
CO$_2$: low	
Pco$_2$: low	
Metabolic alkalosis	Decreased respirations, muscular hypertonicity, tetany
pH: high	
CO$_2$: high	
Pco$_2$: high	

BLOOD TYPES

Group	Red Blood Cell Antigens	Serum Antibodies	Percentage of Population
O	O	Anti-A Anti-B	45%
A$_1$	A$_1$	Anti-B	31%
A$_2$	A$_2$	Anti-B	10%
B	B	Anti-A$_1$ Anti-A$_2$	10%
AB	A, B	None	4%

Glossary

a-, an- Prefix; without, not, negative.

ab- Prefix; from, away from.

abscess A localized collection of pus in a cavity formed as a result of an infectious process.

absorption The uptake of substances into or across tissues; method of removing substances from serum. An absorbed serum is one from which antibodies have been removed.

acanthocyte A distorted erythrocyte characterized by irregular protoplasmic projections that give the cell a thorny appearance on a stained blood smear.

ACD Acid citrate dextrose. The anticoagulant contained in yellow-stoppered tubes that is used for blood bank testing.

acetone A substance found in the blood and urine of diabetic patients that gives the breath a sweet, fruity odor.

acid-fast Designates organisms not easily decolorized by acids after staining (such as *Mycobacterium tuberculosis*, which retains red dyes while other tissues are decolorized).

acidosis Pathologic decrease in the pH of body fluids caused by accumulation of acid in the body (as in diabetic acidosis) or loss of bicarbonate from the body (as in renal disease).

ACP Acid phosphatase. A group of enzymes present in several body tissues, particularly the prostate gland of the male.

ACTH Adrenocorticotropic hormone. An anterior pituitary hormone that regulates the production and secretion of glucocorticosteroids by the adrenal cortex.

acute Having rapid onset, severe symptoms, and a short course; not chronic. That phase during the course of a disease that is most severe and generally of short duration.

Addis count Outdated method for counting red blood cells, white blood cells, epithelial cells, and casts in urine sediment; originally used in the monitoring of renal disease.

adsorption The attachment of one substance to the surface of another.

aerobe A microorganism whose growth and reproduction are promoted by the presence of air or free oxygen.

AFP α-Fetoprotein. A globulin normally present in fetal serum but absent from adult serum. Increased concentrations of AFP appear during certain hepatic malignancies in adults.

713

agglutination Clumping of red blood cells due to the presence of agglutinogen (antigen) on the red blood cell surface and action of the corresponding agglutinin (antibody).

agglutinin Antibody that causes clumping of a specific antigen such as bacteria or red blood cells.

agglutinogen Any substance acting as an antigen that stimulates the production of agglutinin.

agranulocytosis Complete or nearly complete absence of granular leukocytes in the blood and bone marrow. Also known as granulocytopenia.

A/G ratio A ratio between the amount of albumin and the amount of globulin in the serum; formerly used as an index of hepatic function or disease.

AHF Antihemophilic factor. A blood factor (coagulation factor VIII) required for the formation of a blood clot. A cryoprecipitated or lyophilized preparation obtained from whole blood that provides a source of factors VIII and XIII and fibrinogen for the treatment of certain coagulation deficiencies.

aldosterone A mineralocorticoid hormone. The principal electrolyte-regulating steroid produced by the adrenal cortex.

aliquot A portion obtained by dividing the whole into smaller parts. For example, if a 24-hour urine specimen is separated into several smaller containers, each portion is an aliquot of the original sample.

alkalosis Pathologic increase in the pH of body fluids caused by the accumulation of bicarbonate in or loss of acid from the body.

alkaptonuria Excretion of alkapton bodies (usually homogentisic acid) in the urine, causing it to turn dark on standing.

ALP Alkaline phosphatase. A group of enzymes occurring in several organs, primarily the liver and bones.

ALT Alanine aminotransferase. An enzyme, also known as glutamic pyruvic transaminase (GPT), that is present primarily in the liver.

amniocentesis The surgical transabdominal perforation of the uterus to obtain amniotic fluid.

amniotic fluid The intrauterine substance surrounding the fetus that contains material from the fetal urinary and respiratory tracts and secretions from the placental membranes.

amorphous Shapeless; having no definite form and without visible differentiation in structure.

amylase The pancreatic enzyme that aids the metabolism of starch to glucose.

ANA Antinuclear antibodies. A group of immunoglobulins produced against the nuclei of cells in one or more of the host's own tissues; found in patients with various collagen diseases. An immunology test to detect certain autoantibodies.

anaerobe Microorganism whose growth and reproduction are promoted by the complete or almost complete absence of oxygen.

anamnestic response The rapid reappearance of antibodies following administration of an antigen in a subject who previously developed a primary immune response to the same antigen.

androgen   Any substance that possesses masculinizing activities such as testicular hormone.

anemia   Condition in which the number of circulating erythrocytes, the quantity of hemoglobin, or the volume of packed red blood cells is below normal. Anemia is not a disease but a symptom of various diseases.

anion   An ion or particle carrying a negative charge.

aniso   Word element; unequal or dissimilar.

anisocytosis   Condition in which the size of blood cells varies excessively; erythrocytes are particularly susceptible.

anoxemia   Reduction of the oxygen content of blood below physiologic levels.

anoxia   Condition in which body tissues lack sufficient oxygen.

ante-   Prefix; before.

anti-   Prefix; against.

antibiotic susceptibility   Measures the ability of a particular antibiotic or antimicrobial agent to slow or stop the growth of a specific microorganism.

antibody   A specific immunoglobulin produced by the body in response to the introduction of a foreign substance or antigen; antibodies interact only with the antigen that induced their synthesis. Antibody tests are used to determine whether an individual has ever been exposed to the antigen.

anticoagulant   Any substance that prevents or delays the clotting of blood.

antigen   Any substance (such as a pollen, toxin, or bacteria) that, when introduced into the blood or tissues, stimulates antibody formation and reacts specifically with antibodies in some observable way.

antihuman globulin   Any substance that opposes the action of globulin; prepared by immunizing animals with purified human γ-globulin. Also known as antiglobulin or Coombs' serum.

antiserum   Serum that contains antibodies for a specific antigen.

antithrombin   A general term for a naturally occurring or therapeutically administered substance that neutralizes thrombin and thus limits or restricts blood coagulation.

aplasia   Failure of the cellular products of an organ to develop; incomplete or defective blood cell formation.

APTT   Activated partial thromboplastin time. A coagulation test.

asepsis   Free of infection or germs.

ASO   Antistreptolysin O. Antibody developed during infection with streptococcal bacteria that releases a substance (called streptolysin O) that hemolyzes red blood cells. The body develops an antibody that neutralizes streptolysin O to prevent this hemolysis.

AST   Aspartate aminotransferase. An enzyme also known as glutamic oxaloacetic transaminase (GOT), that is present in many tissues, particularly the heart and liver.

atypical antibody   An antibody not regularly present in plasma.

auto-   Prefix; self.

autoantibody   An immunoglobulin formed in response to and reacting against an individual's own normal body constituents.

autoimmunity A condition characterized by a specific immune response against the constituents of the body's own tissues; it may result in hypersensitivity reactions or, if severe, in autoimmune disease.

azotemia An excess of urea or other nitrogenous compounds in the blood.

bacillus A rod-shaped bacterium.

bactericidal Destructive to or destroying bacteria.

bacteriostatic Inhibiting the growth or multiplication of bacteria.

band form A neutrophil in which the nucleus is unsegmented and in a continuous ribbonlike, horsehoe-shaped, twisted, or coiled form. Also known as a stab or non-filamented cell.

BAO Basal acid output. The amount of gastric acid secreted during 1 hour following an overnight fast without any external stimulation.

basophil A white blood cell characterized by large, coarse granules that have an affinity for the basic dye of Wright's stain and appear bluish-black on a stained blood smear. The granules contain histamine and heparin and are involved in immediate hyper-sensitivity reactions.

basophilia The abnormal increase in the blood of immature erythrocytes, which appear grayish-blue on a stained blood smear; basophilic leukocytosis.

basophilic stippling Aggregation of dark granules within erythrocytes on a stained blood smear indicating the presence of underdeveloped erythrocytes.

B cell A lymphocyte that arises from the bone marrow and produces antibodies.

bi- Prefix; two, double, or twice.

bicarbonate Any salt containing the HCO_3^- anion.

bilirubin A product of hemoglobin breakdown; formed in the liver.

-blast Suffix; an immature stage in cellular development.

blood group Classification of blood specimens into phenotypes based on the presence or absence of certain red blood cell agglutinins or antigens, i.e., ABO group, Rh group.

bone marrow The soft material that fills the cavity in most bones and manufactures most of the formed elements of blood.

BSP Bromsulphthalein. A dye used in liver function tests.

buffer A chemical system that maintains the concentration of another chemical substance; most frequently a salt in the blood that helps preserve the original pH despite the addition of an acid or base.

buffy coat A thin, light-colored layer containing mostly white blood cells that appears between the plasma and erythrocytes when whole blood is centrifuged or allowed to stand.

BUN Blood urea nitrogen. The level of nitrogen in the blood in the form of urea; used to assess kidney function.

Burr cells Erythrocytes with abnormal, blunt cytoplasmic projections.

Ca Chemical symbol for calcium; an element found in nearly all tissues that is essential to blood coagulation.

Cabot's rings Lines in the form of loops or figure eights seen in erythrocytes in severe anemia.

calci- Prefix; refers to calcium.

calcitonin A potent hormone, also known as thyrocalcitonin, that is secreted by the parafollicular cells of the thyroid gland.

calculi Abnormal inorganic mass (stone) composed of mineral salts that develops in the kidney, ureter, bladder, or urethra.

capsule Gelatin-like envelope surrounding bacteria.

carbohydrate A group of chemical substances (sugars, glycogen, starches, and celluloses) that provide the basic source of energy.

carbon dioxide A colorless gas that is the final metabolic product of carbon compounds present in food; eliminated through the lungs, in urine, and in perspiration.

cast A cylinder-like structure of precipitated protein that has molded itself to the lumen of renal tubules and is excreted in the urine. Most urinary casts consist of red blood cells, white blood cells, and epithelial cells and indicate renal pathology.

catecholamines A group of hormones (epinephrine and norepinephrine) produced by the adrenal medulla.

cation An ion or particle carrying a positive charge.

CBC Complete blood count. A basic hematology study that includes measurement of hemoglobin, hematocrit, the number of red and white blood cells, differential white blood cell count, mean corpuscular volume (MCV), mean corpuscular hemoglobin (MCH), mean corpuscular hemoglobin concentration (MCHC), and sometimes a platelet count.

CEA Carcinoembryonic antigen. An antigen present in fetal tissues that, when found in adults, is useful in detecting and monitoring colon carcinomas.

centrifuge A device that spins test tubes at high speeds, causing heavier particles to settle to the bottom and lighter particles to rise to the top.

cholesterol A fatlike substance found in animal fats and oils, milk, egg yolks, bile, blood, brain tissues, liver, and kidneys that occurs in atheroma of the arteries.

-chromic Suffix; denotes a relationship to color.

chromosome An intranuclear body containing DNA, thought to be a linear arrangement of genes, that transmits genetic information.

chronic Designating a disease of slow progression and long duration.

chyle A milky fluid consisting of emulsified lymph and fat (chylomicrons) that is removed from the intestine by the lymphatics during digestion.

chylomicrons Small particles of fat in the blood after digestion and absorption of fat in food.

CPK Creatine phosphokinase. An enzyme present in skeletal and cardiac muscle and the brain.

CMV Cytomegalovirus.

CO$_2$ Carbon dioxide.

coagulation The process by which blood clots; coagulation depends on many specialized substances such as prothrombin, thrombin, thrombo-plastin, calcium ions, fibrinogen, and platelets.

cocci Spherical bacteria. When these bacteria appear in chains, they are called strep-tococci; in clusters (like grapes) they are called staphylococci; in pairs they are called diplococci.

cold agglutinins An antibody that reacts best at refrigerator temperatures (4 C).

compatibility testing A series of procedures performed before transfusion, including crossmatch, to ensure the suitability of blood from a particular donor for a specific recipient.

complement A complex series of thermolabile proteins present in fresh normal serum that combine with the antigen-antibody complex and cause lysis of red blood cells that have been sensitized with their specific antibodies.

contaminant Any substance or biologic agent whose presence results in other sub-stances or biologic agents being impure such as foreign organisms developing acci-dentally in a pure culture.

convalescent stage Stage of disease in which the patient is recovering.

Coombs' serum Antiglobulin serum used to detect the presence of antibodies on the surface of red blood cells, as in the test for erythroblastosis fetalis.

coproporphyrin A porphyrin produced in blood-forming organs and the intestines and found in the feces and urine.

cortisol The most abundant steroid hormone produced by the adrenal cortex.

creatine A waste product of muscle contraction that combines with phosphate to yield energy during anaerobic muscle contractions.

creatinine The end product of creatine metabolism.

crenation Abnormal notched appearance, as of the margins of red blood cells after ex-posure to an excessively high-solute concentration.

CRP C-reactive protein. An acute-phase reactant that is elevated in blood during the active phase of certain acute illnesses.

CSF Cerebrospinal fluid. A sterile fluid produced within the brain to nourish the brain and spinal cord and cushion them from trauma.

culture The propagation of microorganisms or living cells in a special nutrient material conducive to their growth, such as agar, to permit the growth and identification of pathogenic organisms.

cylindruria The presence of increased numbers of casts in the urine.

cyst The infective stage in the life cycle of protozoa during which they are enclosed within a protective wall.

-cyto Combining form; denotes relationship to a cell.

DAT Direct antiglobulin test. Study to detect the presence of complement or antibodies absorbed on the red blood cell surface.

di- Prefix; indicates twice, double, or two.

DIC Disseminated intravascular coagulation. A disorder that is secondary to other dis-eases and alters blood coagulation.

differential count   An enumeration of the various types of white blood cells seen on a stained blood smear.

diplococci   Cocci that occur in pairs.

diurnal   Occurring during the day.

dL   Deciliter. A metric measurement for volume that equals 100 mL or 1/10 of a liter.

dys-   Prefix; indicates bad, difficult, or painful.

EBV   Epstein-Barr virus.

EDTA   Ethylenediaminotetraacetate. An anticoagulant that is mixed with blood specimens to prevent them from clotting. EDTA is particularly useful for hematologic examination because it preserves the cellular elements of blood.

electrolyte   A substance that dissociates into ions and is capable of conducting electricity; ionized salts such as sodium, potassium, chloride, and bicarbonate in blood, tissue fluids, and cells.

electrophoresis   A technique for separating materials, such as proteins, into their component parts by the movement of charged particles at different speeds through a medium in an electric field.

-emia   Suffix; pertaining to or within the blood.

endo-   Prefix; indicates within.

enzyme   A complex protein capable of inducing chemical changes and accelerating chemical reactions in other substances without itself being structurally changed.

eosinophil   A granular leukocyte with an affinity for the acid eosin dye of Wright's stain that becomes more active in allergic conditions and appears orange-red on a stained blood smear.

erythro-   Prefix; pertaining to the color red or red blood cells.

erythrocyte   A mature red blood cell that carries oxygen and carbon dioxide and helps regulate acid-base balance (pH).

ESR   Erythrocyte sedimentation rate. A hematology test measuring the rate at which red blood cells fall in a tube within 1 hour to monitor the progress of inflammatory conditions.

estradiol   An estrogen.

estriol   The most physiologically active estrogen.

estrogens   A group of hormones that control the development of female secondary sexual characteristics.

estrone   An estrogen.

etiology   The study of the factors causing disease and the method by which they are introduced to the host.

eu-   Prefix; good, normal, or healthy.

exo-   Prefix; without, outside.

extra-   Prefix; outside of, beyond.

fatty acids   Metabolic degradation products of dietary fats that are absorbed from the intestines with the action of bile salts.

FBS   Fasting blood sugar.

FDP Fibrin-fibrinogen degradation products. The by-products of fibrinolysis.

febrile agglutinins A group of serologic studies used to diagnose enteric fevers, rickettsial diseases, brucellosis, and tularemia.

ferritin The chief form in which iron is stored in the tissues, principally the liver, spleen, and bone marrow.

fibrin An insoluble filamentous protein that forms a meshlike network around blood cells through the action of thrombin on fibrinogen to produce a blood clot.

fibrinogen A protein present in plasma (coagulation factor I) that is essential for coagulation and consumed by thrombin during the formation of fibrin.

fL Femtoliter. A metric unit of volume equal to 1/1000 of a nanoliter (nL).

FSF Fibrin-stabilizing factor. A blood factor (coagulation factor XIII) required to stabilize a blood clot.

FSH Follicle-stimulating hormone. An anterior pituitary hormone that stimulates the development and function of gonads.

FTA-ABS Fluorescent treponemal antibody absorption. Confirms syphilis if the serologic screening test is positive.

g Gram. A metric measurement of mass.

gene The smallest biologic unit of heredity, which is composed of DNA and located at a definite position (locus) on a particular chromosome for each physical or biologic characteristic.

genotype The entire genetic constitution of an individual. Genotype symbols are paired; a capital letter indicates dominance, and a small letter denotes recessive genes.

GGT Gamma-glutamyl transferase. A liver enzyme whose elevation is a sensitive indicator of liver dysfunction.

GH Growth hormone. An anterior pituitary hormone that regulates bone and muscle growth in children and aids adult metabolism.

globulin One of the main classes of proteins.

glucose A simple sugar that is the major carbohydrate in the body.

-glycemia Suffix; pertaining to the presence of glucose in the blood.

glycogen The chief storage form of carbohydrate.

glycohemoglobin An assay used to monitor long-term control of diabetics; its percentage indicates the average glucose concentration in the blood over the previous 2 months.

G-6-PD Glucose-6-phosphate dehydrogenase. An enzyme found in erythrocytes.

Gram's stain A method of staining bacteria to differentiate them in the initial stage of identification. Gram-positive organisms retain the violet stain; gram-negative organisms lose the violet stain but pick up the red counterstain.

granulocyte A white blood cell that contains specific cytoplasmic granules (neutrophilic, eosinophilic, or basophilic).

GTT Glucose tolerance test. A procedure to measure the patient's ability to metabolize glucose.

HAA Hepatitis-associated antigen. A serologic study formerly used to detect the presence of hepatitis B virus.

haptoglobin   A protein that binds free hemoglobin so that it can be recycled; increased in certain inflammatory diseases but decreased in hemolytic disorders.

HAV   Hepatitis A virus.

HBDH   Hydroxybutyric dehydrogenase. An enzyme with the same clinical significance as LDH_1 and LDH_2 isoenzymes.

HBV   Hepatitis B virus; serum hepatitis.

HCG   Human chorionic gonadotropin. The first hormone produced by the placenta following implantation of a fertilized ovum. The substance measured in pregnancy tests.

hct   Hematocrit. The percentage of whole blood volume occupied by erythrocytes.

HDL   High-density lipoprotein. A lipid substance that removes cholesterol from the walls of blood vessels, thus reducing the risk of atherosclerosis and coronary heart disease.

heat labile   Destructible by heat.

Heinz bodies   A red blood cell inclusion observed in the presence of certain abnormal hemoglobins and erythrocytes with enzyme deficiencies.

helminth   General term applied to various species of worms that may be parasitic in humans.

hema-, hemato-   Prefix; blood.

hematology   The branch of medicine dealing with the morphology of the blood and blood-producing tissues, including the manner in which blood cells and organs are affected by disease.

hematoma   A localized collection of blood within an organ, space, or tissue that forms a tumorlike mass and results in swelling, pain, and discoloration.

heme   An iron compound of protoporphyrin that constitutes the pigment portion of hemoglobin.

hemolysis   The destruction of red blood cells with the liberation of hemoglobin that imparts a red color to serum, plasma, or urine.

hemolytic anemia   The type of anemia characterized by excessive intravascular destruction of red blood cells.

hemopexin   A heme-binding serum protein.

hemosiderin   An insoluble storage form of iron.

hemostasis   The arrest of bleeding from a vessel either by vasoconstriction and coagulation or by surgical means; interruption of the flow of blood through any vessel or to any anatomic area, as with a tourniquet.

heparin   A natural anticoagulant, found in many tissues and produced by basophils, that inhibits coagulation by preventing the conversion of prothrombin to thrombin. Heparin may be mixed with blood specimens or administered by therapeutic injection to interfere with blood clotting.

hetero-   Prefix; different.

hgb   Hemoglobin. The iron-containing pigment of red blood cells that carries oxygen from the lungs to the tissues and removes carbon dioxide. There are many abnormal forms of hemoglobin that produce a number of diseases.

5-HIAA   5-Hydroxyindoleacetic acid. A hormone that is the metabolite of serotinin; produced by certain cells of the gastrointestinal tract.

HLA Human leukocyte antigen; histocompatibility locus A antigen. An antigen on the surface of nucleated cells that is important in crossmatching for transplantation procedures.

homo- Prefix; the same as or having a likeness to.

hormone Chemical substance produced by an organ or group of cells that has a specific effect on the activity of a certain organ.

Howell-Jolly bodies Small, round basophilic particles observed within erythrocytes in anemias or leukemias and after splenomegaly.

HPL Human placental lactogen. A hormone normally produced by the placenta during early gestation.

hyaline Glassy and transparent.

hydrometer Instrument used for determining the specific gravity of a fluid.

hyper- Prefix; above, excessive, or beyond.

hyperplasia The abnormal multiplication of cells or increase in the number of normal cells arranged within a tissue.

hypertonic A biologic term denoting a solution with a greater osmotic pressure than blood, with which it is compared. Body cells bathed by a hypertonic solution shrink because of a net flow of water out of the cell.

hypo- Prefix; less than, below, or under.

hypoplasia A decrease in cell formation; incomplete development of an organ.

hypotonic A biologic term denoting a solution having less tonicity or osmotic pressure than blood, with which it is compared. Body cells bathed by a hypotonic solution swell because of a net flow of water into the cell.

idiopathic A pathologic condition of spontaneous origin; of unknown cause, self-originated.

Ig Immunoglobulin. A group of proteins with antibody activity; divided into five major classes—IgG, IgM, IgA, IgE, and IgD.

immunity The body's reaction to foreign substances to protect itself from a particular disease; lack of susceptibility to the pathogenic or toxic effects of antigenic substances.

immunoelectrophoresis A method of electrophoresis that distinguishes between proteins and other materials by means of their electrophoretic mobility patterns and antigenic specificity.

immunohematology The branch of hematology devoted to the study of antigen-antibody reactions related to clinical manifestations of blood disorders; frequently applied to typing and crossmatching blood specimens for transfusion therapy.

intracellular Situated or occurring within a cell or cells.

in vitro Within a glass such as a test tube; in an artificial environment.

in vivo Within the living body.

ion An atom or chemical radical bearing a positive or negative electronic charge.

isoenzyme One of several forms in which an enzyme can exist. These forms differ chemically, physically, and immunologically but catalyze the same reaction.

isotonic Pertaining to solutions having the same tonicity or osmotic pressure as the solution with which it is compared; isotonic (physiologic) saline has the same concentration as blood plasma.

IU International unit. One of the many units of an internationally standardized system of measurement.

jaundice Condition characterized by increased bilirubin and deposition of bile pigment in the skin and mucous membranes, with a resulting yellow appearance of the patient.

K Chemical symbol for potassium.

-kalemia Suffix; potassium in the blood.

kallikrein One of a group of enzymes that become active during the coagulation process.

kg Kilogram. A measure of weight or mass equal to 1000 g or 2.2 lb.

17-KGS 17-Ketogenic steroids. The combination of 17-OHCS and adrenal cortex hormones that can be converted to 17-KS.

17-KS 17-Ketosteroids. A group of organic compounds metabolized from adrenal and testicular androgenic hormones.

L Liter. Metric fluid measure of volume, equal to 1000 mL.

labile Easily altered or decomposed.

LDH Lactate dehydrogenase. An enzyme that exists in different forms within certain tissues, including the lungs and heart.

LDL Low-density lipoprotein.

LE cell Lupus erythematosus cell. A large, mature neutrophil that contains ingested homogenized nuclear material and is characteristic of the chronic collagen disease that affects the skin, joints, kidneys, nervous system, and mucous membranes.

leukemia A progressive, malignant disease of the blood-forming organs that is characterized by increased proliferation and development of leukocytes and their precursors in the blood and bone marrow.

leukemoid reaction Temporary appearance of immature leukocytes in the bloodstream with a marked increase in total white blood cell count; resembles true leukemia to such a degree that initial differentiation may be extremely difficult.

leukocyte White blood cell. There are several varieties of white blood cells—granulated (neutrophils, eosinophils, and basophils) and nongranulated (monocytes and lymphocytes)—each having a different function.

leukocytosis Transient elevation in the number of leukocytes in the blood resulting from a variety of causes, including hemorrhage, fever, or infection.

LH Luteinizing hormone. An anterior pituitary hormone that stimulates the development and function of gonads.

lipase A pancreatic enzyme that aids digestion of triglycerides and phospholipids.

lipemia Abnormal amount of fat or lipid in the blood, giving the serum or plasma a cream-colored appearance.

lipid Any one of a group of organic compounds consisting of fats and other substances with similar properties. They are insoluble in water, soluble in fat solvents and alcohol, and greasy to the touch.

lipoprotein A complex of lipid and protein that transports cholesterol but possesses the general properties of proteins.

L/S ratio The ratio of lecithin to sphingomyelin in the amniotic fluid; used to assess the maturity of the fetal lungs.

lymphocyte A mononuclear, nongranular leukocyte with a round or oval nucleus and sky-blue cytoplasm that is divided into two distinct types: T and B. T-lymphocytes play a role in cell-mediated immunity; B-lymphocytes form antibodies against foreign antigens.

lyse Process of cell destruction that results from the action of specific substances.

macrocyte An erythrocyte that is larger than normal.

macroscopic Refers to gross morphologic characteristics that can be observed and studied with the naked eye.

MAO Maximal acid output. Total amount of gastric acid secreted during 1 hour following intense stimulation of gastric mucosa.

MCH Mean corpuscular hemoglobin. An expression of the average hemoglobin content of a single red blood cell expressed in picograms.

MCHC Mean corpuscular hemoglobin concentration. An expression of the average hemoglobin concentration of a single red blood cell in percent.

MCV Mean corpuscular volume. An expression of the average volume of individual red blood cells in cubic microns.

media A nutritive substance used to support the growth of microorganisms in culture.

megakaryocyte An extremely large cell in the bone marrow from which blood platelets mature.

megaloblast The large nucleated precursor of an abnormal red blood cell found in pernicious anemia.

mEq Milliequivalent. The number of grams of a solute contained in 1 mL of a normal solution. Measure, usually expressed as milliequivalents per liter (mEq/L), to indicate the concentration of electrolytes in a certain volume of solution.

M:E ratio The ratio of myeloid to erythroid cells in the bone marrow.

metamyelocyte Immature white blood cell of granular series that develops between the myelocyte and band form.

meter (m) A linear standard of measurement that equals 39.37 inches.

methemoglobin A form of hemoglobin in which ferrous iron has been changed to ferric iron due to toxic substances or hereditary deficiency of a certain enzyme.

microcyte A red blood cell that is smaller than normal.

microgram (μg) A metric unit of weight measuring 1/1000 of a milligram (mg) or 1/1,000,000 of a gram (g).

micro international unit (μIU) A metric unit equal to 1/1000 of a milli international unit (mIU).

microliter (μL) A metric unit of liquid volume, equal to 1/1000 of a milliliter (mL) or 1/1,000,000 of a liter (L).

micron (μm) Metric unit of linear measure equal to 1/1000 of a millimeter (mm) or 1/1,000,000 of a meter (m).

microorganism   Minute living body invisible to the naked eye, e.g., a bacterium or protozoan.

microscopic   Minute morphologic characteristics that can be observed and studied only under the lens of a microscope.

mg   Milligram. A metric unit of weight measuring 1/1000 of a gram (g).

mIU   Milli international unit. A metric unit equal to 1/1000 of an international unit (IU).

mL   Milliliter. A metric unit of volume measuring 1/1000 of a liter (L).

mm   Millimeter. A metric unit of distance measuring 1/1000 of a meter (m).

mmol/L   Millimoles per liter. The standard metric unit for concentration that can be used in place of mEq/L.

monocyte   A large, ungranulated leukocyte whose main function is to engulf debris that is circulating within the blood (phagocytosis).

morphology   The science of form and structure of an organism without regard to function, principally size and shape.

mOsm   Milliosmoles.

myelocyte   The immature stage in the development of granulocytic leukocytes; characterized by the first appearance of specific granules (neutrophilic, eosinophilic, or basophilic) and followed developmentally by the metamyelocyte.

myeloid cells   Granular leukocytes and their stem cells.

-natremia   Suffix; sodium in the blood.

neutrophil   A type of granular leukocyte that stains easily with neutral dyes; its main function is the ingestion of bacterial invaders. Also known as polymorphonuclear or segmented cells.

ng   Nanogram. A metric unit of weight measuring 1/1000 of a microgram (μg). Formerly called millimicrogram (mμg).

normal flora   Those living forms that normally occur in a given habitat or environment.

normoblast   The nucleated precursor of normal red blood cells.

normochromic   Refers to cells having a normal color as a result of normal hemoglobin content.

normocyte   Red blood cells of normal size, shape, and color.

NPN   Nonprotein nitrogen. A group of nitrogen-containing compounds resulting from the metabolic breakdown of protein.

nucleus   Spheroid body within a cell that controls the cell's vital activities.

occult blood   Blood or hemoglobin that is present in amounts too small for visual observation and that cannot be detected except by special chemical tests.

17-OHCS   17-Hydroxycorticosteroids. A group of compounds metabolized from the adrenocortical steroid hormones.

oliguria   Diminished amount of urine formation in relation to fluid intake.

-osis   Suffix; an increase in the amount of cells or other constituents in the blood.

osmolality   Indication of the concentration or number of particles dissolved in serum or urine. Characteristic of a solution determined by the ionic concentration of the dissolved substances per unit of solvent.

ova   Eggs of parasites.

ovalocyte   An elliptical erythrocyte.

oxalate   A sodium or potassium and ammonium salt of oxalic acid; often used as an anticoagulant for laboratory test specimens.

pancytopenia   A deficiency of all three formed elements of blood (erythrocytes, leukocytes, and thrombocytes). Also known as aplastic anemia.

parasite   Organism that lives within, upon, or at the expense of another organism and depends on that host for essential metabolites without contributing to the host's survival.

pathogen   A microorganism or substance capable of producing disease.

PBI   Protein-bound iodine. An outdated test of thyroid function that has been replaced by T_3, T_4, and T_7 (free thyroxine index) studies.

PCHE   Pseudocholinesterase. An enzyme.

Pco$_2$ Partial pressure of carbon dioxide.

PCT   Prothrombin consumption time. A coagulation study.

-penia   Suffix; lack or deficiency of cells.

petechiae   Small purplish-red pinpoint spots on the skin formed by hemorrhage of blood into the tissues.

pg   Picogram. A metric unit of mass measuring $1/1000$ of a nanogram (ng) or $1/1,000,000,000,000$ of a gram (g). Formerly called micromicrogram ($\mu\mu g$).

pH   Symbol used to express the hydrogen ion concentration of a solution. Pertains to the acidity or alkalinity of a substance. The neutral point where a solution is neither acid nor alkaline is 7. Increasing acidity is expressed as a number less than 7; increasing alkalinity is expressed as a number greater than 7.

phagocyte   Cell that ingests, destroys, and removes organisms and foreign matter, such as bacteria, cells, and cell debris, by a process of envelopment and absorption.

phenotype   The entire physical, biochemical, and physiologic makeup of an individual frequently determined by heredity.

-philia   Suffix; love for, tendency toward, or craving for.

phospholipid   Lipid compounds, such as lecithin and sphingomyelin, that contain phosphorus and can be hydrolyzed to yield glycerin, fatty acids, and a nitrogenous compound.

physiology   The study of chemical and physical processes involved in the function of living organisms.

pipette   A narrow glass tube for transferring and measuring liquids.

PKU   Phenylketonuria. An inborn error of metabolism resulting in mental retardation and neurologic manifestations due to an amino acid defect.

plasma   The liquid portion of whole, unclotted blood.

plasmin   The active portion of the fibrinolytic or clot-lysing system, which has the ability to dissolve formed fibrin clots.

plasminogen   The inactive precursor of plasmin.

platelet   A small disk-shaped structure chiefly known for its role in blood coagulation. Also known as a thrombocyte.

pleocytosis   A greater than normal number of white blood cells in the cerebrospinal fluid.

pleural fluid   A serous effusion produced within the cavity surrounding the lungs.

Po$_2$ Partial pressure of oxygen.

-poiesis   Suffix; making or producing, as in hemopoiesis.

poikilocyte   Erythrocyte showing an abnormal variation in shape.

polychromatophilia   Variation in the hemoglobin content of erythrocytes; detected by the presence of young non-nucleated bluish-staining red blood cells in stained blood smears.

polycythemia   Increase in the total number of erythrocytes in the blood.

polyuria   Passage of abnormally large volumes of urine in a given time.

porphobilinogen   A precursor of porphyrin; an intermediary product in the biosynthesis of heme that characteristically appears in the urine in acute intermittent porphyria.

porphyrins   Group of substances that occur in protoplasm and constitute the basis of the respiratory pigments in humans. Includes coproporphyrin, protoporphyrin, and uroporphyrin.

postprandial   Occurring after a meal.

pregnanediol   The chief urinary metabolite of the progesterone secreted by the ovary and placenta.

PRL   Prolactin. An anterior pituitary hormone that stimulates growth of the mammary gland and regulates postpartum lactation.

proaccelerin   A blood factor (coagulation factor V) required for the formation of a blood clot. Also known as the labile factor.

proconvertin   A blood factor (coagulation factor VII) required for the formation of a blood clot. Also known as the stable factor.

progesterone   A steriod hormone produced by the ovary and adrenal cortex.

promyelocyte   Precursor of the granular leukocyte that contains a few nonspecific cytoplasmic granules; intermediate in development between a myeloblast and myelocyte.

protein   A group of complex nitrogen-containing compounds that form the principal constituents of cell protoplasm in plants and animals. Proteins are essential for building new tissue and repairing injured or broken-down tissue.

proteolysis   Decomposition or digestion of protein by an enzyme or chemical compound.

prothrombin   A blood factor (coagulation factor II) required for the formation of a clot. The inactive precursor of thrombin.

protoporphyrin   The porphyrin that combines with protein to form hemoglobin.

protozoa   Single-celled animals characterized by a body composed of one or more nuclei surrounded by cytoplasm and contained within a limiting cell membrane.

PSP   Phenolsulfonphthalein. A dye used in kidney function tests.

PT   Prothrombin time. A screening test for several coagulation factors.

PTA Plasma thromboplastin antecedent. A blood factor (coagulation factor XI) required for the formation of a clot.

PTC Plasma thromboplastin component. A blood factor (coagulation factor IX) required for the formation of a clot.

PTH Parathyroid hormone. A hormone produced by the parathyroid gland that helps raise calcium levels in the blood. Also known as parathormone.

PTT Partial thromboplastin time. A screening test for almost all coagulation factors.

purpura Extravasation of blood into the tissues, producing ecchymoses and petechiae.

pyuria Presence of pus (white blood cells) in the urine.

qualitative Relating to quality; refers to tests that determine the presence or absence of a substance.

quantitative Relating to quantity; refers to tests that determine the exact amount or concentration of a particular substance.

RBC Red blood cell (erythrocyte) or red blood cell count.

reagent A substance involved in a chemical reaction that is used to detect the presence of another substance.

recessive gene A gene that is incapable of expression unless carried by both members of a pair of corresponding chromosomes.

renin An enzyme secreted by specialized kidney cells involved in controlling blood volume and pressure.

reticulocyte An immature red blood cell containing a basophilic network of filaments or reticulum; immature stage in cellular development between the nucleated red blood cell and the mature erythrocyte.

reticuloendothelial system A system of cells found in bone marrow, liver, spleen, and lungs that is concerned with blood cell formation, bile formation, and phagocytic destruction of particulate matter such as bacteria.

RIA Radioimmunoassay. A sensitive procedure used to measure certain toxic and biologic substances such as drugs and hormones.

rouleau formation A group of red blood cells arranged with their flat surfaces facing so that they resemble stacks of coins.

RPR Rapid plasma reagin. A screening test for syphilis.

saturated Unable to hold in solution any more of a given substance.

schistocytes Fragments of damaged red blood cells that appear as distorted and irregularly shaped particles on a stained blood smear.

sepsis Pathologic state, usually febrile, that is caused by microorganisms or their toxic products in the blood.

serologic test Laboratory test performed on blood serum.

serology The study of antigen-antibody reaction in vitro.

serum The fluid portion of blood after it has clotted. Serum is not the same as plasma because it lacks fibrinogen, an important coagulation protein.

shift to the left Term used to indicate an increase in immature forms of neutrophils in the blood picture.

shift to the right   Term used to indicate an increase in older, hypersegmented neutrophils in the blood picture.

sickle cell   A crescent-shaped erythrocyte characteristic of sickle cell anemia.

siderocyte   An erythrocyte containing nonhemoglobin iron.

siderotic granules   Particles of nonhemoglobin iron appearing as purple-blue specks within erythrocytes on a stained blood smear.

SMA   Sequential Multiple Analyzer. An automated system used to perform 12 chemistry tests simultaneously from a single small blood specimen.

SMAC   Sequential Multiple Analyzer with Computer. An automated system that performs 20–40 chemistry studies simultaneously.

smear   A specimen for microscopic study prepared by spreading the material across a glass slide.

soluble   Capable of being dissolved.

solute   Substance dissolved in a solution.

specific gravity   Weight of a substance compared with the weight of an equal volume of another substance taken as a standard. Water usually is employed as the standard for liquids and has a specific gravity of 1.000.

spherocyte   A red blood cell that is smaller, darker, rounder, and more fragile than normal.

stasis   A stoppage or diminution of the flow of blood or other body fluid in any part.

Stuart-Prower factor   A blood factor (coagulation factor XII) required for the formation of a blood clot.

synovial fluid   A substance produced in joint and tendon spaces to minimize friction between bones during movement.

T$_3$ Triiodothyronine. A thyroid hormone that regulates the general metabolic state of the body.

T$_4$ Thyroxine. A thyroid hormone that regulates the general metabolic state of the body.

T$_7$ Free thyroxine index.

target cell   Abnormally thin erythrocyte that shows a dark center and a peripheral ring of hemoglobin when stained. Also known as a leptocyte.

TBG   Thyroid-binding globulin.

T cell   A lymphocyte produced by the thymus that causes delayed hypersensitivity reactions and the rejection of transplanted tissue. They play a major role in the body's defense against viruses, fungi, and certain bacteria.

testosterone   The primary male sex hormone produced by the testes, ovaries, and adrenal cortex.

TGT   Thromboplastin generation time. A coagulation study.

thoracocentesis   Surgical puncture of the chest wall for the drainage of fluid.

thrombasthenia   Abnormal platelet function.

thrombin   An enzyme manufactured during the clotting process from prothrombin, which converts fibrinogen to fibrin.

thrombocyte   Another word for blood platelet.

thrombocytopathy A qualitative disorder of blood platelets.

thrombocytopenia A decrease in the number of blood platelets.

thrombocytosis An increased number of platelets in the peripheral blood.

thromboplastin A substance that initiates the clotting process and is released from injured tissue or formed by the disintegration of platelets in combination with several plasma factors.

TIBC Total iron-binding capacity. The total amount of iron circulating in the plasma plus the iron that could be bound to transferrin, the iron transport protein.

titer The highest dilution of serum that will demonstrate the antigen-antibody reaction.

TPI *Treponema pallidum* immobilization. A test for syphilis.

transferrin A serum globulin that binds and transports iron.

triglyceride A fat consisting of fatty acid and glycerol that is synthesized from carbohydrates and stored.

trophozoite The active vegetative stage of a protozoa.

TSH Thyroid-stimulating hormone. An anterior pituitary hormone that stimulates thyroid activity.

turbidity Cloudiness or disturbance of sediment in a solution so that it is not clear. Turbidity may be uniform, flocculant, or granular.

two-hour PP Two-hour postprandial. A blood glucose determination performed 2 hours after a meal.

U Unit.

uremia Increased levels of urea in the blood due to deficient renal function.

-uria Suffix; presence in the urine of excessive quantities of a substance.

uric acid The end product of purine metabolism; a common constituent of urinary and renal calculi and gouty concretions.

urinometer Instrument used to measure the specific gravity of urine.

urobilin The oxidized form of urobilinogen; found in the feces and sometimes in urine left exposed to the air.

urobilinogen A colorless derivative of bilirubin that is formed by the action of intestinal bacteria.

urochrome A yellow pigment that gives urine its color.

uroporphyrin One of a group of porphyrins.

vacuole Space or cavity within the cytoplasm of a cell.

vacutainer A general term for vacuum test tubes, which are used in the collection of blood.

VDRL Venereal Disease Research Laboratories. A test for syphilis.

venipuncture The act of puncturing a vein to remove a sample of blood.

VLDL Very low-density lipoprotein.

VMA Vanillylmandelic acid. The chief metabolite of catecholamines secreted by the adrenal medulla.

WBC Abbreviation for white blood cell (leukocyte); white blood cell count.

xanthochromic Yellow pigmentation.

Index

A small "f" following a page number refers to a figure; a "t" refers to a table.

ABO blood groups, 634–637
  agglutinogens/agglutinins in, 635t
  inheritance of, 636–637
  typing of, 637
Abortion
  septic, bacteremia and, 489
  spontaneous
    human placental lactogen and, 338
    pregnanediol and, 340
    rubella and, 629
Acanthocytes, 87
Acanthocytosis, 87
Acetaminophen, 369–370
Acetanilid
  Heinz bodies and, 89
  methemoglobinemia and, 394
  sulfhemoglobinemia and, 396
Acetazolamide, procainamide therapy and, 388
Acetest tablets, ketonuria screening and, 26
n-Acetylprocainamide, 387–389
Acetylsalicylic acid, 370–372; *see also* Salicylates
Achlorhydria, conditions associated with, 464
Acid glycoprotein, 238
Acid phosphatase, 178–179; *see also* Serum acid phosphatase
Acid-base balance, 278–292
Acid-base equilibrium, potassium and, 257
Acid-base imbalances, 289–292
  laboratory indications of, 290t
  urinalysis and, 13
Acid-fast stain, 487

Acidosis, 289
  diabetic, bacteremia and, 489
  metabolic
    differential diagnosis of, 273
    hyperchloremic, 274–275
    signs and symptoms of, 291–292
    partial pressure of carbon dioxide and, 285
    pH and, 283
  respiratory, 289–291
Acne, 504t
Acquired immune deficiency syndrome, blood transfusion and, 667
Acquired porphyria hepatica, 47
Acromegaly, growth hormone secretion and, 323
ACTH; *see* Adrenocorticotropic hormone
Activated coagulation time test, 553
Addison's disease
  intravenous glucose tolerance test and, 163
  plasma cortisol and, 301
  reactive lymphocytes and, 79
Adenohypophysis, hormones of, 319
ADH; *see* Antidiuretic hormone
Adrenal glands, 295
Adrenal hormone studies, 295–311
Adrenocortical insufficiency
  differential diagnosis of, 320
  excessive fluid loss and, 248
  urine concentration test and, 52

Adrenocorticotropic hormone, 320–321
  cortisol synthesis and, 301
  fluid and electrolyte balance and, 250
  free fatty acids and, 211
  functions of, 319
  Thorn test and, 103
AFP; *see* alpha-Fetoprotein
African trypanosomiasis, 527t
Agammaglobulinemia, 235
  B-lymphocytes and, 580
Agglutination, antigen-antibody reactions and, 579
Agglutination tests
  brucellosis and, 597–598
  tularemia and, 598–599
Agglutinins, ABO system and, 635t
Agglutinogens, ABO system and, 635t
Agranulocytosis
  reactive lymphocytes and, 79
  toxic neutrophilic granulation and, 79
A/G ratio, 231
  normal values for, 232
Alanine aminotransferase, 196–198
Albumin, 230–231, 238
  serum, 233
  total, 232–234
Albumin therapy, 660–661
Albuminuria, 21
Alcohol, 360–365; *see also* specific type
  acquired porphyria hepatica and, 47
  acute intermittent porphyria and, 45
  barbiturates and, 380
  benzodiazepines and, 415
  phenothiazines and, 412

Alcohol (*continued*)
  sedative/tranquilizing agents
    and, 417
  tricylic antidepressants and,
    413
Alcoholic cirrhosis; *see also*
    Cirrhosis
  acanthocytosis and, 87
  acquired porphyria hepatica
    and, 47
  porphyria cutanea tarda
    and, 45
Alcoholic liver disease, alanine
    aminotransferase levels
    and, 197
Alcoholism, gamma-glutamyl
    transferase activity and,
    199
Alcohol withdrawal, ben-
    zodiazepines and, 414
Aldolase, 183–185
Aldosterone, 295, 297–298
  renal tubular urine volume
    and, 4
  renin secretion and, 316
Aldosteronism
  conditions associated with,
    298
  differential diagnosis of, 297
  renin-angiotensin system
    and, 316
Alkali denaturation test,
    114–116
Alkaline phosphatase,
    180–182, 238
Alkalosis, 289
  aldosteronism and, 297
  metabolic
    differential diagnosis
      of, 273
    signs and symptoms
      of, 292
  partial pressure of carbon di-
    oxide and, 285
  pH and, 283
  respiratory
    hyperammonemia
      and, 220
    signs and symptoms
      of, 291
Alkaptonuria, homogentisic
    acid excretion and, 58
Allergens, radioallergosorbent
    test and, 582t
ALT; *see* Alanine
    aminotransferase
Amebiasis, 517t
  serologic values for, 608
  tests for, 607

Amebic dysentery, 517t
American trypanosomiasis,
    493t
Amikacin
  activities of, 529
  characteristics of, 366t
  nephrotoxicity of, 366
  therapeutic and toxic con-
    centrations of, 367
Amino acids, 57–58
Aminoaciduria, 57–60
Aminobenzoic esters, pro-
    cainamide therapy and,
    388
Aminoglycosides, 366–367
  adverse reactions to,
    366–367
  characteristics of, 366t
  therapeutic and toxic con-
    centrations of, 367
delta-Aminolevulinic acid,
    128–131
Amitriptyline, 412–413
  characteristics of, 409t
  therapeutic and toxic levels
    of, 413
Ammonia, blood, 220–222
Amniocentesis, 424–425
Amniotic fluid
  alpha-fetoprotein in,
    427–429
  analysis of, 424–434
    specimen collection and
      handling in, 424–425
  bilirubin in, 429–431
  creatinine in, 431–432
    normal values for, 431
  phospholipids in, 433
Amobarbital, 379
  characteristics of, 380t
  therapeutic and toxic levels
    of, 381
Amphetamines, 367–368
  abuse of, 418
Amphetamine sulfate, 367
Amphotericin, activities
    of, 529
Amphotericin B, urinary casts
    and, 40
Ampicillin, activities of, 529
Amylase
  serum, 173–176
  urinary, 173–176
Amyloidosis, monoclonal
    gammopathies and, 235
ANA; *see* Antinuclear
    antibodies
Anabolism, growth hormone
    secretion and, 323

Anacidity, conditions associ-
    ated with, 464
Anaerobic cultures, 488
Anaerobic specimens, 485
Analgesics, 369–372
  characteristics of, 369t
Androgenicity, testosterone
    and, 343
Androgens, 295
  17-ketosteroids and, 307
Anemia; *see also* Megaloblastic
    anemia
  chronic posthemorrhagic,
    hypochromia and, 88
  congenital spheroytic, side-
    rocytes and, 89
  microcytic, hypochromic, 92
  microcytic, normochromic,
    92
  normochromic, macrocytic,
    92
  sickle cell
    basophilic stippling and, 89
    elliptocytosis and, 87
    target cells and, 87
Anencephaly, alpha-feto-
    protein levels and, 242
Angina pectoris, propranolol
    and, 389
Angiotensin, aldosterone se-
    cretion and, 297
Angiotensin II, renin secretion
    and, 316
Aniline, Heinz bodies and, 89
Animal bites, diseases associ-
    ated with, 526t
Anion gap, 272–275
  calculation of, 272
Anion-cation balance, calcula-
    tion of, 272–273
Anions, 248–250
Anisochromia, 87–88
Anisocytosis, 86
Antacids, digoxin levels and,
    383
Anthrax, 493t
Antibiotics, procainamide
    therapy and, 388
Antibiotic susceptibility tests,
    528–530
Antibodies, 579; *see also specific
    type*
  detection of, 642–646
  identification of, 645–646
Antibody deficiency syn-
    drome, immunoelectro-
    phoresis and, 238
Antibody screen, 642,
    644–645

Antibody test, direct, 643–644
Anticoagulants
circulating, 555–556
used in hematology, 65, 152–153
Anticoagulant therapy, 573–576
Anticonvulsants, 372–379
characteristics of, 373t
Antideoxyribonuclease B, 611–612
Antidiuretic hormone
fluid and electrolyte balance and, 250
functions of, 319
renal tubular urine volume and, 4, 14
Antigen-antibody reactions, 579–585
Antigens, 579
Antiglobulin test, direct, 642–644
Antihemophilic factor, 539–540
Antihyaluronidase, 611–612
Antimicrosomial antibodies, 592
Antimitochondrial antibodies, 589–591
Antinuclear antibodies, 586–588
Anti-smooth muscle antibodies, 589–591
Antistreptolysin O titer, 609–611
Antithrombin III, 555, 565–567
Antithyroglobulin, 592
Antitrypsin, 238
Anuria, 8
Anxiety disorders, benzodiazepines and, 414
Appendicitis, anaerobic organisms and, 488
Arsenic, 397–398
acute intermittent porphyria and, 45
Arsenic poisoning, signs and symptoms of, 397
Arteriosclerosis, bacteremia and, 489
Arthritis; see also Rheumatoid arthritis
bacterial, predisposing factors in, 520
differential diagnosis of, 469
infectious, synovial fluid in, 520

septic, synovial fluid glucose in, 477
Arthrocentesis, 470
Arthropod bites, diseases associated with, 527t
Arthropod-borne encephalitis, 527t
Ascites, differential diagnosis of, 213
Ascorbic acid, 214–215
Asiatic cholera, 516t
Aspartate aminotransferase, 194–196
Aspergillosis, 600–601
serologic values for, 601
Aspiration pneumonia, anaerobic organisms and, 488
Aspirin, 370–372; see also Salicylates
AST; see Aspartate aminotransferase
Asthma, bronchial, theophylline and, 407
Atherosclerosis
cholesterol and, 202
lipid concentrations and, 201
lipoprotein distribution and, 207
triglycerides and, 205
Atrial fibrillation
procainamide and, 387
propranolol and, 389
quinidine and, 390
Atrial flutter
propranolol and, 389
quinidine and, 390
Atrial premature beats, propranolol and, 389
Atrial tachycardia
quinidine and, 390
paroxysmal, phenytoin and, 376
Atrophic gastritis, gastric acid secretion and, 462
Autoimmune disease
polyclonal gammopathies and, 236
T-lymphocytes and, 580
Autoimmunity, serologic tests for, 586–593
Azotemia, conditions associated with, 223
B-lymphocytes, 76, 579–580
immunoglobulins and, 235
Bacillary dysentery, 516t
Bacitracin
activities of, 529
urinary casts and, 40

Bacteremia
anaerobic organisms and, 488
clinical significance of, 489–490
Bacteria, urinary, 43
Bacteriology, 481
Bacteriuria, differential diagnosis of, 521–522
Balantidiasis, 517t
BAO; see Basal acid output
Barbiturates, 379–382
abuse of, 418
acquired porphyria hepatica and, 47
acute intermittent porphyria and, 45
characteristics of, 380t
digitoxin concentrations and, 383
ethanol and, 361
intoxication with, signs and symptoms of, 380
narcotic drugs and, 419
phenothiazines and, 412
prothrombin time and, 561
reactive lymphocytes and, 79
sedative/tranquilizing agents and, 417
solubility of, albumin and, 231
Basal acid output, 459, 462
Base excess, 286–287
Basopenia, conditions associated with, 85
Basophilia, conditions associated with, 84–85
Basophilic stippling, 88–89
Basophils, 77
Bence-Jones protein, urinary, 23
Benedict's test, 58
Benzodiazepines, 414–416
Bicarbonate-carbonic acid buffers, 278–279
Biliary cirrhosis, primary, autoimmune immunoglobulins and, 589–590
Bilirubin, 29
amniotic fluid, 429–431
direct, 143, 146
indirect, 143, 146
serum, 143–148
urinary, 29–31
Bilirubinuria, 29–31
Bites, diseases associated with, 526t

Blastomycosis, 510t, 600–601
  serologic values for, 601
Bleeding time, 544–546
Blindness, congenital toxoplasmosis and, 606
Blood
  cultures of, 490–491
  in gastric secretions, 461
  microbiologic examination
    of, 489–491
  normal flora of, 490
  oxalated, keeping time
    of, 66t
  pathogens of, 490
  sequestrinized, keeping time
    of, 66t
  in synovial fluid, 474
Blood component therapy,
    652–661
Blood count, complete, 65–89
  differential white blood cell
    count in, 75–85
  erythrocyte count in, 70–72
  hematocrit in, 68–70
  hemoglobin in, 66–68
  leukocyte count in, 73–75
  stained red blood cell exami-
    nation in, 85–89
Blood donors, selection and
    screening of, 669–671
Blood dyscrasias
  elliptocytosis and, 87
  heparin and, 574
Blood gases, 278–292
  collection and handling of,
    279–283
Blood glucose, 159–163
  Blood smears
  EDTA and, 153
  preparation of, 85
Blood specimens, collection of
  handling of, 63–65,
    152–157
  nursing responsibilities in,
    155–156
  order of draw of, 154
  precautions in, 154–155
  preservation and processing
    of, 156
  precautions in, 156–157
  times for, 153
  tubes for, 153–154
Blood transfusion; see Transfu-
    sion therapy
Blood types, 634–640
  parental, offspring blood
    types and, 636t
Blood urea nitrogen, 53,
    222–224

Blood urea nitrogen/creatinine
    ratio, 227
Blood vessels, hemostasis
    and, 533
Body fluids, 248
  composition of, 249f
  pH of, 283f
Body water balance, po-
    tassium and, 257
Bone disease, metabolic, al-
    kaline phosphatase ac-
    tivity and, 180
Bone marrow
  depression of, carbama-
    zepine and, 372
  differential cell count of,
    normal values for, 117
  examination of, 116–120
  hyperplasia of, conditions
    associated with, 118
  hypoplasia of, conditions as-
    sociated with, 118
  lesions of, nucleated
    erythrocytes and, 88
  transplantation of, methotre-
    xate therapy and, 405
Botulism, 516t
  anaerobic organisms and,
    488
Boutonneuse tick fever, Weil-
    Felix test and, 596
Bowman's capsule, 2
Brain abscess
  anaerobic organisms
    and, 488
  bacteremia and, 489
  cerebrospinal fluid analysis
    and, 434
  cerebrospinal fluid patho-
    gens and, 495
Brain tumor
  cerebrospinal fluid cell
    counts and, 439
  methotrexate therapy
    and, 405
Breast carcinoma
  calcitonin and, 312
  methotrexate therapy and,
    405
  serum ferritin levels and,
    138
Broad casts, conditions associ-
    ated with, 41
Bromide, 404–405
Bronchial asthma, theo-
    phylline and, 407
Brucella antigens, normal val-
    ues for, 598
Brucellosis, 492t

agglutination test for,
    597–598
differential diagnosis of, 490
Buffer base capacity, 286
BUN; see Blood urea nitrogen
Burns
  bacteremia and, 489
  excessive fluid loss and, 248
  mean corpuscular hemoglo-
    bin concentration and, 90
  schistocytes and, 87
  siderotic granules and, 89
Burr cells, 87
Butabarbital, 379
Cabot rings, 89
Calcitonin, 312
Calcium, 265–268
  coagulation and, 538–539
  metabolism of, parathyroid
    hormone and, 268
  normal values for, 48, 266
Calcium oxalate calculi, 56
Calcium phosphate calculi, 56
Calcium pyrophosphate dihy-
    drate crystals, conditions
    associated with, 476
Calciuria, 47–49
Cancer, methotrexate therapy
    and, 405
Candida albicans, in urine, 43
Candidiasis, 505t
  cerebrospinal fluid patho-
    gens and, 495
Cannabinoids, abuse of, 418
Capillary blood specimens,
    63–64
Capillary fragility, 546–547
Carbamazepine, 372–374
  characteristics of, 373t
  phenytoin metabolism and,
    376
Carbenicillin, activities of, 529
Carbohydrates
  metabolism of, cortisol
    and, 295
  tests of, 157–172
Carbon dioxide, 260–262, 285
  partial pressure of, 285–286
Carbon monoxide, 391–394
Carboxyhemoglobin, 392–393
Carcinoembryonic antigen,
    243–244
Carcinoma; *see also specific type*
  bacteremia and, 489
  nucleated erythrocytes
    and, 88
Carcinomatosis, lactate de-
    hydrogenase activity and,
    189

Cardiac anomalies, bacteremia and, 489
Cardiac arrest
  hypokalemia and, 257
  magnesium excess and, 271
Cardiac arrhythmias
  lidocaine and, 385
  phenytoin and, 376
  procainamide and, 387
  propranolol and, 389
  quinidine and, 390
Cardiac drugs, 382–391
Cardiac failure, excessive fluid accumulation and, 248
Cardiovascular system, diseases associated with, 492
Caries, dental, 516t
Carotene, 215–217
Casts
  fatty, 41
  urinary, 40–41
Cat scratch fever, 526t
Cataracts, galactosuria and, 19
Catecholamines, 296, 298–301
  secretion of, vanillylmandelic acid determinations and, 310
Catheterization, complications of, 4
Cations, 248–250
CBC; see Complete blood count
CEA; see Carcinoembryonic antigen
Cefoxitin, activities of, 529
Celiac disease, intravenous glucose tolerance test and, 163
Cell-mediated immunity, T-lymphocytes and, 579
Cellophane tape specimen, 520
Cellulitis
  anaerobic organisms and, 488
  bacteremia and, 489
Central nervous system tumors, IgG/albumin index and, 445
Cephalothin, activities of, 529
Cerebral calcification, congenital toxoplasmosis and, 606
Cerebral infarction, IgG/albumin index and, 445
Cerebrospinal fluid
  analysis of, 434–449

microbiologic examination in, 448
physical examination in, 437–439
specimen collection and handling in, 434–437
cell counts in, 439–442
microbiologic examination of, 491–496
  normal flora of, 495
  pathogens of, 495
  specimens of, 495–496
values of
  normal, 435t
  in selected disorders, 436t
Ceruloplasmin, 217, 238
Chancroid, 503t
Chemical poisoning, toxic neutrophilic granulation and, 79
Chemstrip
  bilirubinuria screening and, 30
  ketonuria screening and, 25
  urinary occult blood screening and, 28
  urinary protein screening and, 23
  urinary sugar screening and, 19
  urinary urobilinogen screening and, 32
Chickenpox, 504t
  atypical lymphocytes and, 79
Childbirth, iron deficiency and, 132
Chloramphenicol
  activities of, 529
  phenytoin metabolism and, 376
Chlorates
  Heinz bodies and, 89
  methemoglobin and, 394
Chlordiazepoxide, 414–415
  acute intermittent porphyria and, 45
  characteristics of, 416t
  ethanol and, 361
  therapeutic and toxic levels of, 415
Chloride, 263–265
Chloroquine, acute intermittent porphyria and, 45
Chlorpromazine, 411
Cholera, 516t
Cholesterol, 202–205
Cholesterol crystals, conditions associated with, 476

Cholestyramine
  digitoxin concentrations and, 383
  digoxin levels and, 383
  type II primary hyperlipemia and, 209
Cholinesterase, 182–183, 238
  true, 182
Choriocarcinoma, methotrexate therapy and, 405
Christmas disease, 560
Christmas factor; see Plasma thromboplastin component
Chromomycosis, 505t
Chvostek's sign, 265
Chylomicrons, 201, 207
Chyluria, 13
Circulating anticoagulants, 555–556
Circulatory overload, signs and symptoms of, 665
Cirrhosis; see also Alcoholic cirrhosis
  alanine aminotransferase levels and, 197
  aspartate aminotransferase levels and, 194
  autoimmune immunoglobulins and, 589
  cholesterol levels and, 202
  excessive fluid accumulation and, 248
  galactosuria and, 19
  hyperammonemia and, 220
  lactic dehydrogenase activity and, 190
  pleural transudates and, 464
  primary biliary, autoimmune immunoglobulins and, 589–590
  target cells and, 87
Clean-catch specimens, 4–5
Clindamycin, activities of, 529
Clinitest tablets, urine sugar screening and, 19–20
Clofibrate, primary hyperlipemias and, 209
Clonazepam, 414
  characteristics of, 416t
  phenytoin metabolism and, 376
  therapeutic and toxic levels of, 415
Clonidine, tricyclic antidepressants and, 413
Clorazepate, 414
  therapeutic and toxic levels of, 415

Clostridium perfringens gastroenteritis, 517t
Clot retraction, 547–548
hemostasis and, 533
Clotting time; *see also* Coagulation time
antihemophilic factor deficiency and, 540
plasma thromboplastin antecedent deficiency and, 541
proaccelerin deficiency and, 539
Coagulation, 534–536
sequence of, 535f
stage I, 534–535
tests of, 558–561
stage II, 536
tests of, 561–568
stage III, 536
tests of, 561–568
stage IV, 536
tests of, 568–573
Coagulation factors, 537–543
Coagulation profile, 543
Coagulation studies, specimen handling and collection in, 543–544
Coagulation time
antihemophilic factor deficiency and, 540
fibrinogen deficiency and, 537
Hageman factor deficiency and, 542
plasma thromboplastin component deficiency and, 540
prothrombin deficiency and, 538
Stuart-Prower factor deficiency and, 541
Cocaine, abuse of, 418
Coccidioidomycosis, 510t, 600–601
serologic values for, 601
Codeine, abuse of, 418
Cold, common, 508t
Cold agglutinins, 602–603
monoclonal gammopathies and, 235
Cold sores, 505t
Colistin, activities of, 529
Colitis, ulcerative
fecal analysis and, 449
reactive lymphocytes and, 79
Collagen, ascorbic acid and, 214

Collagen disease
immunoelectrophoresis and, 238
polyclonal gammopathies and, 236
Colony count, 522
Colorectal adenocarcinoma, carcinoembryonic antigen and, 243–244
Coma
hyperammonemia and, 220
magnesium excess and, 271
Common cold, 508t
Compatibility testing, 646–648
specimen collection and handling in, 647
Complement, 238, 581–585
IgM and, 235
Complement fixation, antigen-antibody reactions and, 579
Complete blood count; *see* Blood count, complete
Component therapy, 652–661
Compound F; *see* Cortisol
Congenital disorders; *see specific disorder*
Congenital malformations, rubella and, 629
Congestive heart failure; *see* Heart failure, congestive
Conjunctivitis, 498t
Connective tissue disease, mixed, antinuclear antibodies and, 587
Contagious conjunctivitis, 498t
Copper, 217–218
Coproporphyria, hereditary, 45
Coproporphyrin, 44, 128–129
increased excretion of, conditions associated with, 44–45
Coronary artery disease, triglycerides and, 205
Coronary insufficiency, aspartate aminotransferase levels and, 195
Corticosteroid crystals, conditions associated with, 476
Corticosteroids
bacterial arthritis and, 520
tricylic antidepressants and, 413
Corticotropin; *see* Adrenocorticotropic hormone
Cortisol, 295, 301–303
adrenocorticotropic hormone secretion and, 320
phenytoin and, 376
transcortin and, 238
Cortisone glucose tolerance test, 164
Coumarin anticoagulants
factor VII and, 539
phenytoin metabolism and, 376
Coumarin derivatives
clinical significance of, 575
drugs interfering with, 576t
therapeutic monitoring of, 575
CPK; *see* Creatine phosphokinase
Cranial epidural abscess, cerebrospinal fluid pathogens and, 495
C-reactive protein, 612–614
Creatine phosphokinase, 185–189
isoenzyme patterns of, 187t
Creatinine, 224–226
amniotic fluid, 431–432
Creatinine clearance test, 50–51
Croup, nasopharyngeal cultures and, 507
CRP; *see* C-reactive protein
Cryoglobulins, 235
Cryoprecipitated antihemophilic factor, 659–660
contraindications for, 659
indications for, 659
side effects of, 660
Cryptococcosis, 494t, 600–601
serologic values for, 601
Cryptogenic cirrhosis, autoimmune immunoglobulins and, 589–590
Crystalluria
clinical significance of, 42
conditions associated with, 42–43
Crystals
cholesterol, 476
corticosteroid, 476
monosodium urate, 476
urinary, 42–43
CSF; *see* Cerebrospinal fluid
Cultures, 488–489; *see also specific type*
Cushing's disease
17-ketogenic steroids and, 306
plasma cortisol and, 301

Cutaneous diphtheria, 508t
Cyanocobalamin; *see* Vitamin
  B$_{12}$
Cylindroids, 41–42
Cylindruria, 40
Cystic fibrosis, fecal trypsin
  and, 456
Cystine stones, 56–57
Cystinuria, 43, 56
Cystitis, 502t
Cytomegalovirus
  atypical lymphocytes
  and, 79
  blood transfusion and,
  667–668
  clinical significance of,
  620–621
  congenital, 620
  increased IgM levels at birth
  and, 235
  normal values for, 621
  serologic tests for, 620–621
Cytomegalovirus IgM test
  reactions
  false-positive, conditions associated with, 621
  serologic tests for, methodology of, 621
Cytomegalovirus inclusion disease, 517t
DAT; *see* Direct antiglobulin test
Deafness, congenital toxoplasmosis and, 606
Dehydration
  hyperchromia and, 88
  mean corpuscular hemo-
  globin concentration
  and, 90
  total protein levels and,
  231–232
Delayed hypersensitivity, T-
  lymphocytes and, 579
Delta base, 286
Dengue, 527t
Dental caries, 516t
Deoxyribonucleic acid antibodies, 588–589
Depressants, abuse of, 418
de Quervain's disease, thyroid
  antibodies and, 593
Dermatomyositis, antinuclear
  antibodies and, 586–587
Desipramine, 412–413
  characteristics of, 409t
  therapeutic and toxic levels
  of, 414
Dexamethasone, phenytoin
  and, 376

Dextroamphetamine, thera-
  peutic and toxic effects of,
  368
Dextroamphetamine sulfate,
  367
Dextrothyroxine, type III primary hyperlipemia and,
  209
Diabetes insipidus, excessive
  fluid loss and, 248
Diabetes mellitus
  acquired porphyria hepatica
  and, 47
  bacterial arthritis and, 520
  coumarin therapy and, 575
  diagnosis of, 158
  urinalysis and, 13
  electrolyte panel for, 274
  fasting blood glucose test
  and, 159
  glucose tolerance test and,
  163, 165
  glycohemoglobin test and,
  168
  ketonuria and, 24
  lipid concentrations and, 201
  lipoprotein electrophoresis
  and, 207
  maternal, amniotic fluid
  analysis and, 424
  opportunistic fungi and, 489
  two-hour postprandial
  glucose and, 161
  urinalysis and, 13
Diabetic acidosis, bacteremia
  and, 489
Diabetic coma, differential diagnosis of, 24
Diabetic ketoacidosis, glycohemoglobin test and, 168
Diarrhea, excessive fluid loss
  and, 248
Diazepam, 414
  characteristics of, 416t
  ethanol and, 361
  phenytoin metabolism and,
  376
  therapeutic and toxic levels
  of, 415
DIC; *see* Disseminated intravascular coagulation
Dicumarol, phenytoin and,
  376
Diethylstilbestrol, acquired
  porphyria hepatica
  and, 47
Differential white blood cell
  count, 75–85
  interpretation of, 79–81

normal values for, 78
variations in, 81–85
DiGeorge's syndrome, T-
  lymphocytes and, 580
Digitalis glycosides, 382–384
  serum potassium concentrations and, 257
Digitalis intoxication, signs and
  symptoms of, 382–383
Digitoxin, 382–384
  phenytoin and, 376
Digoxin, 384
1,25-Dihydroxycalciferol,
  318–319
Diphtheria, 508t
  reactive lymphocytes
  and, 79
  upper respiratory tract cultures and, 507
Direct antibody test, 643–644
Direct antiglobulin test,
  642–644
Disk diffusion tests, 529–530
Disopyramide, 386–387
Disseminated intravascular
  coagulation
  Burr cells and, 87
  clot retraction and, 548
  euglobulin lysis time
  and, 570
  fibrin-fibrinogen degradation
  products and, 569
  paracoagulation studies
  and, 571
  platelet transfusion and, 657
  schistocytes and, 87
  whole blood transfusion
  and, 652
Disseminated lupus erythematosus, C-reactive protein and, 613
Disulfiram, phenytoin metabolism and, 376
Diuretics, thiazide, procainamide therapy and, 388
Diverticulitis, anaerobic organisms and, 488
Dopamine, 296
Down's syndrome
  hypersegmented neutrophils
  and, 79
  mean corpuscular volume
  and, 90
Doxepin, 412
  characteristics of, 409t
  therapeutic and toxic levels
  of, 414
Drug abuse, 418–420
  detection of, 419–42

Drug abuse (*continued*)
laboratory screening tests for, 356
signs and symptoms of, 419
Drug interactions, 359
Drug monitoring, 358–360
Drug reactions, reactive lymphocytes and, 79
Drug response, factors affecting, 358–359
Drug screening, 420–421
Duchenne's muscular dystrophy, creatine phosphokinase levels in, 185
Dwarfism, growth hormone secretion and, 323
Dysentery
amebic, 517t
fecal analysis and, 449
Dysfibrinogenemia, 564
Dysgammaglobulins, 235
Dysproteinemia, paracoagulation studies and, 571
Ear
cultures of, 497
microbiologic examination of, 496–497
normal flora of, 496
pathogens of, 497
EBV; see Epstein-Barr virus
Echinococcosis
serologic values for, 608
tests for, 607
Eclampsia, amniotic fluid analysis and, 424
EDTA, hematologic testing and, 65, 153
Electrolyte panel
balanced, 273
for diabetes mellitus, 274
for hypokalemic, hypochloremic alkalosis, 274
Electrolytes, 248–250; see also Serum electrolytes
Electrophoresis; see also *specific type*
clinical significance of, 238
Elliptocytes, 87
Elliptocytosis, 87
Emergency crossmatch, 648
Emphysema
mean corpuscular volume and, 90
plasma carbon dioxide and, 261
theophylline and, 407
Empyema
anaerobic organisms and, 488

bacteremia and, 489
pleural fluid aspiration and, 464
Encephalitis, 527t
cerebrospinal fluid analysis and, 434, 438–439
pleocytosis and, 439
Endemic murine typhus, 527t
Endocarditis, bacterial, 492t
acute, 492t
differential diagnosis of, 490
subacute, 492t
complement and, 584
Endocrine glands, 296f
Enterococci, antibiotics active against, 529
Enterotoxicosis, 516t
Enzymes, tests of, 172–201
Eosinopenia, conditions associated with, 84, 103
Eosinophil count, 102–104
Eosinophilia, conditions associated with, 84, 103
Eosinophils, 77
in cerebrospinal fluid, 441
Epidemic typhus, 527t
Weil-Felix test and, 596
Epiglottitis, 509t
Epilepsy
carbamazepine and, 372
cerebrospinal fluid cell counts and, 439
congenital toxoplasmosis and, 606
ethosuximide and, 374
phenobarbital and, 374–375
phenytoin and, 376
primidone and, 377
valproic acid and, 378
Epinephrine, 296
blood glucose levels and, 158
free fatty acids and, 211
Thorn test and, 103
Epithelial cells, urinary, 40
Epstein-Barr virus, infectious mononucleosis and, 627–629
Erysipelas, 504t
Erythroblastosis fetalis, nucleated erythrocytes and, 88
Erythrocyte count, 70–72
in cerebrospinal fluid, 438–439
double oxalate mixture and, 152
Erythrocyte indices, 89–93
Erythrocyte osmotic fragility test, 98–100
heparin and, 153

Erythrocyte protoporphyrin, lead poisoning and, 400
Erythrocytes, 85–89
Erythrocyte sedimentation rate, 93–96
double oxalate mixture and, 152
Erythrocytosis, secondary, leukocyte alkaline phosphatase stain and, 106
Erythromycin
activities of, 529
theophylline therapy and, 407
Erythropoiesis, 70
Erythropoietin, 70
Escherichia coli gastroenteritis, 517t
Esophageal varices, blood ammonia and, 220
ESR; see Erythrocyte sedimentation rate
Estradiol, 331
follicle-stimulating hormone and, 321
levels of, variations in, conditions associated with, 334
Estriol, 331
levels of, variations in, conditions associated with, 334
Estrogen fractions
determinations of, 334–335
normal values for, 332–333
Estrogens, 331–335
follicle-stimulating hormone and, 321
luteinizing hormone and, 324
Estrone, 331
Ethacrynic acid, urinary casts and, 40
Ethanol, 360–363
phenytoin metabolism and, 376
Ethanol gelation test, 571
Ethanol intoxication
blood concentrations producing, 362
signs and symptoms of, 361
Ethchlorvynol, 416–418
characteristics of, 416t
Ethosuximide, 373–374
Ethyl alcohol; see Ethanol
Ethylenediaminetetraacetate; see EDTA
Euglobulin lysis time, 570–571
Extracellular fluid reservoir, 248

Extrinsic pathway, 534
Eye
    cultures of, 499
    diseases associated with,
        498t
    microbiologic examination
        of, 497–499
    normal flora of, 499
    pathogens of, 499
Fasting blood glucose,
    159–161
Fasting volume, conditions as-
    sociated with, 461
Fatty casts, conditions associ-
    ated with, 41
FDP; see Fibrin degradation
    products
Febrile agglutinins, serologic
    tests for, 593–599
Febrile transfusion reactions,
    665–666
    signs and symptoms of, 666
Fecal analysis, 449–458; see
    also Feces
    physical examination in,
        450–452
    specimen collection and
        handling in, 449–450
Fecal fat analysis, 452–454
Fecal occult blood, 454–456
Feces
    microbiologic examination
        of, 514–520
    pathogenic organisms
        and, 518
Ferric chloride screening, 59
Ferritin, serum, 137–139
Fetal death, pregnanediol
    and, 340
Fetal distress, amniotic fluid
    analysis and, 424
Fetal growth retardation,
    rubella and, 629
Fetal hemoglobin, 115
Fetal hemolytic disease, am-
    niotic fluid bilirubin
    and, 430
Fetal maturity
    amniotic fluid bilirubin
        and, 429
    amniotic fluid creatinine
        and, 431
Fetoplacental function, estriol
    and, 331
alpha-Fetoprotein, 242–243
Fever; see also Rheumatic fever
    excessive fluid loss and, 248
Fever of unknown origin, feb-
    rile agglutination tests
    and, 593–594

Fibrin degradation products,
    536
Fibrin stabilizing factor, 542
Fibrinase; see Fibrin stabilizing
    factor
Fibrin-fibrinogen degradation
    products, 568–570
Fibrinogen, 537
    clot formation and, 536
Fibrinogen assay, 567–568
Fibrinolysis, 536
    euglobulin lysis time
        and, 570
    Hageman factor and, 542
    hemostasis and, 533–534
    paracoagulation studies
        and, 571
    plasminogen and, 572
Fibrinolytic system, 536
Fibrous thyroiditis, thyroid
    antibodies and, 593
Fletcher factor, 538, 542–543
Fluid and electrolyte balance,
    248–277
    aldosterone and, 295
    clinical significance of, 252t
Fluid and electrolyte imbalance
    osmolality determinations
        and, 275
    urinalysis and, 13
    urine concentration test
        and, 52
Fluorescent treponemal anti-
    body absorption test,
    618–619
Flurazepam, 414
    characteristics of, 416t
Foam stability test, 432
Folate, 127–128
    hematopoiesis and, 127
    phenytoin metabolism
        and, 376
Folic acid, 127–128
Folic acid deficiency, mean
    corpuscular volume
    and, 90
Follicle-stimulating hormone,
    321–323
    functions of, 319
Follitropin; see Follicle-
    stimulating hormone
Formaldehyde, urine preser-
    vation and, 7
Formalin 40%, urine preserva-
    tion and, 7
Francisella antigens, normal
    values for, 599
Free fatty acids, 211–213
Free thyroxine index,
    352–353

Fresh-frozen plasma, 660
Frozen red blood cells, 654
    administration of, indications
        for, 655
Fructosuria, 19
FSF; see Fibrin stabilizing
    factor
FSH; see Follicle-stimulating
    hormone
FTA-ABS; see Fluorescent
    treponemal antibody ab-
    sorption test
FTI; see Free thyroxine index
Fungal infections, serologic
    tests for, 599–601
Fungi
    antibiotics active against,
        529
    cultures of, 488
    specimens of, 485–486
Furosemide, urinary casts
    and, 40
Galactorrhea, 327
Galactosuria, 19
Gamma-glutamyl transferase,
    198–200
Gangrene, 526t
Gas gangrene, anaerobic orga-
    nisms and, 488
Gastric acidity, 462–464
Gastric analysis, 458–464
    gastric acidity in, 462–464
    physical examination in,
        460–462
    specimen collection and
        handling in, 458–460
Gastric resection, intravenous
    glucose tolerance test
    and, 163
Gastritis, atrophic, gastric acid
    secretion and, 462
Gastroenteritis, 516t, 517t
Gastrointestinal system,
    diseases associated
    with, 516t
Gastrointestinal tract
    bleeding in, fecal analysis
        and, 449
    hemorrhage of
        basophilic stippling and, 89
        heparin and, 574
    malignancy of, fecal occult
        blood and, 455
    normal flora of, 515
    obstruction of, fecal analysis
        and, 449
Genetic defects, amniotic fluid
    analysis and, 424
Genital herpes, 503t

Genitourinary system, diseases associated with, 502t
Genitourinary tract
infection of, catheterization and, 4
inflammation of, urinalysis and, 13
normal flora of, 500
pathogens of, 500–501
secretions of, microbiologic examination of, 500–501
specimens of, 501
Gentamicin
activities of, 529
characteristics of, 366t
nephrotoxicity of, 366
therapeutic and toxic concentrations of, 367
urinary casts and, 40
German measles, 505t
GFR; see Glomerular filtration rate
GGT; see Gamma-glutamyl transferase
GH; see Growth hormone
Giardiasis, 517t
Glass contact factor; see Hageman factor
Globulin, 231, 238
serum, 234
total, 232
alpha-Globulin, 238
levels of, variations in, conditions associated with, 239
beta-Globulin, 238
levels of
in cerebrospinal fluid, 447
variations in, conditions associated with, 239–240
gamma-Globulin, 238
levels of
in cerebrospinal fluid, 447
variations in, conditions associated with, 241
Glomerular filtration, 2
Glomerular filtration rate, creatinine clearance and, 50
Glomerulonephritis, 502t
anti-DNase B and, 612
antinuclear antibodies and, 586
antistreptolysin O titer and, 609
complement and, 584
upper respiratory tract cultures and, 507
Glucagon, blood glucose levels and, 158

Glucocorticoid metabolism, 17-ketogenic steroids and, 306
Glucose
blood, 159–163
cerebrospinal fluid, 442–443
pleural fluid, 467
synovial fluid, 477–478
urinary, 18–20
Glucose-6-phosphate dehydrogenase, normal values for, 108
Glucose-6-phosphate dehydrogenase deficiency
clinical significance of, 108
Heinz bodies and, 89
test for, 108–109
Glucose tolerance curves, 165f
Glucose tolerance test, 163–168
cortisone, 164
interpretation of, 165–166
intravenous, 163–164
oral, 163
Glutethimide, 416–417
abuse of, 418
acute intermittent porphyria and, 45
characteristics of, 416t
determinations of, 418
ethanol and, 361
prothrombin time and, 561
therapeutic and toxic levels of, 417
Glycohemoglobin, 168–169
Glycosuria, 18–19
screening for, 19–20
Goiter, thyroid antibodies and, 593
Gonadal dysfunction, estradiol and, 331
Gonadotropins, functions of, 319
Gonococcemia, differential diagnosis of, 490
Gonorrhea, 502t
clinical diagnosis of, 500
Gonorrheal ophthalmia, neonatal, 498t
Gout, C-reactive protein and, 613
Graft rejection, T-lymphocytes and, 579
Gram-negative bacteria, antibiotics active against, 529
Gram-positive bacteria, antibiotics active against, 529
Gram's stain, 487
Granular casts, conditions associated with, 41

Granulocyte concentrate, 656–657
Granulocytes, bone marrow, conditions associated with, 118
Granuloma inguinale, 503t
Graves' disease
T-lymphocytes and, 580
thyroid antibodies and, 593
Griseofulvin
activities of, 529
acute intermittent porphyria and, 45
prothrombin time and, 561
urinary casts and, 40
Growth deficit, thyroxine deficiency and, 348
Growth hormone, 323–324
blood glucose levels and, 158
free fatty acids and, 211
functions of, 319
Guanethidine
ethanol and, 361
tricylic antidepressants and, 413
Gynecologic infection, anaerobic organisms in, 488
Hageman factor, 542
Hair
microbiologic examination of, 501–506
pathogens on, 506
specimens of, 506
Half-life, 359
Hallucinogens
abuse of, 418
intoxication with, signs and symptoms of, 419
Haptoglobin, 141–143, 238
Hashimoto's disease
antinuclear antibodies and, 586
thyroid antibodies and, 593
Hashish, abuse of, 418
HBDH; see Hydroxybutyric dehydrogenase
HCG; see Human chorionic gonadotropin
HDLs; see High-density lipoproteins
Heart disease
alanine aminotransferase elevations in, 194t
aspartate aminotransferase elevations in, 194t
cholesterol levels and, 202
congestive, nucleated erythrocytes and, 88
coronary, lipoprotein distribution and, 207

Heart failure, congestive
aspartate aminotransferase
levels and, 195
pleural transudates and, 464
theophylline therapy
and, 407
Heavy metals, 397–404
intoxication with, acquired
porphyria hepatica
and, 47
Heavy-chain disease, monoclonal gammopathies
and, 235
Heinz bodies, 89
Hemagglutination, antigen-
antibody reactions and,
579
Hemarthrosis, 474
Hematocrit, 68–70
double oxalate mixture
and, 152
Hematopoiesis
copper and, 217
folates and, 127
folic acid and, 127
vitamin B_{12} and, 125
Hematuria, 26
clinical significance of, 38
conditions associated with,
38–39
renal calculi and, 55
screening for, 27–28
Heme, hemopexin and, 238
Hemochromatosis, siderotic
granules and, 89
Hemodialysis, methanol intoxication and, 365
Hemoglobin
abnormal, 110–112
breakdown of, 29f, 124f
tests of, 139–149
carbon monoxide saturation
of, 392t
concentrations of, clinical
significance of, 66–67
copper and, 217
derivatives of, 391–397
determinations of, 66–68
electrophoresis of, 109–113
fetal, 115
hemopexin and, 238
levels of, 67–68
metabolism of, tests of, 120
normal values for, 110
plasma, 139–141
synthesis of, 124f
tests of, 125–139
urinary, 26–28
Hemoglobin C, 112

Hemoglobin C disease, target
cells and, 87
Hemoglobin D, 112
Hemoglobin E, 112
Hemoglobin H, 112
Hemoglobin S, 110–112
Hemoglobinemia, 26, 140
Hemoglobin-haptoglobin
complex, metabolism
of, 125
Hemoglobinopathies
fetal hemoglobin and, 115
Heinz bodies and, 89
hemoglobin electrophoresis
and, 109
microcytosis and, 86
schistocytes and, 87
Hemoglobinuria, 26–28
conditions associated
with, 27
screening for, 27–28
Hemolytic anemia
acanthocytosis and, 87
autoimmune
complement and, 584
direct antiglobulin test
and, 643
glucose-6-phosphate de-
hydrogenase deficiency
and, 108
Heinz bodies and, 89
hemolytic jaundice and, 144
Howell-Jolly bodies and, 89
schistocytes and, 87
total iron-binding capacity
and, 134
urinary urobilinogen and,
31
Hemolytic disease of newborn
amniotic fluid analysis and,
424
direct antiglobulin test and,
643
Hemolytic jaundice; see Jaundice, hemolytic
Hemolytic transfusion reactions, acute, 663–664
Hemopexin, 125, 238
Hemophilia
bleeding time and, 545
classification of, 540
differential diagnosis of, 560
Hemophilia A
cryoprecipitated antihemophilic factor and, 659
whole blood transfusion
and, 652
Hemophilic factor B; see
Plasma thromboplastin
component

Hemophilic factor C; see
Plasma thromboplastin
antecedent
Hemophilus influenzae meningitis, 494t
Hemostasis, 533–534
Hemothorax, pleural fluid aspiration and, 464
Heparin, 573–574
acanthocytosis and, 87
antithrombin III and,
565–566
hematologic testing and, 65,
153
therapeutic monitoring of,
574
Hepatic coma, blood ammonia
and, 220
Hepatic insufficiency
bacteremia and, 490
coumarin therapy and, 575
Hepatic jaundice; see Jaundice,
hepatic
Hepatic porphyrias, types of,
45–47
Hepatitis
alanine aminotransferase
levels and, 197
aspartate aminotransferase
levels and, 194
autoimmune immuno-
globulins and, 589
blood transfusion and, 668
cholesterol levels and, 202
chronic active, autoimmune
immunoglobulins and,
589
complement and, 584
hyperammonemia and, 220
lactic dehydrogenase activity
and, 190
lupoid, autoimmune immu-
noglobulins and, 590
polyclonal gammopathies
and, 235
target cells and, 87
viral
atypical lymphocytes
and, 79
autoimmune immuno-
globuins and, 590
normal values for,
624–625
polyclonal gammopathies
and, 235
serologic test for, 624–625
Hepatitis A, 517t, 621–622
Hepatitis A antibody, 623
Hepatitis B, 493t, 621–622

Hepatitis B core antigen antibody, 623
Hepatitis B "e" antigen, 624
Hepatitis B "e" antigen antibody, 624
Hepatitis B surface antigen, 623
Hepatitis B surface antigen antibody, 623
Hepatobiliary obstruction, 5'-nucleotidase and, 200
Hepatocellular carcinoma, alpha-fetoprotein levels and, 242
Hepatocellular dysfunction, alpha-fetoprotein levels and, 242
Hepatomegaly, differential diagnosis of, 213, 242
Heroin, abuse of, 418
Herpes, increased IgM levels at birth and, 235
Herpes antibodies, 626
Herpes simplex, 505t
Herpes simplex virus
  normal values for, 626
  serologic tests for, 625–627
Herpetic keratitis, 498t
Heterophil antibody test
  false-positive, conditions associated with, 628–629
  infectious mononucleosis and, 627–629
  methodology of, 629
High-density lipoproteins, 207
Hirsutism, female, testosterone and, 343
Histoplasmosis, 510t, 600–601
  serologic values for, 601
HLA antigens
  diseases associated with, 641t
  platelet transfusion and, 657–658
HLA system, 640
Hodgkin's disease, T-lymphocytes and, 580
Homogentisic acid
  ascorbic acid and, 214
  clinical significance of, 58
  screening for, nursing responsibilities in, 58
Hormone balance, blood glucose levels and, 158
Hormones; see specific type
Howell-Jolly bodies, 89
HPL; see Human placental lactogen

HSV; see Herpes simplex virus
Human chorionic gonadotropin, 335–338
Human placental lactogen, 338–339
Hyaline casts, conditions associated with, 41
Hydatidosis, 510t
Hydrocephaly, congenital toxoplasmosis and, 606
Hydrocortisone; see also Cortisol
  blood glucose levels and, 158
Hydronephritis, urine concentration test and, 52
Hydronephrosis, renal calculi and, 55
Hydroxybutyric dehydrogenase, 192–193
25-Hydroxycholecalciferol, 318–319
17-Hydroxycorticosteroids, 303–305
5-Hydroxyindoleacetic acid, urinary, 313–314
Hyperalbuminemia, conditions associated with, 233
Hyperaldosteronism, differential diagnosis of, 316
Hyperammonemia, 220
Hyperbilirubinemia, conditions associated with, 146
Hypercalcemia, 265
  calcitonin and, 312
  conditions associated with, 266
  differential diagnosis of, 314
  vitamin A and, 216
Hypercalcemic crisis, calcium excess and, 265
Hypercalciuria, conditions associated with, 48, 56
Hyperchloremia, 263
  conditions associated with, 263–264
Hyperchloremic metabolic acidosis, classification of, 274–275
Hyperchlorhydria, conditions associated with, 464
Hypercholesterolemia, conditions associated with, 203
Hyperchromic cells, 88
Hypercupremia, conditions associated with, 217
Hyperfibrinogenemia, paracoagulation studies and, 571

Hyperfibrinolysis, euglobulin lysis time and, 570
Hyperglobulinemia, conditions associated with, 234
Hyperglycemia
  conditions associated with, 159–160
  pleural fluid glucose and, 467
Hyperkalemia, 257
  conditions associated with, 258
Hyperlipemia, 209
  coumarin therapy and, 575
Hyperlipoproteinemia
  lipid changes in, 208t
  lipoprotein electrophoresis and, 201–202, 207
  secondary, conditions associated with, 209–210
Hypermagnesemia, 270
  conditions associated with, 271
Hypernatremia, 251
  aldosteronism and, 297
  conditions associated with, 251–255
Hyperparathyroidism, parathyroid hormone and, 314
Hyperphosphatemia, 268
  conditions associated with, 269
Hyperprolactinemia, 327
Hyperproteinemia, conditions associated with, 232
Hypersensitivity, delayed, T-lymphocytes and, 579
Hypersensitivity states, antinuclear antibodies and, 586
Hypersensitivity transfusion reactions, 666–667
Hypertension
  aldosteronism and, 297
  propranolol and, 389
Hyperthyroidism
  differential diagnosis of, 329
  thyroxine and, 347
  triiodothyronine and, 346
Hyperuricemia, conditions associated with, 228–229
Hyperventilation
  hyperammonemia and, 220
  plasma carbon dioxide and, 261
Hypervitaminosis A, conditions associated with, 216

Hypnotics, acquired porphyria hepatica and, 47
Hypoalbuminemia, conditions associated with, 233
Hypocalcemia, 265
conditions associated with, 267
parathyroid hormone and, 314
Hypocalciuria, conditions associated with, 48
Hypochloremia, 263
conditions associated with, 264
Hypochlorhydria, conditions associated with, 464
Hypocholesterolemia, conditions associated with, 204
Hypochromic anemia, fecal occult blood and, 455
Hypochromic cells, 88
Hypocupremia, conditions associated with, 217
Hypofibrinogenemia
paracoagulation studies and, 571
plasminogen and, 572
Hypogammaglobulinemia, 235
Hypoglobulinemia, conditions associated with, 234
Hypoglycemia
conditions associated with, 160
growth hormone secretion and, 323
pleural fluid glucose and, 467
Hypokalemia, 257
aldosteronism and, 297
conditions associated with, 258–259
Hypokalemic, hypochloremic alkalosis, electrolyte panel for, 274
Hypomagnesemia, 270
conditions associated with, 271–272
Hyponatremia, 251
conditions associated with, 255–256
Hypoparathyroidism, parathyroid hormone and, 314
Hypophosphatemia, 268
conditions associated with, 269
Hypopituitarism
clinical symptoms of, 320

growth hormone and, 323
intravenous glucose tolerance test and, 163
Hypoplasia, thymic, T-lymphocytes and, 580
Hypoprolactinemia, 327
Hypoproteinemia
conditions associated with, 232–233
pleural transudates and, 464
Hypothyroidism
differential diagnosis of, 329
intravenous glucose tolerance test and, 163
lipid concentrations and, 201
lipoprotein electrophoresis and, 207
macrocytosis and, 86
thyroxine and, 347–348
Hypoxia
conditions associated with, 287
lactic dehydrogenase activity and, 189
Hypoxyapatite crystals, conditions associated with, 477
Icotest tablets, bilirubinuria screening and, 30
ICSH; see Interstitial cell-stimulating hormone
IgA, 235, 580–581
IgD, 235, 581
IgE, 235, 581
IgG, 235, 580
in cerebrospinal fluid, 445, 447
IgG/albumin index, cerebrospinal fluid and, 445
IgM, 235, 581
FTA-ABS, 618
IM; see Mononucleosis, infectious
Imipramine, 412–413
characteristics of, 409t
therapeutic and toxic levels of, 414
Immunodeficiency disease, T- and B-lymphocytes and, 580
Immunodiffusion, antigen-antibody reactions and, 579
Immunoelectrophoresis, 235, 237–241
antigen-antibody reactions and, 579
Immunoglobulins, 235–237, 580–581

Immunohematology, 634
Immunology, 579
Immunosuppression, opportunistic fungi and, 489
Impetigo, 504t
Impotency, testosterone and, 343
Inborn errors of metabolism, 58
Inclusion conjunctivitis, 498t
Indomethacin, prothrombin time and, 561
Infectious mononucleosis; see Mononucleosis, infectious
Infertility, luteinizing hormone assay and, 325
Influenza, 510t
INH; see Isoniazid
Insulin
blood glucose levels and, 157–158
growth hormone and, 323
Interstitial cell-stimulating hormone, 325
Interstitial fluid, 248
Intracellular fluid reservoir, 248
Intracerebral hemorrhage, cerebrospinal fluid and, 438–439
Intracranial hemorrhage, heparin and, 574
Intravascular fluid, 248
volume of, renin secretion and, 316
Intravenous glucose tolerance test, 163–164
Intrinsic pathway, 535–536
Iron, 398–400
serum, 132–134
Iron deficiency anemia
anisocytosis and, 86
elliptocytosis and, 87
erythrocyte porphyrin concentrations and, 129
hypochromia and, 88
mean corpuscular volume and, 90
microcytosis and, 86
poikilocytosis and, 87
polychromatophilia and, 88
target cells and, 87
Iron overload
serum ferritin and, 137
total iron-binding capacity and, 134
Isoenzymes, 172–173
Isoniazid
activities of, 529

Isoniazid (*continued*)
ethanol and, 361
phenytoin metabolism
and, 376
urinary casts and, 40
Isopropanol, 363–364
Isopropyl alcohol; *see*
Isopropanol
Jaundice
bilirubinuria and, 29–30
differential diagnosis of,
29–31, 143–145, 144t,
213, 242
hemolytic, 144–145
bilirubinuria and, 29
hepatic, 144–145
bilirubinuria and, 29–30
cholesterol levels and, 202
obstructive, 144–145
bilirubinuria and, 29–30
cholesterol levels and, 202
fecal analysis and, 449
fecal urobilinogen and, 457
lactate dehydrogenase ac-
tivity and, 190
target cells and, 87
urinary urobilinogen
and, 31
Joint disease, classification of,
469–470
Joint effusions, conditions associated with, 476
Kallikrein, 534–535
Kanamycin
activities of, 529
characteristics of, 366t
nephrotoxicity of, 366
therapeutic and toxic concentrations of, 367
urinary casts and, 40
Kaolin, digoxin levels and, 383
Keratoconjunctivitis, epidemic,
498t
Ketoacidosis, diabetic,
glycohemoglobin test
and, 168
17-Ketogenic steroids,
305–307
Ketones, urinary, 24–26
Ketonuria, 24–25
17-Ketosteroids, 307–309
Kidney
acid-base balance and,
278–279
glomerular filtration in, 2
tubular reabsorption in, 2
tubular secretion in, 4
Kidney dialysis, blood urea ni-
trogen/creatinine ratio
and, 227

Kidney disease
creatinine clearance and, 50
excessive fluid loss and, 248
heparin and, 574
polycystic, urine concentration test and, 52
serum amylase and, 173
serum creatinine and, 225
tubular reabsorption and,
51–52
Kidney function tests, 49–57
Kidney stones; *see* Renal
calculi
Klebsiella pneumonia, 509t
Labile factor; *see* Proaccelerin
Lactate dehydrogenase, 189–
192, 238
Lactation
lactosuria and, 19
prolactin and, 326–327
Lactic acid, cerebrospinal
fluid, 443–444
Lactose tolerance test,
171–172
Lactosuria, 19
LDH; *see* Lactate
dehydrogenase
LDLs; *see* Low-density
lipoproteins
Lead, 400–402
Lead poisoning
basophilic stippling and,
88–89
Cabot rings and, 89
erythrocyte porphyrin concentrations and, 129
siderotic granules and, 89
signs and symptoms of, 400
Lecithin/sphingomyelin ratio,
432–434
Lee-White coagulation time;
see Whole blood clotting
time
Legionnaires' disease, 509t
Leprosy, 494t
antinuclear antibodies
and, 586
polyclonal gammopathies
and, 235
Leptocytes, 87
Leptospirosis, 502t
Weil-Felix test and, 597
Leucinuria, 43
Leukemia
acute lymphocytic, metho-
trexate therapy and, 405
anisocytosis and, 86
basophilic stippling and, 89
cerebrospinal fluid analysis
and, 434

chronic granulocytic, leukocyte alkaline phosphatase
stain and, 106
granulocytic, immature neutrophils and, 79
Howell-Jolly bodies and, 89
hypochromia and, 88
lymphocytic, 580
methotrexate therapy
and, 405
nucleated erythrocytes
and, 88
plasma cell, monoclonal
gammopathies and, 235
Leukemoid reactions
immature neutrophils
and, 79
leukocyte alkaline phos-
phatase stain and, 106
Leukocyte alkaline phos-
phatase stain, 106–107
Leukocyte count, 73–75; *see
also* Differential white
blood cell count
in cerebrospinal fluid,
438–440
Leukocyte-poor red blood
cells, 654
administration of, indications
for, 655
Leukocytes
immature, 77–79
types of, 76f
LH; *see* Luteinizing hormone
Lidocaine, 385–386
Lincomycin, activities of, 529
Lipase, serum, 176–177
Lipemia, 209
Lipids, tests of, 201–213
Lipoprotein electrophoresis,
201–202
hyperlipemia and, 207–209
alpha-Lipoprotein, 238
beta-Lipoprotein, 238
beta-Lipoproteinemia, acanthocytosis and, 87
Lipoproteins, 201, 207–211
Lipuria, 13
Listeriosis, 493t
cerebrospinal fluid pathogens and, 495
Lithium, 409–411
characteristics of, 409t
Liver
abscess of, anaerobic organisms and, 488
carcinoma of, alpha-fetoprotein levels and, 242

disease of
  alanine aminotransferase
    elevations in, 194t
  aminoaciduria of, 58
  aspartate aminotransferase
    elevations in, 194t
  blood ammonia and, 220
  gamma-glutamyl trans-
    ferase and, 199
  heparin and, 574
  hypersegmented neu-
    trophils and, 79
  immunoelectrophoresis
    and, 238
  macrocytosis and, 86
  5′-nucleotidase and, 200
  polyclonal gammopathies
    and, 235−236
  serum bilirubin and, 143
  toxic neutrophilic granula-
    tion and, 79
  urine concentration test
    and, 52
  dysfunction of, theophylline
    therapy and, 407
Liver function tests, 213−214,
    214t
Low-density lipoproteins, 207
LSD; see Lysergic acid
  diethylamine
L/S ratio; see Lecithin/sphin-
  gomyelin ratio
Lung
  abscess of
    anaerobic organisms
      and, 488
    bacteremia and, 489
  carcinoma of, calcitonin
    and, 312
Lupus erythematosus; see
  also Systemic lupus
  erythematosus
  polyclonal gammopathies
    and, 236
Lupus erythematosus cells,
  conditions associated
  with, 105
Lupus erythematosus cell test,
  104−106
  clinical significance of,
    104−105
  heparin and, 153
  methodology of, 105
  normal values for, 105
  nursing responsibilities in,
    106
  precautions in, 105
Lupus erythematosus plasma
  factor, 104

Lupus erythematosus rosettes,
    105
Luteinizing hormone,
    324−326
Lutropin; see Luteinizing
  hormone
LVG; see Lymphogranuloma
  venereum
Lymphatic system, diseases associated with, 492
Lymphocytes, 76−77
  atypical, 79
  in cerebrospinal fluid, 441
Lymphocytosis, conditions associated with, 82−83
Lymphogranuloma venereum,
    503t
  polyclonal gammopathies
    and, 235
Lymphoma
  B-lymphocytes and, 580
  methotrexate therapy and,
    405
  monoclonal gammopathies
    and, 235
  T-lymphocytes and, 580
Lymphopenia, 80
  conditions associated
    with, 83
Lymphoproliferative disorders,
  opportunistic fungi and,
  489
Lymphoproliferative malignancy, B-lymphocytes
  and, 580
Lysergic acid diethylamine,
  abuse of, 418
Macrocytes, 86
Macrocytic, normochromic
  anemia, conditions associated with, 92
Macrocytosis, 86
Macroglobulin, 235, 238
Macroglobulinemia, immu-
  noelectrophoresis
  and, 238
Maduromycosis, 505t
Magnesium, 270−272
Malabsorption syndrome
  fecal trypsin and, 456
  glucose tolerance test
    and, 163
Malaria, 527t
  blood transfusion and,
    668−669
  complement and, 584
  reactive lymphocytes
    and, 79

serologic values for, 608
tests for, 607
Manic-depressive disorders,
  lithium and, 409
MAO; see Maximal acid
  output
Maple syrup urine disease, 58
Marijuana, abuse of, 418
Maximal acid output, 459,
    462
  normal values for, 463
MCH; see Mean corpuscular
  hemoglobin
MCHC; see Mean corpus-
  cular hemoglobin
  concentration
MCV; see Mean corpuscular
  volume
Mean corpuscular hemo-
  globin, 90
  calculation of, 93
Mean corpuscular hemoglobin
  concentration, 90
  calculation of, 93
Mean corpuscular value,
  double oxalate mixture
  and, 152
Mean corpuscular volume, 90
  calculation of, 92
Measles, 505t
Medicolegal specimens, collection and handling of, 357
  nursing responsibilities in,
    357−358
Medullary thyroid tumors,
  calcitonin and, 312
Megakaryocytes, bone mar-
  row, conditions associ-
  ated with, 119
Megaloblastic anemia
  folate deficiency and, 127
  Howell-Jolly bodies and, 89
  hypersegmented neutrophils
    and, 79
  lactic dehydrogenase activity
    and, 189
  mean corpuscular volume
    and, 90
  nucleated erythrocytes
    and, 88
  poikilocytosis and, 87
  primidone and, 377
  vitamin B_{12} deficiency and,
    125
Megaloblastosis
  differential diagnosis of, 127
  folate deficiency and, 127
Melena, 454

Meningitis, 494t
anaerobic organisms and, 488
bacterial
cerebrospinal fluid cultures and, 495
cerebrospinal fluid glucose and, 442
cerebrospinal fluid lactic acid and, 444
pleocytosis and, 439
bacteremia and, 489
causative organisms in, 495
cerebrospinal fluid analysis and, 434, 439
cerebrospinal fluid culture and, 491–495
differential diagnosis of, 490, 613
fungal, cerebrospinal fluid lactic acid and, 444
IgG/albumin index and, 445
meningococcal, 494t
otogenic, anaerobic organisms and, 488
pleocytosis and, 439
tuberculous
cerebrospinal fluid clarity and, 438
cerebrospinal fluid glucose and, 442
cerebrospinal fluid lactic acid and, 444
cerebrospinal fluid specimen collection and, 435
pleocytosis and, 439
viral
cerebrospinal fluid glucose and, 442
cerebrospinal fluid lactic acid and, 444
Menstruation
acute intermittent porphyria and, 45
iron deficiency and, 132
pregnanediol excretion and, 339
Mental retardation
congenital toxoplasmosis and, 606
galactosuria and, 19
thyroxine deficiency and, 348
Meperidine
abuse of, 418
phenothiazines and, 412
Mephenytoin, reactive lymphocytes and, 79
Meprobamate, 416–418

acute intermittent porphyria and, 45
characteristics of, 416t
ethanol and, 361
therapeutic and toxic levels of, 417
Mercury, 402–404
Mescaline, abuse of, 418
Metabolic acidosis
differential diagnosis of, 273
hyperchloremic, classification of, 274–275
signs and symptoms of, 291–292
Metabolic alkalosis
differential diagnosis of, 273
signs and symptoms of, 292
Metabolic bone disease, alkaline phosphatase activity and, 180
Metabolic factor, 278
Metanephrine, 310–311
catecholamine metabolism and, 298
Methadone, abuse of, 418
Methamphetamine hydrochloride, 367
Methanol, 364–365
Methaqualone, 416–418
abuse of, 418
characteristics of, 416t
Methemoglobin, 394–395
in cerebrospinal fluid, 438
Methemoglobinemia, 394–395
Methicillin, activities of, 529
Methotrexate, 405–407
Methyl alcohol; see Methanol
Methyldopa
acute intermittent porphyria and, 45
tricylic antidepressants and, 413
Methylphenidate, tricyclic antidepressants and, 413
Methyprylon
acute intermittent porphyria and, 45
therapeutic and toxic levels of, 417
Metyrapone, phenytoin and, 376
Mexican hat cells, 87
MIC; see Minimum inhibitory concentration
Microbiology
specimen collection and handling in, 482–486

specimens for examination in, 489–528
stained smear examination in, 486–489
Microcephaly, congenital toxoplasmosis and, 606
Microcytes, 86
Microcytosis, 86
Minimum inhibitory concentration, 529
Monoclonal gammopathies, 235
immunoelectrophoresis and, 238
Monocytes, 77
Monocytosis, conditions associated with, 83–84
Mononucleosis, infectious, 493t
antinuclear antibodies and, 586
atypical lymphocytes and, 79
autoimmune immunoglobulins and, 590
latent cytomegalovirus and, 620
normal values for, 628
polyclonal gammopathies and, 236
serologic tests for, 627–629
Monosodium urate crystals, 476
Morphine
abuse of, 418
phenothiazines and, 412
Morphine addiction, pentosuria and, 19
Morphine derivatives, barbiturates and, 380
Mouth, diseases associated with, 516t
Mucin clot formation, in synovial fluid, 474–475
Mucous strands, urinary, 43
Mucus, gastric, 461
Multiple myeloma
B-lymphocytes and, 580
monoclonal gammopathies and, 235
nucleated erythrocytes and, 88
Multiple sclerosis
cerebrospinal fluid analysis and, 434, 439
cerebrospinal fluid protein electrophoresis and, 445
myelin basic protein and, 445

N-Multistix
  bilirubinuria screening
    and, 30
  ketonuria screening and, 25
  urinary occult blood screen-
    ing and, 28
  urinary protein screening
    and, 23
  urinary sugar screening and,
    19
  urinary urobilinogen screen-
    ing and, 32
Mumps, 517t
  atypical lymphocytes
    and, 79
Murine typhus, Weil-Felix test
  and, 596
Muscular dystrophy, Duch-
  enne's, creatine phos-
  phokinase levels in, 185
Myasthenia gravis, antinuclear
  antibodies and, 586
Mycology, 481
Mycoplasmal antibodies,
  603–604
Mycoplasmal pneumonia,
  509t
  serologic tests for, 602–603
Mycotic infections, specimens
  in, 485–486
Myelofibrosis
  Cabot rings and, 89
  nucleated erythrocytes
    and, 88
  poikilocytosis and, 87
Myeloid-erythroid ratio, 118
  variations in, conditions as-
    sociated with, 118–119
Myeloma, immunoelectro-
  phoresis and, 238
Myocardial infarction
  alanine aminotransferase
    levels and, 197
  aspartate aminotransferase
    levels and, 195
  cholesterol levels and, 202
  C-reactive protein and, 613
  creatine phosphokinase ac-
    tivity in, 185–186
  erythrocyte sedimentation
    rate and, 93
  gamma-glutamyl transferase
    activity and, 199
  hydroxybutyric dehydro-
    genase levels and, 193
  lactic dehydrogenase activity
    and, 190
  lidocaine and, 385

reactive lymphocytes and,
  79
  serum enzyme activity after,
    190t
Myocarditis, 493t
Myoglobinuria, 26
  conditions associated
    with, 27
Nails
  microbiologic examination
    of, 501–506
  pathogens on, 506
NAPA; see n-Acetylpro-
  cainamide
Narcotic analgesics, abuse of,
  418
Narcotic intoxication, signs
  and symptoms of, 419
Nasopharyngeal cultures, 507
Nasopharynx
  microbiologic examination
    of, 506–512
  normal flora of, 507
  pathogens of, 511
Needle and syringe aspiration,
  485
Neomycin
  activities of, 529
  digoxin levels and, 383
  urinary casts and, 40
Neoplasms
  monoclonal gammopathies
    and, 235
  pleural exudates and, 464
Nephrons, 2, 3f
Nephropathies, bacteremia
  and, 489
Nephrotic syndrome
  excessive fluid accumulation
    and, 248
  lipid concentrations and, 201
  lipoprotein electrophoresis
    and, 207
Nervous system, diseases associated with, 494
Neural tube defects, alpha-
  fetoprotein levels and, 242
Neuroblastoma
  catecholamine secretion
    and, 299
  metanephrine excretion
    and, 310
  vanillylmandelic acid excre-
    tion and, 310
Neurohypophysis, hormones
  of, 319
Neuroleptics, tricylic antidepressants and, 413

Neurosyphilis, pleocytosis
  and, 439
Neutropenia
  conditions associated
    with, 82
  granulocyte transfusion
    and, 656
Neutrophilia, 80
  conditions associated with,
    81–82
Neutrophilic leukemoid reactions, immature neu-
  trophils and, 79
Neutrophils, 75–76
  in cerebrospinal fluid,
    440–441
NGU; see Urethritis,
  nongonococcal
Nicotinic acid
  primary hyperlipemia and,
    209
  primary lipemia and, 209
Nitrates
  methemoglobin and,
    394–395
  sulfhemoglobinemia
    and, 396
Nitrites
  methemoglobin and,
    394–395
  sulfhemoglobinemia
    and, 396
  urinary, 33–37
Nitrofurantoin, activities
  of, 529
Nitrogen, urea, 222–223
Nitroglycerine, methemo-
  globin and, 394
Nonprotein nitrogen com-
  pounds, 219–230
Nontoxic goiter, thyroid antibodies and, 593
Nontreponemal antibody tests,
  615–618
Norepinephrine, 296
  ascorbic acid and, 214
Normoblasts, 88
  bone marrow, conditions as-
    sociated with, 119
Normochromic cells, 85
Normocytes, 85
Normocytic, normochromic
  anemia, 91
Nortriptyline, 412–413
  characteristics of, 409t
  therapeutic and toxic levels
    of, 413–414
Novobiocin, activities of, 529

NPN compounds; *see* Nonprotein nitrogen compounds
Nucleated red blood cells, 88
5′-Nucleotidase, 200–201
Nystatin, activities of, 529
Obstructive biliary disease, 5′-nucleotidase and, 200
Obstructive jaundice; *see* Jaundice, obstructive
Occult blood
  fecal, 454–456
  urinary, 26–28
Oleandomycin, activities of, 529
Oligoclonal bands, 445
  conditions associated with, 447
Oliguria, 8
  conditions associated with, differentiation of, 14
Ophthalmia, neonatal gonorrheal, 498t
Opiates, abuse of, 418
Oral glucose tolerance test, 163
Ornithosis, 509t
Osmolality, 275–277
Osteogenic sarcoma, methotrexate therapy and, 405
Osteomyelitis, bacteremia and, 489
Otitis externa, 504t
Otitis media, 508t
Ovalocytes, 87
Ovaries, hormones of, 330
Ovulation
  pregnanediol and, 330, 339
  progesterone and, 341
Oxalates, hematologic testing and, 65, 152
Oxalosis, conditions associated with, 56
Oxycodone, abuse of, 418
Oxygen, partial pressure of, 287–288
Oxygen saturation, 288–289
Oxytocin, functions of, 319
Packed cell volume; *see* Hematocrit
Packed red blood cells, 654
  administration of, indications for, 655
Palsy, congenital toxoplasmosis and, 606
Pancreatic disease
  serum amylase and, 173
  serum lipase and, 176
Pancreatic insufficiency, fecal trypsin and, 456

Pancreatitis
  serum amylase and, 173
  serum lipase and, 176
PAO; *see* Peak acid output
Para-aminosalicylic acid
  activities of, 529
  reactive lymphocytes and, 79
Paracoagulation tests, 571–572
Paragonimiasis, 510t
Parasites, urinary, 43
Parasitic infections, serologic tests for, 605–609
Parasitic infestations
  fecal analysis and, 449
  polyclonal gammopathies and, 235
Parasitology, 481
Parathormone; *see* Parathyroid hormone
Parathyrin; *see* Parathyroid hormone
Parathyroid hormone, 314–316
  calcitonin and, 312
  calcium metabolism and, 268
  phosphorus metabolism and, 268
  total calcium concentration and, 266
Paratyphoid fever, Widal test for, 594–596
Paroxysmal atrial tachycardia, phenytoin and, 376
Paroxysmal tachycardia, procainamide and, 387
Partial pressure of carbon dioxide, 285–286
Partial pressure of oxygen, 287–288
Partial thromboplastin time, 556–557
  antihemophilic factor deficiency and, 540
  fibrinogen deficiency and, 537
  Fletcher factor deficiency and, 543
  Hageman factor deficiency and, 542
  plasma thromboplastin antecedent deficiency and, 541
  plasma thromboplastin component deficiency and, 540–541
  proaccelerin deficiency and, 539

prothrombin deficiency and, 538
  Stuart-Prower factor deficiency and, 541
PAS; *see* Para-aminosalicylic acid
Pasteurellosis, 526t
Paul-Bunnell test, infectious mononucleosis and, 627–628
PCT; *see* Prothrombin consumption time
Peak acid output, 462
  normal values for, 463
Pectin, digoxin levels and, 383
Penicillin
  activities of, 529
  urinary casts and, 40
Penicillin G
  acquired porphyria hepatica and, 47
  activities of, 529
Pentobarbital, 379
Pentosuria, 19
Peptic ulcer disease, gastric acidity and, 462
Percent saturation, 134–137
Pericarditis, 492t, 493t
Periodontal disease, 516t
Peritonitis
  anaerobic organisms and, 488
  bacteremia and, 489
Pernicious anemia
  anisocytosis and, 86
  Cabot rings and, 89
  elliptocytosis and, 87
  hypersegmented neutrophils and, 79, 125
  macrocytosis and, 86
  polychromatophilia and, 88
  siderotic granules and, 89
  vitamin B12 deficiency and, 125
Peyote, abuse of, 418
pH, 283–285
  pleural fluid, 467–468
  urinary, 16–18
Phagocytosis, 76
  complement and, 581
Pharyngitis, C-reactive protein and, 613
Phenacetin
  Heinz bodies and, 89
  methemoglobin and, 394
  sulfhemoglobinemia and, 396
Phenistix, phenylketonuria screening and, 60

Phenmetrazine hydrochloride, 367
  therapeutic and toxic effects of, 368
Phenobarbital, 374–376
  characteristics of, 373t, 380t
  phenytoin and, 376
  therapeutic and toxic concentrations of, 375, 381
  tricylic antidepressants and, 413
Phenolsulfonphthalein test, 53–54
Phenothiazines, 411–412
  Heinz bodies and, 89
  narcotic drugs and, 419
Phenylbutazone
  digitoxin concentrations and, 383
  phenytoin metabolism and, 376
  prothrombin time and, 561
  reactive lymphocytes and, 79
Phenylpyruvic acid, 59–60
Phenytoin, 376–377
  acute intermittent porphyria and, 45
  characteristics of, 373t
  digitoxin concentrations and, 383
  digoxin levels and, 383
  ethanol and, 361
  reactive lymphocytes and, 79
  therapeutic and toxic concentrations of, 377
Pheochromocytoma
  catecholamine secretion and, 299
  metanephrine excretion and, 310
  vanillylmandelic acid excretion and, 310
Phosphate resorption, parathyroid hormone and, 314
Phospholipids, 211–213
  amniotic fluid, 433
Phosphorus, 268–270 metabolism of, parathyroid hormone and, 268
Pituitary hormones, 319–330
PKU; see Phenylketonuria
Placenta, hormones of, 330
Placental dysfunction
  estriol and, 331
  pregnanediol and, 340
Placenta previa, amniotic fluid analysis and, 424

Plague, 527t
Plasma cells, 76–77
  bone marrow, conditions associated with, 118–119
  immunoglobulins and, 235
Plasma clotting time; see Plasma recalcification time
Plasma coagulation factors; see Coagulation factors
Plasma infusion, 660–661
Plasma recalcification time, 557–558
Plasma specimens, 152
Plasma thromboplastin, 534, 536, 538
Plasma thromboplastin antecedent, 541
Plasma thromboplastin component, 540–541
Plasmacytosis, conditions associated with, 83
Plasminogen, 238, 536, 572–573
Plasminogen activators, euglobulin lysis time and, 570
Platelet adhesion, 551–552
Platelet adhesion studies, 550–552
Platelet aggregation, 550–556
  response in selected conditions, 551t
  thrombin and, 536
Platelet count, 100–102, 548–550
  EDTA and, 153
Platelet function
  drugs interfering with, 553t
  tests of, 544–553
Platelet preparations, 657–658
  contraindications for, 658
  indications for, 658
  side effects of, 658
Platelets, hemostasis and, 533
Pleocytosis, 439
  conditions associated with, 440–441
Pleural exudates, 464
Pleural fluid
  analysis of, 464–469
    microbiologic examination in, 469
    physical examination in, 465–466
    specimen collection and handling in, 465
  aspiration of, 464
  cell counts in, 466–467

glucose in, 467
pH of, 467–468
specific gravity of, 468
total protein in, 468
volume of, conditions associated with, 465–466
Pleural transudates, 464
Pneumonia, 509t
  bacteremia and, 489
  cerebrospinal fluid pathogens and, 495
  fungal, 510t
  mycoplasmal, 509t
    serologic tests for, 602–613
  nasopharyngeal cultures and, 507
  pleural exudates and, 464
  pneumococcal, 509t
    C-reactive protein and, 613
  Pneumocystis, 510t
  viral, 510t
    atypical lymphocytes and, 79
Pneumonitis, serologic tests for, 602–603
Poikilocytosis, 86–87
Poliomyelitis, 494t
  cerebrospinal fluid cell counts and, 439
  pleocytosis and, 439
Polychromatophilia, 88
Polyclonal gammopathies, 235–236
  immunoelectrophoresis and, 238
Polycystic kidney disease, urine concentration test and, 52
Polycythemia vera, leukocyte alkaline phosphatase stain and, 106
Polymyositis, antinuclear antibodies and, 587
Polymyxin B, activities of, 529
Polyuria, 7–8
  aldosteronism and, 297
Porphobilinogen, 44, 128–131
Porphyria cutanea tarda, 45
Porphyria erythropoietica, 45
Porphyrias, 44–47, 129
  acute intermittent, 45
  clinical and laboratory findings in, 46t
  hepatic, 45–47
Porphyrins, 44, 128–131
Porter-Silber chromogens; see 17-Hydroxycorticosteroids

Posthemorrhagic anemia, chronic, hypochromia and, 88
Potassium, 257–260
reabsorption of, renin-angiotensin-aldosterone system and, 316
Precipitation, antigen-antibody reactions and, 579
Preeclampsia, amniotic fluid analysis and, 424
Pregnancy
acute intermittent porphyria and, 45
C-reactive protein and, 613
human chorionic gonadotropin and, 335–336
iron deficiency and, 132
lactosuria and, 19
pregnanediol and, 339
prolactin and, 327
serial estriol measurements and, 331
urine concentration test and, 52
Pregnanediol, 339–341
ovulation and, 330
Prekallikrein, 534–535, 542–543
Primary hyperlipemia, 209
Primary lipemia, 209
Primidone, 377–378
characteristics of, 373t
PRL; see Prolactin
Proaccelerin, 539
Probucol, type II primary hyperlipemia and, 209
Procainamide, 387–389
tricylic antidepressants and, 413
Procaine
acquired porphyria hepatica and, 47
procainamide therapy and, 388
Prochlorperazine, 411
Procoagulants; see Coagulation factors
Proconvertin, 539
Progesterone, 341–342
luteinizing hormone and, 324
pregnanediol and, 339
Prolactin, 326–328
functions of, 319
Promazine hydrochloride, 411
Promethazine hydrochloride, 411
Propoxyphene, abuse of, 418

Propranolol, 389–390
Prostate gland
carcinoma of, serum acid phosphatase and, 178
normal flora of, 500
Prosthetic heart valves, schistocytes and, 87
Protamine sulfate test, 571
Protein
cerebrospinal fluid, 444–448
C-reactive, 612–614
disturbances in, diagnostically significant, 233t
myelin basic, 445–447
serum, 230–241
total, 231–234
urinary, 21–24
Proteinuria, 21–24
Proteus antigens
normal values for, 596
Weil-Felix test and, 596–597
Prothrombin, 538
Prothrombin consumption time, 558–560
antihemophilic factor deficiency and, 540
Hageman factor deficiency and, 542
plasma thromboplastin antecedent deficiency and, 541
plasma thromboplastin component deficiency and, 541
Stuart-Prower factor deficiency and, 541
Prothrombin time, 561–563
drugs affecting, 562t
fibrinogen deficiency and, 537
proaccelerin deficiency and, 539
proconvertin deficiency and, 539
prothrombin deficiency and, 538
Stuart-Prower factor deficiency and, 541
Protoporphyrin, 128–129
Protriptyline, 412
characteristics of, 409t
therapeutic and toxic levels of, 414
Pseudocholinesterase, 182–183
Pseudohypoparathyroidism, parathyroid hormone and, 314
Psilocybin, abuse of, 418

Psittacosis, 509t
Psoriasis, methotrexate therapy and, 405
Psychedelics, abuse of, 418
Psychomotor retardation, congenital toxoplasmosis and, 606
Psychotherapeutic agents, 409–414
characteristics of, 409t
PT; see Prothrombin time
PTA; see Plasma thromboplastin antecedent
PTC; see Plasma thromboplastin component
Pteroylglutamic acid; see Folic acid
PTH; see Parathyroid hormone
PTT; see Partial thromboplastin time
Puerperal sepsis, 492t
anaerobic organisms and, 488
Pulmonary infarction, pleural exudates and, 464
Purine metabolism, uric acid and, 228
Pyelonephritis, 502t
catheterization and, 4
pyuria and, 39
urine concentration test and, 52
Pyelonephrosis, renal calculi and, 55
Pyoderma, anti-DNase B and, 612
Pyridine, Heinz bodies and, 89
Pyruvate kinase deficiency
acanthocytosis and, 87
Burr cells and, 87
schistocytes and, 87
Pyuria, 13
bacterial infection and, 43
clinical significance of, 39
conditions associated with, 39
Q fever, 509t
Quantitative dilution tests, 530
Queensland tick fever, Weil-Felix test and, 596
Quinidine, 390–391
tricylic antidepressants and, 413
Quinine, abuse of, 418
Rabies, 494t
Radial immunodiffusion, 235
Radioallergosorbent test, 581
allergens detected by, 582t

Radiographic agents, urinary
   casts and, 40
Rapid plasma reagin, blood
   donor screening and, 669
RAST; *see* Radioallergosorbent
   test
Rat bite fever, 526t
Raynaud's syndrome, anti-
   nuclear antibodies and,
   587
RBC; *see* Erythrocyte count
Reagin, 615–616
Red blood cell casts, conditions
   associated with, 41
Red blood cell count; *see*
   Erythrocyte count
Red blood cells
   frozen, 654–655
   nucleated, 88
   urinary, 38–39
   washed, 655
Red blood cell therapy,
   653–656
   contraindications for, 655
   indications for, 655
   side effects of, 656
Refractometry, urine specific
   gravity and, 15
Refrigeration, urine preservation and, 6
Relapsing fever, 527t
Renal allograft rejection,
   creatinine clearance
   and, 50
Renal calculi, 55–57
   calcium oxalate, 56
   calcium phosphate, 56
   conditions associated with,
   55–57
   cystine, 56–57
   xanthine, 57
Renal disease; *see* Kidney
   disease
Renal epithelial casts, conditions associated with, 41
Renal failure, Burr cells
   and, 87
Renal function tests, 49–57
Renal insufficiency, creatinine
   clearance and, 50
Renin, 316–317
Renin-angiotensin-aldosterone
   system, 316
Renin-angiotensin system,
   aldosterone secretion
   and, 297
Reproductive hormones,
   330–344
Reptilase time test, 564

Reserpine, barbiturates and,
   380
Resorcinol, Heinz bodies
   and, 89
Respiratory acidosis, 289–291
Respiratory alkalosis
   hyperammonemia and, 220
   signs and symptoms of, 291
Respiratory arrest, hypo-
   kalemia and, 257
Respiratory factor, 278
Respiratory system, diseases
   associated with, 508t
Reticulocyte count, 96–98
Reticulocytes, 96
Reticulocytopenia, conditions
   associated with, 97
Reticulocytosis
   conditions associated
   with, 97
   macrocytosis and, 86
   mean corpuscular volume
   and, 90
Reticuloendothelial system,
   hemoglobin-haptoglobin
   complex and, 125
Retinitis pigmentosa, acanthocytosis and, 87
Retinochoroiditis, congenital
   toxoplasmosis and, 606
Reye's syndrome, hyperam-
   monemia and, 220
Rh blood types, inheritance
   of, 639
Rh genotypes, 638t
Rh phenotypes, 638t
Rh sensitivity, amniotic fluid
   bilirubin and, 429–430
Rh system, 637–640
Rh typing, 639–640
Rheumatic fever, 492t
   antistreptolysin O titer
   and, 609
   C-reactive protein and, 613
   complement and, 584
   erythrocyte sedimentation
   rate and, 93
   upper respiratory tract cultures and, 507
Rheumatoid arthritis
   antinuclear antibodies
   and, 586
   C-reactive protein and,
   613
   complement and, 584
   erythrocyte sedimentation
   rate and, 93
   polyclonal gammopathies
   and, 236

synovial fluid glucose
   and, 477
Rheumatoid disease, pleural
   exudates and, 464
Rheumatoid factor, 591–592
Rickettsial diseases, Weil-Felix
   test for, 596–597
Rickettsialpox
   reactive lymphocytes and, 79
   Weil-Felix test and, 597
Ringworm, 505t
Rocky Mountain spotted fever,
   527t
   Weil-Felix test and, 596–597
Routine crossmatch, 647–648
   antiglobulin phase of, 648
   protein phase of, 647
   thermo phase of, 648
RPR; *see* Rapid plasma reagin
Rubella, 505t
   atypical lymphocytes and, 79
   increased IgM levels at birth
   and, 235
   serologic tests for, 629–630
Rubella antibodies, 629–630
Rubeola, 505t
Russell's viper venom assay,
   563–564
Salicylates; *see also* Acetylsalicylic acid
   characteristics of, 369t
   prothrombin time and, 561
Salmonella antibodies, Widal
   test and, 594–596
Salmonella antigens, normal
   values for, 595
Salmonellosis, 516t
   cerebrospinal fluid pathogens and, 495
   differential diagnosis of, 490
   stool specimens and,
   514–515
Sarcoidosis
   methotrexate therapy and,
   405
   polyclonal gammopathies
   and, 236
Scarlet fever, 508t
   reactive lymphocytes and,
   79
   upper respiratory tract cultures and, 507
Schistocytes, 87
Schistosoma haematobium, in
   urine, 43
Schistosoma mansoni, in urine,
   43
Schistosomiasis, 493t
   serologic values for, 608
   tests for, 607

Scleroderma, antinuclear antibodies and, 586–587
Scrub typhus, Weil-Felix test
and, 596
Scurvy, 215
Secobarbital, 379
characteristics of, 380t
therapeutic and toxic levels
of, 381
Sedative/tranquilizing agents,
416–418
acquired porphyria hepatica
and, 47
characteristics of, 416t
Seizures; see Epilepsy
Septicemia, cerebrospinal fluid
pathogens and, 495
Sequestrene; see EDTA
Serologic tests
autoimmunity and,
586–593
febrile agglutinins and,
593–599
fungal infections and,
599–601
mycoplasmal infections and,
602–604
parasitic infections and,
605–609
specimen collection for,
585–586
streptococcal infections and,
609–614
syphilis and, 614–619
TORCH diseases and, 619
viral infections and,
620–630
Serology, 579
Serum electrolytes
normal concentrations
of, 273t
responses in selected conditions, 255t
Serum prothrombin time; see
Prothrombin consump-
tion time
Serum sickness, reactive lymphocytes and, 79
Serum specimens, 152
Sex hormones; see specific type
Shigellosis, 516t
stool specimens and,
514–515
Shock, lactic dehydrogenase
activity and, 189
Siberian tick fever, Weil-Felix
test and, 596
Sickle cell anemia
basophilic stippling and, 89

elliptocytosis and, 87
target cells and, 87
Sickle cell crisis, nucleated
erythrocytes and, 88
Sickle cell test, 113–114
Sickledex, 110
Sickling phenomenon, 113
Siderotic granules, 89
Single-donor plasma, 660
Sinusitis, anaerobic organisms
and, 488
Sjogren's syndrome, anti-
nuclear antibodies
and, 587
Skin
diseases associated with,
504t
microbiologic examination
of, 501–506
pathogens on, 506
specimens of, 506
Smallpox, 504t
Sodium, 250–256
reabsorption of, renin-
angiotensin-aldosterone
system and, 316
Sodium citrate, hematologic
testing and, 65, 153
Somatotropins, functions
of, 319
Spasticity, congenital toxoplasmosis and, 606
Specimens; see also specific type
anaerobic, 485
fungal, 485–486
general examination of,
482–484
stained smear, 484
viral, 486
Spermatogenesis, testosterone
and, 330
Spermatozoa, in urine, 43
Spherocytes, 87
Spherocytosis, hereditary, 87
erythrocyte osmotic fragility
and, 98
mean corpuscular hemo-
globin concentration
and, 90
microcytosis and, 86
Spina bifida, alpha-fetoprotein
levels and, 242
Spinal epidural abscess, cerebrospinal fluid pathogens
and, 495
Spinal puncture, traumatic,
cerebrospinal fluid and,
438–439

Splenectomy
acanthocytosis and, 87
siderotic granules and, 89
target cells and, 87
Sprue, intravenous glucose
tolerance test and, 163
Sputum
cultures of, 513–514
microbiologic examination
of, 512–514
normal flora of, 513
pathogens of, 513
Stained erythrocyte examination, 85–89
Stained smears
microscopic examination of,
486–487
specimens for, 484
Staphylococcal food poisoning, 516t
Status epilepticus, phenobarbital and, 375
Steatorrhea
fecal analysis and, 449
idiopathic, macrocytosis
and, 86
Stones, kidney; see Renal
calculi
Stools
microbiologic examination
of, 514–520
pathogenic organisms and,
518
specimens of, 518–520
Streptococcal infections,
serologic tests for,
609–614
Streptococcal pharyngitis, C-
reactive protein and, 613
Streptococcal sore throat, 508t
upper respiratory tract cultures and, 507
Streptococcus MG agglutinins,
604
Streptomycin
activities of, 529
urinary casts and, 40
Streptozyme (STZ) procedure,
611
Stuart-Prower factor, 541
Stypven time, 563–564
Subacute bacterial endocarditis, 492t
complement and, 584
Subarachnoid hemorrhage,
cerebrospinal fluid analysis and, 434, 438
Subdural empyema, anaerobic
organisms and, 488

Sugars; *see* Urine, sugars in
Sulfa drugs, acute intermittent porphyria and, 45
Sulfapyridine, Heinz bodies and, 89
Sulfasalazine, digoxin levels and, 383
Sulfhemoglobin, 396–397
Sulfonamides
  acquired porphyria hepatica and, 47
  activities of, 529
  intoxication with, abnormal urinary crystals and, 42
  methemoglobin and, 394
  prothrombin time and, 561
  solubility of, albumin and, 231
  sulfhemoglobinemia and, 396
  urinary casts and, 40
Sulkowitch test, urinary calcium and, 49
Surgical drainage, excessive fluid loss and, 248
Sydenham's chorea, anti-DNase B and, 612
Synovial fluid
  analysis of, 469–478
    microbiologic examination in, 478
    physical examination in, 470–475
    specimen collection and handling in, 470
  characteristics in selected disorders, 472t
  glucose in, 477–478
  microbiologic examination of, 520–521
  normal flora of, 520
  pathogens of, 521
  specimens of, 521
Synovial fluid cell counts, 475–476
  methodology of, 476
  normal values for, 475
  variations in, conditions associated with, 476
Synovial fluid crystals, 476–477
Syphilis, 503t
  acquired porphyria hepatica and, 47
  blood transfusion and, 668–669
  congenital, 614–615
  intrauterine, polyclonal gammopathies and, 235

polyclonal gammopathies and, 235
reactive lymphocytes and, 79
serologic findings in, 615t
serologic tests for, 448–449, 614–619
Systemic lupus erythematosus
  antinuclear antibodies and, 586–587
  complement and, 584
  deoxyribonucleic acid antibodies and, 588
  lupus erythematosus cell test and, 104, 104–105
  T-lymphocytes and, 580
T-lymphocytes, 76, 579–580
Tachycardia; *see* Atrial tachycardia, Paroxysmal tachycardia, Ventricular tachycardia
Tapeworm infestation, 517t, 518–519
Target cells, 87
Testes, hormones of, 330
Testicular function, testosterone and, 343
Testicular tumors, testosterone and, 343
Testosterone, 342–344
  follicle-stimulating hormone and, 321
  luteinizing hormone and, 325
Tetanus, 526t
  anaerobic organisms in, 488
Tetany
  aldosteronism and, 297
  calcium depletion and, 265
Tetracycline, activities of, 529
TGT; *see* Thromboplastin generation time
Thalassemia
  basophilic stippling and, 89
  elliptocytosis and, 87
  erythrocyte porphyrin concentrations and, 129
  fetal hemoglobin and, 115
  Heinz bodies and, 89
  hypochromia and, 88
  macrocytosis and, 86
  mean corpuscular volume and, 90
  microcytosis and, 86
  nucleated erythrocytes and, 88
  siderocytes and, 89
  target cells and, 87
Theophylline, 407–408

Therapeutic drug monitoring, 358–360
  specimen collection and handling in, 360
  test interpretation in, 359–360
Thioridazine, 411
  tricylic antidepressants and, 413
Thoracic empyema, anaerobic organisms in, 488
Thoracocentesis, 465
Thorn test, 102–104
Throat
  normal flora in, 507
  pathogens in, 511
  secretions and discharges from, microbiologic examination of, 506–512
Thrombasthenia
  bleeding time and, 544–545
  clot retraction and, 547
  platelet transfusion and, 657
Thrombin, platelet aggregation and, 536
Thrombin clotting time, 564
Thrombin time, 564–565
  fibrinogen deficiency and, 537
Thrombocytopathy, bleeding time and, 544–545
Thrombocytopenia
  bleeding time and, 544
  conditions associated with, 549–550
  heparin and, 574
  platelet transfusion and, 657
  whole blood transfusion and, 652
Thrombocytosis, conditions associated with, 549
Thrombophlebitis, septic, cerebrospinal fluid pathogens and, 495
Thromboplastin, 538
  plasma, 534, 536, 538
  tissue, 534, 538
Thromboplastin generation time, 560
  antihemophilic factor deficiency and, 540
  Hageman factor deficiency and, 542
  plasma thromboplastin antecedent deficiency and, 541
  plasma thromboplastin component deficiency and, 541

Thrombotic thrombocytopenic
purpura, Burr cells
and, 87
Thrush, upper respiratory tract
cultures and, 507
Thymol, urine preservation
and, 7
Thymus, hypoplasia of, T-
lymphocytes and, 580
Thyrocalcitonin; *see* Calcitonin
Thyroid antibodies, 592–593
Thyroid carcinoma, thyroid
antibodies and, 593
Thyroid hormones, 344–353
values in selected conditions,
345t
Thyroid-binding globulin, 238
Thyroid-stimulating hormone,
329–330
Thyrotoxicosis
coumarin therapy and, 575
intravenous glucose tolerance test and, 163
Thyrotropin; *see also* Thyroid-
stimulating hormone
free fatty acids and, 211
Thyrotropin-releasing hormone, 329
thyroid hormone synthesis
and, 344
Thyroxine, 347–350; *see also*
Free thyroxine index
blood glucose levels and,
158
Thyroxine uptake, 350–352
Thyroxine uptake ratio,
350–352
TIBC; *see* Total iron-binding
capacity
Tic douloureux; *see* Trigeminal
neuralgia
Tinea nigra, 505t
Tissue thromboplastin, 538
activation of, 534
Tobramycin
activities of, 529
characteristics of, 366t
nephrotoxicity of, 366
therapeutic and toxic concentrations of, 367
Toluene, urine preservation
and, 6
Tophi, 228
TORCH diseases, serologic
tests for, 619
Total albumin, 232–234
Total body fluid, 248
composition of, 249f

Total iron-binding capacity,
134–137
Total lipids, 211–213
Tourniquet test, 546–547
Toxemia of pregnancy
immature neutrophils
and, 79
toxic neutrophilic granulation and, 79
Toxic granulation, 79
Toxicology, 356–358
Toxoplasmal antibody test,
605–606
Toxoplasmosis, 493t, 605–606
increased IgM levels at birth
and, 235
Trachoma, 498t
Tranquilizing agents, 414–418
barbiturates and, 380
Transcortin, 238
Transferrin, 134–137, 238
Transfusion reactions,
661–669
acute hemolytic, 663–664
bacterial, 664–665
circulatory overload
and, 665
delayed, 662
febrile, 665–666
hypersensitivity, 666–667
immediate, 661–662
investigation of, nursing
responsibilities in,
662–663
nucleated erythrocytes
and, 88
Transfusion therapy, 649–652
anticoagulants and, 152–153
blood administration in,
650–651
donor selection in, 649–650
massive, 651–652
Transplant rejection, T-
lymphocytes and, 579
Trauma, pleural exudates
and, 464
Treponema pallidum immobilization (TPI) test, 618
Treponemal antibody tests,
618–619
TRH; *see* Thyrotropin-releasing
hormone
Trichinosis, 517t
serologic values for, 608
tests for, 607
Trichomonas vaginalis, in urine,
43
Trichomoniasis, 503t

Tricyclic antidepressants,
412–414
Trifluoperazine, 411
Trigeminal neuralgia, car-
bamazepine and, 372
Triglycerides, 205–207
Triiodothyronine, 346–347
functions of, 344
Troleandomycin, theophylline
therapy and, 407
Trousseau's sign, 265
Trypanosomiasis, 493t, 527t
serologic values for, 608
tests for, 608
Trypsin, fecal, 456
TSH; *see* Thyroid-stimulating
hormone
Tsutsugamushi disease, Weil-
Felix test and, 596
Tubercle bacilli, antibiotics active against, 529
Tuberculosis, 509t
C-reactive protein and, 613
cerebrospinal fluid patho-
gens and, 495
erythrocyte sedimentation
rate and, 93
pleural exudates and, 464
polyclonal gammopathies
and, 235
reactive lymphocytes
and, 79
Tuberculous meningitis; *see*
Meningitis, tuberculous
Tularemia, 492t
agglutination test for,
598–599
differential diagnosis of, 490
Tumor immunity, T-lympho-
cytes and, 579
Tumor markers, 241–244
Tumors; *see specific type*
Two-hour postprandial glucose, 161–163
Two-tube swab system, 485
Typhoid fever, 516t
differential diagnosis of, 490
Widal test for, 594–596
Typhus, 527t
reactive lymphocytes and, 79
Weil-Felix test and, 596–597
Tyrosinosis, 58
Tyrosinuria, 43
Ulcerative colitis
fecal analysis and, 449
reactive lymphocytes and,
79
Upper respiratory tract cul-
tures, 507

Urea nitrogen, urinary, 222–223

Uremia
Burr cells and, 87
schistocytes and, 87

Urethra, normal flora of, 500

Urethritis, nongonococcal, 503t

Uric acid, 228–230

Uric acid stones, 56

Urinalysis, 13–37
nursing responsibilities in, 13–14

Urinary casts, 40–41

Urinary obstruction, bacteremia and, 489

Urine
amino acids in, 57–60
bilirubin in, 29–31
collection of
methodology of, 523
nursing responsibilities in, 4–6, 523–524
procedures for, 4–5
times for, 5–6
color of, 9, 10t
formation of, 2–4
ketones in, 24–26
microbiologic examination of, 521–524
microscopic examination of, 37–43
microscopic examination of, normal values for, 37
nitrites in, 33–37
normal flora of, 522
occult blood in, 26–28
odor of, 9
osmolality of, 275–277
pathogens of, 523
pH of, 16–18
physical examination of, 7–13
preservation of, 6–7
protein in, 21–24
screening of, methods for, 34t
specific gravity of, 14–16
sugars in, 18–20
turbidity of, 12–13
urobilinogen in, 31–33
volume of, 7–8
normal values for, 7

Urine concentration, 51–53

Urinometry, specific gravity measurements and, 15

Urobilinogen, 31–33, 148–149
fecal, 456–458

Uroporphyrin, 44, 128–129

Vagina, normal flora of, 500

Valproic acid, 378–379

Valvular stenosis, schistocytes and, 87

Vancomycin, activities of, 529

Vanillylmandelic acid, 310–311
catecholamine metabolism and, 298

Varicella, 504t

Variegate porphyria, 45

Variola, 504t

Vascular function tests, 544–553

Vasculitis, antinuclear antibodies and, 586

Vasopressin; see Antidiuretic hormone

VDRL reactions
false-negative, conditions associated with, 617
false-positive, conditions associated with, 448

VDRL screening tests, 616–618

Vegetarianism, vitamin B12 deficiency and, 125

Venipuncture, 64–65, 154
precautions in, 154–155

Ventricular arrhythmias
disopyramide and, 386
lidocaine and, 385

Ventricular ectopic rhythms, phenytoin and, 376

Ventricular fibrillation, hyperkalemia and, 257

Ventricular premature beats, propranolol and, 389

Ventricular tachycardia
ectopic, propranolol and, 389
procainamide and, 387
quinidine and, 390

Versene; see EDTA

Very low-density lipoproteins, 207

Vibrio parahaemolyticus gastroenteritis, 516t

Viral infections, serologic tests for, 620–630

Virology, 481–482

Virus specimens, 486

Vitamin A, 215–217

Vitamin B$_{12}$, 125–126
deficiency of, mean corpuscular volume and, 90

Vitamin C; see Ascorbic acid

Vitamin C deficiency, 215

Vitamin D, 317–319
calcitonin and, 312
parathyroid hormone and, 314

Vitamin K, coumarin therapy and, 575

VLDLs; see Very low-density lipoproteins

VMA; see Vanillylmandelic acid

Vomiting, excessive fluid loss and, 248

Vulvovaginal candidiasis, 503t

Waldenstrom's macroglobulinemia
B-lymphocytes and, 580
monoclonal gammopathies and, 235

Warts, 504t

Washed red blood cells, 654
administration of, indications for, 655

Water intoxication, total protein levels and, 231

WBC; see Leukocyte count

Weil-Felix test, 596–597

White blood cell casts, conditions associated with, 41

White blood cell count; see Leukocyte count

White blood cells, urinary, 39

Whole blood clotting time, 553–554

Whole blood therapy (transfusion), 652–653
contraindications for, 653
indications for, 653
side effects of, 653

Whooping cough, 508t
nasopharyngeal cultures and, 507

Widal test, 594–596

Wilson's disease, copper metabolism and, 217

Wiskott-Aldrich syndrome, T-lymphocytes and, 580

Wound exudates and drainage, microbiologic examination of, 524–528

Wound infections
anaerobic organisms and, 488
pathogens of, 525

Wound specimens

Wounds, diseases associated with, 526t

Xanthine stones, 57

Xanthinuria, 43, 57

Xanthochromia, 438

X-ray irradiation, toxic neutrophilic granulation
and, 79
D-Xylose absorption test,
170–171

Yeast, in urine, 43
Yellow fever, 527t
Zinc, 218–219
Zollinger-Ellison syndrome,
gastric acidity and, 462